Clinical Cases in Eye Care

Clinical Cases in Eye Care

Mark Rosenfield, MCOptom, PhD, FAAO
Professor
SUNY College of Optometry
New York, NY

Eunice Myung Lee, OD, FAAO
Assistant Professor
Southern California College of Optometry at Marshall B. Ketchum University
Fullerton, CA

Denise Goodwin, OD, FAAO
Professor
Pacific University College of Optometry
Forest Grove, OR

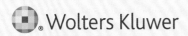. Wolters Kluwer

Philadelphia • Baltimore • New York • London
Buenos Aires • Hong Kong • Sydney • Tokyo

Acquisitions Editor: Chris Teja
Editorial Coordinator: Jeremiah Kiely
Development Editor: Sean McGuire
Marketing Manager: Rachel Mante Leung
Production Project Manager: Bridgett Dougherty
Design Coordinator: Holly McLaughlin
Manufacturing Coordinator: Beth Welsh
Prepress Vendor: Newgen Knowledge Works Pvt. Ltd., Chennai, India

First Edition

Library of Congress Cataloging-in-Publication Data
Names: Rosenfield, Mark, editor. | Lee, Eunice Myung, editor. | Goodwin, Denise, editor.
Title: Clinical cases in eye care / [edited by] Mark Rosenfield, Eunice Myung Lee, Denise Goodwin.
Description: First edition. | Philadelphia, PA : Wolters Kluwer, [2019] | Includes bibliographical references.
Identifiers: LCCN 2018026805 | ISBN 9781496385345 (pbk.)
Subjects: | MESH: Eye Diseases—therapy | Vision Disorders—therapy | Case Reports
Classification: LCC RE46 | NLM WW 166 | DDC 617.7—dc23
LC record available at https://lccn.loc.gov/2018026805

Preface

Many branches of higher education have adopted problem-based learning (PBL) strategies. Frequently, healthcare teaching institutions (such as schools and colleges of medicine, dentistry, and optometry) introduce PBL at the very beginning of the professional curriculum and continue that approach throughout the entire program. An effective method of presenting PBL within medical education is to use clinical case examples of specific conditions to stimulate discussion. Often, the same cases are threaded throughout the curriculum and are considered in varying amounts of detail depending on the degree of knowledge of the reader. However, there is no universal source of optimal case examples. Many clinicians use their own personal patient encounters as teaching tools, but they may not provide a sufficiently wide scope to cover the range of topics required within a comprehensive curriculum.

Accordingly, the aim of this book is to provide a broad range of case examples to illustrate the contemporary practice of eye and vision care. The initial impetus for this work came from a meeting of the Clinical Optometric Methods and Procedures Special Interest Group. At its yearly meeting, the instructors discussed the need to develop a bank of cases to serve as good examples for teaching purposes. The 3 editors of this volume have all been active within this group. We asked experts in the field to submit examples of conditions encountered on a regular basis in the clinical setting.

While perhaps less exciting than more esoteric cases, we believe that they have greater value as teaching tools, as they are more likely to be encountered on a regular basis. The "once-in-a-lifetime" occurrence may be more exhilarating, but might never be seen by most practitioners. We also asked each author to include "Clinical Pearls" as a summary of the critical points brought up by that case.

We are delighted to include contributions from authors around the world, even though the scope and methods of practice may vary with physical location. Indeed, irrespective of geography, it is quite likely that the reader will disagree with some of the proposed treatment plans. In many ways, this is to be encouraged since the goal of this work is to stimulate discussion. It is rare that there is only 1 way of managing a particular condition. This can be frustrating to students, who frequently ask for the definitive method of treatment. However, one of the joys of patient care is to realize that there are often multiple viable management options. The task of the clinician is to select the one that has the best likelihood of success for the specific patient in front of them.

Finally, we would like to thank all of our authors, and we hope they will forgive us for all the nagging e-mails and annoying editorial changes that managing a text such as this entails. Despite what some of our communications may have implied, we are truly grateful for your contributions to the book and your efforts to advance eye and vision care.

Mark Rosenfield
Eunice Myung Lee
Denise Goodwin

Contributors

Roya Attar, OD, MBA, FAAO
Department of Ophthalmology
The University of Mississippi Medical
    Center
Jackson, Mississippi

Alexandra Bavasi, OD
Pacific University College of Optometry
Forest Grove, Oregon

Anna K. Bedwell, OD, FAAO
Clinical Assistant Professor
School of Optometry
Indiana University
Bloomington, Indiana

**Gurpreet K. Bhogal-Bhamra, MCOptom,
PhD, FHEA**
Lecturer in Optometry
Aston University
Birmingham, UK

Adam B. Blacker, OD, MS
Assistant Professor
Arizona College of Optometry
Midwestern University
Glendale, Arizona

Aaron Bronner, OD, FAAO
Staff Optometrist
Pacific Cataract and Laser Institute
Adjunct Faculty
Pacific University College of Optometry
Forest Grove, Oregon

Ryan Bulson, OD, MS, FAAO
Associate Professor
Pacific University College of Optometry
Forest Grove, Oregon

Evan Canellos, OD, FAAO
Adjunct Associate Clinical Professor
SUNY College of Optometry
New York, New York

Harriette Canellos, OD, FAAO
Associate Clinical Professor
SUNY College of Optometry
New York, New York

Julia Canestraro, OD, FAAO
Associate Clinical Instructor
SUNY College of Optometry
New York, New York

Joanne Caruso, OD
Adjunct Associate Professor
New England College of Optometry
Boston, Massachusetts

Rebecca Charlop, OD, FAAO
Behavioral Optometry
ODA Primary Health Care Network
Brooklyn, New York

Marlena A. Chu, OD, FAAO
Chief of Low Vision Services
UC Berkeley School of Optometry
Berkeley, California

Michelle Chun, OD, FAAO
Optometrist
UC Berkeley School of Optometry
Berkeley, California

Naomi Chun, OD, FAAO
Optometrist
Michael E. DeBakey Veterans Hospital
Houston, Texas

Kenneth J. Ciuffreda, OD, PhD, FAAO, FCOVD
Distinguished Teaching Professor
SUNY College of Optometry
New York, New York

Marcelline A. Ciuffreda, OD, FAAO
Optometrist
San Diego, California

Dawn K. DeCarlo, OD, MS, MSPH, FAAO
Professor
School of Medicine
University of Alabama at Birmingham
Birmingham, Alabama

Kathryn Deliso, OD
Assistant Professor
School of Optometry
MCPHS University
Worcester, Massachusetts

Andrew J. Di Mattina, OD, FAAO
Adjunct Clinical Faculty
New England College of Optometry
Boston, Massachusetts

Tracy Doll, OD, FAAO
Assistant Professor
Pacific University College of Optometry
Forest Grove, Oregon

Erin M. Draper, OD, FAAO
Assistant Professor
Pennsylvania College of Optometry
Salus University
Elkins Park, Pennsylvania

Kyla S. Duchin, OD, MS, FAAO
Staff Optometrist
VA Maine – Lewiston CBOC
Lewiston, Maine

Jennifer Elgin, MSOT, OTR/L, CDRS
Occupational Therapist
Department of Ophthalmology
University of Alabama at Birmingham
Birmingham, Alabama

Daniel Epshtein, OD, FAAO
Adjunct Assistant Clinical Professor
SUNY College of Optometry
NY Vision Group
New York, New York

Graham B. Erickson, OD, FAAO
Professor
Pacific University College of Optometry
Forest Grove, Oregon

Louis Frank, OD, FAAO
Associate Professor
School of Optometry
MCPHS University
Worcester, Massachusetts

Marcela Frazier, OD, MPH, FAAO
Associate Professor
School of Medicine
University of Alabama at Birmingham
Birmingham, Alabama

Nadine M. Furtado, OD, MSc, FAAO
Assistant Clinical Professor
School of Optometry & Vision Science
University of Waterloo
Waterloo, Ontario

Janet Garza, OD
Clinical Assistant Professor
University of Houston College of Optometry
Houston, Texas

Kelly Glass, OD
Clinical Assistant Professor
Oklahoma College of Optometry
Northeastern State University
Tahlequah, Oklahoma

Daniel B. T. Goh, MSc, BSc (Hons), MCOptom
Senior Optometrist
Department of Optometry
Moorfields Eye Hospital
London, UK

Denise Goodwin, OD, FAAO
Professor
Pacific University College of Optometry
Forest Grove, Oregon

Lacey Haines, BSc, OD, FIACLE
Clinical Assistant Professor
School of Optometry and Vision Science
University of Waterloo
Waterloo, Ontario, Canada

Ami R. Halvorson, OD, FAAO
Clinic Director
Pacific Cataract and Laser Institute
Portland, Oregon

Kirk L. Halvorson, OD
Staff Optometrist
VA Portland Health Care System
Portland, Oregon

M. H. Esther Han, OD, FCOVD, FAAO
Associate Clinical Professor
SUNY College of Optometry
New York, New York

Jessica Haynes, OD, FAAO
Consulting Faculty
Southern College of Optometry
Memphis, Tennessee

Amiee Ho, OD
Assistant Professor
Pacific University College of Optometry
Forest Grove, Oregon

Gregory R. Hopkins, OD, MS, FAAO
Clinical Assistant Professor
College of Optometry
The Ohio State University
Columbus, Ohio

Cheyenne Huber, OD, FAAO
Assistant Clinical Professor
UC Berkeley School of Optometry
Berkeley, California

Isabel Kazemi, OD
Assistant Clinical Professor
UC Berkeley School of Optometry
Berkeley, California

Lucy E. Kehinde, OD, PhD
Clinical Assistant Professor
University of Houston College of Optometry
Houston, Texas

Alia N. Khalaf, OD
Assistant Professor
School of Optometry
MCPHS University
Worcester, Massachusetts

Jeung Hyoun Kim, OD, PhD
Assistant Professor
Pacific University College of Optometry
Forest Grove, Oregon

Beth Kinoshita, OD, FAAO
Associate Professor
Pacific University College of Optometry
Forest Grove, Oregon

Britney Kitamata-Wong, OD, FAAO
Associate Optometrist
Lamorinda Optometry
Lafayette, California

Len V. Koh, OD, FAAO
Staff Optometrist
Mann-Grandstaff VA Medical Center
Spokane, Washington

Sai Kolli, MA(Cantab), MBBChir, FRCOphth, PhD
Consultant Opthalmic Surgeon
Queen Elizabeth Hospital
Birmingham, UK

Marjean Taylor Kulp, OD, MS, FAAO
Distinguished Professor
College of Optometry
The Ohio State University
Columbus, Ohio

Kaira Kwong, OD, FAAO
Assistant Clinical Professor
SUNY College of Optometry
New York, New York

Susan J. Leat, FCOptom, PhD, FAAO
Professor
School of Optometry and Vision Science
University of Waterloo
Waterloo, Ontario, Canada

John H. Lee, OD
Assistant Professor
Southern California College of Optometry at
   Marshall B Ketchum University
Fullerton, California

Priscilla A. Lenihan, OD, FAAO
Staff Optometrist
VA Maine - Lewiston CBOC
Lewiston, Maine

Alejandro León, OD, MSc
Associate Professor
Facultad Ciencias de la Salud
Universidad de la Salle
Bogotá, Colombia

Jennifer Long, B. Optom (Hons), M. Safety Sc, PhD, FAAO
Conjoint Senior Lecturer
School of Optometry and Vision Science
University of New South Wales
Sydney, NSW, Australia

Paula Luke, OD, FAAO
Associate Professor
Pacific University College of Optometry
Forest Grove, Oregon

Sarah MacIver, OD, FAAO
Clinical Associate Professor
School of Optometry and Vision Science
University of Waterloo
Waterloo, Ontario, Canada

Ashley Kay Maglione, OD, FAAO
Assistant Professor
Pennsylvania College of Optometry
Salus University
Elkins Park, Pennsylvania

Kelly A. Malloy, OD, FAAO
Associate Professor
Pennsylvania College of Optometry
Salus University
Elkins Park, Pennsylvania

Catherine McDaniel, OD, MS, FAAO
Associate Professor
College of Optometry
The Ohio State University
Columbus, Ohio

Alan G. McKee, MS, OD, FAAO
Professor
Oklahoma College of Optometry
Northeastern State University
Tahlequah, Oklahoma

Sandra Milena Medrano, OD, MSc
Associate Professor
Facultad Ciencias de la Salud
Universidad de la Salle
Bogotá, Colombia

Rebekah Montes, OD, FAAO
Visiting Assistant Professor
University of Houston College of Optometry
Houston, Texas

Kelsey L. Moody, OD, FAAO
Instructor
Pennsylvania College of Optometry
Salus University
Elkins Park, Pennsylvania

Susana C. Moreno, OD
Visiting Clinical Assistant Professor
University of Houston College of Optometry
Houston, Texas

A. Mika Moy, OD, FAAO
Health Sciences Clinical Professor
UC Berkeley School of Optometry
Berkeley, California

Eunice Myung Lee, OD, FAAO
Assistant Professor
Southern California College of Optometry at
    Marshall B. Ketchum University
Fullerton, California

Jason S. Ng, OD, PhD, FAAO
Associate Professor
Southern California College of Optometry at
    Marshall B. Ketchum University
Fullerton, California

Rosalynn H. Nguyen-Strongin, OD
Assistant Professor
Southern California College of Optometry at
    Marshall B. Ketchum University
Fullerton, California

Caroline M. Ooley, OD, FAAO
Assistant Professor
Pacific University College of Optometry
Forest Grove, Oregon

Reena A. Patel, OD, FAAO
Assistant Professor
Southern California College of Optometry at
    Marshall B. Ketchum University
Fullerton, California

Neil A. Pence, OD, FAAO
Associate Dean
Indiana University School of Optometry
Bloomington, Indiana

Jeffrey D. Perotti, OD, MS
Clinical Associate Professor
Indiana University
School of Optometry
Bloomington, Indiana

Tamara Petrosyan, OD
Associate Clinical Professor
SUNY College of Optometry
New York, New York

Joan K. Portello, OD, MPH, MS, FAAO
Associate Professor
SUNY College of Optometry
New York, New York

Tina Porzukowiak, OD, FAAO
Optometrist
Spindel Eye Associates
Derry, New Hampshire

Jeff C. Rabin, OD, MS, PhD, FAAO
Professor & Assistant Dean for Graduate
    Studies, Research and Assessment
The Rosenberg School of Optometry
University of the Incarnate Word
San Antonio, Texas

Mohammad Rafieetary, OD, FAAO
Adjunct Faculty
Southern College of Optometry
Memphis, Tennessee

Elaine C. Ramos, OD
Clinical Assistant Faculty
College of Optometry
Western University of Health Sciences
Pomona, California

Dashaini Retnasothie, OD, MS, FAAO
Assistant Professor
Southern California College of Optometry at
    Marshall B. Ketchum University
Fullerton, California

Doug Rett, OD, FAAO
Attending Optometrist
VA Boston
Boston, Massachusetts

Mark Rosenfield, MCOptom, PhD, FAAO
Professor
SUNY College of Optometry
New York, New York

Navjit Kaur Sanghera, OD, FAAO
Assistant Professor
Illinois College of Optometry
Chicago, Illinois

Shannon K. Santapaola, OD, FAAO
Optometry Attending
VA Medical Center
West Haven, Connecticut

Alana M. Santaro, OD, FAAO
Adjunct Clinical Faculty
New England College of Optometry
Boston, Massachusetts

Kathryn J. Saunders, BSc, PhD, FHEA, FCOptom
Professor of Optometry and Vision Science
School of Biomedical Sciences
University of Ulster
Northern Ireland, UK

Bhagya Segu, OD, FAAO
Optometrist
Michael E. DeBakey Veterans Affairs
    Medical Center
Houston, Texas

Padhmalatha Segu, OD, FAAO
Clinical Associate Professor
University of Houston College of Optometry
Houston, Texas

Angela V. Shahbazian, OD
Clinical Instructor
UC Berkeley School of Optometry
Berkeley, California

Munish Sharma, MD, OD, FAAO
Chief of Optometry
Kaiser Permanente San Bernardino
    County
Southern California Permanente
    Medical Group
Fontana, California

Jerome Sherman, OD, FAAO
Distinguished Teaching Professor
SUNY College of Optometry
New York, New York

Jared Staats, OD
Eye Specialists of Indiana
Indianapolis, Indiana

Andre Stanberry, OD
Associate Clinical Professor
School of Optometry & Vision Science
University of Waterloo
Waterloo, Ontario

Ira Strenger, OD, FAAO
SeeClear Associates LLC
Summit, New Jersey

Sosena Tsz-Wei Tang, BSc (Hons), MSc
Senior Optometrist
Department of Ophthalmology
The Queen Elizabeth II Hospital
Welwyn Garden City, Hertfordshire, UK

Barry Tannen, OD, FCOVD, FAAO
Associate Clinical Professor, Emeritus
SUNY College of Optometry
New York, New York

Noah M. Tannen, OD
Eyecare Professionals, PC
Hamilton Square, New Jersey

John D. Tassinari, OD, FAAO
Associate Professor
College of Optometry
Western University of Health Sciences
Pomona, California

Jacqueline M. Theis, OD, FAAO
Clinical Instructor
UC Berkeley School of Optometry
Berkeley, California

Marsha Thomas, OD, FAAO
Berkeley Eye Center
Pearland, Texas

Jeffrey J. Walline, OD, PhD, FAAO
Associate Dean for Research
College of Optometry
The Ohio State University
Columbus, Ohio

Barry A. Weissman, OD, PhD, FAAO
Professor of Optometry
Southern California College of Optometry at
    Marshall B. Ketchum University
Fullerton, California

James S. Wolffsohn, BSc, MBA, PhD, FAAO
Associate Pro Vice Chancellor
Optometry, Life and Health Sciences
Aston University
Birmingham, UK

Joanne M. Wood, BSc (Hons), PhD, FAAO
Professor
School of Optometry and Vision Science
Queensland University of Technology
Brisbane, Australia

Lorne Yudcovitch, OD, MS, FAAO
Professor
Pacific University College of Optometry
Forest Grove, Oregon

Phillip T. Yuhas, OD, MS, FAAO
Clinical Instructor
College of Optometry
The Ohio State University
Columbus, Ohio

Jillian F. Ziemanski OD, MS, FAAO
Clinical Assistant Professor
School of Optometry
University of Alabama at Birmingham
Birmingham, Alabama

Contents

SECTION 1

Refraction, Perceptual and Binocular Vision

Lead section editor: Mark Rosenfield

1.1   Astigmatism   3
Eunice Myung Lee

1.2   Presbyopia   7
John H. Lee

1.3   Anisometropia   11
Catherine McDaniel and Marjean Taylor Kulp

1.4   Pseudophakia   15
John H. Lee

1.5   Myopia Control   19
Jeffrey J. Walline

1.6   Sports Vision: Lens Tints   23
Jacqueline M. Theis

1.7   Dispensing Issues With Progressive Addition Lenses: Adaptational Issues When Switching From Conventional to Free-Form Progressive Addition Lenses   27
Alan G. McKee

1.8   Dispensing Anomalies: Disorientation Following Prescription Change   30
Alan G. McKee

1.9   Dispensing Issues With Progressive Addition Lenses: Adaptation Issues   33
Alan G. McKee

1.10   Prescribing for Musicians   36
Jennifer Long

1.11   Prescribing for a Computer User   40
Jennifer Long

1.12   Eye Protection   44
Jennifer Long

1.13   Low Vision Management of a Patient With Choroideremia   48
Gregory R. Hopkins

1.14   Age-Related Macular Degeneration   52
Cheyenne Huber

1.15   Oculocutaneous Albinism: Low Vision Case Using Simple Magnification   57
Marlena A. Chu

1.16   Use of a Bioptic Telescope for Driving   61
Dawn K. DeCarlo, Jennifer Elgin, and Joanne M. Wood

1.17   Management of the Geriatric Patient   65
Harriette Canellos and Evan Canellos

1.18   A Complex Case of Accommodative Insufficiency   69
John D. Tassinari

1.19   Convergence Excess   74
Paula Luke

1.20   Convergence Insufficiency   78
Graham B. Erickson

1.21   Divergence Excess   87
Alejandro León and Sandra Milena Medrano

1.22   Clinical Use of Fixation Disparity   90
Sosena Tsz-Wei Tang

1.23   Vision Therapy in an Adult With Congenital Nystagmus   95
Ira Strenger, Barry Tannen, and Kenneth J. Ciuffreda

1.24   Management of Convergence Insufficiency With Prism   101
Dashaini Retnasothie

1.25   Vertical Heterophoria   106
Paula Luke

1.26　Amblyopia　109
Marcela Frazier

1.27　Neuro-Optometric Rehabilitation of a
Post-concussion Patient　114
Barry Tannen, Noah M. Tannen, and
Kenneth J. Ciuffreda

1.28　Intermittent Exotropia, Divergence
Excess Type　118
Elaine C. Ramos and M. H. Esther Han

1.29　Duane Retraction Syndrome　122
Rebecca Charlop and M. H. Esther Han

1.30　Pseudomyopia　127
Reena A. Patel

1.31　Comprehensive Color Vision
Evaluation　130
Jason S. Ng

1.32　Color Vision Occupational
Questions　136
Jason S. Ng

1.33　Hereditary Color Vision Deficiency in a
Young Child　141
Jeff C. Rabin

1.34　Acquired Color Vision
Deficiency　144
Jeff C. Rabin

1.35　Infant Hyperopia　147
Susan J. Leat

1.36　High Refraction in Infancy　152
Susan J. Leat

1.37　Down Syndrome　157
Kathryn J. Saunders

1.38　Retinoblastoma　163
Alexandra Bavasi

SECTION 2
Anterior Segment
Lead section editor: Eunice Myung Lee

2.1　Use of Gas Permeable Versus Soft
Contact Lenses　171
Lacey Haines

2.2　Monovision Contact Lenses　176
Isabel Kazemi

2.3　Multifocal Gas Permeable Contact
Lenses　180
Louis Frank

2.4　Management of Keratoconus With Gas
Permeable Contact Lenses　184
Beth Kinoshita

2.5　Contact Lens Noncompliance:
Medico-legal　190
Barry A. Weissman

2.6　Contact Lens Noncompliance:
Therapeutic　193
Kathryn Deliso

2.7　Hordeolum　196
Padhmalatha Segu, Janet Garza,
Marsha Thomas, and Bhagya Segu

2.8　Chalazia　199
Tamara Petrosyan

2.9　Blepharitis　203
Daniel B. T. Goh and Sosena Tsz-Wei Tang

2.10　Ectropion　207
Kathryn Deliso

2.11　Blepharospasm　210
Nadine M. Furtado and Andre Stanberry

2.12　Dacryocystitis　213
Anna K. Bedwell

2.13　Dry Eye Disease　216
Tracy Doll

2.14　Dry Eye Disease Associated With
Secondary Sjögren Syndrome　223
Jillian F. Ziemanski

2.15　Preseptal Cellulitis　227
Phillip T. Yuhas

2.16　Papilloma　230
Kelly Glass

2.17　Molluscum Contagiosum　233
Bhagya Segu and Padhmalatha Segu

2.18　Adult Inclusion Conjunctivitis　236
Kaira Kwong

2.19　Epidemic Keratoconjunctivitis　239
Navjit Kaur Sanghera

2.20　Vernal Keratoconjunctivitis　244
Kaira Kwong

2.21　Giant Papillary Conjunctivitis　249
Rebekah Montes, Lucy E. Kehinde,
Susana C. Moreno, and Naomi Chun

2.22　Ocular Rosacea　253
Nadine M. Furtado and Andre Stanberry

2.23   Childhood Ocular Rosacea   257
A. Mika Moy and Michelle Chun

2.24   Phlyctenule   262
A. Mika Moy

2.25   Conjunctival Cysts   265
Len V. Koh

2.26   Subconjunctival Hemorrhage   268
Lucy E. Kehinde, Rebekah Montes, and Susana C. Moreno

2.27   Pinguecula   271
Britney Kitamata-Wong

2.28   Pterygium   274
Aaron Bronner

2.29   Herpes Simplex Keratitis   278
Julia Canestraro

2.30   Peripheral Corneal Ulcer   281
Neil A. Pence

2.31   Recurrent Corneal Erosion   285
Aaron Bronner and A. Mika Moy

2.32   Ocular Effects of Amiodarone   289
Kelly Glass

2.33   Cataract   294
Adam B. Blacker

2.34   Toric Multifocal Intraocular Lenses   297
Gurpreet K. Bhogal-Bhamra, Sai Kolli, and James S. Wolffsohn

2.35   Multifocal Intraocular Lenses   303
Gurpreet K. Bhogal-Bhamra, Sai Kolli, and James S. Wolffsohn

2.36   Lens Subluxation   307
Julia Canestraro

2.37   Episcleritis   313
Susana C. Moreno, Padhmalatha Segu, and Rebekah Montes

2.38   Herpetic Anterior Uveitis   316
Rosalynn H. Nguyen-Strongin

2.39   Toxoplasmosis   320
Jerome Sherman

2.40   Sarcoidosis   324
Sarah MacIver

2.41   Iris Melanoma   329
Lorne Yudcovitch

2.42   Ciliary Body Melanoma   333
Joanne Caruso

SECTION 3
Posterior Segment, Neuro-Ophthalmic, and Systemic Conditions
Lead section editor: Denise Goodwin

3.1   Dry Age-Related Macular Degeneration   339
Angela V. Shahbazian

3.2   Wet Age-Related Macular Degeneration   344
Kelly Glass

3.3   Diabetic Retinopathy   348
Munish Sharma

3.4   Cystoid Macular Edema   355
Munish Sharma

3.5   Central Serous Retinopathy   361
Amiee Ho

3.6   Hydroxychloroquine Retinopathy   365
Anna K. Bedwell and Jared Staats

3.7   Vitreomacular Traction   371
Daniel Epshtein

3.8   Angioid Streaks   375
Jessica Haynes and Mohammad Rafieetary

3.9   Retinitis Pigmentosa   380
Jeung Hyoun Kim

3.10   Retinal Vein Occlusion   385
Jessica Haynes, Roya Attar, and Mohammad Rafieetary

3.11   Retinal Artery Occlusion   389
Jeffrey D. Perotti

3.12   Peripheral Retinal Lesions   394
Kyla S. Duchin and Priscilla A. Lenihan

3.13   Rhegmatogenous Retinal Detachment   398
Amiee Ho

3.14   Horner Syndrome   402
Kirk L. Halvorson

3.15   Tonic Pupil   407
Kelly A. Malloy

3.16   Light–Near Disassociation   412
Kelsey L. Moody

3.17   Optic Nerve Drusen   416
Ryan Bulson

3.18 Demyelinating Optic Neuritis 422
Erin M. Draper

3.19 Nonarteritic Anterior Ischemic Optic Neuropathy 427
Alana M. Santaro and Andrew J. Di Mattina

3.20 Idiopathic Intracranial Hypertension 433
Caroline M. Ooley

3.21 Minocycline-Induced Pseudotumor Cerebri 439
Marcelline A. Ciuffreda and Kenneth J. Ciuffreda

3.22 Pituitary Adenoma 444
Denise Goodwin

3.23 Cranial Nerve III Palsy 452
Kirk L. Halvorson

3.24 Cranial Nerve IV Palsy 456
Mark Rosenfield

3.25 Cranial Nerve VI Palsy 459
Erin M. Draper

3.26 Internuclear Ophthalmoplegia 463
Ashley Kay Maglione

3.27 Intracranial Tumor 466
Kelsey L. Moody

3.28 Pansinusitis 473
Ami R. Halvorson and Kirk L. Halvorson

3.29 Nonorganic Vision Loss 476
Kelly A. Malloy

3.30 Primary Open Angle Glaucoma 480
Lorne Yudcovitch

3.31 Pseudoexfoliation Glaucoma 489
Priscilla A. Lenihan and Kyla S. Duchin

3.32 Angle Closure Glaucoma 495
Joan K. Portello

3.33 Corneal Foreign Body 502
Lorne Yudcovitch

3.34 Ocular Trauma 506
Navjit Kaur Sanghera

3.35 Ocular Effects of Hypertension 510
Tamara Petrosyan

3.36 Sarcoid Optic Neuropathy 514
Ashley Kay Maglione

3.37 Ocular Toxoplasmosis 521
Jeung Hyoun Kim

3.38 Thyroid Eye Disease 524
Len V. Koh and Tina Porzukowiak

3.39 Myasthenia Gravis 531
Doug Rett

3.40 Acute Leukemia With Roth Spots 535
Joanne Caruso

3.41 Ocular Lymphoma 543
Shannon K. Santapaola

3.42 Human Immunodeficiency Virus Retinopathy 547
Alia N. Khalaf

Index 553

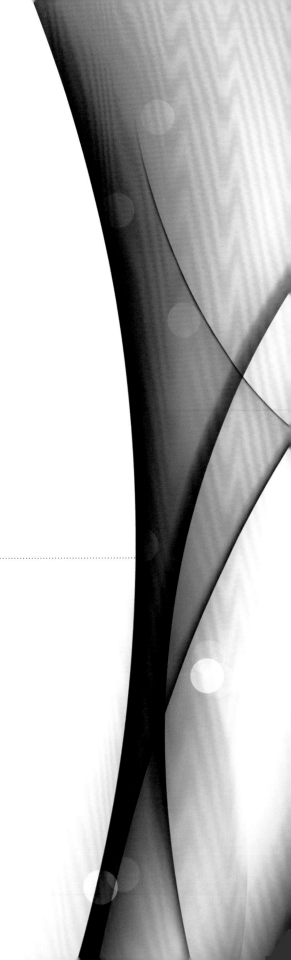

SECTION 1

Refraction, Perceptual and Binocular Vision

Lead section editor: MARK ROSENFIELD

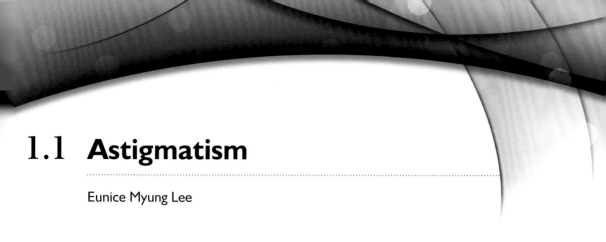

1.1 Astigmatism

Eunice Myung Lee

Jason, a 19-year-old Hispanic male, presented with continuous, slight blur in his left eye when viewing distant objects. He first noticed the problem several months ago when he took his driving test. Although he was able to pass the vision screening, he realized that he was having more difficulty reading the letters with his left eye than with his right. Jason was concerned because his job required him to drive. He had not had an eye examination before, nor had he worn a refractive correction. He was in good health and did not take any prescribed medication. His last physical examination was 3 or 4 years ago. He reported having seasonal allergies, which were worse in the spring, and took over-the-counter loratadine (Claritin) as needed. There was also a family history of allergies, and his maternal grandfather had a corneal problem, although the exact diagnosis was unknown.

Clinical Findings

Unaided distance VA	OD: 20/40 (pinhole 20/25); OS: 20/50 (pinhole 20/25); OU: 20/30^{-2}
Unaided near VA	OD: 20/30; OS: 20/30; OU: 20/30
Cover test (unaided)	Distance: ortho; near: 6Δ XP
Near point of convergence	To the nose
Confrontation visual fields	Full to finger counting OD and OS
Stereopsis	20 s of arc
Pupil evaluation	PERRL; no RAPD
Keratometry	OD: 48.50 @ 77/45.00 @ 167; OS: 48.00 @ 83/44.25 @ 173 Mires clear and slightly irregular OD and OS
Retinoscopy	OD: −0.50 −2.50 × 170; OS: −0.50 −3.00 × 180 No scissor motion OD or OS
Subjective refraction	OD: −0.50 −2.00 × 170 (20/25); OS: −0.50 −3.25 × 175 (20/25)
NRA/PRA	+2.50/−4.00
Near phoria (through subjective Rx)	4Δ exo
Intraocular pressure (iCare)	OD: 12 mm Hg; OS: 11 mm Hg at 2:15 PM
Slit-lamp examination	Unremarkable; no ptosis, pterygium, chalazion, or Fleischer ring OU
Fundus examination	Unremarkable

Corneal topography	OD: regular with-the-rule toricity limbus to limbus
	OS: with-the-rule toricity with slight irregularity (possible inferior steepening)

Abbreviations: NRA, negative relative accommodation; OD, right eye; OS, left eye; OU, both eyes; PERRL, pupils equal, round, reactive to light; PRA, positive relative accommodation; RAPD, relative afferent pupillary defect; Rx, prescription; VA, visual acuity; XP, exophoria.

Comments

To determine if there was corneal irregularity, particularly in the left eye, a gas-permeable (GP) contact lens was placed on each eye to create a regular anterior surface. While both the pinhole test and subjective refraction had already established an improvement in visual acuity (VA) to 20/25, this simple test narrows the locus of any vision loss to the anterior corneal surface. Any reasonably fitting GP lens can be used, although in this case, the selected base curve was the average keratometry reading in diopters minus 0.75 D. Good movement and centration were observed, and the distance VA through the trial contact lenses was OD: 20/25; OS: 20/25, with a plano over-refraction in each eye.

In order to determine the prescription that would provide the best acuity and optimal comfort, trial frame verification was performed. The following findings were obtained: OD: $-0.75 - 1.50 \times 170$ (20/25); OS: $-0.75 - 2.25 \times 175$ (20/25[−]).

Discussion

It was presumed that Jason had long-standing, moderate astigmatism in each eye, although he had only recently noticed the blur (particularly in his left eye). If VA had indeed been reduced through his entire life, then he may not have realized it until his first examination as part of his driving test. Alternatively, a small increase in myopia might have occurred recently. The slightly reduced, best-corrected VA in each eye appears more likely to have been caused by bilateral meridional amblyopia, rather than a corneal abnormality such as keratoconus.

Depending on the threshold selected, up to 85% of the general population has astigmatism. While there is evidence for a hereditary component whereby 1 major autosomal dominant locus is responsible,[1] this genetic link is not predictable, and environmental factors may also make a contribution.[2] Astigmatism is more prevalent in infants and young children than adults, with the magnitude decreasing significantly during the first 2 years of life.[3] The cornea makes the largest contribution to astigmatism, and typically the highest amount of corneal astigmatism occurs between birth and around 4 years of age. The most common axis orientation in this age group is against-the-rule. Between 4 and 18 years of age, corneal astigmatism generally reduces, but small degrees of with-the-rule astigmatism frequently remain. From 18 to 40 years of age, the corneal shape is generally stable, and again small degrees of with-the-rule astigmatism are most prevalent. After 40 years of age, the cornea steepens slightly in the horizontal meridian, causing a shift toward against-the-rule astigmatism.[4] Although smaller in magnitude, age-related changes in the crystalline lens may also contribute to the astigmatic shift in older patients. There are also some prevalent differences among racial groups. In an observational study of children between 5 and 17 years of age from 4 ethnic groups within the United States, a higher prevalence of astigmatism was observed in Hispanic and Asian populations compared with whites and African Americans.[5] In addition, Native American schoolchildren and adults had an increased prevalence of high astigmatism (≥3D) when compared with the general US population.[6,7]

Some individuals are able to adapt to habitual uncorrected astigmatism via a perceptual learning effect. Additionally, uncorrected astigmats appear to have an increased tolerance to overall blur.[8] Although the size of the effect varies with the orientation of the correcting cylinder axis, astigmatic patients often squint to improve their visual resolution.[9] Occasionally, patients complain of brow ache or headache from squinting. Unlike myopia, VA is less predictable in astigmatism due to the interaction of cylinder power and axis orientation.

The age of the patient should be considered when prescribing a first-time astigmatic correction. In adults, the sudden correction of astigmatism may cause distortion and/or visual discomfort. Before finalizing the prescription, trial frame verification should be performed to determine the cylindrical power that can be tolerated with the least reduction in VA. In higher amounts of astigmatism, frequently only a partial astigmatic correction will be tolerated. While there is no definitive amount, a reasonable starting point is around 50% of the measured astigmatism. If the reduced cylinder power provides good comfort without distortion, incremental increases can be demonstrated. In order to keep the circle of least confusion on the retina, the decreased cylindrical component may warrant an increase in minus sphere power, especially if there is perceived blur. Generally, children can adapt well to a full astigmatic correction. In young children, the risk of amblyopia development may also play a role in prescribing decisions (see Chapter 1.36).

It is important to discuss potential issues in adapting to the new correction with the patient. Most individuals are able to adapt within 1 to 2 weeks if they wear the spectacles full-time. If symptoms of dizziness or distortion persist or worsen, then the patient should be advised to return so that the prescription and spectacle fit can be rechecked. In addition, if only a partial astigmatic correction has been provided, then the patient should be warned that an increase in lens power may be necessary in the future. They should be reassured that this is not necessarily because their prescription has increased.

Astigmatism may also be corrected with soft, GP, or specialty contact lenses. With the amount of astigmatism found in Jason's left eye (3.25 D), an extended-range, soft contact lens may be required, but a custom-made lens is unlikely to be necessary. The resulting VA would probably be similar to (or possibly slightly worse than) the spectacle correction. Gas-permeable lenses provide superior optics to soft contact lenses and are likely to provide a visual outcome that is at least as good as spectacles. In addition, all contact lenses provide an improved field of view when compared with spectacles, especially for higher ametropias. Jason was happy with the demonstrated spectacle correction, and expressed no interest in trying contact lenses. He was told that he could return for a contact lens fitting in the future if desired.

Eyelid pathology (eg, chalazia or ptosis), conjunctival/corneal pathology (eg, pterygia or keratoconus), or trauma can also cause adult-onset astigmatism. Iatrogenic astigmatism may also arise following corneal or eyelid surgery. Less commonly, ocular pathology related to Down syndrome, spina bifida, and Treacher Collins syndrome can lead to corneal distortion and astigmatism.[10] In Jason's case, it was unclear whether the blur appeared suddenly or was long-standing, and so the possibility that it was secondary to a pathological condition must be considered. Jason's examination findings, including a positive personal and family history of allergy, slight corneal irregularity in the left eye, and reduced best-corrected VA is weakly supportive of keratoconus or other corneal abnormality. However, the typically found keratometry values at regular axes, lack of a scissor motion on retinoscopy, and absence of pathognomonic slit lamp findings do not support a diagnosis of keratoconus. Nevertheless, Jason should be monitored for inferior corneal steepening and irregular astigmatism using corneal topography.

CLINICAL PEARLS

- The effect of astigmatism on VA is not always predictable, because it varies with both magnitude and axis orientation.

- When prescribing a first-time astigmatic correction, always demonstrate the lenses to the patient using a trial frame. Comfort may be as important as good VA. The patient should be educated that a partial prescription may be necessary in order to satisfy both of these parameters.

- If there is a suspicion of keratoconus or other corneal irregularity, over-refraction through a GP contact lens may be helpful.

REFERENCES

1. Clementi M, Angi M, Forabosco P, Di Gianantonio E, Tenconi R. Inheritance of astigmatism: evidence for a major autosomal dominant locus. *Am J Hum Genet.*1998;63(3):825-830.
2. Teikari JM, O'Donnel JJ. Astigmatism in 72 twin pairs. *Cornea.* 1989;8(4):263-266.
3. Gwiazda J, Grice K, Held R, McLellan J, Thorn F. Astigmatism and the development of myopia in children. *Vision Res.* 2000;40:1019-1026.
4. Read SA, Collins MJ, Carney LG. A review of astigmatism and its possible genesis. *Clin Exp Optom.* 2007;90(1):5-19.
5. Kleinstein RN, Jones LA, Hullett SH, et al. Refractive error and ethnicity in children. *Arch Ophthalmol.* 2003;121:1141-1147.
6. Pensyl CD, Harrison RA, Simpson P, et al. Distribution of astigmatism among Sioux Indians in South Dakota. *J Am Optom Assoc.* 1997;68(7):425-431.
7. Benjamin W, ed. *Borish's Clinical Refraction.* 2nd ed. St Louis, MO: Butterworth-Heinemann; 2006.
8. Vinas M, de Gracia P, Dorronsoro C, et al. Astigmatism impact on visual performance: meridional and adaptational effects. *Optom Vis Sci.* 2013;90(12): 1430-1442.
9. Brookman K, ed. *Refractive Management of Ametropia.* Boston, MA: Butterworth-Heinemann; 1996.
10. Read SA, Vincent SJ, Collins MJ. The visual and functional impacts of astigmatism and its clinical management. *Ophthalmic Physiol Opt.* 2014;34:267-294.

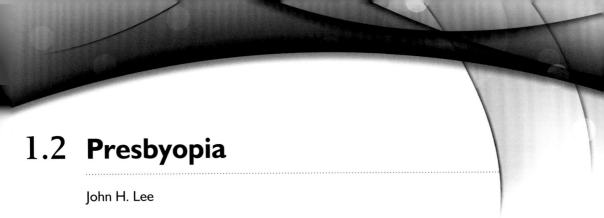

1.2 Presbyopia

John H. Lee

Janet, a 43-year-old female law clerk, presented with tired eyes, tearing, and headaches when working on her laptop computer. These symptoms were less severe when viewing her larger desktop computer monitor. In addition, the small print on some legal documents was difficult to read. Janet stated that these symptoms began 2 months ago and occurred every day, especially in the afternoon while at work. She reported frequent "raging" headaches around the eyes at the end of the workday. Accordingly, she reduced the amount of time she used her tablet computer at home, and had stopped trying to read e-mails on her phone. Janet could no longer read novels for pleasure, which she regarded as a significant loss. She was able to function better when using a magnifying lens or with improved lighting.

Janet's last eye examination was 6 years ago and found to be unremarkable. She wore single-vision glasses full time, containing a prescription from that examination. Janet had worn glasses for about 30 years and stated that she could not function without them. She was found to be in good health at her last physical examination performed 2 years ago. Janet was not taking any medications and had no known allergies. Her hobbies included watching movies and running marathons.

Clinical Findings

Current Rx	OD: −2.00 −0.50 × 90 (20/20); OS: −2.00 −0.50 × 90 (20/20)
Near VA (with current Rx)	OD: 20/30; OS: 20/30; OU: 20/30
Cover test (with current Rx)	Distance: ortho; near: 8Δ XP
Near point of convergence	4 cm/7 cm
Ocular motility	Full and unrestricted OU
Confrontation visual fields	Full to finger counting OD and OS
Pupil evaluation	PERRL; no RAPD
Retinoscopy	OD: −2.00 −0.50 × 90; OS: −2.00 −0.50 × 90
Subjective refraction	OD: −2.00 −0.50 × 90 (20/20); OS: −2.00 −0.50 × 90 (20/20)
Tentative add (binocular cross-cylinder)	+0.75 D OU (OD: 20/20; OS: 20/20; OU: 20/20)
Near phoria (Von Graefe)	Horizontal: 8Δ XP; vertical: ortho
Gradient AC/A ratio	3Δ/D
Near vergence ranges	BI: x/7/4; BO: x/18/9
NRA/PRA	+1.50/−0.75
Amplitude of accommodation (push-up method)	OD: 4.00 D; OS: 4.00 D; OU: 4.00 D

Tear break-up time	OD: 12 s; OS: 12 s
Final Rx prescribed (see Discussion section)	OD: $-2.00 -0.50 \times 090$; OS: $-2.00 -0.50 \times 090$ ADD: $+1.00$ OU

Abbreviations: AC/A, accommodative convergence to accommodative ratio; D, diopters; NRA, negative relative accommodation; OD, right eye; OS, left eye; OU, both eyes; PERRL, pupils equal, round, reactive to light; PRA, positive relative accommodation; RAPD, relative afferent pupillary defect; Rx, prescription; VA, visual acuity; XP, exophoria.

Discussion

Janet presented with classical symptoms of presbyopia. While the most obvious symptom is a gradual increase in blur at near, there are a variety of other complaints related to the diagnosis, such as only being able to read for short periods, double vision at near, unable to read small or low-contrast print, tearing, need for increased lighting, headache, or drowsiness.[1] Presbyopia is an age-related, chronic visual condition that usually becomes symptomatic in the fifth decade of life. All individuals can expect to be presbyopic in their early to mid-40s.

When analyzing this case, with a presumed diagnosis of presbyopia, it is important to verify that the best-corrected, near visual acuity (VA) is reduced without a near add. Janet did indeed have decreased near VA through her distance glasses. It is important to note that as a myopic patient, she did not take off her glasses to read. A tentative near add should be determined, which will improve her performance at near. This can be quantified using a variety of methods, including balancing the negative relative accommodation/positive relative accommodation (NRA/PRA) findings, using tables that predict the required add based on the patient's age, plus buildup, dynamic retinoscopy, sustaining a proportion (typically 50%) of their amplitude, or the binocular cross cylinder.[1-3] In this case, a tentative ADD of +0.75 D was determined using the binocular cross-cylinder test, through which NRA and PRA findings of +1.50 and −0.75, respectively, were determined. As these are unbalanced, the tentative add was modified. An add of +1.12 will balance the relative accommodation results. This revised add was placed in a trial frame

to confirm the range of clear vision. Excessive plus power should be avoided in the near add, as this will bring the range of near vision closer to the eye, which may be uncomfortable and/or unsuitable for the patient's visual requirements. Their preferred working distance and visual requirements must be taken into account when determining the final near add. For Janet, an ADD of +1.00 was determined to be appropriate.

Rather than wearing a multifocal lens (bifocal or progressive addition lens) or single-vision reading glasses, this patient (a moderate myope) had the option of taking off her distance glasses to see at near. Some patients, including Janet, are unaware that they can do this, or may believe that it could damage their eyes. Her spherical equivalent refractive correction of −2.25 D meant that she would not have to accommodate more than 0.25 D to see clearly at 40 cm. Even that may not be required based on the depth of focus of the eye. However, Janet did not like the option of removing her glasses to see at near, as she felt that she would put them down and forget where they were.

A complicating factor in this case was that Janet had 8$^\Delta$ exophoria at near through her distance glasses. Although her compensating base-out range at near was x/18/9, which satisfied Sheard's criterion,[4] a large exophoria at near can cause symptoms. Given a gradient accommodative convergence to accommodative (AC/A) ratio of 3Δ/D, increasing the add (and thereby reducing the accommodative response) will increase the near exophoria. While the add will reduce blur at near, the accompanying increase in heterophoria may lead to asthenopia, including tired eyes, tearing, and headaches. Other symptoms, including diplopia or words moving on the page, may also become apparent. The patient should be counseled on these symptoms and told to return if they become manifest.

Differential diagnoses for presbyopia include accommodative insufficiency, convergence insufficiency, and dry eye. The age of the patient usually confirms the diagnosis of presbyopia, although age-related norms for the amplitude of accommodation can also be used for reference. In Janet's case, convergence insufficiency can be ruled out by evaluating the near point of convergence, near lateral heterophoria and the base-out (compensating) vergence range.[2,3] Her near point of convergence was normal, while her near lateral heterophoria was very close to the expected range of 0 to 6Δ of exophoria.[5] Janet's base-out vergence range at near satisfies Sheard's criterion, and therefore this is unlikely to be a case of convergence insufficiency. Furthermore, her presenting symptoms are not consistent with the more severe clinical findings associated with convergence insufficiency.[6] Finally, dry eye is typically assessed in the primary care setting by quantifying the tear breakup time. Because the tear breakup time here was greater than 10 seconds, this does not indicate a case of dry eye.[7]

There are a myriad of both optical and surgical treatment options for presbyopia. Spectacle options include single-vision lenses (at distance, near, or both), bifocals, trifocals, variable focus, and progressive addition lenses. Contact lens options include distance contact lenses with near spectacles, as well as monovision and multifocal contact lenses. Surgical treatments include corneal alterations, such as refractive surgery, to correct distance refractive error with spectacles for near vision, monovision refractive surgery, and corneal inlays. Surgical interventions on the crystalline lens, such as premium intraocular lenses (both multifocal and "accommodating") or lens extraction are also available.[7,8] Follow-up visits may be necessary depending on the method of treatment, especially with contact lenses and surgical therapies. Finally, patient education regarding the advantages and limitations of the available treatment options should be provided, so that the patient has reasonable expectations, and is aware of the changes that will occur concurrent with further age-related loss of accommodation.

CLINICAL PEARLS

- Do not prescribe excessive plus at near for presbyopic patients. The lowest amount necessary to provide comfort and clarity at the preferred viewing distance should be prescribed. The required addition is highly predictable based on the patient's age and working distance.

- Monitor symptoms after a presbyopic correction has been dispensed. If they persist, then evaluate the patient's binocular status for conditions such as convergence insufficiency.

- There are multiple modalities to treat presbyopia. Pick the one that is most appropriate for the patient's lifestyle and visual requirements.

- Although not discussed here, patients with higher adds (+2.00 and higher) should be monitored for any occupational or avocational visual needs at intermediate distance, such as a desktop computer monitor, artist's canvas, sheet music placed at an intermediate distance, or cookbook stand. In such situations, consider prescribing an addition for these intermediate distances (as well as the required prescription [Rx] for both distance and near).

REFERENCES

1. American Optometric Association. *Optometric Clinical Practice Guideline. Care of the Patient With Presbyopia.* http://www.aoa.org/documents/optometrists/CPG-17.pdf. 1995. Accessed August 30, 2017.
2. Yazdani N, Khorasani AA, Moghadam HM, Yekta AA, Ostadimoghaddam H, Shandiz JH. Evaluating three different methods of determining addition in presbyopia. *J Ophthalmic Vis Res.* 2016;11:266-281.
3. León A, Estrada JM, Rosenfield M. Age and the amplitude of accommodation measured using dynamic retinoscopy. *Ophthalmic Physiol Opt.* 2016; 36:5-12.
4. Sheard C. Zones of ocular comfort. *Am J Optom Physiol Opt.* 1930;7:9-25.

5. Morgan MW. The clinical aspects of accommodation and convergence. *Am J Optom Arch Am Acad Optom*. 1944;21:301-313.

6. Teitelbaum B, Pang Y, Krall J. Effectiveness of base in prism for presbyopes with convergence insufficiency. *Optom Vis Sci*. 2009;86:143-156.

7. Lee JH, Kee CW. The significance of tear film breakup time in diagnosis of dry eye syndrome. *Kor J Ophthalmol*. 1988;2:69-71.

8. Charman WN. Developments in the correction of presbyopia 1: spectacle and contact lenses. *Ophthalmic Physiol Opt*. 2013;34:8-29.

9. Papadopoulos PA, Papadopoulos AP. Current management of presbyopia. *Middle East Afr J Ophthalmol*. 2014;21:10-17.

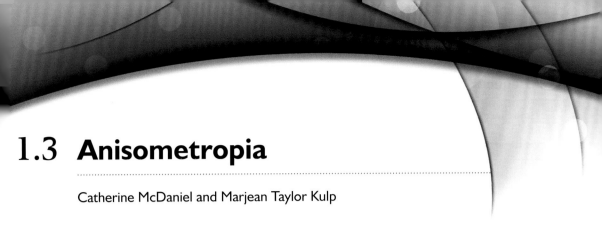

1.3 Anisometropia

Catherine McDaniel and Marjean Taylor Kulp

Jenna, a 5-year-old Caucasian female, presented after failing a school vision screening. She was doing well in school and had not complained of blur, double vision, or eyestrain. Her parents had not noticed an eye turn. Her last physical examination was 6 months ago with no significant abnormal health findings. She was not taking any medications and had no known drug allergies. There was no family history of amblyopia or strabismus.

Clinical Findings

Unaided distance VA	OD: 20/30; OS: 20/150; OU: 20/30
Unaided near VA	OD: 20/40; OS: 20/200
Extraocular motility	Full range of motion OD and OS
Pupil evaluation	PERRL; no RAPD
Hirschberg test	Reflexes 0.5-mm nasal to pupil center OD and OS
Stereopsis	None reported with either Randot Stereotest circles (local/contour) or random dot targets (global)
Dry retinoscopy	OD: +1.75 sph; OS: +6.75 −1.00 × 30
Cover test (through dry retinoscopy finding)	Distance: 4Δ XP; near: 12Δ XP
Wet retinoscopy (1 drop 1% cyclopentolate OU)	OD: +2.00 sph; OS: +7.50 −1.25 × 30
Slit lamp and fundus examination	Unremarkable OD and OS
Final spectacle Rx	OD: +1.00 sph; OS: +6.50 −1.25 × 30 (for full-time wear)

Abbreviations: OD, right eye; OS, left eye; OU, both eyes; PERRL, pupils equal, round, reactive to light; RAPD, relative afferent pupillary defect; Rx, prescription; sph, sphere; VA, visual acuity; XP, exophoria.

Follow-up Visit (2 Months After the Initial Examination)

History	Jenna's mother reported that Jenna had been wearing her glasses on a full-time basis since her evaluation.
Aided distance VA	OD: 20/20; OS: 20/50
Aided near VA	OD: 20/20; OS: 20/60
Cover test	Distance: 4Δ XP; near: 8Δ XP
Near point of convergence	2 cm
Stereopsis	100" with Randot Stereotest circles (local/contour); no random dot (global)
MEM retinoscopy	OD: 0.75 lag; OS: 0.75 lag

Abbreviations: MEM, monocular estimate method (retinoscopy); OD, right eye; OS, left eye; VA, visual acuity; XP, exophoria.

Subsequent Follow-up Visits

Time Since Initial Visit, mo	Distance VA OS	Rx Update	Stereopsis (L, Local; G, Global)	Treatment Initiated (in Addition to Full-Time Spectacle Wear)
5	20/40		100″L	
9	20/40		100″L	2-h patching OD daily
12	20/30		500″G, 100″L	2-h patching OD daily
14	20/30	Cycloplegic retinoscopy: OD: +1.75 sph OS: +6.75 −1.00 × 30 Final Rx: OD: +1.00 sph OS: +6.00 −1.00 × 30	250″G, 100″L	2-h patching OD daily
17	20/30		250″G, 70″L	30-min anti-suppression activities daily
19	20/25		250″G, 30″L	30-min anti-suppression activities daily
22	20/25		250″G, 30″L	30-min anti-suppression activities daily
24	20/25	Manifest refraction: OD: +1.00 sph (20/20) OS: +5.50 −1.25 × 30 (20/25+) Cycloplegic retinoscopy: OD: +1.75 sph OS: +6.25 −1.50 × 30 Final Rx = manifest refraction	250″G, 25″L	30-min anti-suppression activities daily
25	20/20		250″G, 25″L	Contact lenses 30-min anti-suppression activities daily

Abbreviations: OD, right eye; OS, left eye; Rx, prescription; sph, sphere; VA, visual acuity.

Discussion

Anisometropia of at least 1 D is found in approximately 2% to 6% of children.[1-3] In children, this condition presents a particular challenge because it must often be treated using objective rather than subjective findings. Cycloplegic refraction is essential to determine the full amount of hyperopia and anisometropia. Atropine may be needed if a stable retinoscopy reflex is not achieved with 1% cyclopentolate.

Anisometropia is often associated with amblyopia and decreased stereoacuity.[4,5] The patient will generally have reduced acuity in the eye with higher refractive error. It is important to remember that patients with the following amounts of anisometropia are at risk of developing refractive amblyopia[6]:

Anisometropic Refractive Errors Associated With Amblyopia

Refractive Error Type	Interocular Difference in Refractive Error, D
Hyperopia	1.00
Myopia	2.00
Astigmatism	1.50

Abbreviation: D, diopters.

Proper prescribing for anisometropia will ensure the best visual outcome for the patient. In this case, Jenna had 5.50 D of hyperopic anisometropia at the initial evaluation. To have clear retinal images bilaterally, it was important to leave the same amount of uncorrected hyperopia in each eye. Jenna did not present with strabismus and was exophoric when first corrected; hence it was not necessary to correct the total hyperopia for her. However, if a patient presents with esotropia, the final prescription should include full correction for the anisometropia while also increasing the plus spherical power to minimize the strabismus.

Lenses having equal base curves and center thickness can help minimize the difference in spectacle magnification between the 2 eyes. The use of high-index materials and frames with a small eye size can improve cosmesis. Nevertheless, patients with anisometropia corrected with glasses would be expected to report aniseikonia, that is, a perceived difference in image size between the 2 eyes.

In addition, the differential vertical prism induced when looking above, or more commonly below, the optical center of the spectacle lens must be considered. The size of the prismatic effect can be calculated using Prentice's rule. If patients cannot fuse the vertically disparate images, they may experience diplopia, asthenopia, and/or reduced stereopsis.

The simplest way of minimizing both the difference in image size and induced prism is to fit the patient with contact lenses, and this was done at the 25-month visit. Jenna was nervous about wearing contact lenses prior to this time. Had the patient been unwilling or unable to wear contact lenses, alternative methods of minimizing the differential vertical prism, such as slab-off or partial correction, should be considered.

In patients with anisometropic amblyopia, acuity should be assessed using crowded optotypes with a logarithm of the minimum angle of resolution (LogMAR) size progression. Child-friendly single-surrounded optotypes (Lea symbols or HOTV chart) and a response card should be used to improve testability in children. An ETDRS chart with crowding bars should be used for adults.

Initial treatment for amblyopia is full-time correction and monitoring of visual acuity (VA) every 4 to 6 weeks. The results of the recent Amblyopia Treatment Study showed that with glasses alone, most children showed improvement in VA over the course of the first 15 weeks, although 1 child continued to improve with glasses alone for up to 30 weeks.[7,8] In the majority of cases, VA improved at least 2 lines, and the acuity of the amblyopic eye was within 1 line of the better eye in 27% of patients. Therefore, spectacles alone will eliminate the need for further treatment in some patients. Even in those children where amblyopia does not resolve completely with spectacles, the improved VA will reduce the demand placed on any subsequent amblyopia therapy (such as patching or atropine), and may improve patient compliance with these treatments.[8] The Pediatric Eye Disease Investigator Group (PEDIG) and others[8,9] have recently conducted extensive research on amblyopia therapy. Because amblyopia is a binocular disorder, the effect of binocular treatments is also being investigated.[9] In this particular case, red–green anaglyphs were used to provide binocular therapy.

CLINICAL PEARLS

- Any reduction in hyperopic correction should be equal between the 2 eyes to fully correct for anisometropia.

- Visual acuity should be tested using optotypes with crowding bars to improve detection of amblyopia.

REFERENCES

1. Borchert M, Tarczy-Hornoch K, Cotter SA, et al. Anisometropia in Hispanic and African American infants and young children the multi-ethnic pediatric eye disease study. *Ophthalmology.* 2010;117(1):148-153.e1.
2. Deng L, Gwiazda JE. Anisometropia in children from infancy to 15 years. *Invest Ophthalmol Vis Sci.* 2012;53(7):3782-3787.
3. Giordano L, Friedman DS, Repka MX, et al. Prevalence of refractive error among preschool children in an urban population: the Baltimore Pediatric Eye Disease Study. *Ophthalmology.* 2009;116(4):739-746, 746.e1-4.
4. Tarczy-Hornoch K, Varma R, Cotter SA, et al. Risk factors for decreased visual acuity in preschool children: the multi-ethnic pediatric eye

disease and Baltimore pediatric eye disease studies. *Ophthalmology*. 2011;118(11):2262-2273.

5. Ying GS, Huang J, Maguire MG, et al. Associations of anisometropia with unilateral amblyopia, interocular acuity difference, and stereoacuity in preschoolers. *Ophthalmology*. 2013;120(3):495-503.

6. Weakley DR Jr. The association between nonstrabismic anisometropia, amblyopia, and subnormal binocularity. *Ophthalmology*. 2001;108(1):163-171.

7. Cotter SA, Pediatric Eye Disease Investigator Group, Edwards AR, et al. Treatment of anisometropic amblyopia in children with refractive correction. *Ophthalmology*. 2006;113(6):895-903.

8. Repka MX, Holmes JM. Lessons from the amblyopia treatment studies. *Ophthalmology*. 2012;119(4): 657-658.

9. Birch EE. Amblyopia and binocular vision. *Prog Retin Eye Res*. 2013;33:67-84.

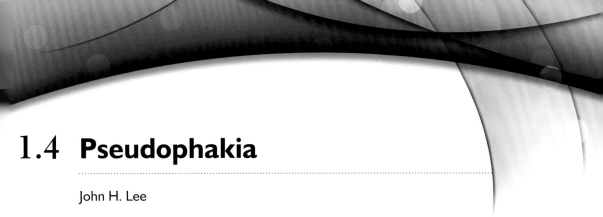

1.4 Pseudophakia

John H. Lee

Jean, a 66-year-old female, presented with a complaint of constant blurred vision at both distance and near. She was concerned with driving safely (especially at night), and was worried that she would not be able to continue reading the newspaper and novels from her favorite author. This problem started during the past year. Jean had difficulty navigating dark environments such as movie theaters. Her last eye examination was 4 years ago. At that time, she was told that everything was fine, and she did not need a change in her spectacle prescription. Jean wore progressive addition lenses, and the current prescription was 10 years old. She was in good health and not taking any medications. She had no allergies to medications, food, or the environment.

Clinical Findings

Present Rx	OD: +2.25 −1.00 × 85 (20/80: no improvement with pinhole); OS: +3.00 −1.25 × 95 (20/80: no improvement with pinhole); ADD: +3.00 OU (near VA OD: 20/100; OS: 20/100; OU: 20/100)
Cover test (with present Rx)	Distance: ortho; near: 4^Δ XP
Near point of convergence	4 cm/6 cm
Ocular motility	Full and unrestricted OU
Confrontation visual fields	Full to finger counting OD and OS
Pupil evaluation	PERRL; no RAPD
Keratometry	OD: 45.75/46.25 @85; OS: 45.50/46.12 @90 Mires clear and regular OD and OS
Autorefraction	OD: +1.00 −0.50 × 75; OS: +1.75 −0.50 × 105
Subjective refraction	OD: +1.00 −0.50 × 75 (20/60: no improvement with pinhole) OS: +1.75 −0.50 × 105 (20/60: no improvement with pinhole)
Near addition	+3.00 sph OU (OD: 20/60; OS: 20/60; OU: 20/60)
Von Graefe test at near	Poor subjective responses
Vergence ranges at near	Poor subjective responses
NRA/PRA	Poor subjective responses
Stereopsis	200 s (Wirt circles); 250 s (random dot stereograms)
Intraocular pressure (GAT)	OD: 14 mm Hg; OS: 15 mm Hg at 2:59 PM

Slit-lamp examination	OD: mild arcus; 3+ nuclear sclerotic cataract, trace anterior cortical cataract; grade 1 Van Herrick anterior chamber angle width; otherwise unremarkable
	OS: mild arcus; 3+ nuclear sclerotic cataract, trace anterior cortical cataract; grade 1 Van Herrick anterior chamber angle width; otherwise unremarkable
Fundus examination	OD: 0.35/0.35 CD ratio; healthy rim tissue with distinct disc margins; slight peripapillary atrophy; fovea flat and dry; normal vasculature; periphery intact;
	OS: 0.35/0.35 CD ratio; healthy rim tissue with distinct disc margins; slight peripapillary atrophy; fovea flat and dry; normal vasculature; periphery intact
Brightness acuity meter	Poor responses
Retinal acuity meter[1]	OD: 20/25; OS: 20/25

Abbreviations: CD, cup to disc; GAT, Goldmann applanation tonometry; NRA, negative relative accommodation; OD, right eye; OS, left eye; OU, both eyes; PERRL, pupils equal, round, reactive to light; PRA, positive relative accommodation; RAPD, relative afferent pupillary defect; Rx, prescription; sph, sphere; VA, visual acuity; XP, exophoria.

Discussion

Jean's symptoms were primarily due to moderate-to-severe nuclear sclerotic cataracts in each eye. These left her with reduced best-corrected visual acuity (VA) at distance and near, which could not be corrected with lenses. She was presented with multiple treatment options that included monitoring the progression of the cataracts without changing her correction, updating the spectacle prescription with limited improvement in VA, or improving her vision by cataract surgery. She chose to pursue cataract surgery. Jean was referred for a preoperative surgical evaluation where the risks, benefits, and alternative treatments were reviewed. Surgery was performed first on the right eye, followed by the left eye 1 week later. After phacoemulsification of each lens and insertion of a single-vision intraocular lens (IOL), Jean had unaided distance VA of 20/20 OD, OS, and OU. She was provided with near-vision spectacles (+2.50 sph OU), which gave her 20/20 vision in each eye at 40 cm. It is important to note that Jean was happy and could perform her tasks of daily living.

The decision to recommend cataract surgery is dependent on the patients' lifestyle and daily activities. Any functional loss of vision that interferes with their occupation or lifestyle must be considered.[1] If VA is better than 20/40, factors such as disability glare, decrease in contrast sensitivity, monocular diplopia, or task-specific difficulties should be taken into account. Most practitioners recommend a surgical consultation when the VA reaches 20/40 or worse. If patients decline surgery, they should be advised that their VA is likely to worsen without intervention.

The retinal acuity meter is often a good predictor of the expected postoperative VA, especially if the preoperative VA is 20/100 or better.[2] If there are confounding factors, such as retinal or corneal disease contributing to the decreased VA, then cataract surgery would likely result in minimal improvement in VA. Macular, corneal, or other organic diseases are the most likely causes. Evaluation and treatment of the causative condition responsible for the decreased vision would give patients a greater improvement in VA, thereby providing improved visual satisfaction.

The current standard procedure for cataract surgery is lens phacoemulsification with implantation of a foldable IOL.[3] Although the new femtosecond laser-assisted cataract surgery is more precise for removing the anterior capsule and reduces the amount of ultrasonic energy required to eliminate the cataract, the success rates are equivalent in terms of safety, efficiency, or recovery time when compared with phacoemulsification. Other procedures may be used for cataract excision including large-incision extracapsular cataract extraction

(ECCE) or small-incision cataract surgery (SICS).[4]

Pseudophakia describes the condition where an acrylic or silicone IOL is implanted in place of the natural crystalline lens. On occasion, "premium" toric (to correct up to 3 D of astigmatism) or multifocal (for the correction of presbyopia) IOLs may be used. The IOL is most commonly placed in the lens capsule within the posterior chamber. However, other options include anterior chamber or iris-fixated IOLs. A higher rate of secondary complications, particularly ocular hypertension or glaucoma, have been associated with these alternative options.[5]

Postoperative, follow-up care is critical after cataract surgery. While topical antibiotics, corticosteroids, NSAIDS, and oral analgesics are usually prescribed after surgery, there are no controlled studies specifying a particular regimen. Therefore, treatment schedules vary by practitioner. Complications from postoperative medications may include elevated IOP from corticosteroids and allergic reactions to antibiotics. Rarely, nonsteroidal anti-inflammatory drugs (NSAIDS) may cause epithelial defects, stromal ulceration, and melting. The first postoperative visit is commonly within 48 hours of surgery for patients not considered to be high risk or having signs or symptoms of possible complications following SICS. Subsequent visits are based on the refractive error, visual function, and medical condition of the eye. If patients are functionally monocular, intraoperative complications occur, or there is a high risk of postoperative complications such as an IOP spike, then they should be seen within 24 hours of surgery. Furthermore, subsequent postoperative visits should be scheduled more frequently than for a patient at lower risk of complications. All patients should be instructed to contact their surgeon promptly if they experience significant reduction in vision, increasing pain, progressive redness, or periocular swelling as these may indicate the onset of endophthalmitis.[4]

The postoperative examination should consist of a history of medication use, determination of any new symptoms, and the patients' impression of the quality of their vision. VA should be tested, along with IOP measurement and slit-lamp biomicroscopy. The placement of the IOL should be evaluated, together with examination of the posterior lens capsule for opacification. A dilated fundus examination should be performed if there is a high risk of posterior segment problems, such as cystoid macular edema. If the improvement in VA is less than anticipated, then additional diagnostic testing may be performed. For example, suspected maculopathy could be evaluated with ocular coherence tomography or fluorescein angiography. Corneal topography can be used to diagnose irregular astigmatism, while visual fields may be performed to show the presence of a suspected neuro-ophthalmic abnormality.[4] A spectacle prescription is generally provided 1 to 4 weeks following SICS, and between 6 and 12 weeks after sutured large-incision cataract extraction.[6]

Anisometropia and aniseikonia are potential concerns after cataract surgery, especially if the patient either had a relatively high refractive error before surgery, or the procedure was only carried out on 1 eye. A significant difference in refractive error and/or perceived image size may also cause problems with sensory fusion. A contact lens that corrects the difference in refractive error may minimize these difficulties. The remaining refractive error (at both distance and near) can then be corrected with spectacles. If cataract surgery of the second eye is scheduled within a short period of time after the first procedure, proper patient education and the temporary visual disturbances will be eliminated quickly. Variable focus spectacles have also been used in these situations.

CLINICAL PEARLS

- Loss of vision due to cataracts can be dramatic as it may affect activities of daily living. Proper management is essential.

- Although cataract surgery is a relatively common and safe procedure, postsurgical follow-up care is important for proper recovery.

- Patients with high refractive error may experience size and fusion problems after uniocular surgical removal. Proper management is important.

REFERENCES

1. Milia M, Giannopoulos T, Asteriades S, Vakalis T, Stavrakas P, Tranos P. Predictability of postoperative visual acuity in patients with dry age-related macular degeneration using the retinal acuity meter. *J Cataract Refract Surg*. December 2012;38(12):2198-2199.

2. American Optometric Association. *Optometric Clinical Practice Guideline. Care of the Patient with Cataract*. http://www.aoa.org/documents/optometrists/CPG-8.pdf. 1995. Accessed August 30, 2017.

3. Chang MA, Airiani S, Miele D, Braunstein RE. A comparison of the potential acuity meter (PAM) and the illuminated near card (INC) in patients undergoing phacoemulsification. *Eye (Lond)*. 2006;20:1345-1351.

4. American Academy of Ophthalmology. *Preferred Practice Pattern Guideline. Cataract in the Adult Eye PPP – 2016*. http://www.aao.org/preferred-practice-pattern/cataract-in-adult-eye-ppp-2016. 2016. Accessed August 30, 2017.

5. Apple DJ, Mamalis N, Olson RJ, Kincaid MC. *Intraocular lenses: evolution, designs, complications and pathology*. Baltimore, MD: Williams & Wilkins; 1989:230-233.

6. Masket S, Tennen DG. Astigmatic stabilization of 3.0 mm temporal clear corneal cataract incisions. *J Cataract Refract Surg*. 1996;22:1451-1455.

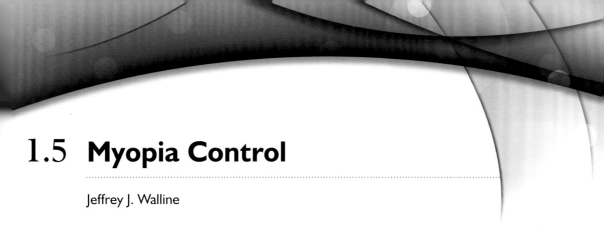

1.5 Myopia Control

Jeffrey J. Walline

Jenny, a 10-year-old female, presented for her yearly eye examination. She complained of poor distance vision in each eye for the past few months. There were no visual problems at near. Jenny's myopia had increased by over 1.00 D during the previous year, so she was referred for myopia control. Her glasses were updated 6 months ago for progressing myopia. Her mother reported that Jenny had no significant medical conditions and was not taking any medications. Jenny was allergic to dogs (causing red, itchy eyes and a runny nose), but no medical therapy was necessary because they did not have any dogs at home.

Clinical Findings

Current spectacles (6 months old)	OD −4.00 −0.50 × 180 (20/25) OS −3.75 −0.75 × 180 (20/30)
Manifest refraction	OD −4.50 −0.50 × 180 (20/15−) OS −4.25 −0.75 × 180 (20/20+)
Cover test	Distance: orthophoria; Near: 4Δ exophoria
Keratometry (simulated keratometry readings)	OD 40.50 sph (mires clear) OS 40.25 sph (mires clear)
Amplitude of accommodation (push-up)	OD: 12 D, 10 D, 12 D OS: 10 D, 10 D, 12 D
Slit-lamp examination	Unremarkable OD and OS
Intraocular pressure (Tonopen)	OD 14 mm Hg OS 15 mm Hg (at 4:15 PM)

Abbreviations: D, diopters; OD, right eye; OS, left eye; sph, sphere.

Three myopia control options were discussed with the parent and child, namely corneal reshaping contact lenses,[1,2] soft multifocal contact lenses,[3,4] and 0.01% atropine.[5-7] Neither the parent nor the child wanted to instill eye drops every day, so atropine was eliminated from the list of treatment alternatives. It was explained to the parent that, on average, orthokeratology and soft multifocal contact lenses each slow the progression of myopia by approximately 40%, so they provide similar levels of myopia control. The desired lifestyle with contact lenses was the most important factor in determining which contact lens modality may be best. A summary of the primary factors used to decide the preferred contact lens modality is shown in Table 1.5-1.

Table 1.5-1   Factors Used to Determine Which Contact Lens Modality (ie, Orthokeratology or Soft Multifocals) May Be More Desirable As a Myopia Control Treatment for a Particular Patient

Factor	Orthokeratology	Soft Multifocal	Comment
Wants to wear glasses sometimes		X	Soft contact lenses can be worn only when desired
Swims every day	X		Orthokeratology contact lenses allow clear vision in the pool without contact lens wear
Parent wears soft contact lenses		X	Parent will know how to deal with issues of soft contact lens wear
May have issues with contact lens handling	X		Orthokeratology contact lenses are only worn at home
Contact lens–related dry eye	X		Orthokeratology contact lenses may result in fewer symptoms of dryness
Less than 1.50 D myopia		X	Soft multifocal may provide more myopic defocus, which may result in better myopia control
More than 4.00 of myopia		X	Orthokeratology fits become more difficult over 4.00 D, especially with flat corneas
Significant astigmatism		X	Orthokeratology is more difficult for against-the-rule astigmatism

Abbreviation: D, diopters.

Because the parent wore soft contact lenses, and the patient liked wearing glasses and had over 4.00 D of myopia, it was decided to fit Jenny with center-distance design, soft multifocal contact lenses with a +2.50 D ADD, as described in the following table:

Contact lenses (center-distance design, soft multifocal, +2.50 D ADD)	OD −4.50 sph (20/25) OS −4.50 sph (20/30)
Spherical over-refraction	OD −0.50 (20/20^{+2}); OS: −0.75 (20/20^{-1})
Lenses dispensed	OD −5.00 sph (20/20) OS −5.25 sph (20/20) VA OU 20/15

Abbreviations: D, diopters; OD, right eye; OS, left eye; OU, both eyes; sph, sphere; VA, visual acuity.

Jenny was told to wear the contact lenses to the follow-up visit in 1 week. She was told not to wear her contact lenses for more than 8 hours per day during the first week of wear, then wear during all waking hours if desired.

At the 1-week follow-up visit, Jenny had no visual or asthenopic complaints. She reported the ability to apply both contact lenses in less than 5 minutes each day, and she could remove them on the first try every night.

Contact lenses (center-distance design, soft multifocal, +2.50 D ADD)	OD −5.00 sph (20/20) OS −5.25 sph (20/20)
Spherical over-refraction	OD −0.25 (20/20^{+2}); OS: plano (20/20)
Lenses dispensed	OD −5.25 sph (20/20^{+2}) OS −5.25 sph (20/20) VA OU 20/15

Abbreviations: D, diopters; OD, right eye; OS, left eye; OU, both eyes; sph, sphere; VA, visual acuity.

To adjust for the spherical over-refraction, the right lens was changed to −5.25 sph. It was also beneficial to have the same power in each eye, so the patient would not have to concern herself with which lens goes in which eye. The patient was told to wear her contact lenses to the next visit in 3 weeks.

At a 1-month follow-up visit, Jenny had no visual or asthenopic complaints, and she wore contact lenses every day but 1. The lens in the right eye was 3 weeks old, and the lens in the left eye was 4 weeks old.

Contact lenses (center-distance design, soft multifocal, +2.50 D ADD)	OD −5.25 sph (20/20) OS −5.25 sph (20/20⁻¹)
Spherical over-refraction	OD +0.25 (20/20); OS: plano (20/20)
Lenses dispensed	OD −5.25 sph (20/20) OS −5.25 sph (20/20) VA OU 20/15

Abbreviations: D, diopters; OD, right eye; OS, left eye; OU, both eyes; sph, sphere; VA, visual acuity.

Although the over-refraction in the right eye was +0.25 D, the benefit of having the same prescription for each eye outweighed the desire to lower the prescription based on the over-refraction. The patient was asked to return in 5 months for a checkup.

Six-Month Follow-up

Approximately 5 months after the last appointment, Jenny reported no change in vision or comfort. She also reported wearing the contact lenses almost every day.

Contact lenses (center-distance design, soft multifocal, +2.50 D ADD)	OD −5.25 sph (20/20⁺¹) OS −5.25 sph (20/20⁺¹)
Spherical over-refraction	OD: plano (20/20⁺²); OS: plano (20/20⁺¹)
Lenses dispensed	OD −5.25 sph (20/20⁺¹) OS −5.25 sph (20/20⁺¹)

Abbreviations: D, diopters; OD, right eye; OS, left eye; sph, sphere.

Jenny exhibited excellent care of her contact lenses, and she was told to continue daily wear with monthly replacement. She was asked to return for a comprehensive eye examination in a further 6 months. At the subsequent examination, she reported no visual or asthenopic complaints, and exhibited no change in prescription or ocular health. She continued in the contact lenses for 18 months, with no change in prescription being required.

Summary

This young patient enjoyed the visual[8] and non-visual[9] benefits of soft multifocal contact lens wear. This type of contact lens has been shown to slow myopia progression by about 40%.[3,4] Center-distance design soft multifocal contact lenses are thought to slow myopia progression by focusing the peripheral light rays in front of the retina, which may act as a signal to slow eye growth. Animal studies have shown that blur placed behind the retina increases eye growth, even when the hyperopic blur is isolated to the peripheral retina or when the macula is ablated.[10] In humans, the amount of myopic blur in the periphery is related to axial elongation of the eye,[11] and a contralateral control trial showed slowed myopia progression only in the eye wearing multifocal contact lenses.[12] If the myopia control effect were due to reduced accommodative effort or lag, then myopia control would have been effective in both of the eyes, because accommodation is yoked. All of this evidence illustrates peripheral myopic blur (light focused in front of the retina) as a putative cue for slowed eye growth.

Contact lens wear can improve how children feel about their physical appearance, athletic competence, and social acceptance.[9] After the initial fitting, this young patient was motivated to wear the contact lenses, which made lens care easier to teach, with a higher likelihood of success. Some children are not motivated to wear contact lenses, because they believe that they will hurt, so motivation should not be considered as the sole factor in the fitting process until the child has experienced contact lens wear.

Few parents know about myopia control, and should be educated about the possibility of using soft multifocal contact lenses, corneal reshaping contact lenses, and/or low-concentration atropine. Even if the child is not yet mature enough for elective contact lens wear, the parent may opt for eye drops at bed time or consider myopia control in the future.

CLINICAL PEARLS

- Children are frequently nervous about contact lens wear, but once they experience them, they understand the benefits and often become full-time contact lens wearers.

- Patients can only be told about the average rate of myopia control. One cannot predict the degree of myopia control for a specific individual because we do not know how much they would have progressed without control therapy.

- On average, soft multifocal and orthokeratology contact lenses both slow myopia progression by approximately 40%, so the parent can determine the most appropriate treatment based on lifestyle.

- Low-concentration atropine eye drops slow myopia progression by about 60%, they do not sting when instilled, and they cause only minor changes in accommodation or pupil size that is typically well tolerated by patients.[5]

- No evidence exists about the combination therapy of atropine and contact lenses, but combination therapy may provide additive benefit because, in theory, atropine provides a pharmacologic treatment mechanism and contact lenses provide an optical treatment mechanism.

- To provide optimal treatment with soft multifocal contact lenses, one must perform an over-refraction to optimize distance vision. Lowering the add power to provide optimal vision should rarely be necessary.

- All parents of myopic children, regardless of age, should be educated about the possibility of myopia control. They can decide when their child is ready for such therapy.

REFERENCES

1. Charm J, Cho P. High myopia-partial reduction ortho-k: a 2-year randomized study. *Optom Vis Sci.* 2013;90(6):530-539.
2. Cho P, Cheung SW. Retardation of myopia in orthokeratology (ROMIO) study: a 2-year randomized clinical trial. *Invest Ophthalmol Vis Sci.* 2012;53(11):7077-7085.
3. Aller TA, Liu M, Wildsoet CF. Myopia control with bifocal contact lenses: a randomized clinical trial. *Optom Vis Sci.* 2016;93(4):344-352.
4. Lam CS, Tang WC, Tse DY, Tang YY, To CH. Defocus incorporated soft contact (DISC) lens slows myopia progression in Hong Kong Chinese schoolchildren: a 2-year randomized clinical trial. *Br J Ophthalmol.* 2014;98(1):40-45.
5. Chia A, Chua WH, Cheung YB, et al. Atropine for the treatment of childhood myopia: safety and efficacy of 0.5%, 0.1%, and 0.01% doses (atropine for the treatment of myopia 2). *Ophthalmology.* 2012;119(2):347-354.
6. Chia A, Chua WH, Wen L, Fong A, Goon YY, Tan D. Atropine for the treatment of childhood myopia: changes after stopping atropine 0.01%, 0.1% and 0.5%. *Am J Ophthalmol.* 2014;157(2):451-457.e1.
7. Chia A, Lu QS, Tan D. Five-year clinical trial on atropine for the treatment of myopia 2: myopia control with atropine 0.01% eyedrops. *Ophthalmology.* 2016;123(2):391-399.
8. Rah MJ, Walline JJ, Jones-Jordan LA, et al. Vision specific quality of life of pediatric contact lens wearers. *Optom Vis Sci.* 2010;87(8):560-566.
9. Walline JJ, Jones LA, Sinnott L, et al. Randomized trial of the effect of contact lens wear on self-perception in children. *Optom Vis Sci.* 2009;86(3):222-232.
10. Smith EL III, Hung LF, Huang J. Relative peripheral hyperopic defocus alters central refractive development in infant monkeys. *Vision Res.* 2009;49(19):2386-2392.
11. Sankaridurg P, Holden B, Smith E III, et al. Decrease in rate of myopia progression with a contact lens designed to reduce relative peripheral hyperopia: one-year results. *Invest Ophthalmol Vis Sci.* 2011;52(13):9362-9367.
12. Anstice NS, Phillips JR. Effect of dual-focus soft contact lens wear on axial myopia progression in children. *Ophthalmology.* 2011;118(6):1152-1161.

1.6 Sports Vision: Lens Tints

Jacqueline M. Theis

John, a 65-year-old African American male, was referred by his primary care optometrist for a comprehensive sports vision examination. He wanted to know whether there was anything he could do to improve his ability to play tennis. Recently retired, he played tennis every day and noticed that he had trouble seeing the ball when it was in motion, especially on foggy days. He reported that he was able to see a stationary tennis ball clearly in the distance with his current glasses. Most commonly, he played in the morning or afternoon using standard yellow tennis balls on a red clay court with a green boundary. John preferred playing in daylight as he had trouble seeing under the standard metal halide outdoor lighting fixtures at night.

His ocular health history was unremarkable, with a normal dilated fundus examination performed 1 month ago according to the records he brought with him. John was healthy, did not take any medications, and denied any allergies.

Clinical Findings

All "distance" testing was performed at a physical distance of 12.8 ft (3.9 m) using a chart calibrated for a 20-ft (6 m) viewing distance.

Current Rx (nylon rimless frame with single-vision distance photochromic, polycarbonate lenses)	OD: −1.75 sph (20/20); OS: −1.75 −0.50 × 180 (20/15)
Unaided static near VA	OD: 20/20; OS: 20/20; OU: 20/20
Cover test (aided)	Distance: orthophoria; near: orthophoria
Near point of convergence	To the nose
Pupil evaluation	PERRL; no RAPD
Confrontation visual fields	Full to finger counting OD and OS
Eye movements (assessed by direct observation)	Fixation: steady, no nystagmus, no abnormal head movement Saccades: fast and accurate horizontally and vertically, with no abnormal head movement Pursuits: smooth and accurate horizontally and vertically, with no abnormal head movement
Subjective refraction	OD: −1.75 sph (20/20); OS: −1.75 −0.50 × 180 (20/15)
Distance VA with −0.25 ADD OU	OD: 20/20; OS: 20/15
Aided dynamic VA (at 10 cm/ms) (measured using the M&S Sports Performance Software at distance)	OU: 20/16
Distance vergence ranges	BI *x*/6/4; BO *x*/12/10

23

Near vergence ranges	BI x/10/8; BO x/15/12
Distance stereopsis (measured using the M&S Sports Performance Software)	20 s of arc
Slit-lamp examination	Trace nuclear sclerosis OU; otherwise unremarkable
Undilated fundus examination	No abnormalities observed OD and OS

Abbreviations: BI, base in; BO, base out; OD, right eye; OS, left eye; OU, both eyes; PERRL, pupils equal, round, reactive to light; RAPD, relative afferent pupillary defect; Rx, prescription; sph, sphere; VA, visual acuity.

Supplementary Testing

Using the M&S Sports Performance Software (M&S Technologies, Niles, Illinois)

Contrast threshold[a] (with habitual distance Rx)	OD: 10%; OS: 8%; OU: 8%
Contrast threshold with −0.25 ADD OU	OD: 8%; OS: 6%; OU: 4%
Tachistoscope— Perceptual speed[b]	72.5 percentile, best 40 ms (see description in the Discussion section)

[a] This refers to the lowest level of contrast perceived by the observer. The manufacturer indicated that the average monocular and binocular findings were 5.8% (SD ±3.0) and 3.3% (SD ±1.36), respectively.
[b] Performed at 40 cm.

Using the Senaptec Sensory Performance Software (Synaptec, Beaverton, Oregon)

This software uses data analytics to compare the patient's performance with a large database that includes youth to professional level athletes within a wide range of sports and positions. The patient's performance data are represented as a percentile ranking. An area where the performance fell below the 50th percentile is one for improvement, whereas a ranking greater than the 50th percentile is considered an area of relative strength. In this case, the data were compared with other recreational tennis players of all ages. At the time of writing, age-based normative data for these metrics have not been established.

The tests denoted in the following table were performed either at a 10-ft (3 m) "distance" or 2-ft (0.61 m) "near" working distance.

Contrast sensitivity *At distance*	10th percentile
Hart chart[1] *At distance and near*	46th percentile
Multiple object tracking *At near*	49th percentile
Eye–hand reaction time *At near*	95th percentile

Discussion

John had excellent static distance visual acuity (VA) with his current glasses. However, that test measures the ability to resolve stationary targets, whereas sports like tennis require the resolution of moving targets, while the athlete may also be moving, that is, dynamic VA. Because John was complaining of difficulty seeing the ball in motion, it was important to test both static and dynamic parameters. Dynamic VA can be measured using specialized computerized charts or rotating discs.[2] In this case, John's dynamic VA was measured using the M&S Sports Performance program. Here, a single letter moved horizontally across the screen at a constant speed, while gradually increasing in size until the patient is able to identify it. John had excellent dynamic VA (20/16) at distance.

Ocular alignment, vergence function, and eye movements were normal. Accommodative testing was not performed because of his manifest presbyopia. Additional sports vision performance metrics showed that John's higher level visual processing skills, that is, near-far speed, multiple object tracking, eye–hand coordination, and visual perception speed were at or above the age-expected normative values.

In any sports vision examination, measurement of contrast sensitivity is fundamental.[3] Although John had normal VA using a high-contrast Snellen chart, reduced contrast sensitivity was also found. This is consistent with his difficulties in seeing the ball depending on the level and type of illumination. Contrast sensitivity may be improved optically, either through additional refractive power or by prescribing tinted lenses.[2] While an additional −0.25 sph OU did not alter his static VA, it improved contrast sensitivity. If additional 0.25 sph minus lens power is provided to athletes to enhance their contrast sensitivity, it is important to inform the patient that this prescription is for sportswear only, and that daily use of this prescription could lead to eye-strain over time. One must also demonstrate this prescription to a presbyopic patient using a trial frame, to ensure their visual comfort at distance.

In addition, John was advised to try either yellow- or amber-tinted lenses in an attempt to improve his contrast sensitivity. Yellow tints can improve low-contrast VA, with no adverse effects on vision performance. However, dark gray lenses, commonly used by athletes, may actually have an adverse effect on sports performance by reducing hand–eye coordination and contrast sensitivity.[4] Amber tints have also been shown to improve visual performance for high-speed ball sports.[5] It is believed that amber and yellow tints, by blocking out shorter wavelength light, will reduce chromatic aberration and intraocular light scatter, thereby resulting in improved VA and contrast sensitivity.[2] The practitioner should test contrast sensitivity through yellow- and amber-tinted lenses to confirm any perceived changes. However, a true test of sports performance under varying luminance levels is difficult to simulate in an office setting, and can really only be tested in the actual environment where the sport is performed. Given this patient's age and ocular health findings, it seems likely that the

reduced contrast sensitivity could have been caused by increased intraocular light scatter from his cataracts. While difficulties with glare can prompt a patient to be interested in cataract surgery, in view of his excellent VA (20/20), the possible risks of the surgery probably outweigh its benefits at this time. It is best to counsel John that the cataracts are probably responsible for his problems with glare, and to discuss the options for removal in the future should they worsen.

John presented wearing single-vision lenses in a nylon rimless fashion eyewear frame. In addition to prescribing lenses for optimal sports performance, the practitioner must also educate the patient regarding impact-resistant lenses and frame materials. Spectacle-related eye injuries are one of the most preventable causes of ocular and facial trauma. The use of a nonimpact-resistant frame and lens materials puts the patient at greater risk, were he to be hit by a flying object (like a tennis ball) or fall while wearing the eyewear. Improper eyewear can shatter and cause penetrating eye injuries.[6,7] Practitioners should be aware of the appropriate standards for protective eyewear (eg, in the United States, referral should be made to the American National Standards Institute [ANSI] and American Society for Testing and Materials International [ASTM] standards).

This case is an example of how a sports-vision optometrist can enhance visual performance by means of a refractive correction, irrespective of the patient's age.

CLINICAL PEARLS

- Contrast sensitivity is a critical visual skill in sports vision.

- Optometrists must provide impact-resistant frames and lenses to protect the athletic patient.

REFERENCES

1. Scheiman M, Wick B. *Clinical Management of Binocular Vision: Heterophoric, Accommodative, and Eye Movement Disorders*. Philadelphia, PA: Lippincott Williams & Wilkins; 2014:25-27.
2. Erickson GB. Visual performance evaluation. In: Erickson G, ed. *Sports Vision: Vision Care for*

the Enhancement of Sports Performance. St. Louis, MO: Butterworth-Heinemann; 2007:45-83.

3. Zimmerman AB, Lust KL, Bullimore MA. Visual acuity and contrast sensitivity testing for sports vision. *Eye Contact Lens*. 2011;37:153-159.

4. Kohmura Y, Murakami S, Aoki K. Effect of yellow-tinted lenses on visual attributes related to sports activities. *J Hum Kinet*. 2013;36:27-36.

5. Erickson GB, Horn FC, Barney T, Pexton B, Baird R. Visual performance with sport-tinted contact lenses in natural sunlight. *Optom Vis Sci*. 2009;86:509-516.

6. Dain SJ. Sports eyewear protective standards. *Clin Exp Optom*. 2016;99:4-23.

7. Hoskin AK, Philip S, Dain SJ, Mackey DA. Spectacle-related eye injuries, spectacle-impact performance and eye protection. *Clin Exp Optom*. 2015;98:203-209.

1.7 Dispensing Issues With Progressive Addition Lenses: Adaptational Issues When Switching From Conventional to Free-Form Progressive Addition Lenses

Alan G. McKee

Andrew, a 50-year-old male university professor, returned 3 days after the dispensing of his new spectacles complaining of "difficulty getting used to my new glasses." He stated that his vision was clear at both distance and near, and that he had no problems with the required head position, field of view, image distortion, or general comfort. Andrew could only say that compared with his old glasses, "the vision was clearer but something doesn't seem right." His previous glasses were 2 years old, and he reported increasing difficulty with reading with this prescription. His hobbies included woodworking and playing the guitar.

Clinical Findings

Previous Rx: conventionally surfaced, standard corridor length, PAL (2 years old)	OD: +2.00 −0.50 × 175 (20/15) (base curve +6.00); OS: +1.50 −0.50 × 176 (20/15) (base curve +6.00); ADD: +2.00 OU (20/20 at 40 cm with moderate effort)
New Rx: free-form backside, optimized for Rx PAL	OD: +2.50 −0.50 × 175 (20/15) (nominal base curve +6.00); OS: +2.00 −0.50 × 176 (20/15) (nominal base curve +6.00); ADD: +2.00 OU (20/20 at 40 cm)

Abbreviations: OD, right eye; OS, left eye; OU, both eyes; Rx, prescription; PAL, progressive addition lens.

Comments

Both the old and new glasses were made with the same model, size and shape rimless frame having the same distance monocular interpupillary distances, fitting heights, pantoscopic tilt, and face wrap. Free-form "optimized for Rx" progressive addition lenses (PALs) (ie, free-form lenses that have an optimized back-surface geometry to minimize specific lens aberrations) were chosen for the new glasses to enhance the field of view through all zones of the lens. It was thought that reducing aberrations would also improve vision under low-light conditions.

On examination, it was confirmed that other than a slight difference in the vertex distance between the 2 pairs of glasses, the frame adjustments were identical. Even when the vertex distances of the 2 pairs were equalized, Andrew still reported that his vision did not feel right. The fitting crosses and distance and near areas of each pair were re-marked using the manufacturer's PAL layout guide. All measurements were within the American National Standards Institute (ANSI) Z80.1 tolerances.[1] The nominal base curves for each lens were found to be similar between the old and new glasses.

Andrew was asked to continue wearing the new spectacles and to return in a week. He was also asked not to wear his old glasses. However, he did not return for this follow-up visit. Andrew was called to see how he was adapting to the new eyewear. He stated that for 2 more days after he left the office (5 days after dispensing), he continued to notice the sensation of uneasiness while wearing the new eyewear. However, this feeling gradually diminished. In an additional 3 days (8 days after dispensing), the sensation was no longer present, and he was doing well with his new spectacles.

Discussion

Modern PALs have patient acceptance rates of 90% and higher.[2] The most common reasons for dissatisfaction with PALs are improper fitting measurements (particularly when the frame is not adjusted properly before fitting), poor frame selection, and incorrect add power.[3] Modern lens designs ease the initial adaptation as long as the lens is positioned correctly before the eye.[4] Management of this case is made more difficult by the patient's vague complaint that "something doesn't seem right" when switching from a conventional to a free-form backside PAL (ie, a customized lens with the progressive curve on the rear surface).

While a number of patients have presented to our institution with similar complaints on switching from conventional PALs to newer free-form PALs, most only needed reassurance that they will adapt to the new and improved optics of free-form PALs. Ultimately they wore the new lens designs successfully. Based on our data, only 2 out of 2000 (0.1%) patients who switched from a conventional to a free-form PAL had to revert back to a conventionally surfaced lens. This corresponds to a 99.9% success rate. Both of these nontolerance cases involved add powers greater than +1.75 D.

The precise reason for Andrew's uneasiness with the new lens, or the rare inability to change successfully from a conventional to free-form lens designs is unclear. One possible explanation is that having become accustomed to the aberrations found in a conventionally surfaced lens, discomfort may arise when first wearing a free-form lens design in which aberrations no longer exist. When a patient has adapted to a lens with aberrations, suddenly removing them may be perceptually similar to experiencing the opposite aberrations. Alternatively, the altered spatial perception could be due to changes in spectacle magnification resulting from differences in the front-surface geometry of conventional versus free-form lens designs.

To maximize the likelihood of success when dispensing any type of PAL:

1. Always adjust the frame to the patient's face before taking any fitting measurements. Just as conventional PALs require more precise positioning when compared with lined multifocals, free-form PALs are even more dependent on proper positioning.

2. Periodically check the calibration of digital pupillometers and/or computerized frame measurement systems. Many modern computerized dispensing instruments such as the iTerminal 2 (Carl Zeiss Vision, San Diego, California), VisiOffice 2® (Essilor, Dallas, Texas), and the Spectangle® Pro/Optikam (HOYA Vision Care, Lewisville, Texas) can automate the frame and lens fitting measurements. An instrument that is not calibrated correctly can lead to lens-positioning errors and patient discomfort.

3. Before dispensing a PAL, verify the prescription (either compared with the original prescription, or with a modified version of the prescription if customized for frame fit and personalized lenses) and that the monocular interpupillary distance and fitting heights are correct.

4. At the time of dispensing, verify the placement of the optics, distance and near visual acuities (VAs), right and left fields of view and head posture during both distance and near viewing. If required, make appropriate frame and/or fitting measurement adjustments.

5. For patients for whom a change in prescription (Rx) and/or lens design occurs, demonstrate the improvement in distance and/or near vision.

6. Tell first-time, free-form PAL wearers that vision in dim light and night vision will be enhanced because of improvements in the optics of the lenses.

7. Tell the patients that a few days may be required to become fully accustomed to the new glasses. During that time, they should avoid any potentially hazardous tasks where misjudging distances could result in injury to themselves or others. Encourage them to call or return if they are noticing any issues after the first week of wearing new spectacles. Ask them not to wear the old spectacles until they are fully adapted to the new eyewear, as switching between the 2 may slow down the adjustment to the change in optical design.

8. Be empathetic to patients having adaptational issues. Verify frame adjustment and the Rx (lenses sometimes rotate within the frame). Be aware of other issues that might interfere with adaptation such as a significant change in Rx, base curve, lens thickness or lens design.

9. As a last resort, consider returning to a conventionally surfaced lens for the rare patient who cannot adapt successfully to a free-form design.

CLINICAL PEARLS

- When switching patients form a conventional to a free-form PAL, inform them that a few days may be required to become fully accustomed to the new glasses.

- Increase the likelihood of success with PALs by assuring proper frame adjustment, calibrating measuring equipment, verifying lens parameters, and educating the patient about adaptation.

REFERENCES

1. ANSI Z80.1-2015. *American National Standard for Ophthalmics – Prescription Ophthalmic Lenses – Recommendations*. Alexandria, VA: The Vision Council; 2015.
2. Fannin T, Grosvenor T. *Clinical Optics*. 2nd ed. Waltham, MA: Butterworth-Heinemann; 1996:261-262.
3. Brooks CW, Borish IM. *System for Ophthalmic Dispensing*. 2nd ed. St. Louis, MO: Butterworth-Heinemann; 2007:454-467.
4. Han S, Graham A, Lin M. Clinical assessment of a customized free-form progressive add lens spectacle. *Optom Vis Sci*. 2011;88(2):234-243.

1.8 Dispensing Anomalies: Disorientation Following Prescription Change

Alan G. McKee

Robert, a 63-year-old retired male farmer, presented for an annual diabetic eye examination and refraction with a chief complaint of blurred vision with his current glasses. The blur was more apparent at near than distance. His hobbies included hunting and fishing. He had received conventional progressive addition lenses (PALs) 5 years ago, and was happy with them at that time.

Clinical Findings

Previous Rx: conventionally surfaced, tall-corridor PAL (5 years old)	OD: +0.75 sph (20/50) (base curve +4.50); OS: +1.00 −0.25 × 54 (20/40) (base curve +4.50); ADD: +2.50 OU (20/25 @ 40 cm)
New findings: free-form PAL (Rx1)	OD: +2.50 −0.50 × 175 (20/15) (base curve +4.50); OS: +2.00 −0.50 × 176 (20/15) (base curve +4.50); ADD: +2.50 OU

Abbreviations: OD, right eye; OS, left eye; OU, both eyes; PAL, progressive addition lens; Rx, prescription; sph, sphere.

Comments

A significant increase in plus power was found in both eyes, and the style of PAL was changed from a conventional tall-corridor PAL to a free-form optimized for prescription (Rx) (ie, free-form lenses that have an optimized back-surface geometry to minimize specific lens aberrations) PAL so as to sharpen night vision and increase the field of view of the distance, intermediate, and near zones of his lenses (Rx1).

Follow-up Visit (1 Month Following Initial Examination)

Robert returned reporting "blurry distance vision that improves when I tilt my head down." The plus power was reduced in each eye (Rx2), and the glasses were remade as shown in overleaf.

Rx2: free-form PAL	OD: +2.00 −0.75 × 120 (20/15) (base curve +4.50); OS: +1.50 −0.75 × 60 (20/15) (base curve +4.50); ADD: +2.50 OU (20/20 at 40 cm)

Abbreviations: OD, right eye; OS, left eye; OU, both eyes; PAL, progressive addition lens; Rx, prescription.

Follow-up Visit (2.5 Months Following Initial Examination)

Some 6 weeks after Rx2 had been dispensed, Robert returned complaining of having to "tilt my head back to see clearly at distance and near." During the visit his refractive error was found to be more plus than at the earlier follow-up visit, and nearly identical to the Rx prescribed 10 weeks before. Robert's most recent fasting blood glucose and HbA1c levels (recorded 1 week earlier) were verified to be well controlled at 102 mg/dL and 5.6%, respectively. Spectacles were remade with the modified Rx (Rx3) as shown in table below.

Rx3: free-form PAL	OD: +2.50 −0.75 × 120 (20/15) (base curve +6.50 aspheric); OS: +2.00 −0.75 × 60 (20/15) (base curve +6.50 aspheric); ADD: +2.50 OU (20/20 at 40 cm)

Abbreviations: OD, right eye; OS, left eye; OU, both eyes; PAL, progressive addition lens; Rx, prescription.

Follow-up Visit (3.5 Months Following Initial Examination)

One month later Robert returned complaining of feeling "off-balance when walking" with Rx3, although his distance and near vision were clear. The frame adjustment, lens powers, and fitting measurements were verified to be correct. However, on consultation with the manufacturing lens laboratory, a decision was made to return to a conventional PAL (Rx4) so that the base curves could be matched to his original spectacles (Rx1).

Rx4: conventionally surfaced tall-corridor PAL	OD: +2.50 −0.75 × 120 (20/15) (base curve +4.50); OS: +2.00 −0.75 × 60 (20/15) (base curve +4.50); ADD: +2.50 OU (20/20 at 40 cm)

Abbreviations: OD, right eye; OS, left eye; OU, both eyes; PAL, progressive addition lens; Rx, prescription.

At the time when Rx4 was dispensed, Robert noted immediately that he could walk without feeling "off-balance."

Discussion

At least 4 distinct clinical issues were considered for this patient: First, poorly controlled diabetes with changes in blood glucose levels can cause marked shifts in refractive error.[1] If this is suspected, then the patient should be refracted 2 or 3 times over a 4- to 6-week period until a stable result is found. Unfortunately, many patients either do not want to return for multiple examinations, or have lost or damaged their spectacles and need an immediate replacement for work or school. In this particular case, changes in blood glucose did not appear to be the issue.

Second, patients may have difficulty accepting modified prescriptions. The prescribing clinician must determine how much of a prescription change will be tolerated by the patient. Here, the initial prescription change was significant, but this was ultimately accepted by the patient as it provided improved VA at both distance and near.

Third, based on the increased prescription, the lens manufacturer recommended a change in the base curve. Increased plus power generally requires a steeper base curve. However, a steeper base curve creates higher spectacle magnification,[2] which may make objects appear to be closer than when viewed through lenses with a flatter base curve. This seemed to be the major contributing factor for Robert. The previous lenses were made with a flatter base curve, and when the prescription was increased, a steeper base curve was incorporated in the lens design by the manufacturing laboratory. Although this would not be a problem for most patients, changes in magnification can be problematic for some, especially individuals with oblique astigmatism.

Fourth, the patient was switched from a conventional PAL design to a free-form, optimized for Rx, design. In most cases, patients prefer free-form, optimized for Rx designs over conventional PALs as a result of decreased aberrations and improved performance in dim illumination.[3] However, on occasion, patients may report a sensation of "vague uneasiness" with the lens, particularly with higher add powers. This may be caused by differences in the shape of the progression corridor, magnification differences between lens designs, or the reduction in aberrations commonly found in more conventional lenses.

This patient was switched back to a conventional PAL design to allow a specific base curve to be selected. Free-form, optimized lens designs require a specific base curve. When a different base curve is required, the lenses must be conventionally surfaced.

CLINICAL PEARLS

- Improvements in vision by tilting the head up or down can occur because of spherical power changes within the intermediate and near portions of a PAL. Alternatively, a more complex interaction between the astigmatism induced by tilting a lens and the unwanted astigmatism adjacent to the PAL corridor may also be responsible.

- For patients with a high Rx ($> \pm 6.00$ D), moderate astigmatism (> 2.00 D), and/or greater than normal amounts of pantoscopic tilt or frame wrap, the clinician should consider free-form PALs customized to maximize the useable areas of the lens.

REFERENCES

1. Li H, Lou G, Gou J, Liang Z. Effects of glycemic control on refraction in diabetic patients. *Int J Ophthalmol.* 2010;3(2):158-160.
2. Brooks CW, Borish IM. *System for Ophthalmic Dispensing.* 3rd ed. St. Louis, MO: Butterworth-Heinemann; 2007:493-494.
3. Han S, Graham A, Lin M. Clinical assessment of a customized free-form progressive add lens spectacle. *Optom Vis Sci.* 2011;88(2):234-243.

1.9 Dispensing Issues With Progressive Addition Lenses: Adaptation Issues

Alan G. McKee

Matt, a 55-year-old male handyman, returned 1 week after the dispensing of new free-form, optimized to prescription (Rx), progressive addition lenses (PALs), that is, a free-form lens that has an optimized back-surface geometry to minimize the aberrations present in a conventionally surfaced lens of the same prescription. Matt complained of difficulty finding the correct head position for comfortable viewing of his home computer for an extended period of time with the new Rx.

Although he agreed that both his distance and near vision were improved with the new glasses, he stated that he did not have the same problem viewing his computer with his old pair. He used a desktop computer with a 24-in display. While seated at a similar computer in the examination room, he was asked to adopt the same working position. The viewing distance was determined to be 56 cm from the spectacle plane, with a gaze angle 15° below primary gaze. Matt had worn PALs successfully for the past 15 years.

Clinical Findings

Previous Rx: fixed-length corridor free-form optimized for Rx PAL with a minimum fitting height of 17 mm Metal frame with B-dimension of 33 mm	OD: −4.50 −0.50 × 177 (20/20); OS: −4.75 −0.75 × 6 (20/20) ADD: +1.75 OU (20/20 @ 40 cm)
New Rx: variable-length free-form optimized for Rx PAL with a minimum fitting height of 13 mm Metal frame with B-dimension of 30 mm	OD: −4.25 −0.25 × 178 (20/20); OS: −4.25 −0.25 × 178 (20/20) ADD: +2.00 OU (20/20 @ 40 cm)

Abbreviations: OD, right eye; OS, left eye; OU, both eyes; PAL, progressive addition lens; Rx, prescription.

Comments

The monocular pupillary distances, fitting heights, distance prescription, and near adds were verified to lie within the current American National Standards Institute (ANSI) Z80.1 standards.[1] Adjusting the new frame to alter the fitting height, pantoscopic tilt, face wrap, and vertex distance each failed to improve the performance of the spectacles at the required intermediate distance. Using the manufacturer's PAL layout guide, the fitting crosses and distance and near areas of each lens were re-marked. While the patient was able to find 1 position where the computer screen was clear, maintaining this head position for an extended period of time remained difficult.

In consultation with the manufacturer, lenses were reordered with a fixed-length corridor design and a corridor length that was 2 mm shorter than the previous PAL's minimum fitting height of 17 mm.

All of the remaining fitting measurements were kept as before. The resulting 15 mm fixed corridor length PAL was dispensed. Matt was able to find an acceptable head position for computer work while retaining the improved distance and near vision with the new glasses.

Discussion

For the particular type of PAL selected, the manufacturer provided 4 fixed-length and 1 variable-length corridor designs. In the latter design, the lens laboratory makes the corridor length as long as possible for the B-dimension of the selected frame. The fixed-length corridor designs allow the practitioner to customize the corridor length as needed for a particular patient's visual requirements. The recommendation from the laboratory was to use the variable-length design unless a specific corridor length was indicated for a particular task. In this case, the slight decrease in the B-dimension of the frame, combined with the variable-length corridor PAL resulted in a more rapid power progression from distance to near, and a narrower intermediate corridor, when compared with Matt's previous PALs. The solution was to match the corridor length to his previous lenses to achieve a similar rate of power increase in downgaze. In addition, increasing the corridor length also results in a wider intermediate corridor,[2] as shown in Figure 1.9-1.

This case illustrates the importance of a thorough case-history to identify whether the patient requires a gradual or more rapid power progression, and to determine the appropriate widths of the distance, intermediate, and near vision zones. Variable length PAL designs have been marketed as optimizing the distance and near zones for a specific frame size. Although this is true, it does not eliminate the need for careful frame selection to meet the patient's specific needs. For extended intermediate visual tasks, such as viewing a desktop computer monitor, a longer corridor length is helpful to allow a larger range of head positions.[3]

In an ideal world, patients should have a pair of spectacles customized specifically for extended, intermediate tasks such as using a desktop computer. Although general-purpose PALs provide clear vision at all distances, they may not be optimal for extended intermediate visual needs. Specialized lenses, such as so-called computer PALs with small distance and larger intermediate zones, can better satisfy these requirements, but may not be optimal for driving or other daily activities. If the patient is unwilling to purchase a pair of spectacles designed primarily for intermediate tasks, then the practitioner should select lenses that provide optimal vision at the most important viewing distance. Patients should understand that compromise will likely be needed at other distances. Individuals falling into this category include athletes, artists, computer users, hunters, and musicians. They may attempt to use a single pair of spectacles for both everyday wear and their specific occupation or avocation.

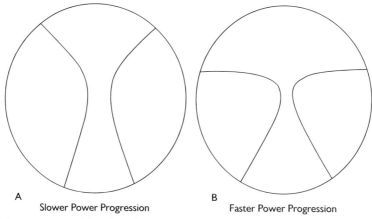

A   Slower Power Progression

B   Faster Power Progression

Figure 1.9-1   The progressive addition lens depicted on the left (A) has a longer corridor resulting in a slower power progression, wider intermediate corridor, and smaller distance and near zones. The lens illustrated on the right (B) shows the effect of a shorter corridor length, namely a more rapid power progression, narrowing of the intermediate corridor, and wider distance and near zones.

CLINICAL PEARLS

- When evaluating the patient's visual requirements, consider the B-dimension of the frame and whether the power progression of the PAL should be rapid or gradual for the particular task. All recommendations should be recorded on the spectacle Rx and conveyed to the staff as the patient transitions to the optical area to choose glasses.

- Both the eyecare practitioner and optical staff must be aware of any potential unwanted side effects when switching from a fixed-length to a variable-length corridor design. Careful attention to the patient's visual requirements at distance, intermediate, and near should guide frame and multifocal lens selection.

REFERENCES

1. ANSI Z80.1-2015. *American National Standard for Ophthalmics – Prescription Ophthalmic Lenses – Recommendations*. Alexandria, VA: The Vision Council; 2015.
2. Meister D, Fisher S. Progress in the spectacle correction of presbyopia. Part 1: design and development of progressive lenses. *Clin Exp Optom*. 2008; 91(3):245.
3. Jaschinski W, Konig M, Mekontso T, Ohlendorf A, Welscher M. Comparison of progressive addition lenses for general purpose and for computer vision: an office field study. *Clin Exp Optom*. 2015;98:234-243.

1.10 Prescribing for Musicians

Jennifer Long

Monica, a 48-year-old female musician, played both the piano and the pipe organ. Although she had natural monovision, Monica preferred clear vision in both eyes for tasks requiring concentration (such as driving and reading). She often experienced headaches when the vision in 1 eye was blurry. Therefore, she wore her spectacles most of the time. Monica had 2 pairs of single-vision spectacles: distance spectacles for driving and watching television and near spectacles for reading books, playing the piano, and practicing the pipe organ.

While playing the organ during church services, Monica needed to see her music as well as look into the distance to watch the service proceedings and the choir conductor. She viewed these distance tasks in a mirror, which was located above head height on the organ console (Figure 1.10-1). Monica did not wear either of her spectacles during church services because they only provided clear vision at a single-viewing distance. She had tried wearing her near spectacles low on her nose (so that she can look over the top to see in the distance) but needed to tip her head slightly forward to look over the frame. She was self-conscious that this posture made her look old. Consequently, Monica relied on her unaided vision, even though she often experienced frontal headaches when trying to focus on the various tasks.

Monica wanted to simplify her spectacles and enquired about wearing multifocal spectacles full time. She did not want to wear contact lenses.

Clinical Findings

Unaided distance VA	OD: 20/70; OS: 20/20^{-2}; OU: 20/20^{-2}
Unaided near VA	OD: 20/20; OS: 20/40; OU: 20/20
Dominant eye	Left eye
Present Rx	OD: −1.25 sph (20/15); OS: −0.25 sph (20/15); (OU: 20/15) ADD: +1.25 OU (20/20)
Near point of convergence	8 cm
Confrontation visual fields	Full to finger counting OD and OS
Pupil evaluation	PERRL; no RAPD
Retinoscopy	OD: −1.00 −0.25 × 90; OS: −0.25 sph
Subjective refraction	OD: −1.25 sph (20/15); OS: −0.25 sph (20/15)
Distance phoria (through subjective)	1Δ exophoria, 0 vertical phoria
Near add	+1.25 OU (near VA = 20/20)
Range of clear vision through near add	35-70 cm
Near phoria (through near addition)	4Δ exophoria

| Intraocular pressure (GAT) | OD: 16 mm Hg; OS: 17 mm Hg (at 10:30 AM) |
| Slit lamp and fundus examination | Unremarkable |

Abbreviations: GAT, Goldmann applanation tonometry; OD, right eye; OS, left eye; OU, both eyes; PERRL, pupils equal, round, reactive to light; RAPD, relative afferent pupillary defect; Rx, prescription; sph, sphere; VA, visual acuity.

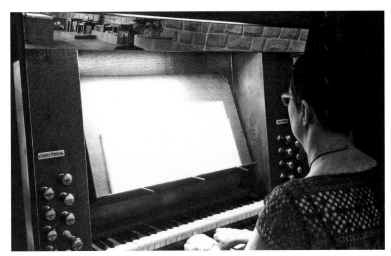

Figure 1.10-1   Monica at the pipe organ console. Note the mirror above Monica's head, which allows her to view the church service while playing the organ.

Comments

General-purpose progressive addition lenses (PALs) will simplify Monica's spectacle wear for daily activities such as driving, watching television, and reading books. However, there is a risk that she will be uncomfortable wearing these spectacles while playing the piano and the organ because the music stand on these instruments is usually located in the straight-ahead position and at an intermediate distance, whereas the reading zone in general-purpose PALs is designed for a downward gaze and a near distance. Wearing general-purpose PALs for these tasks could promote an awkward head and neck posture (head tipped back, chin thrust forward) similar to postures adopted by people using desktop computers while wearing general-purpose bifocals[1] or general-purpose PALs (see Chapter 1.11).

The optimal lens design for playing the pipe organ during church services will depend on the actual viewing distance and height while seated at the organ console. Monica did not

know these exact parameters and agreed to measure them and return for a follow-up consultation so that task-specific lenses could be prescribed (eg, special-purpose occupational bifocals). Meanwhile, Monica was keen to purchase general-purpose PALs for everyday use, which she ordered at the conclusion of this consultation.

At a follow-up visit, 6 weeks after the initial consultation, Monica had been successfully wearing her general-purpose PALs for 4 weeks, and reported that her overall visual comfort was better and her headache frequency had reduced. She continued to wear her single-vision near spectacles while playing the piano because she could "see the music more clearly" than with the PALs. Monica tried wearing the PALs while playing the organ at church, but as predicted, found that she tipped her head back to see the music. Therefore, she reverted to unaided vision for this task.

Monica's colleague took some photographs of her playing the piano (Figure 1.10-2) and the pipe organ (Figure 1.10-1) and measured

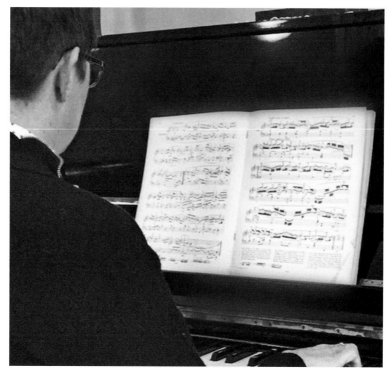

Figure 1.10-2   Monica playing the piano.

her viewing distances at both instruments with a tape measure. The viewing distance to the music stand on the piano was 58 cm and the top of the music was approximately 8 cm below Monica's eye level. Her single-vision near spectacles provide clear vision at this distance (range of clear vision was 35 to 70 cm) and allowed a straight-ahead posture. This explained why Monica was comfortable wearing single-vision spectacles for this task.

The pipe organ was more complex. The music stand was 66 cm from Monica's eyes and the top of the music was located 0 to 5 cm below eye level, depending on the size of the music book (Figure 1.10-1). Monica used the entire width of the music stand (74 cm). Above her head was a mirror that allowed her to see the church service proceedings and the choir conductor without twisting her body or her head (18 cm above eye height). On each side of the organ keyboard were registration stops that enabled a change in the sound of the organ (eg, trumpet or flute sound), and Monica often changed these mid-piece (ie, while she was playing). Monica was familiar with the location of the various registration stops so only needed

to glance at them. The viewing distance to the registration stops was about 70 cm.

After conducting a mock-up and discussing various lens options, Monica decided to order 28-mm flat top bifocal lenses set 3 mm above the top of her pupil to allow her to see the music in a straight-ahead posture. The distance zone in the top portion of the lenses was only 9 mm high, but was of sufficient size for her to be able to gaze upward into the mirror for viewing the church service and choir conductor. Monica was advised not to use these spectacles for driving.

Discussion

It was a challenge to comprehend the task and viewing requirements necessary for playing the pipe organ. Once the requirements were understood, and Monica became engaged in the prescribing process (eg, by taking photographs and measuring viewing distances and viewing heights), it was possible to develop an elegant optical solution.

The task demands of musicians can vary widely. For example, some guitarists look at the fretboard while playing, while others do not.

The demands can also vary between playing conditions (eg, playing the violin at home is different from playing in an orchestra where the violinist needs to read their music and watch the conductor) and between different instruments (eg, pipe organs may have up to 7 keyboards and hundreds of registration stops, which will affect the location of the music stand and mirrors). Therefore, it is important to ask specific questions about how patients play their instruments and where they need to look while playing. It may also require creative thinking to devise an optical solution for the patient, for example, extra high bifocal segments as in this case, or bifocal segments set at a 45° angle for a harpist as described by Kadrmas et al.[2]

When patients present with complex task requirements, it is often useful to simulate the various task locations and confirm the correct prescription for the different viewing distances using a trial frame and lenses. It is also possible to illustrate the proposed viewing zones by drawing a line with a marking pen on the lenses of an existing pair of spectacles. This process facilitates a more in-depth conversation with the patient about the task, helps refine what type of spectacle lens may be required, and allows discussion with the patient about various spectacle lens options.

Contact lenses are also an option for presbyopic musicians who need to look in unconventional gaze positions. This could include multifocal lenses, monovision, and single-vision near spectacles worn over the top of single-vision distance contact lenses. As in this case study, the best option will depend on the task requirements as well as patient expectations for their vision.

CLINICAL PEARLS

- When prescribing for musicians, ask specific questions about how they play their instrument and where they need to look while playing.

- It can be useful to simulate (mock-up) the various task locations and confirm the correct prescription for the various viewing distances using a trial frame and trial lenses.

REFERENCES

1. Martin D, Dain S. Postural modifications of VDU operators wearing bifocal spectacles. *Appl Ergon.* 1988;19:293-300.
2. Kadrmas E, Dyer J, Bartley G. Visual problems of the aging musician. *Surv Ophthalmol.* 1996;40:338-341.

1.11 Prescribing for a Computer User

Jennifer Long

Margaret, a 60-year-old female, presented wearing general-purpose progressive addition lenses (PALs) in her spectacles. For 15 years she worked in a retail store where she dealt with customers, worked with stock in the store, and used the computer to process sales transactions. Four months ago, she was transferred to a clerical position within the company, and now she works half time at the head office and half time at home. Since taking on this new desktop computer–based role, Margaret had been experiencing headaches at the end of her workdays. At first, she attributed the headaches to the stress associated with learning a new role, and had been taking over-the-counter analgesics to relieve the pain. Her employer arranged an assessment of her workstations to ensure that they were set up correctly for her. These were conducted by a work health safety officer within the company. Despite this, and the fact that she was no longer stressed about her work, her headaches had become more intense. She visited her general medical practitioner, who confirmed that her blood pressure medication was appropriate. He suggested that she have her eyes examined. If all was well with her eyes, then the next step would be to instigate further tests, including a referral to a neurologist.

Clinical Findings

Unaided distance VA	OD: 20/40; OS: 20/60^{-1}; OU: 20/30^{-1}
Present Rx	OD: +0.75 sph (20/20); OS: +1.00 sph (20/20); ADD: +2.50 OU (20/20)
Near point of convergence	12 cm
Confrontation visual fields	Full to finger counting OD and OS
Pupil evaluation	PERRL; no RAPD
Retinoscopy	OD: +1.00 sph; OS: +1.25 sph
Subjective refraction	OD: +1.00 sph (20/15^{-1}); OS: +1.25 sph (20/15^{1})
Distance phoria (through subjective Rx)	Horizontal: 2Δ exophoria; Vertical: 0Δ
Near add	+2.50 OU (near VA = 20/20)
Near phoria (through subjective near addition)	Horizontal: 6Δ exophoria; Vertical: 0Δ
Intraocular pressure (GAT)	OD: 17 mm Hg; OS: 17 mm Hg at 3:00 PM
Slit-lamp examination	Unremarkable OD and OS
Dilated fundus examination	Unremarkable OD and OS

Abbreviations: GAT, Goldmann applanation tonometry; OD, right eye; OS, left eye; OU, both eyes; PERRL, pupils equal, round, reactive to light; RAPD, relative afferent pupillary defect; Rx, prescription; sph, sphere; VA, visual acuity.

Comments

There was a small increase in Margaret's hyperopia, which, when corrected, provided her with slightly clearer vision for distance and near tasks. More significant was the fact that Margaret had changed job tasks, and that her headaches commenced about the same time that she started her new job.

There is evidence in the scientific literature that viewing a desktop computer monitor while wearing general-purpose PALs can contribute to an altered head posture[1] and increased musculoskeletal load in the neck and shoulders.[2] Although Margaret wore general-purpose PALs in the retail store, her computer use was only transient when processing sales transactions. After changing job responsibilities, she was using a desktop computer for the majority of her working day. When asked if she had neck or shoulder pain, Margaret confirmed that she had headaches that started at the base of her skull and radiated to the frontal and temporal regions of her head. Further questioning revealed that Margaret had trouble finding the "sweet spot" in her spectacles when viewing the computer monitor, and that she had to tip her head back and move her head from side to side to find a clear zone of vision.

Alternative spectacle lens designs that could help Margaret maintain a more neutral head posture at work included single-vision near spectacles and computer PALs.[3] Margaret's work involved multiple viewing distances, for example, referring to hardcopy documents (viewing distance approximately 40 cm) and reading from the computer monitor (viewing distance approximately 80 cm). She decided to purchase computer PALs because these lenses provided a wider range of focus than single-vision near spectacles. Margaret did not update her general-purpose PALs, but planned to continue wearing these for non-work tasks.

The computer PALs were ordered from a lens laboratory by supplying the distance and near prescription; the laboratory then calculated the optical adjustments for the lens design. It is wise to confirm what information the lens laboratory requires (such as fitting heights, format of the prescription) before placing an order, because there may be different requirements between lens designs and laboratories.

Two weeks after receiving her new spectacles, Margaret telephoned to say that her headaches have resolved and that she can see her work more comfortably and easily. A letter was written to Margaret's primary physician thanking him for the referral, and explaining how alternative spectacle lenses had solved Margaret's headaches.

Discussion

Margaret was a successful wearer of general-purpose PALs, so the lens design could easily be overlooked as the cause of her headaches. It was only by questioning Margaret about her work tasks that the cause of her headaches was discovered. Changing the lens design was a relatively simple intervention and averted costly medical investigations, such as neurologic assessments, which would not have solved Margaret's headache problem.

Computer work is performed by people of all ages, so it is wise to ask patients about their use of digital devices, including patients who are not employed, children, and retirees. Office work using a desktop computer is not the only mode of computer use. Other devices in common usage include laptop computers, tablets, and smartphones, and these may be used in a myriad of combinations such as multiple desktop monitors, laptops on a desktop docking station, and concurrent use of a tablet and a smartphone. Computers are used across a range of industries, such as retail, heavy industry, health, education, security, and transport. Questions that could be asked of patients include the following:

- How much time do you spend viewing the display?
- How often do you take rest breaks from computer work during your work day?
- What are the number, location, and size of the display(s)?
- What are the viewing distances and viewing heights of the display(s)?

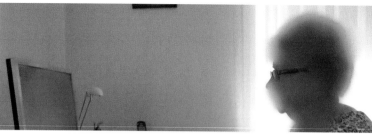

Figure 1.11-1   Margaret, as she initially sits at her computer workstation.

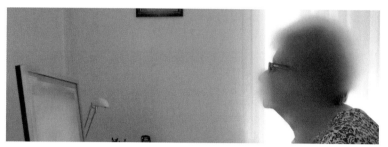

Figure 1.11-2   Margaret leaning forward and tipping her head back to view the computer display while wearing general-purpose progressive addition lens spectacles.

- What do you view on the display, for example, text, spreadsheets, video, or pictures?
- Are there any other tasks that you perform at work, for example, talking to customers, walking around, and watching presentations in meetings?

These questions are particularly important for presbyopic patients, because it will help the eye care professional understand the task requirements and assist in prescribing the appropriate spectacle lens designs. It may also mean that the presbyopic patient requires alternative spectacles for different tasks. For example, Margaret now has general-purpose PAL spectacles for everyday use and computer PAL spectacles to use at her desktop computer.

Margaret's computer workstations were assessed by a work health safety officer within the company, and the setup was deemed correct. It is possible that Margaret adopted an upright posture because she was aware of being observed (Figure 1.11-1) and this was not her habitual posture during the working day when wearing her general-purpose PALs (Figure 1.11-2). Eye care professionals are accustomed to working with other health care practitioners to manage ocular problems in patients. There is a need to expand the range of professionals with whom they interact to include ergonomists and work health safety personnel[4,5] and to educate the broader community about the important relationship between vision and posture.

CLINICAL PEARLS

- Presbyopic patients may require alternative spectacles for different tasks.

- General-purpose PALs are not always suitable for prolonged use at a desktop computer.

- Computer PALs may be a better option because the wearer can adopt a more comfortable head and neck posture while viewing the desktop computer display.

REFERENCES

1. Becker M, Rothman J, Nelson A, et al. The effects of multifocal refractive lenses on occipital extension and forward head posture during a visual task. *Ergonomics.* 2007;50:2095-2103.

2. Horgen G, Aaras A, Fagerthun H, Larsen S. Is there a reduction in postural load when wearing progressive lenses during VDT work over a three-month period? *Appl Ergon.* 1995;26:165-171.

3. Horgen G, Aaras A, Thoresen M. Will visual discomfort among visual display unit (VDU) users change in development when moving from single vision lenses to specially designed VDU progressive lenses? *Optom Vis Sci.* 2004;81:341-349.

4. Long J, Helland M. A multidisciplinary approach to solving computer related vision problems. *Ophthalmic Physiol Opt.* 2012;32:429-435.

5. Long J. Forging partnerships between optometrists and ergonomists to improve visual comfort and productivity in the workplace. *Work.* 2014;47:365-370.

1.12 Eye Protection

Jennifer Long

John, a 51-year-old male office worker, presented for a comprehensive eye examination. He was wearing high index plastic (refractive index 1.67), general-purpose progressive addition lenses (PALs). He reported that he enjoyed gardening, and spent about 10 hours per week tending to plants, vegetables, and fruit trees. Twelve years ago, John suffered a corneal abrasion to his left eye when a tree branch poked between his face and the temporal portion of his spectacles. At that time, his vision was reduced to 20/60, and he was treated with antibiotic eye drops (brand and dose unknown) for 1 week and over-the-counter ocular lubricants for about 2 months. Subsequently, his eye and vision recovered fully, and he has not required any further treatment for this condition.

Most of John's gardening was performed in shadowed sunlight wearing nonprescription, clear eye protectors over his untinted PALs (Figure 1.12-1), and a brimmed hat for additional UV radiation and glare protection. When working in full sunlight, John sometimes wore prescription sunglasses (approximately 75% gray tint polarized general-purpose PALs with UV protection) underneath the clear, nonprescription eye protectors (Figure 1.12-2).

Although the nonprescription eye protectors fitted John's face well, he reported that having 2 frame temples on his ear was uncomfortable for more than about an hour or in hot weather. He enquired about alternative options for eye protection that would be more comfortable for prolonged wear. John did not want to wear contact lenses in place of his prescription spectacles. He has attempted to wear contact lenses previously, but had difficulty inserting and removing the lenses.

Clinical Findings

Unaided distance VA	OD: 20/400; OS: 20/400; OU: 20/400
Present Rx	OD: −3.50 −0.25 × 180 (20/15^{-2}); OS: −3.50 −0.50 × 170 (20/15^{-1}); ADD: +1.50 OU (20/20)
Near point of convergence	6 cm
Confrontation visual fields	Full to finger counting OD and OS
Pupil evaluation	PERRL/no RAPD
Retinoscopy	OD: −3.75 sph; OS: −3.75 −0.25 × 180
Subjective refraction	OD: −3.75 −0.25 × 180 (20/15); OS: −3.75 −0.25 × 170 (20/15)
Distance phoria (measured through subjective Rx)	Horizontal 2Δ EP; vertical 0Δ
Near add	+1.75 OU (20/20 at near)
Near phoria through add	Horizontal and vertical: 0Δ
Intraocular pressure (Perkins handheld applanation tonometer)	OD: 14 mm Hg; OS: 14 mm Hg (at 3:00 PM)

Slit-lamp examination	Unremarkable OD and OS
Fundus examination	OD: 0.5/0.5 CD ratio; healthy rim tissue with distinct disc margins; fovea is flat and dry; normal vasculature; periphery intact

Abbreviations: CD, cup to disc; EP, esophoria; OD, right eye; OS, left eye; OU, both eyes; PERRL, pupils equal, round, reactive to light; RAPD, relative afferent pupillary defect; Rx, prescription; VA, visual acuity.

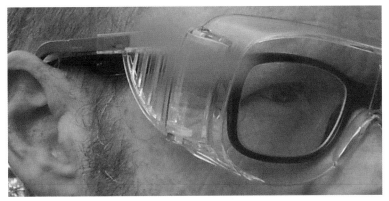

Figure 1.12-1   Eye protectors worn on top of prescription spectacles.

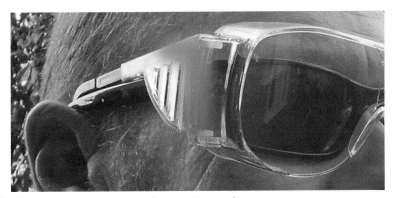

Figure 1.12-2   Eye protectors worn on top of prescription sunglasses.

Discussion

John is an office worker who spends a significant amount of his leisure time gardening. During the eye examination, John asked specifically about eye protection options for use in the garden. Not all patients talk about their hobbies or non-work activities, especially if the case history questions only inquired about work-related activities. It is incumbent on the practitioner to ask about both work- and non–work-related tasks that may pose a risk of eye injury.

There are many hazards associated with horticulture and gardening (see Table 1.12-1). To address John's request for alternative eye protection, it is important to understand the hazards to which John is exposed. This will indicate the required level of eye protection

Table 1.12-1   Examples of Hazards and Risks associated With Horticulture and Gardening Tasks

Type of Hazard	Example of Hazard	Example of Ocular Risk
Mechanical	Tree branch	Corneal abrasion
Mechanical	A stone that flies out from underneath the lawn mower	Corneal foreign body injury
Chemical	Pesticides	Burn to the anterior eye and adnexa
Biological	Plant material and manure	Irritation, infection
Radiation	Ultraviolet radiation	Increased risk of pterygium, cataract, age-related macular degeneration, skin cancer
Visible light	Sun glare	Discomfort glare, disability glare
Visible light	Blue light	Age-related macular degeneration

and guide advice for the optimal type of appliance.

When more detailed questions were asked about his gardening, John reported that the tasks he spent most time on were planting, pruning, and handling manure. Secondary tasks (performed regularly but less frequently) were mowing and edging lawns.

The subsequent paragraphs make reference to the Australian/New Zealand (AS/NZS) eye protection standards because John was examined in Australia. Eye care practitioners should refer to the relevant standards, guidelines, and legislative requirements in their own jurisdiction when applying the principles of this case to their own clinical practice.*

AS/NZS1336[1] recommends at least medium impact protection for gardening and horticultural tasks. Features of a medium impact eye protector include lateral protection (eg, fixed side shields and a wraparound design) and the ability to withstand impact from low mass, high velocity particles. These appliances are labeled either "I" or "F" to indicate medium impact protection. AS/NZS1336 also recommends outdoor clear (labeled "O" to indicate that they provide UV protection) or tinted lenses (offering both UV and sun glare protection).

AS/NZS1336[1] was consulted to determine the types of eye protectors that will meet these requirements. Recommended options include wide vision spectacles and goggles, face shields, and hoods or helmets that incorporate a face or eye shield. Some of these products can be worn in conjunction with prescription eyewear. Prescription eye protector options include powered lenses glazed into a carrier that sits behind a nonprescription eye protector and prescription lenses glazed into a safety frame.[3] In Australia and New Zealand, the latter needs to comply with the medium impact requirements outlined in AS/NZS1337.6.[4]

The advantages and disadvantages of these prescription and nonprescription options were discussed with John, and it was determined that he needed three different types of eye protection. Medium impact eye protectors compliant with AS/NZS1337.6 were prescribed to address John's presenting request for improved comfort (Figure 1.12-3). The frame has an elasticized strap that holds the eye protectors in place. Clear, polycarbonate,

---

* **A note about eye protection standards:** Eye protection prevents eye injuries and may protect against mechanical, chemical, thermal, radiation, and biological hazards. Standards and guidelines provide recommendations for the most appropriate type of eye protector for different hazards. In Australia and New Zealand AS/NZS 1336:2014,[1] the AS/NZS1337 series (eye and face protection) and the AS/NZS1338 series (filters for eye protectors) are used, whereas Z87.1-2015[2] is used in North America.

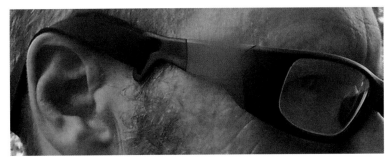

Figure 1.12-3   Medium impact prescription eye protectors.

general-purpose PALs with UV protection up to approximately 400 nm (ie, providing both UV-A and UV-B protection) were fitted to the frame. These are suitable to wear for all gardening tasks.

John tended not to wear sunglasses while gardening because his work was performed in shadowed sunlight. On those occasions when he needed additional sun protection (eg, when mowing lawns), he agreed that he could wear his current clear, nonprescription eye protectors (labeled either "I" or "O") over the top of his prescription sunglasses (Figure 1.12-2), rather than purchase an additional pair of tinted prescription eye protectors.

An alternative option would have been to prescribe medium impact prescription eye protectors with photochromic lenses that automatically adjust the tint density according to the ambient light conditions. This option was discussed with John, but he preferred to purchase untinted lenses for his prescription eye protector spectacles.

John liked the idea of wearing a full face shield over the top of his spectacles or his medium impact eye protectors when necessary. He recalled that when using a lawn edger, a stone once hit him in the face. Although he was not hurt at that time, a face shield would have offered additional protection. Face shields can be purchased from home hardware stores, and may offer low, medium, or high impact

protection. Since AS/NZS1336 recommends at least medium impact protection for gardening tasks, John was instructed to look for products which are labeled medium impact ("I" or "F") or high impact ("V" or "B").

CLINICAL PEARLS

- During an eye examination, ask the patient about both work-related and non–work-related tasks that may pose a risk of eye injury.

- It is possible to provide an untinted eye protector with UV protection to patients who do not want to wear tinted lenses when working outdoors.

REFERENCES

1. Australian/New Zealand Standard AS/NZS 1336:2014. *Eye and face protection – Guidelines.* Sydney, Australia: SAI Global Limited.
2. American National Standards Institute. ANSI/ISEA Z87.1-2015. *American National Standard for Occupational and Educational Personal Eye and Face Protection Devices.* Arlington, Virginia: International Safety Equipment Association.
3. Long J. What every ergonomist needs to know about . . . New choices for medium impact eye protection. *Ergon Aust.* 2007;21:20-25.
4. Australian/New Zealand Standard AS/NZS 1337.6: 2012. Personal eye protection. Part 6: Prescription eye protectors against low and medium impact. Sydney, Australia: SAI Global Limited.

1.13 Low Vision Management of a Patient With Choroideremia

Gregory R. Hopkins

Frederick, a 15-year-old white male with a history of retinal dystrophy, previously diagnosed as choroideremia, presented for a comprehensive eye examination. He was a student at a State School for the Blind (SSB). School records indicated that he had been under the care of a retinal specialist over the past 5 years.

Although there was no family history of retinal dystrophy, Frederick presented with symptoms of eyestrain, headaches, and night blindness. The record indicated that he had been complaining of eyestrain since he was 8 years old. At that time, Frederick's best-corrected visual acuity (VA) was 20/40 in each eye. Mid-peripheral pigment mottling and attenuated blood vessels were noted, as well as mid-peripheral visual field loss in each eye.

In addition, Frederick reported dry skin, nasal congestion, occasional cluster headaches, attention deficit hyperactivity disorder (ADHD), and bipolar disorder. He was taking Dextroamphetamine-Amphetamine (Adderall) (20 mg) and fluoxetine (Prozac) (20 mg) daily. An auditory screening was found to be normal, as were his vocabulary comprehension, working memory, reading, writing, and word problem-solving skills.

Frederick was in the eighth grade at the SSB, and various adaptations had been made to help him with his schoolwork. He had access to an iPad whose font was set to 70-point print (the largest available). He achieved optimal function when electronic text was displayed as a yellow font on a blue background. He could read comfortably for up to 2 hours with these accommodations. When working on desktop computers, he would use 28- to 32-point Arial black font. He reported that ZoomText magnification software was available on the computers at the SSB.

Frederick did not wear his glasses as he felt they caused headaches, but he was willing to try a pair of magnifying glasses for reading. He had a long white cane, but only used it in bright conditions or total darkness. He felt his color vision might be worsening since his previous visit 4 months ago. Regarding his distance vision, Frederick was introduced to handheld monocular telescopes in his orientation and mobility class at the SSB. He found them useful for looking at street signs and other signage. He did not have a telescope of his own at the present time.

The goals for the examination included the following:

1. to obtain reading glasses or appropriate magnification devices for brief near work;
2. to obtain sunglasses to assist with minimizing glare;
3. to assess his peripheral vision;
4. to obtain a monocular telescope for distance visual tasks; and
5. to retest his color vision.

Clinical Findings

Frederick's current glasses were OD: −2.00 −1.50 × 20 (20/300); OS: −2.00 −1.00 × 10 (20/160). His binocular visual acuity (VA) was 20/80. Because these values were consistent with the findings obtained 4 months earlier, neither retinoscopy nor trial frame refraction was repeated. Contrast sensitivity using a Mars chart was 0.76 (11 times worse than normal).

Color vision testing was performed using a fully saturated, D-15 cap arrangement test. Several minor cap-order reversal errors were made, but no major crossing errors were found (Figure 1.13-1). Unfortunately, this test was not repeated, nor was a desaturated cap test performed to search for a more subtle color vision defect.

An unaided reading assessment found that Frederick held the MN reading card (Precision Vision Inc., Woodstock, Illinois) at 25 cm (4 D), where he could read 5M print comfortably. He preferred to hold the card at 20 cm (5 D) to read 6.3M print, and could bring the card into 10 cm (10 D) using his accommodation to read 2.5M print. These findings

predict a range of lenses between 20 D and 31.5 D that would enable Frederick to read 1M (or 8 point) print. These lens powers are derived by multiplying the working distance (in diopters) by the critical print size magnification required to read 1M print. Thus, "4 D × 5M" gives a value of 20 D, while "5 D × 6.3M" and "10 D × 2.5M" give powers of 31.5 D and 25 D, respectively. However, Frederick would have to hold the print at the focal point of the lens, namely, 5, 3.2, or 4 cm. This would allow him to bring printed material 5×, 6.3×, and 2.5× closer than his original working distances of 25, 20, and 10 cm, respectively. Many children with visual impairments have reduced accommodative responsivity due to their decreased VA. Practitioners need to assess the accommodative demands of pediatric low vision patients, and ensure that they can meet the accommodation and convergence requirements of the reading add or optical device.[1,2]

Goldmann perimetry revealed irregularly constricted visual fields in each eye using the largest stimulus (V4e) (Figure 1.13-2). These results imply that Frederick was probably using his right eye for orientation and mobility, because this was affected only moderately in normal lighting conditions. However, the III4e isopter showed a circular constriction at a level qualifying for legal blindness.

These clinical findings are consistent with Frederick's report of difficulties with mobility in darkened environments. Ordinarily, the separation between isopters is not so dramatic. When a significant radial spread between the V4e and III4e isopters is observed, the patient is likely to have compromised rod function.

Low Vision Device Trials

Frederick was shown 16 D (4×) Coil Microscopic reading glasses, which provided an effective add of approximately 19 D (since his myopic prescription had a spherical equivalent of approximately −3.00 OU). He was able to read 2M print comfortably with these glasses at 5 cm using his left eye. Frederick was willing to try these glasses for both brief and sustained reading tasks.

In addition, he was shown 16 D (5×), 20 D (6×), and 23 D (7×) illuminated handheld

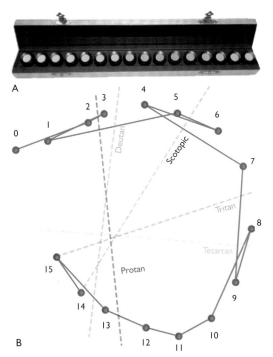

Figure 1.13-1 A. Fully saturated Farnsworth D-15 test caps. B. Color cap arrangement results in color space.

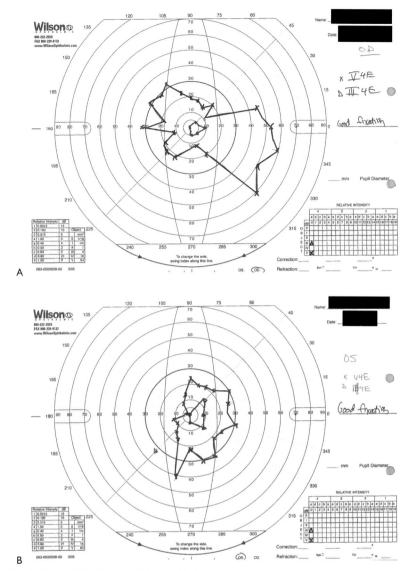

Figure 1.13-2   Goldmann V4e (shown in blue) and III4e (shown in red) visual field results for the right (top figure) and left (bottom figure) eyes.

magnifiers. Frederick was able to read 2M comfortably with the first 2 lenses, and 1.6M with the third magnifier. However, he found it difficult to maintain the appropriate viewing distance when reading, as the magnifier tended to sink toward the printed page. Frederick was also shown an illuminated 20 D (5×) slide-out, pocket magnifier, and was able to read 0.8M at a relatively quick reading speed, compared with the larger handheld magnifiers. His enthusiasm for the compact-size pocket magnifier may explain the improved reading performance

when compared with the larger devices of similar strength described earlier. He was also able to read 0.8M print comfortably with a 7× illuminated stand magnifier, but preferred the compact slide-out pocket magnifier as his primary optical device. He already had access to video and electronic magnification systems for other prolonged reading tasks.

To address the glare-control issues, Frederick was taken outside to a brightly lit space, and various no infrared (NoIR) fit-over sunglasses were demonstrated. This began with neutral gray shades, and then proceeded to brown filters of similar density. Finally, he was shown other lens colors. He preferred the NoIR medium brown (U40) fit-overs. While outside, he also tried a 4× Walters handheld monocular telescope, remarking that "I can't believe this little thing makes me see that clearly." Back in the examination room, VA through the telescope with his left eye was 20/25. Note that he obtained slightly greater than 4× magnification due to his myopic eye working in concert with the plus lens eyepiece of this Keplerian telescope.

Assessment and Plan

Frederick's visual status was similar to that found at his previous examination and his visual fields were quantified. Color vision testing continued to be inconclusive. A summary letter was sent to his school principal, with a copy to his parents. It was recommended that he continue to be followed by the retinal specialist.

Authorization was sought from his insurance plan for a 16 D (4×) Coil Microscopic reading glass fitted over the left eye. A plano lens was ordered for the right lens to avoid the high convergence demand created by attempting binocular viewing at working distances of less than 8 cm. In addition, a 20 D (5×) Mattingly pocket slide-out magnifier and a 4×12 Walters monocular telescope were also ordered. However, the cost of the NoIR U40 medium brown fit-overs was not covered by his insurance plan.

Summary and Conclusions

Frederick's diagnosis of choroideremia made him susceptible to night blindness (which he overcame by avoiding going out at night), peripheral vision loss (he was receiving white cane training), and reduced central VA (for which optical and electronic low vision devices were prescribed). His complaint of changes in color vision may be justified, because his VA was poorer than typically found in most young patients with choroideremia (he had suffered

greater inner-retinal damage). The reduced contrast sensitivity was expected given the increased intraocular light scatter, resulting from the reduced amount of retinal pigment epithelium available to absorb stray light.

Frederick was able to attempt close working distances for brief reading but, similar to an early presbyope, he found it difficult to maintain his desired working distance without significant eyestrain. With technologies such as a ZoomText enabled computer, iPad or CCTV, Frederick would be able to assume more comfortable viewing distances (since the print could be enlarged). It is hoped that the proposed interventions will alleviate the symptoms from his reduced accommodation and subsequent eyestrain. It can sometimes be a challenge to get young students to "open up" when they are questioned about their visual comfort while reading. Fortunately, Frederick was placed in an appropriate educational setting to give him the tools and training necessary to cope with any further vision loss.

CLINICAL PEARLS

- Assessment of contrast sensitivity and the impact of glare, as well as visual fields, color vision, and reading performance are important components of managing low vision patients of all ages.

- Individuals with low vision often report eyestrain (due to reduced accommodative responsivity) when adopting close working distances. This can be helped by prescribing a near-vision addition lens.

REFERENCES

1. Alabdulkader B, Leat SJ. Do reading additions improve reading in pre-presbyopes with low vision? *Optom Vis Sci.* 2012;89:1327-1335.
2. Leat SJ, Mohr A. Accommodative response in pre-presbyopes with visual impairment and its clinical implications. *Invest Ophthalmol Vis Sci.* 2007;48:3888-3896.

1.14 Age-Related Macular Degeneration

Cheyenne Huber

Terry, a 79-year-old Caucasian female, presented to the clinic for a low vision evaluation. Terry was pseudophakic and had geographic atrophy associated with dry age-related macular degeneration (AMD) in each eye. Her chief concern was difficulty reading with her current progressive addition lenses (PALs), and she was interested in glasses or low vision devices to help her read. She also reported difficulty seeing in dim light and when walking in unfamiliar places.

Terry saw a retinal specialist every 6 months, and took nutritional supplements for AMD. Her hobbies were going to movie theaters and operas. She used opera glasses as needed and felt these were satisfactory. She lived alone and had a part-time assistant. There were no difficulties in cooking, cleaning, or shopping. Her assistant accompanied her to the clinic.

Clinical Findings

Retinoscopy and trial frame refraction	OD: +0.50 −1.50 × 90 OS: +1.00 −0.50 × 76
Best-corrected VA (back-illuminated Bailey-Lovie chart)	OD: logMAR = 0.34 (20/40⁻²); OS: logMAR = 0.50 (20/63)
VA using a 4% transmission neutral density filter (NoIR U23) to simulate dim lighting conditions (Figure 1.14-1)	OU: logMAR = 0.60 (20/80)
Contrast sensitivity (Mars test)	OU: substantially reduced to 1.0 log unit (10% Weber) in standard room lighting and profoundly reduced to 0.2 log units (63% Weber) when wearing the NoIR U23 filter
Confrontation visual fields:	Full to finger counting OD and OS
Near tangent screen used to measure central 10° visual field of the better-seeing eye (8-mm black target against a white background at 50 cm—see Figure 1.14-2)	OD: small paracentral scotoma that became significantly larger when retinal illuminance was reduced (Figure 1.14-3) OS: not tested

Abbreviations: logMAR, logarithm of the minimum angle of resolution; NoIR, no infrared; OD, right eye; OS, left eye; OU, both eyes; VA, visual acuity.

Discussion

Terry did not bring her opera glasses to the clinic, but most opera glasses have a magnification of around 2× to 3×. Given the relatively good distance visual acuity (VA) of logMAR = 0.34 (20/40⁻²) in the better eye, and her report that the opera glasses worked well, we did not consider stronger telescopes at this examination.

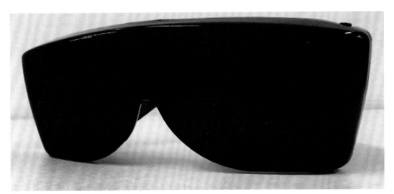

Figure 1.14-1   No infrared U23 gray fit-over sunglasses with 4% transmission.

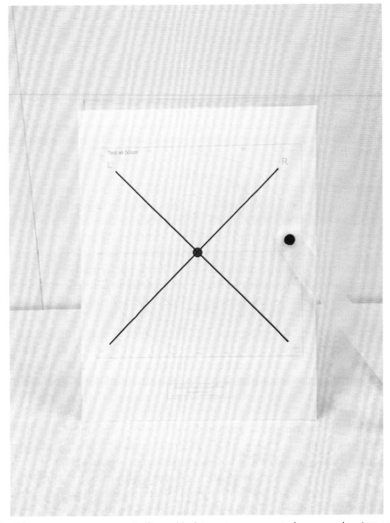

Figure 1.14-2   Near tangent screen test. An 8-mm black target was presented on a wand against a white background at 50 cm.

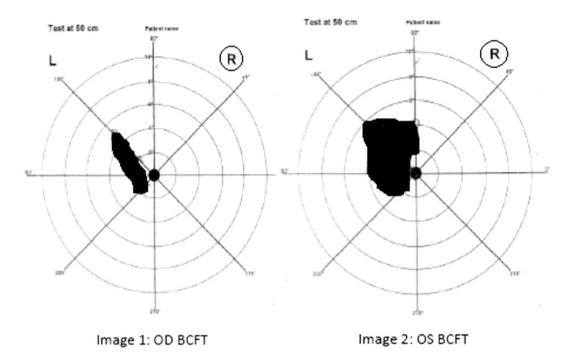

Image 1: OD BCFT   **Image 2: OS BCFT**

Figure 1.14-3 Central visual field test results for the right eye in room lighting (left) and with 4% gray filter (right). The narrow paracentral scotoma superior temporal to fixation expands with low luminance conditions to extend to approximately 4° of that quadrant.

Reading VA was measured using a trial frame and Bailey-Lovie reading card in normal room lighting. With a +3.25 D effective ADD, 1.6M print was read efficiently at 32 cm, and she could just read 1.25M print (her reading acuity threshold) with difficulty at the same distance.

When considering visual performance with low vision devices, 1.0M print is commonly taken as a reading goal, because it is representative of average newsprint and other common reading materials. Given that Terry could read 1.6M print efficiently at 32 cm, by proportion it was predicted that she would be able to read 1.0M print efficiently at an equivalent viewing distance of 20 cm (32 cm × [1.0/1.6] = 20 cm). This 20-cm viewing distance required a +5.00 D addition.

Reading performance was tested with both optical and nonoptical low vision devices. With the +5.00 D addition, Terry read 1.0M print with reasonable efficiency, but felt uncomfortable with the close working distance of 20 cm. Reading performance was also assessed with a Mattingly 2.5×/8 D handheld magnifier (equivalent viewing power of +5.7 D) with an embedded light-emitting diode (LED) light. She was able to read 0.8M print comfortably with this device, and the field of view seemed satisfactory. We considered this magnifier to be suitable for short-term reading tasks.

Terry performed some reading tasks with electronic magnifiers including the portable Ruby XLHD and the 24″ Merlin HD desktop video magnifier. She was able to read the *New York Times* (print size approximately 1.0M) comfortably with both video magnifiers. Terry compared the video image with enhanced contrast (black letters on a white background) and reversed contrast (white letters on a black background). While she reported little difference between them, she had a marginal preference for the white background with enhanced contrast. Her preferred setting was at minimum magnification.

Terry used both an iPad and a desktop computer at home on occasions. We discussed the available options for modifying the visual display, as well as the possibility of using speech output options. We recommended that she experiment with the magnification and enhanced contrast options. At the end of the examination, the clinic's rehabilitation specialist met with her and demonstrated most of the "Accessibility" and "Display and Brightness" controls on the iPad, as well as some of the accessibility features on the desktop computer.

Audiobooks were discussed as a nonvisual option for accessing books, and Terry was given information regarding sources of audiobooks as well as the Library of Congress Talking Books Program that provides audiobooks free of charge to the visually impaired. The rehabilitation specialist also raised the possibility for orientation and mobility training, but Terry was not interested in these options.

However, she was well aware that her visual difficulties became worse in dim environments, and the importance of good lighting was emphasized. Terry was encouraged to continue care with her ophthalmologist and to return to the clinic for low vision care as needed.

Age-Related Macular Degeneration

Age-related macular degeneration is a bilateral, progressive retinal disease that impairs central vision. It is the main cause of visual impairment in Western society. Approximately 1.75 million people in the United States have AMD, with 80% having the dry form of the disease.[1] Dry AMD is characterized by reduced function and atrophy of photoreceptors, retinal pigment epithelium and choriocapillaris as a result of drusen deposition in Bruch's membrane.

As is common in AMD, Terry's VA at near (1.25M at 32 cm, equivalent to a minimum angle of resolution of 4 minutes of arc) was significantly worse than at distance (20/40; or a minimum angle of resolution of 2 minutes of arc). This occurs because a reading task is more congested and complex than identifying spaced letters on a distance acuity chart. With disturbed macula function, there can be pronounced differences between reading text and isolated letters. Reading efficiency or speed is often reduced in macular degeneration where more fixations per word are required to read across a row of printed text.[2] While we did not formally measure reading speed, it was estimated at approximately 80 to 100 words per minute when reading aloud at the larger print sizes. This is about half the speed of normally sighted individuals when reading from the same test cards.

With AMD, it is common for patients to report greater difficulties in dim light. In Terry's case, her distance VA decreased from $20/40^{-2}$ to $20/80$ when retinal illuminance was reduced using the very dark NoIR U23 fit-over sunglasses. A more pronounced change was observed with contrast-sensitivity testing. Here, reduced retinal illuminance produced a decline from moderately impaired (1.0 log unit, 10% Weber) to profoundly impaired (0.20 log unit, 63% Weber). Furthermore, the paracentral scotoma in the right eye became substantially larger in dim illumination. Difficulties with mobility and reduced visual performance in dim light were thought to be due mainly to the reduced contrast sensitivity.

The Mattingly 2.5×/8D LED illuminated, handheld magnifier was prescribed. This has an equivalent power of +5.7 D lens and a diameter of 100 mm. It should help the patient with short-term reading tasks, especially when viewing small- and/or low-contrast materials. Terry will also benefit from the illumination in the device. We did not recommend a change in spectacles, but did emphasize the importance of good lighting.

Terry became acquainted with both portable and tabletop video magnifiers. She occasionally uses an iPad and a desktop computer but was unfamiliar with the available range of magnification and display variables. The low vision clinic's rehabilitation specialist discussed available services and resources, including audiobooks, mobility training, information technology accessibility options, luminaires, and environmental modifications to enhance contrast.

Prognosis

Age-related macular degeneration is a progressive condition, but it can be difficult to predict its development, which can be gradual or episodic. At this time, the illuminated, handheld, low-power magnifier and the opera glasses are Terry's only optical magnifiers. Although not required at the time of examination, we did make a point of acquainting her with video magnifiers, talking books, mobility training, and rehabilitation services, as they may be needed later should additional visual deterioration occur.

CLINICAL PEARLS

- Macular degeneration is a condition that can severely affect visual functions including VA, contrast sensitivity, and the central visual field. Difficulty reading is a common problem for patients with this disease.

- Patients with macular degeneration can benefit greatly from magnification, and often require stronger powers to enable them to read small print.

REFERENCES

1. Friedman DS, O'Colmain BJ, Munoz B, et al. Prevalence of age-related macular degeneration in the United States. *Arch Ophthalmol*. 2004;122:564-572.
2. Bullimore MA, Bailey IL. Reading eye-movements and age related maculopathy. *Optom Vis Sci*. 1995; 72:125-138.

1.15 Oculocutaneous Albinism: Low Vision Case Using Simple Magnification

Marlena A. Chu

Roy, an 11-year-old Caucasian male who had been diagnosed with oculocutaneous albinism, presented for his first low vision evaluation. Both parents accompanied him to the examination. There was no previous family history of oculocutaneous albinism, and his ocular health was monitored annually by a pediatric ophthalmologist. Roy was an active, curious child in sixth grade at a private school. He did not have an Independent Education Program (IEP) in place, nor was he assigned a Teacher of students with Visual Impairment (TVI). He wore single-vision spectacles full time, and did not feel a need to wear glare protection indoors or out. At the time of the examination, Roy was not using any low vision devices. Both he and his parents felt that the school provided adequate accommodations for his needs, such as sitting him closer to the white board and providing large print material (reported as 16 point) for homework and tests. Roy did not seem particularly sensitive to light, as he had prescription sunglasses (approximately 30% transmission gray) but rarely wore them. He occasionally wore a baseball cap on sunny days. While no specific presenting complaints were stated at this first visit, the goal of both Roy and his parents was to learn more about available low vision devices and services, hoping there might be something to help with schoolwork and activities of daily living.

Clinical Findings

Current Rx (VA measured with a back-illuminated, Bailey-Lovie chart at 3 m)	OD: $+1.50 -1.75 \times 175$ (0.82 logMAR ($20/125^{-1}$); OS: $+1.25 -1.25 \times 005$ (0.78 logMAR ($20/125^{+1}$)
VA using a 4% transmission neutral density filter (NoIR U23) over the current Rx to simulate dim lighting conditions	OU: 0.74 logMAR ($20/100^{-2}$)
Contrast sensitivity (Mars test)	OU: 1.8 log units (1.6% Weber) in standard room lighting; no change with NoIR U23 filters
Confrontation visual fields	Full in each meridian to a transilluminator, OD and OS
Retinoscopy and trial frame refraction	OD: $+1.50 -2.25 \times 175$ (0.82 logMAR, $20/125^{-1}$); OS: $+1.00 -1.75 \times 005$ (0.76 logMAR, $20/125^{+2}$)
Reading acuity limit (Bailey-Lovie reading card at 16 cm [patient's preferred distance])	OU: 1.0 M
Good reading efficiency (Bailey-Lovie reading card at 16 cm [patient's preferred distance])	OU: 1.6 M

Abbreviations: logMAR, logarithm of the minimum angle of resolution; OD, right eye; OS, left eye; OU, both eyes; Rx, prescription; VA, visual acuity.

Discussion

Most street and other signs are designed for 20/40 acuity, and given Roy's distance visual acuity (VA) of 0.78 logMAR (equivalent to 20/125[+1]), the 4×13 Eschenbach Microlux monocular telescope (Figure 1.15-1) allowed easy reading of the 20/40 line. The simplicity and "click-in" case design makes this fixed-focus telescope easy to use for children.

Regarding printed materials, most small newsprint is around 1.0M in size, and this is commonly taken as a print size goal for reading. Roy's preferred and most comfortable reading efficiency was measured at 16 cm with 1.6M print; therefore, using simple proportions, the equivalent viewing distance of 10 cm was calculated as follows:

$$\frac{0.16}{1.6 \text{ M}} = \frac{0.10}{1.0 \text{ M}}$$

The equivalent viewing distance is the distance at which the original object subtends an angle equal to that subtended by the magnified image at the observer's eye. For Roy, directly reading at the equivalent viewing distance of 10 cm would allow him to read 1M print with the same reading efficiency that he had with 1.6M print at the 16-cm distance.

Alternatively, Roy could use an optical system that would allow him to adopt an equivalent viewing distance of 10 cm or closer. In this situation, the equivalent viewing power would have to be at least +10.00 D. While he is 11 years of age, and has abundant accommodation that would allow him to adopt a viewing distance of 10 cm, such close viewing may not be comfortable for sustained viewing of relatively small print (see Chapter 1.13). Accordingly, additional magnification may be beneficial in enhancing the visibility of small print, and to help with comfort during sustained reading.

Handheld or pocket magnifiers having low dioptric powers can easily provide an equivalent viewing distance of 10 cm. Many incorporate light sources that provide task lighting as required. Roy's reading performance was tested both with a Mattingly Advantage 4×/12 D LED illuminated handheld magnifier (70 mm diameter) and a Peak 16 D (50 mm diameter) foldout lens. These magnifiers were determined to have equivalent powers (F_e) of +10.6 D and +10 D. Manufacturer's labels can be misleading, and devices may be labeled with different dioptric powers, even within the same line of magnifiers. After evaluating these magnifiers, Roy preferred to read without either of these handheld devices, although he did express a preference for the lens with the larger diameter.

Stand magnifiers, which are moved across the page for reading, were also considered. Hemispheric dome magnifiers enlarge print by 1.5× (equal to the refractive index), and the image is in the same plane as the object. Dome magnifiers are especially suitable for children, because they get the benefit of using their own accommodation, and obtain a larger field of view than with other stand magnifiers. For hemispherical domes, the field of view is equal to the lens diameter divided by 1.5. Due to their light gathering properties, dome magnifiers make the brightness of the image appear greater than that of the object. In addition, dome magnifiers can function as place markers when reading. An equivalent viewing distance of 10 cm can be achieved with a dome magnifier when the eye-to-page distance is 15 cm (ie, 10 × 1.5). Roy liked the 65 mm Optelec dome magnifier (Figure 1.15-2). With a diameter of 65 mm, the field of view was 43 mm (ie, 65/1.5). Roy read with good facility with this device using a viewing distance of 12 to 16 cm.

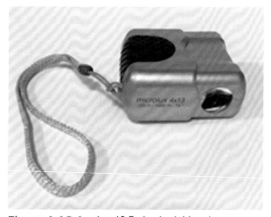

Figure 1.15-1   4 × 13 Eschenbach Microlux monocular telescope.

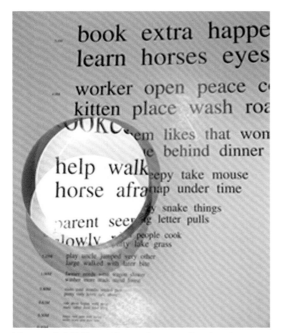

Figure 1.15-2 A 65 mm diameter Optelec dome magnifier.

A Mattingly Advantage 4×/12 D LED illuminated stand magnifier was also tested. This has a 70 mm round, +10.4 D lens, and provided a 2.9× enlargement ratio with the image located 17 cm below the lens. With 2.9× magnification, a 10 cm equivalent viewing distance can be achieved with an eye-to-image distance of 29 cm or closer. This requires an eye-to-lens distance of approximately 12 cm, and the accommodation demand would be modest. However, Roy preferred the simpler dome magnifier.

In addition, Roy and his parents were shown some electronic magnifiers. He could read quite easily with a portable video magnifier, but these were not considered suitable for him at this time. The field of view was too restricted even when using minimum magnification. Both Roy and his parents liked the idea of video magnification, and felt that this technology might become useful as his educational demands increased.

With this in mind, we gave him a short experience using an Onyx HD portable closed circuit television (CCTV) that provides magnification for both distance and near. Such devices have a video camera that connects with a laptop computer, and they allow magnification and other image manipulations for viewing displays on a chalkboard or a projector screen. They can also be used to read from books or documents.

In summary, we recommended the 4 × 13 Eschenbach Microlux monocular telescope and 65 mm Optelec dome magnifier for Roy, and his parents planned to obtain these devices through their vision insurance plan. We also discussed the process of establishing an IEP with the school authorities. Through the IEP, it is probable that Roy would be assigned a TVI. This individual would serve as his advocate in the classroom and ensure that he is receiving appropriate accommodations. These might include large print classroom materials, extended time on tests, avoiding the use of multiple-choice tests with "bubble" answer forms, the use of low vision aids, sitting closer to the board, and reading with laptop or tablet computers. A TVI might also provide some training in orientation and mobility, as well as travel skills. The availability of rehabilitation services beyond high school was also discussed. Finally, both Roy and his parents were reminded to continue regular evaluations by his pediatric ophthalmologist.

Oculocutaneous albinism is an autosomal recessive disorder affecting melanin biosynthesis.[1] It results in hypopigmentation of the skin and hair. The lack of ocular melanin during fetal development leads to foveal hypoplasia and misalignment of the optic nerves.[2] Clinically, oculocutaneous albinism patients present with reduced VA, nystagmus, and iris transillumination. Strabismus and astigmatism are usually present.[3] The condition is found in all ethnic groups, is distributed equally in males and females, and has a prevalence of 1 in 17 000 in the United States. It has been extrapolated that 1 in 70 individuals carry the gene for oculocutaneous albinism.[1]

Roy was typical of a young patient with oculocutaneous albinism. Reduced VA was the primary visual problem. Most oculocutaneous albinism patients have excellent contrast sensitivity and unrestricted visual fields. Reading speed is often quite good provided the angular print size is sufficiently large. Roy had no hypersensitivity to light or any degree of photophobia. Oculocutaneous albinism patients may exhibit a wide range of light sensitivities.

Sometimes very dark filters, protective side shields, and visors are essential, while others may only need moderate protection from bright light. However, since Roy did not complain of sensitivity to light, these were not considered necessary in this case.

CLINICAL PEARLS

- Magnification is prescribed based on the equivalent viewing distance, or the angle subtended at the viewing distance where the patient reads most comfortably.

- Clinicians should keep in mind the optical properties of specific devices, and if the use of adds are necessary to account for accommodative demands.

- Integrated, rehabilitative care of low vision children with TVI, or other rehabilitative providers, is essential to their academic success.

REFERENCES

1. Summers CG. Albinism: classification, clinical characteristics, and recent findings. *Optom Vis Sci.* 2009;86(6):659-662.
2. Cronin CA, Ryan AB, Talley EM, Scrable H. Tyrosinase expression during neuroblast divisions affects later path finding by retinal ganglion cells. *J Neurosci.* 2003;23(37):11692-11697.
3. Lee KA, King RA, Summers CG. Stereopsis in patients with albinism: clinical correlates. *J AAPOS* 2001;5:98-104.

1.16 Use of a Bioptic Telescope for Driving

Dawn K. DeCarlo, Jennifer Elgin, and Joanne M. Wood

Ryan, a 19-year-old white male college student with dominant optic atrophy, presented to the low vision service with the goal of obtaining a restricted driving license. He had no prior experience with bioptic telescopes, although he did use near magnification devices and he had no previous driving experience.

Clinical Findings

Refractive correction	OD: −2.50 −0.75 × 135 (20/200); OS: −2.50 −0.75 × 65 (20/200)
Color vision	Mildly abnormal, with 2 errors on the Panel D-15 test
Fundus examination	Temporal pallor of the optic nerve OD and OS
Visual field (Goldmann)	Full OD and OS

Abbreviations: OD, right eye; OS, left eye.

In Ryan's state of residence, bioptic driving is permitted when visual acuity (VA) in each eye is 20/200 or better and the visual field is at least 110°. In addition, VA must be at least 20/60 through the bioptic telescope. Therefore, Ryan was a potential candidate for driving with a bioptic telescope.

Eye dominance testing revealed left eye dominance. A series of bioptic telescopes were demonstrated before the left eye, several of which met the 20/60 requirement. Ryan selected 2 bioptic telescopes for further trials, based on image clarity and field of view, namely the Ocutech 4X VES-K and the Designs for Vision 4X BIO I telescopes. He achieved a VA of 20/40 through each device. The Ocutech is a Keplerian telescope with a 12.5° field of view and is longer, heavier, and more expensive than the Designs for Vision BIO I, which is a Galilean telescope having a 6° field of view. Both bioptic telescopes were demonstrated to Ryan on the street where multiple real-world traffic lights and signs were visible. He preferred the Ocutech 4X VES-K, primarily due to its larger field of view.

Measurements were made to customize the VES-K. The monocular pupillary distance was measured both in primary gaze for the left eye and when viewing straight ahead with the chin depressed, to simulate bioptic telescope use. Frame selection for the VES-K is limited to the manufacturer's frames, as the bioptic telescope is mounted to a double bridge. However, for other bioptic telescope designs, sturdy frames with adjustable nose pads and spring hinges should be selected. Lens material, antireflective coating, and tint are determined for the carrier lenses as for any spectacle prescription. As Ryan had only moderate photosensitivity outdoors, a slip-behind sun filter was recommended. However, for patients who have greater light sensitivity, a wraparound fit over shield may be appropriate (Figure 1.16-1).

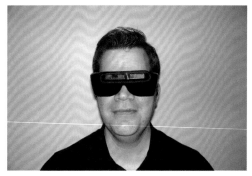

Figure 1.16-1   Example of a wraparound fit-over shield fitted over the bioptic telescope of a patient who reported light sensitivity.

Follow-up Visits

Ryan had monocular and binocular VA of 20/200 through the carrier lenses, and 20/40 through the bioptic telescope. The telescope was adjusted so that the lower edge was located just above the upper lid margin, and set with the maximum upward tilt that the device allowed (Figure 1.16-2A), so that it would be parallel to the ground when the chin was depressed. When adjusting the bioptic telescope, if the view through the telescope is incomplete, adding a slight amount of retroscopic tilt to the frame can be beneficial.

Once the bioptic telescope was adjusted, Ryan proceeded to occupational therapy training to ensure proper techniques for viewing through the telescope. The emphasis of training is to practice using the carrier lenses to search for objects, and then switching to the telescope for identification purposes. This is known as "dipping" or "spotting," because the head is

tilted downward slightly to view through the telescope; however, the "dip" should not last longer than 2 seconds (Figure 1.16-2B).

Some training should take place outdoors so that the response to glare can be assessed. A variety of stationary and moving objects are "spotted." Subjective comfort and function outdoors with the prescribed glare shields are determined, and if needed, changes are made to enhance glare protection. Ryan was instructed to practice using the bioptic telescope to read road signs and observe traffic patterns as a passenger in moving vehicles, and he was referred for an on-road assessment of his bioptic skills with a certified driving rehabilitation specialist before taking the written test for his learner's driving permit.

Supplementary Testing: Driver Training With the Certified Driving Rehabilitation Specialist

Ryan completed several training sessions as a passenger, where he was required to provide a narrative description of the driving environment, including traffic lights, stop signs, vehicles turning, and the presence of pedestrians. Intersections or other road conditions were identified through the carrier lens, with Ryan "dipping" to identify traffic light colors and road signs through the telescope. He continued to use his bioptic telescope for other mobility tasks, such as navigating around his college campus on his bicycle or riding in the car with friends, until he received his learner's permit and began on-road driver training.

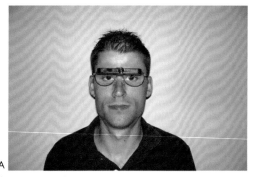
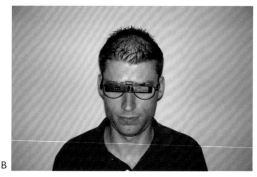

A

B

Figure 1.16-2   An example of a patient with a bioptic telescope (A) viewing through the carrier lens (left) and (B) dipping their head to view through the bioptic telescope (right).

Ryan completed several driving training sessions with the driving rehabilitation specialist in an empty parking lot, including mirror adjustment, location of various vehicle controls, basic acceleration, braking skills, and lane keeping. Once proficient in these skills, training progressed into a low traffic neighborhood. The difficulty of the driving environment was increased as his skills progressed. Importantly, during the initial driver training sessions, the use of the bioptic telescope was limited until he was proficient in all basic driving skills, with the driving rehabilitation specialist verbally providing information regarding the driving environment. Once proficient, vehicle control was demonstrated in a variety of traffic and roadway conditions, and the bioptic telescope was incorporated into the driver training during daylight hours for a range of traffic conditions and roadways, including multiple opportunities for lane changes in high traffic conditions and on higher speed roads. Several sessions focused on anticipating traffic lights in a variety of road conditions and speeds. Ryan completed approximately 75 hours of training with the driving rehabilitation specialist, and successfully gained a daytime-only restricted license. It should be noted that he completed all of his driving practice hours with the driving rehabilitation specialist, whereas many patients only have the opportunity to practice their driving skills with family members. Indeed, Dougherty et al[1] reported that the median (interquartile range) duration of training with the driving rehabilitation specialist before testing was 21 (17) hours. Following licensure, Ryan subsequently drove accident free for 2 years, and following 10 hours of additional driver training at night, the daytime-only restriction was removed from his license.

Additional Follow-up

Ryan returned to the low vision clinic for his annual follow-up appointment. The telescope fitted well, but he no longer met the vision requirements through the carrier lenses due to increased myopia. He wished to change to contact lenses so the bioptic telescope carrier lenses were remade with plano power. Ryan has been recertified annually for bioptic driving over the past 11 years, and has not been involved in any motor vehicle collisions. He continues to wear contact lenses and drives with an Ocutech VES-K mounted before the left eye.

Discussion

A bioptic telescope can facilitate driving for individuals with stable vision impairment who fail to meet vision licensing standards. This may be critical for younger individuals, since the lack of a driver's license can be associated with reduced employment options, as well as other economic and social ramifications.[2] A bioptic telescope can provide additional information at longer distances, thereby enabling patients to make appropriate and timely driving decisions, such as preparing to merge or slowing down for a red light, provided they have adequate vision to maintain lane control and basic navigation through the carrier lens.

The literature on bioptic driving is sparse, and most studies have significant limitations that prevent generalizability.[3] Nonetheless, bioptic driving is now permitted in 45 states within the United States, and in other countries, such as the Netherlands and Canada. However, the legal requirements vary across jurisdictions, so local regulations should be determined before fitting a patient with a bioptic telescope for driving.

Most bioptic telescope drivers consider the telescope to be very helpful for driving, including enabling recognition of traffic lights, pedestrians, and roadway obstacles.[4] Importantly, 85% of patients who are younger than 65 years use their bioptic telescope to get to work,[5] as was the case for this patient. Therefore, bioptic telescopes can enhance the employability of individuals with low vision by making it easier for them to reach their place of work independently.

In a recent study of motor vehicle crashes and bioptic driving,[6] inexperienced drivers with bioptic telescopes were more likely to crash compared with individuals who had driven before becoming a bioptic driver. However, after 10 years of driving experience, the crash rate of those who first learned to drive with a bioptic telescope was similar to those with non-bioptic driving experience. This is an important point to remember, as novice drivers with normal vision are also more likely to be involved in crashes.[7] Therefore, the collision rate is probably due to driver inexperience, rather than the bioptic telescope itself.

The only on-road study of bioptic drivers reported that 96% were rated as safe by back-seat raters using a standardized scoring system.[8] Bioptic drivers could detect pedestrians, maintain speed, and judge gaps as well as age-matched controls, although they had more problems in lane positioning and steadiness of steering, as well as lower rates of sign and traffic signal recognition.

In summary, bioptic driving is a viable option for patients with adequate vision through their carrier lenses. Although more research is needed in the area of bioptic driving, clinicians can assist their patients by providing a selection of bioptic telescopes to choose from, and fitting them properly, with the selection of appropriate carrier lenses and glare filters also being critical for success.

CLINICAL PEARLS

- Always evaluate multiple telescopes suitable for bioptic mounting so that patients can choose the one that they are most comfortable using. Field of view is extremely important for bioptic driving.

- Allow patients to use the 2 telescopes that were most preferred in the examination room in an outdoor location, so that road signs and traffic lights can be viewed. This enables them to choose their device while using it for tasks relevant to bioptic driving.

REFERENCES

1. Dougherty BE, Flom RE, Bullimore MA, Raasch TW. Vision, training hours, and road testing results in bioptic drivers. *Optom Vis Sci.* 2015;92:395-403.
2. Crudden A, McBroom LW. Barriers to employment: a survey of employed persons who are visually impaired. *J Vis Impair Blind.* 1999;93:341-350.
3. Owsley C. Driving with bioptic telescopes: organizing a research agenda. *Optom Vis Sci.* 2012;89:1249-1256.
4. Owsley C, McGwin G Jr, Elgin J, Wood JM. Visually impaired drivers who use bioptic telescopes: self-assessed driving skills and agreement with on-road driving evaluation. *Invest Ophthalmol Vis Sci.* 2014;55:330-336.
5. Bowers AR, Apfelbaum DH, Peli E. Bioptic telescopes meet the needs of drivers with moderate visual acuity loss. *Invest Ophthalmol Vis Sci.* 2005;46:66-74.
6. Dougherty BE, Flom RE, Bullimore MA, Raasch TW. Previous driving experience, but not vision, is associated with motor vehicle collision rate in bioptic drivers. *Invest Ophthalmol Vis Sci.* 2015;56:6326-6332.
7. Mayhew DR, Simpson HM, Pak A. Changes in collision rates among novice drivers during the first months of driving. *Accid Anal Prev.* 2003;35:683-691.
8. Wood JM, McGwin G Jr, Elgin J, Searcey K, Owsley C. Characteristics of on-road driving performance of persons with central vision loss who use bioptic telescopes. *Invest Ophthalmol Vis Sci.* 2013;54:3790-3797.

1.17 Management of the Geriatric Patient

Harriette Canellos and Evan Canellos

Ben, an 87-year-old white male, presented with a longstanding history of burning and irritation in each eye. He was unable to respond to specific questions regarding the presenting complaint. In addition, Ben complained of blurred vision in both eyes at distance and near, but could not remember when it first started. He did state that he preferred more light when reading. Ben was quite forgetful during the examination. Despite wearing hearing aids, some questions had to be repeated due to hearing loss. He walked slowly, and needed additional time to get into and out of the examination room.

There was a positive history of floaters in each eye, but no history of flashes of light, diplopia, pain, redness, or photophobia.

The rest of the history was reported by Ben's son, who accompanied him on the visit. Ben's last eye examination was 1 year ago. At that time, he was told that he had cataracts, but they were not ready for surgery. His son reported that his father's vision did not seem to impact his activities of daily living. Ben did not drive and he lived with his son. He had hypertension, high cholesterol, early Parkinson disease, early dementia, and hearing loss. Medications included atenolol and simvastatin. His blood pressure was 130/90, recorded 2 weeks ago.

Clinical Findings

Distance VA (with present Rx)	OD: 20/70− (no improvement with pinhole); OS: 20/60 (no improvement with pinhole)
Present Rx	OD: −1.50 −0.50 × 99; OS: −0.50 −0.50 × 90; ADD: +2.50 OU
Pupil evaluation	PERRL; no RAPD; small, sluggish pupils OU
Ocular motility	Full range of motion OU
Cover test	Distance: ortho; near: 6Δ exophoria
Near point of convergence	13 cm/18 cm
Confrontation visual fields	Full OD and OS
Retinoscopy	Dull reflex observed in each eye
Subjective refraction	OD: −2.00 −0.50 × 90 (20/60); OS: −1.00 −0.50 × 90 (20/50)
Trial frame	Patient did not perceive any difference in distance vision from the current Rx
Near add	+3.00 OU (20/50)
Subjective binocular testing	The patient was unable to perform these tests

65

Slit-lamp examination	OD and OS: clogged meibomian glands with corrugated lid margins; age related eyelid ectropion; conjunctivochalasis; conjunctival hyaline plaques nasally; arcus 360°; inferior superficial punctate keratitis OD > OS; 2+ nuclear sclerosis and 2+ anterior cortical cataract; shallow anterior chamber angle; otherwise unremarkable
Intraocular pressure (GAT)	OD: 16 mm Hg; OS: 15 mm Hg at 2:45 PM
Gonioscopy	Open to trabecular meshwork 360° OD and OS, convex iris approach, Grade 1 TM pigment 360° OD and OS
Fundus examination	OD: 0.4/0.4 CD ratio; healthy rim tissue with distinct disc margins; fovea is flat and dry with dull foveal reflex; arteriolar attenuation; mild reticular pigmentary degeneration peripherally;
	OS: 0.35/0.35 CD ratio; healthy rim tissue with distinct disc margins; fovea is flat and dry with dull foveal reflex; arteriolar attenuation; mild reticular pigmentary degeneration peripherally

Abbreviations: CD, cup to disc; GAT, Goldmann applanation tonometry; OD, right eye; OS, left eye; OU, both eyes; PERRL, pupils equal, round, reactive to light; RAPD, relative afferent pupillary defect; Rx, prescription; VA, visual acuity.

Discussion

Ben had multiple ocular and systemic issues that needed to be addressed. His symptoms of ocular burning and irritation were felt to be due to meibomian gland dysfunction and dry eye. He was educated regarding lid hygiene and the use of warm compresses. In addition, lipid-based artificial tears and a thicker lubricating ointment for use at bed time were prescribed. He was instructed on how to instill artificial tears and was observed performing this task. Because Ben had difficulty with drop instillation, his son was also instructed on this task. All instructions were also given in writing.

Ben's cataracts were causing significant visual impairment and surgery was recommended. Although he was informed of the anticipated benefits, he did not wish to proceed with surgery at this time. Ben was advised that his cataracts were likely to progress. His spectacle prescription was updated, and he was given instructions regarding optimal lighting for use when reading. A 6-month follow-up appointment was recommended to check visual acuity (VA) and his performance with activities of daily living.

The geriatric patient requires a multifaceted multidisciplinary approach and assessment. The goal was to evaluate and potentially improve the patient's functional abilities while taking into consideration their physical and mental health, as well as social and environmental factors.[1] For instance, when examining geriatric patients, the practitioner often has to deal with ambulatory, hearing, and cognitive issues, as well as ocular and systemic disease. It is imperative to communicate and comanage with the primary care physician and other relevant health care providers.

The prevalence of hearing loss increases with age. Approximately 50% of patients older than 75 years have disabling hearing loss.[2] Dementia also increases with age and is highest in individuals older than 85 years.[3] Ben had both conditions. Communicating with a family member or caregiver can be extremely beneficial when discussing the diagnosis and treatment. Giving written instructions is also helpful. Health care providers are permitted, in most circumstances, to communicate with the patients' family, friends, or others involved in their care. In the United States, communication with others must follow the Health Insurance Portability and Accountability Act (HIPAA) guidelines.[4]

Mobility also declines with age. Falls are the leading cause of injury-related death in persons older than 75 years.[1] Ben walked slowly, and it was important that he took his time when moving into and out of the examination room.

Equally, providers must allow the patient as much time as required to move around during the examination. Walkers, motorized scooters, and wheelchairs may require additional space in the examination room. It can be very difficult and time-consuming to move these patients into and out of the examination room. A second examination lane may be valuable so that the patient does not have to be moved while dilating drops are taking effect.

Older patients should be given longer appointment times because of the prolonged examination process. Taking a case history is more time-consuming. These patients often have numerous (but sometimes vague) complaints. It is useful to ask problem-oriented questions (eg, are you able to read all the things that you want to?), and repeat inquiries as needed. The practitioner should speak slowly and give the patients sufficient time to consider their answers. History questionnaires are often helpful, as they can be completed prior to the appointment. It is important that the case history includes questions regarding activities of daily living.

Many parts of the eye examination, such as refraction, will require additional time. One should consider the slower reaction and response times, as well as delayed visual and auditory processing. During subjective refraction, the just noticeable difference (JND) may need to be increased. Trial frame refraction, or a refractive assessment over their existing spectacles using Jannelli or Halberg clips, can be helpful. On occasion, it may not be possible to obtain accurate subjective refraction findings and objective results must be used. This is difficult in cases like Ben's where media opacities were present.

Bifocal or multifocal lenses can confuse or disorient the patient even when they have been worn previously. Indeed, Supuk et al[5] observed that the rate of falls in elderly patients switching into multifocal glasses (30%) was twice that of patients who discontinued multifocal wear (15%). Polycarbonate lenses and sturdy plastic frames may be helpful to avoid injury and frame breakage if falls do occur.

Many of Ben's ocular findings were expected with increasing age, such as small, sluggish pupils, senile ectropion, dry eye, hyaline plaques, conjunctivochalasis, cataracts, posterior vitreous detachment, and retinal degeneration.

Eye drop instillation can be challenging for older patients. This is especially true for individuals who are unable to tilt their head back, as well as those with a tremor.[6] Difficulty with drop instillation can lead to poor compliance.[7] The patient may need help instilling topical ocular medications. Ben's son lived with him, and so was able to assist. However, approximately 30% of noninstitutionalized, older persons live alone.[8] It is important to be aware of the patients' home environment.

Depending on the level of visual function, these patients can have difficulty with other routine daily activities. The assistance of family members and, on occasion, social workers should be considered if the eye care practitioner believes that the visual capabilities of the patient, when combined with any cognitive and ambulation issues, place them in danger when living alone.

At the end of the examination, it is important to ask the patients if they have any outstanding questions. Reassure them that they can return if existing problems get worse or if new difficulties arise. Depending on the particular circumstances, suggesting more frequent follow-up visits to monitor compliance can be valuable.

Each older patient is unique and must be evaluated accordingly. Some are highly active, while others are more sedentary. Some are relatively healthy, while others are frail. As a result, it is important to evaluate each geriatric patient as an individual, and to recognize that older patients have a wide range of health care needs.[9]

CLINICAL PEARLS

- Perform problem-oriented examinations on geriatric patients so as not to overwhelm them.

- It is important that your geriatric patient can hear and understand you. Written instructions can be very helpful.

- When prescribing eye drops, provide instruction in drop instillation. If the patient is unable to perform this task, ask if he or she has someone who can assist them.

REFERENCES

1. Elsawy B, Higgins K. The geriatric assessment. *Am Fam Phys*. 2011;83(1):48-54.
2. National Institute on Deafness and Other Communication Disorders. Quick Statistics About Hearing. www.nidcd.nih.gov/health/ statistics/Pages/quick.aspx. December 16, 2016. Accessed April 2018.
3. Alzheimer's Association. 2016 Alzheimer's disease facts and figures. *Alzheimer's Dement*. 2016;12(4):6-8.
4. *A Health Care Provider's Guide to the HIPAA Privacy Rule*. U.S. Department of Health and Human Services. https://www.hhs.gov/sites/default/files/provider. Accessed March 2017.
5. Supuk E, Alderson A, Davey CJ, et al. Dizziness, but not falls rate, improves after routine cataract surgery: the role of refractive and spectacle changes. *Ophthal Physiol Opt*. 2016;36:183-190.
6. Van Santvliet L, Ludwig A. Determinants of eyedrop size. *Surv Ophthalmol*. 2004;49:197-213.
7. Winfeld AJ, Jessiman D. A study of the causes of non-compliance by patients prescribed eye drops. *Br J Ophthalmol*. 1990;74:477-480.
8. U.S. Census Bureau. Statistical Brief. Sixty-five Plus in the United States. http://www.census.gov/population/socdemo/statbriefs/age i.brief.html. 1995. Accessed February 2017.
9. *Talking With Your Elderly Patient. A Clinician's Handbook*. Baltimore, MD: National Institute on Aging. February 2016; No. 16-7105.

1.18 A Complex Case of Accommodative Insufficiency

John D. Tassinari

Nancy, an 8-year-old girl, presented for a second opinion regarding a complaint of intermittent blur at near. She stated that her eyes hurt and became tired when reading. These symptoms began 6 months ago, namely at the start of the school year (third grade), and became manifest every time she read. Her parents asked if Nancy would benefit from vision therapy.

Three months before this examination, Nancy underwent a comprehensive eye examination by her family optometrist and was prescribed reading glasses to "help her eyes focus up close." These helped "a little bit," although Nancy's parents reported that she had to be reminded to wear them. They did not think her reading had improved when wearing the correction. Nancy also reported momentary blur at both distance and near while working (without her glasses) in the classroom. She would also lose her place when reading, and often skip words or entire lines of text. Her parents reported that Nancy's reading was "smoother" if she used a bookmark to keep her place. Nancy's general health was unremarkable, and she was not taking any medication.

Clinical Findings

Unaided distance VA	OD: 20/20; OS: 20/20
Unaided near VA	OD: 20/25; OS: 20/25
Present Rx[a]	OD: +1.00 sph; OS: +1.00 −0.25 × 170
Cover test (unaided)	Distance: orthophoria; near: 3Δ XP
Near point of convergence	7 cm/12 cm; diplopia noted
Confrontation visual fields	Full to finger counting OD and OS
Pupil evaluation	PERRL; no RAPD
Dry retinoscopy	OD: +0.25 sph; OS: plano
Subjective refraction	OD: plano (20/20); OS: plano (20/20)
Distance phoria	Horizontal: 1Δ XP; vertical: ortho
Distance vergence ranges	BI: x/3/2; BO: 8/10/8
Near phoria	Horizontal: 5Δ XP; vertical: ortho
Binocular cross cylinder	+0.50
Near vergence ranges	BI: 10/16/8; BO: 8/18/2
NRA / PRA	+1.25/−2.25
Push-up amplitude of accommodation	OD: 9.0 D; OD: 9.0 D
Calculated AC/A ratio	3.9 Δ/D
Vergence facility (3Δ BI/12Δ BO)	8 cpm (BO and BI equally difficult)

MEM retinoscopy (unaided)	OD: +0.25; OS: +0.25
MEM retinoscopy (with current Rx)	OD: −0.25; OS: −0.25
Cycloplegic retinoscopy	OD: +0.25 sph; OS: +0.25 sph
Intraocular pressure (non-contact tomometry)	OD: 14 mm Hg; OS: 14 mm Hg at 4:15 PM
Slit-lamp examination	Unremarkable OD and OS
Dilated fundus examination	Unremarkable OD and OS
Developmental eye movement test	Vertical: 41 s (62nd percentile) Horizontal adjusted time: 66.3 s (14th percentile) Errors: 10 omissions (6th percentile) Ratio: 1.62 (2nd percentile)
NSUCO saccade	Ability: 5; body: 5; head: 3; accuracy: 3
NSUCO pursuit	Ability: 5; body: 5; head: 4; accuracy: 4

Abbreviations: AC/A, accommodative convergence to accommodative ratio; BI, base in; BO, base out; MEM, monocular estimate method (retinoscopy); NRA, negative relative accommodation; OD, right eye; OS, left eye; PERRL, pupils equal, round, reactive to light; PRA, positive relative accommodation; RAPD, relative afferent pupillary defect; Rx, prescription; sph, sphere; VA, visual acuity; XP, exophoria.

[a] It can be assumed that the presenting Rx included a plus add at the time of prescribing given the cycloplegic result at this examination. To know for sure, we would have to look at the refractive findings from the eye examination that occurred 3 months ago. This information was not available at the time of this consultation.

Discussion

Nancy's chief concern of near point blur, coupled with a low amplitude of accommodation is consistent with a diagnosis of accommodative insufficiency. This condition is said to exist when the patient has difficulty stimulating accommodation, and is generally defined as an amplitude of accommodation below Hofstetter's minimum expected value, that is, 15 − [0.25 × patient's age].[1] At 8 years of age, Nancy would be expected to have an accommodative amplitude of at least 13 D. As noted earlier, she falls well below this level (push-up amplitudes were 9 D in each eye). While a reduced monocular amplitude of accommodation is the hallmark finding in accommodative insufficiency, there are other low test scores that *may* accompany the diagnosis. For example, low positive relative accommodation (PRA) and difficulty clearing the minus lenses during accommodative facility testing are also reported as possible findings in accommodative insufficiency.[1] In Nancy's case, both the PRA and minus portion of the monocular accommodative facility test were normal, whereas the minus portion of the binocular accommodative facility test was low. This incomplete fit of clinical findings with the classic textbook description of a condition is common in clinical care.

An important consideration with a diagnosis of accommodative insufficiency is whether it could be secondary to a general illness or a side effect of systemic medication. There is no support from the case history for such a conclusion.

Further consideration should be given to Nancy's performance on other tests that also support a diagnosis of accommodative insufficiency. The chief concern of near point blur, coupled with low accommodative amplitude, supports a straightforward diagnosis. At first glance, a plus add for near work is a reasonable treatment strategy, and indeed she was prescribed an add 3 months ago. However, this treatment failed to provide benefit here, because Nancy had a multitude of visual problems that complicated the case analysis. A list of findings that either supported or contraindicated the use of a near add is shown in Table 1.18-1. Nancy had other conditions that were not amenable to treatment with a near add, namely convergence insufficiency (ie, greater exophoria at near than distance[2]), fusional vergence dysfunction (vergence

Table 1.18-1 Clinical Findings for Nancy's Case That Either Support or Oppose the Use of a Near-Vision Addition Lens

Support the Use of a Near-vision Add	Mild Contraindication	Definite Contraindication to the Use of a Near-vision Add
Low amplitude of accommodation	Hyperopia absent	Low NRA
Low divergence range at near	Normal PRA	Difficulty clearing plus on accommodative facility
	Normal binocular (dynamic) crossed cylinder	Accommodative lead (from MEM retinoscopy) with an add in place
	Normal lag of accommodation (from MEM retinoscopy)	Low convergence range at near
		Receded near point of convergence
		Near exophoria

Abbreviations: MEM, monocular estimate method; NRA, negative relative accommodation; PRA, positive relative accommodation.

abnormalities that do not fit into Duane's classification), accommodative infacility (inadequate accommodative accuracy, facility, and flexibility), and oculomotor dysfunction (a deficiency of saccadic or pursuit eye movement). The test results that support these diagnoses (based on the initial evaluation) are shown in Table 1.18-2.

The diagnosis of oculomotor dysfunction is based on low scores in two tests. First, the NSUCO test assesses saccadic and pursuit eye movements using a standard protocol.[3] The examiner grades the performance on a scale from 1 to 5. This score is compared with the age-expected finding to impart a conclusion of low, satisfactory, or high oculomotor function. In Nancy's case, 6 slight undershoots were observed during the 10 performed saccades resulting in an accuracy rating of 3. This rating is less than the expected value of 4 for her age range. The second oculomotor test performed was the developmental eye movement test.[4] This required the patient to read printed numbers aloud. The numbers were presented in either vertical columns or horizontal rows. The time to complete reading the 16 rows is divided by the time taken to read the 4 columns. This

quotient is called the ratio score and can be assigned a percentile rank score. As shown in Table 1.18-2, Nancy's ratio score of 1.62 fell at the 2nd percentile level.

In considering an effective treatment plan for this case, vision therapy may result in a long-term or permanent cure,[1] whereas plus lenses will only compensate for some of the abnormal accommodative findings. Accordingly, an office-based, vision therapy program was recommended for Nancy. It comprised 16 office visits coupled with daily, home therapy. A progress evaluation was included at the 8th and 16th visit. By the final visit, her visual skills had normalized and all visual symptoms, including the principal complaint of blur at near had abated. Encouragingly, Nancy, her parents, and her classroom teacher all described her reading as being more fluent. Clinical findings measured after vision therapy are shown in Table 1.18-2.

This case is prototypical of many vision therapy cases. A patient presented with several visual complaints, and had multiple associated functional vision problems that responded to vision therapy. Nancy had deficiencies in accommodation, vergence, and

Table 1.18-2 Abnormal Initial Findings That Point to Various Binocular Vision Disorders

Diagnosis	Clinical Test	Initial Evaluation	After Vision Therapy
Accommodative insufficiency	Push-up amplitude of accommodation	OD **9 D**; OS **9 D**	OD 20 D; OS 20 D
Accommodative infacility	Accommodative facility (±2.00 flippers)	OD 5 cpm; OS 6 cpm; OU 6 cpm	OD 12 cpm; OS 12 cpm; OU 13 cpm
Convergence insufficiency	Near point of convergence	7 cm/**12 cm**	To the nose
	Distance BO vergence range	8/**10**/8	8/20/12
	Near BO vergence range	8/**18**/2	20/36/30
	NRA	**+1.25**	+2.25
	Cover test	Orthophoria at distance, 3XP at near	Not done
Fusional vergence dysfunction	Distance BI vergence range	x/**3**/2	x/6/3
	Vergence facility	8 cpm	17 cpm
	Binocular accommodative facility	6 cpm	13 cpm
Oculomotor dysfunction	NSUCO saccade accuracy	3	4
	Developmental eye movement test	Ratio **1.62**/2nd percentile, errors **−10**/6th percentile	1.20/57th percentile, −5/31st percentile

Abbreviations: BI, base in; BO, base out; D, diopters; NRA, negative relative accommodation; OD, right eye; OS, left eye; OU, both eyes; XP, exophoria.

Test scores that are ≥1 standard deviation below the mean value are shown in bold.[1] The right column shows the findings for these parameters after the office-based vision therapy had been completed.

saccadic ability. One of the diagnoses, namely accommodative insufficiency, was emphasized in this report.

Accommodative insufficiency, typically identified by a low age-related amplitude of accommodation, is a common visual dysfunction that may be treated with plus addition lenses or vision therapy.[1,5,6] If it occurs in isolation or is accompanied by a high accommodative convergence to accommodative (AC/A) ratio and/or near esophoria, then a plus add is a good first treatment option. However, if other findings either fail to support or contraindicate the use of a plus add (Table 1.18-1), then office-based vision therapy is the optimal treatment regimen. Rarely, accommodative dysfunction may be an ocular manifestation of a systemic disease,[7] while it may occasionally result from an adverse reaction to a systemic medication.[8] A comprehensive evaluation is indicated to rule organic etiologies.

CLINICAL PEARLS

- Accommodative insufficiency is usually a straightforward diagnosis based on a comparison from age-expected amplitude of accommodation. In many non-presbyopic patients, it may be treated with vision therapy, rather than using plus addition lenses.

- Accommodative dysfunction often occurs alongside other functional visual problems such as convergence insufficiency and oculomotor dysfunction.

REFERENCES

1. Scheiman M, Wick B. *Clinical Management of Binocular Vision*. 3rd ed. Philadelphia, PA: Lippincott Williams & Wilkins; 2008.
2. Rouse MW, Borsting E, Hyman L, et al. Frequency of convergence insufficiency among fifth and sixth graders. *Optom Vis Sci*. 1999;76:643-649.
3. Maples WC. *NSUCO Oculomotor Test*. Santa Ana, CA: Optometric Extension Program Foundation Inc; 1995.
4. Richman JE, Garzia RP. *Developmental Eye Movement Test Version 1. Examiner's Booklet*. Mishawaka, IN: Bernell; 1987.
5. Rouse MW. Management of binocular anomalies: efficacy of vision therapy in the treatment of accommodative deficiencies. *Am J Optom Physiol Opt*. 1987;64:415-420.
6. Cooper JS. Burns CR, Cotter SA, Daum KM, Griffin JR, Scheiman MM. *American Optometric Association Clinical Practice Guideline. Care of the Patient With Accommodative and Vergence Dysfunction*; 2010.
7. Rutstein R, Daum K. *Anomalies of Binocular Vision*. St. Louis, MO: Mosby; 1997.
8. London R. Accommodation. In: Baressi BJ, ed. *Ocular Assessment: The Manual of Diagnosis for Office Practice*. Boston, MA: Butterworth-Heinemann; 1984:123-130.

1.19 Convergence Excess

Paula Luke

Debbie, a 15-year-old female, presented with general visual discomfort while doing schoolwork. These symptoms occurred only when she was undertaking near tasks. She had experienced these symptoms since she was 6 years old. The discomfort started after reading for just a couple of minutes. She often felt sleepy when reading and believed that she read more slowly than her classmates. She wore glasses for 1 to 2 years when she was about 7 years of age, but was later told she did not need to wear them anymore. She denied diplopia, redness, or headaches. Her last eye examination was 2 years ago, and the findings were unremarkable. She was taking a daily multi-vitamin and had no known allergies to medications. Both her medical and family ocular history were unremarkable. Her father was diagnosed with hypertension 25 years ago, which was well controlled with medication.

Clinical Findings

Unaided distance VA	OD: 20/20; OS 20/30^{-2}; OU 20/20^{-1}
Unaided near VA	OD: 20/20; OS: 20/30^{-1}
Unaided cover test	Distance: orthophoria; near: 6Δ esophoria
Near point of convergence	To the nose
Unaided prism bar vergences	Distance: BI: x/6/2; BO: 8/16/6 Near: BI: x/8/6; BO: x/40/35
Confrontation visual fields	Full to finger counting OD and OS
Pupil evaluation	PERRL; no RAPD
Interpupillary distance	62/59
Retinoscopy	OD: +0.25 −0.25 × 5; OS: +0.25 −0.75 × 5
Subjective refraction	OD: +0.25 −0.50 × 155 (20/20) OS: Pl −0.75 × 7 (20/20)
Von Graefe phorias	Distance: ortho; near: 5Δ eso
Near vergence ranges (through distance subjective Rx)	BI: 12/14/6; BO: x/28/12
NRA/PRA	+2.25/−1.50
Fused crossed cylinder	+1.25
Phoria through fused cross cylinder	2Δ exo
Near base	+1.25 ADD
Near vergence ranges (through +1.25 ADD)	BI: x/24/18; BO: 16/40/35
Minus lens amplitude	OD: 6.75 D; OS: 6.50 D
Accommodative facility (±2.00 D)	Monocular: OD: 15 cpm; OS: 16 cpm; Binocular: 0 cpm (unable to clear minus)

Calculated AC/A	Using cover test finding: 6.2 + 0.4 (6 − 0) = 8.6:1
	Using Von Graefe finding: 6.2 + 0.4 (5 − 0) = 8.2:1
Gradient AC/A	5 + (2/1.25) = 5.6:1
Intraocular pressure (Goldmann)	OD: 14 mm Hg; OS: 15 mm Hg at 9:57 AM
Slit lamp examination	Mild blepharitis OU; otherwise unremarkable OD and OS
Fundus examination	Unremarkable OD and OS

Abbreviations: AC/A, accommodative convergence to accommodative ratio; D, diopters; NRA, negative relative accommodation; OD, right eye; OS, left eye; OU, both eyes; PERRL, pupils equal, round, reactive to light; Pl, plano; PRA, positive relative accommodation; RAPD, relative afferent pupillary defect; Rx, prescription; VA, visual acuity.

Comments

The patient's trial frame refraction was OD: +0.25 −0.50 × 155 OS: Pl −0.75 × 7; ADD: +1.25 OU. She confirmed clear and comfortable vision (20/20) at both distance and near.

Debbie was offered three different options for correction: single-vision lenses for use at near, flat-top bifocals, or progressive addition lenses (PALs). She chose a PAL for the convenience of having clear vision at distance and near without having to take them off, and she preferred the cosmetic appearance over a flat top bifocal.

At the comprehensive vision examination performed 1 year following the initial consultation, Debbie had no concerns. Her visual symptoms were relieved with the glasses. A cover test through the habitual prescription revealed orthophoria at distance and 4Δ exophoria at near through the +1.25 ADD.

Discussion

A pre-presbyopic patient presenting with visual discomfort during near work suggests an accommodative or vergence disorder. Accordingly, both oculomotor systems must be assessed carefully during the primary care examination. In addition, the possibility of spasm of accommodation due to an underlying systemic condition (or medication) with secondary esophoria must also be considered.[1]

Debbie demonstrated a lag of accommodation on the fused dynamic cross-cylinder test, which would appear to rule out accommodative spasm (where a lead of accommodation would be expected). Comparison of the monocular and binocular accommodative facility findings can be used to identify whether the primary problem is due to accommodation or vergence. She had excellent monocular but poor binocular accommodative facility. As she was unable to clear the minus lenses binocularly, this indicates difficulty with disparity divergence. This is also consistent with the low positive relative accommodation (PRA) finding (−1.50 D). While the minus lens amplitudes are also low for a 15-year-old patient (the minimum expected is 11.25 D based on Hofstetter's equations),[2] Debbie was able to clear 4.25 and 4.00 D of additional minus lens power when viewing with her right and left eyes, respectively. Comparison of the BI blur (12Δ) and the gradient accommodative convergence to accommodative ratio (AC/A) (5.6:1) findings also supports the conclusion of difficulty with disparity divergence. Using the gradient AC/A ratio, 5.6Δ of fusional divergence will be accompanied by a 1.00 D reduction in the accommodative response. Because clear and single vision was first lost during the base-in vergence range test when viewing through 12Δ base-in, one would expect the PRA finding to be no more than −2.14 D [12 Δ/5.6 (Δ/D) = 2.14 D]. Given that the PRA was actually −1.50, this is consistent with the notion that the patient's symptoms were caused by poor divergence ability.

In addition to ruling out accommodative dysfunction, divergence insufficiency and basic esophoria should also be eliminated as potential diagnoses. Divergence insufficiency patients will have a larger esophoria at distance compared with near, and a low AC/A ratio. Individuals with basic esophoria will have approximately equal esophoria at distance and near with an average AC/A ratio. Debbie exhibited a high calculated AC/A ratio, near, esophoria, reduced PRA and base-in ranges at near, and a lag of accommodation on the binocular dynamic cross-cylinder test. These findings are consistent with a diagnosis of convergence excess.

The prevalence of convergence excess ranges from 1.5% to 15%.[3-7] Indeed, Scheiman et al[6] observed that the prevalence of convergence excess exceeded that of convergence insufficiency. Convergence excess may present with symptoms of asthenopia, headache, diplopia, and/or blurred vision. Alternatively, some patients with this condition may be asymptomatic, especially if they employ strategies to avoid nearwork. Any diagnosis of convergence excess must be followed up with questions regarding avoidance or reports of falling asleep during reading as potential "symptoms."

Treatment should begin with the maximum tolerated plus lens power that provides optimal distance visual acuity (VA). At near, plus addition lenses relax accommodation and accommodative convergence, thereby reducing the esophoria. This will be most effective in a patient with a high AC/A ratio. Vision therapy to improve divergence at near may also be a useful therapeutic option. The high AC/A ratio in this case makes a plus addition lens an excellent treatment option. Generally speaking, the lowest amount of plus that alleviates the patient's symptoms should be prescribed. The appropriate add power can be determined from the midpoint of the negative relative accommodation (NRA) and PRA results, the fused cross-cylinder finding, near (dynamic) retinoscopy, or use of the AC/A ratio.

In Debbie's case, the practitioner started with the add determined from the fused cross-cylinder test. With a gradient AC/A of 5.6:1, the lens power required to bring the near phoria (5Δ eso) to ortho would be +1.00 if rounded to the nearest diopter (5/5.6 = 0.89 D). Ultimately, the near lens determination should be based on the patient's subjective comfort

when the lenses are placed in a trial frame. This improvement should be supported by reduced phoria at near and improved divergence ability. Debbie preferred a reading distance of approximately 35 cm (accommodative demand ≈ 2.87 D). When shown +1.00 and +1.25 adds at her habitual working distance, she preferred the +1.25 near addition lens. This may be prescribed as a single-vision lens for nearwork only, a traditional bifocal or a PAL. Debbie chose the PAL, and when returning for a comprehensive eye examination 1 year later, she was 4Δ exophoric at near through the PAL and asymptomatic when reading.

In those cases with a large esophoria at near where divergence ability is significantly reduced and a plus addition lens does not eliminate symptoms, vision therapy to improve divergence should be recommended. Vision therapy can be used alone or in combination with a near add. A high success rate (84%) has been reported.[8]

Convergence excess is a common binocular vision dysfunction, and can be managed successfully with ophthalmic lenses in most instances. It is important to rule out any accommodative disorder secondary to an underlying systemic condition (or medication).

CLINICAL PEARL

- When evaluating a patient with convergence excess, begin near testing though the maximum tolerated plus lens power that provides the optimal distance VA.

REFERENCES

1. Scheiman M, Wick B. *Clinical Management of Binocular Vision. Heterphoric, Accommodative and Eye Movement Disorders*. 4th ed. Philadelphia, PA: Lippincott Williams & Wilkins, 2014.
2. Rosenfield M. Clinical assessment of accommodation. In: Rosenfield M, Logan N, eds. *Optometry: Science, Techniques and Clinical Management*. 2nd ed. Edinburgh, Scotland: Butterworth Heinemann; 2009: 229-240.
3. Dwyer P. The prevalence of vergence accommodation disorders in a school-age population. *Clin Exp Optom*. 1992;75:10-18.
4. Lara F, Cacho P, García A, Megías R. General binocular disorders: prevalence in a clinic population. *Ophthalmic Physiol Opt*. 2001;21:70-74.

5. Porcar E, Martinez-Palomera A. Prevalence of general binocular dysfunctions in a population of university students. *Optom Vis Sci*. 1997;74:111-113.

6. Scheiman M, Gallaway M, Coulter R, et al. Prevalence of vision and ocular disease conditions in a clinical pediatric population. *J Am Optom Assoc*. 1996;67:193-202.

7. García-Muñoz Á, Carbonell-Bonete S, Cantó-Cerdán M, Cacho-Martínez P. Accommodative and binocular dysfunctions: prevalence in a randomised sample of university students. *Clin Exp Optom*. July 2016;99(4):313-321.

8. Gallaway M, Scheiman M. The efficacy of vision therapy for convergence excess. *Optometry – J Am Optom Assoc*. 1997;68:81-86.

1.20 Convergence Insufficiency

Graham B. Erickson

Jed, a 12-year-old male, presented with a history of fatigue and sleepiness after reading or studying for more than 15 minutes. These symptoms first began 1 year ago (at the start of sixth grade), and occurred whenever Jed read for more than 15 minutes. He rated the severity of the symptoms as between 6 and 7 on a scale from 0 to 10. However, if he took a 5- to 10-minute break, the symptoms disappeared. This was his first eye examination. His parents reported that he was an excellent student, but struggled to complete his homework in the evenings. He enjoyed playing soccer, basketball, tennis, and video games, but did not report any symptoms associated with these activities. His medical history was unremarkable and he was not currently taking any medications. His maternal grandmother had age-related macular degeneration (AMD).

Clinical Findings

Unaided distance VA	OD: 20/15; OS: 20/15; OU: 20/15
Unaided near (40 cm) VA	OD: 20/20; OS: 20/20
Pupil evaluation	PERRL; no RAPD
Confrontation visual fields	Full, OD and OS
Cover test	Distance: ortho; near: 10Δ exophoria
Near point of convergence	10/18 cm
Subjective refraction (dry)	OD: +0.25 −0.25 × 175 (20/15); OS: +0.25 sph (20/15)
Binocular cross-cylinder	+0.50
Von Graefe phoria (through subjective Rx)	Distance: ortho; near:12Δ exophoria
Near vergence ranges	BO: 8/14/4; BI: 10/16/6
PRA/NRA	−2.75/+1.50
Fundus examination	Unremarkable, OD and OS

Abbreviations: BI, base in; BO, base out; NRA, negative relative accommodation; OD, right eye; OS, left eye; OU, both eyes; PERRL, pupils equal, round, reactive to light; PRA, positive relative accommodation; RAPD, relative afferent pupillary defect; Rx, prescription; sph, sphere; VA, visual acuity.

Comments

Jed was diagnosed with convergence insufficiency (CI) based on the large exophoria at near and the receded near point of convergence. No spectacle prescription was indicated. Office-based vision therapy (VT) was recommended, although alternative treatments, such as home-based VT and prism reading glasses were also discussed with Jed and his parents. They were informed that the likely prognosis with the latter 2 treatment approaches was similar to that of placebo lenses.[1] Accordingly, a vision skills evaluation was scheduled 3 weeks later.

Vision Skills Evaluation

Push-up amplitude of accommodation	OD: 14 D; OS: 16 D
MEM retinoscopy	OD: +0.50; OS: +0.50
Accommodative facility (±2 D)	OD: 12 cpm; OS: 14 cpm; OU: 5.5 cpm (difficulty with plus, no suppression)
Near point of convergence (Capobianco method[4])	12 cm with white light; 20 cm with red filter
8Δ BI/BO vergence facility	4 cpm (BO harder, intermittent OS suppression)
Score on Convergence Insufficiency Symptom Survey (Figure 1.20-1)	26
NSUCO oculomotor test[2,3]	5 out of 5 for ability, accuracy, and head and body movement on both saccade and pursuit testing

Abbreviations: BI, base in; BO, base out; D, diopters; MEM, monocular estimate method; OD, right eye; OS, left eye; OU, both eyes.

It was estimated that Jed would require approximately 10 to 15 sessions of office-based VT, each of which would last about 60 minutes. A summary of the VT procedures employed during the first 5 therapy sessions is shown in Table 1.20-1. In addition, daily home VT activities lasting approximately 15 to 30 minutes were recommended. Regarding the home VT, the patient/family was encouraged to: (a) perform the activities twice daily, (b) do them at a consistent time of day, (c) maximize efficacy with parental involvement, and (d) develop a reward system for effort and cooperation. An interim evaluation was carried out after 5 in-office VT sessions (Table 1.20-2). A summary of the VT procedures employed during

		Never	(not very often) Infrequently	Sometimes	Fairly often	Always
1.	Do your eyes feel tired when reading or doing close work?				✓	
2.	Do your eyes feel uncomfortable when reading or doing close work?				✓	
3.	Do you have headaches when reading or doing close work?		✓			
4.	Do you feel sleepy when reading or doing close work?					✓
5.	Do you lose concentration when reading or doing close work?				✓	
6.	Do you have trouble remembering what you have read?			✓		
7.	Do you have double vision when reading or doing close work?			✓		
8.	Do you see the words move, jump, swim or appear to float on the page when reading or doing close work?	✓				
9.	Do you feel like you read slowly?		✓			
10.	Do your eyes ever hurt when reading or doing close work?		✓	✗		
11.	Do your eyes ever feel sore when reading or doing close work?			✓		
12.	Do you feel a "pulling" feeling around your eyes when reading or doing close work?			✓		
13.	Do you notice the words blurring or coming in and out of focus when reading or doing close work?			✓		
14.	Do you lose your place while reading or doing close work?	✓				
15.	Do you have to re-read the same line of words when reading?	✓				
		3 x 0	3 x 1	5 x 2	3 x 3	1 x 4

TOTAL SCORE 2 6

Figure 1.20-1 Jed's Convergence Insufficiency Symptom Survey at the initial evaluation.

Table 1.20-1 Vision Therapy Procedures Employed During the First 5 Treatment Sessions. A Brief Description of Some of These Procedures Appears Underneath the Table

	Week 1	Week 2	Week 3	Week 4	Week 5
Accommodative Therapy					
Monocular lens sorting (in-office only)[a]	Up to +3.00 D in 0.50 D steps. Up to −6.00 D in 0.50 D steps				
Monocular loose lens rock[14]	Loose lenses +2 D and −6 D				
Monocular Hart chart[15]	Near chart at near point. Far chart at 3 m				
Binocular Hart chart[15]		Near chart at near point. Far chart at 3 m			
Binocular accommodative facility[15]		±1.75 D	±2.50 D	±2.50 D	
Binocular sustained reading through lenses[b]			±1.75 D	±2.00 D	±2.00 D
Vergence Therapy					
Pencil pushups[14,15]	Emphasized clarity to break				
Brock string[14,15]	Bead pushup and jumps	Bead jumps and bug walk	Bug walk + gaze pursuits	Bug walk + gaze pursuits	
Three dot (barrel) card[14,15]		Emphasized fusion	Fusion with look-aways[c]	Look-aways[c] and +2.00 D rocks	
Computer Orthoptics vergence (Random Dot Stereo)—in office only[d 14,15]	Computer Orthoptics with multiple choice vergence	Computer Orthoptics with multiple choice vergence	Computer Orthoptics with multiple choice vergence	Computer Orthoptics with multiple choice vergence	Computer Orthoptics with multiple choice vergence
Vectograms (in office only)[14,15]		BO and BI amplitudes	BO and BI amplitudes	BO and BI amplitudes and look-aways	Look-aways and BIM/BOP[c]
Variable tranaglyphs[14,15]				BO and BI amplitudes	BO and BI amplitudes and look-aways

(Continued)

Table 1.20-1 (Continued)				
	Week 1	**Week 2**	**Week 3**	**Week 4**	**Week 5**
Vergence Therapy					
Sustained reading through prism					6Δ Base out

Abbreviations: BI, base in; BO, base out; D, diopters.

[a] Monocular lens sorting: To help the patient gain awareness of subtle changes in accommodative effort and clarity via an appreciation changes in blur. The patient is asked to put a series of lenses in order by perceived power based on his or her perception of clarity/blur and effort. The lens series starts with large incremental differences, and then proceeds to smaller increments.[2]

[b] Sustained reading tasks requiring the patient to maintain clarity and fusion while alternating between reading for 2 minutes with plus lenses, followed by 2 minutes viewing through minus lenses having the same dioptric power. This procedure is typically performed for a period of 20 minutes.

[c] These tests use the Lifesaver card. Base-in minus/base-out plus (BIM/BOP) uses ±1.50 flippers. Once fusion is achieved and held for between 5 and 10 seconds, the patient places the lens flipper in front of his or her eyes and attempts to regain fusion and clarity. The plus lenses are used for chiastopic (convergence) fusion, and minus lenses for orthopic (divergence) fusion. The procedure is repeated 5 to 10 times for each target separation.

[d] Computer Orthoptics Liquid Crystal Automated Vision Therapy System is a computer- based system of diagnostic tests and therapy programs. The multiple choice vergence program asks the patient to find the depth feature in a random dot stereogram and respond with the direction of the target displacement (up, down, left, or right). The vergence demand is increased with correct responses, and reduced with incorrect responses.[2]

the second 5 therapy sessions is shown in Table 1.20- 3.

DISCUSSION

Convergence insufficiency is a binocular vision disorder that causes symptoms during prolonged reading or other near work. Common symptoms include fatigue, eyestrain, headaches, diplopia, blurred vision, and reduced comprehension. The Convergence Insufficiency Symptom Survey (CISS)[5] has been shown to be a valid and reliable method for quantifying symptoms associated with CI.[5] Symptomatic CI is associated with a symptom score of at least 16 and 21 for individuals younger than and older than 18 years, respectively. The prevalence of CI varies depending on the precise criteria used for classification and the age of the population being studied. Using stringent diagnostic criteria, the prevalence of definitive CI in school and university student populations has been found to be approximately 4% and 7.7%, respectively.[6,7]

Common criteria used for the diagnosis of CI include: (a) exophoria that is significantly larger at near than distance (typically a difference of at least 4Δ is required), (b) a receded near point of convergence (break value ≥6 cm), and (c) reduced positive fusional vergence (base-out range) at near (either failing to satisfy Sheard's criterion that the blur value should be at least twice the phoria, or a blur finding of less than 15 to 20Δ). It is also common to find reduced NRA, a low accommodative convergence to accommodative (AC/A) ratio and poor accommodation and vergence facility findings. In addition, there is evidence of reduced vergence velocity in CI patients.[8,9] To support a diagnosis of CI, there should be a preponderance of these findings, although not all of them are always found.

The treatment of CI has recently been the focus of several multicenter clinical trials. Previously, home-based pencil pushups was the most commonly prescribed treatment for children with symptomatic CI.[10] However, the findings of the Convergence Insufficiency Treatment Trial (CITT) demonstrated that a 12-week period of office-based vergence/accommodative therapy was significantly more effective in improving both symptoms and

Table 1.20-2   Clinical Findings at the Progress Evaluations

	Visit 5 Progress Evaluation	Visit 10 Progress Evaluation	3-Month Post-VT Progress Evaluation	11-Month Post-VT Progress Evaluation
Symptoms	Can read/study for an hour before symptoms occur. Getting homework done much faster.	Can read/study without symptoms. Teachers have commented on significantly improved performance in the classroom and homework.	No return of symptoms. CISS score = 5 (see Figure 1.20-2). Can read for 3-4 h without symptoms.	No return of symptoms. CISS score = 7 (see Figure 1.20-3). Excellent performance in school.
Distance cover test	Ortho	Ortho	Ortho	Ortho
Near cover test	10Δ XP	8Δ XP	10Δ XP	10Δ XP
Distance phoria (von Graefe)	Ortho	Ortho	Ortho	Ortho
Near phoria (von Graefe)	10Δ XP	10Δ XP	12Δ XP	10Δ XP
Near point of convergence (Capobianco method[4])	4 cm with white light; 6 cm with red filter	4 cm with white light; 4 cm with red filter	2 cm with white light; 2 cm with red filter	2 cm with white light; 4 cm with red filter
Near BO range	14/18/12	22/36/20	20/34/22	18/28/20
Near BI range	10/16/8	16/24/18	14/24/16	12/20/16
PRA/NRA	−5.50/+2.75			
Binocular accommodative facility (±2.00 D)	14 cpm (difficulty with plus, no suppression)			
Assessment and plan	Excellent progress	Convergence insufficiency was resolved. Prescribed maintenance VT 3×/wk. To return in 3 mo.	Convergence insufficiency remains resolved. Discontinue maintenance VT. To return in 6 mo.	Convergence insufficiency remains resolved. To return for comprehensive eye examination with referring practitioner in 1 y.

Abbreviatons: BI, base in; BO, base out; CISS, Convergence Insufficiency Symptom Survey; D, diopters; NRA, negative relative accommodation; PRA, positive relative accommodation; VT, vision therapy; XP, exophoria.

Table 1.20-3 Vision Therapy Procedures Employed During the Second 5 Treatment Sessions

	Week 6	Week 7	Week 8	Week 9	Week 10
Vergence Therapy					
Computer Orthoptics (Random Dot Stereogram): in office only[14,15]	Computer Orthoptics with jump duction	Computer Orthoptics with jump duction	Computer Orthoptics with jump duction	Computer Orthoptics with jump duction and BIM/BOP[a]	
Vectograms: in office only[14,15]	Look-aways[b] and BIM/BOP				
Variable Tranaglyphs[14,15]	Look-aways and BIM/BOP (±1.25 D)				
Sustained reading through prism[c]	12Δ Base out	12Δ Base out			
Aperture rule trainer[14,15]	BO and BI amplitudes (in-office only)	BO and BI amplitudes	BO and BI amplitudes and look-aways	Look-aways and BIM/BOP (±1.50 D)	
Non-variable Tranaglyphs[14,15]		Look-aways and BIM/BOP (±1.75 D)	BIM/BOP (±1.75 D)— in office only		
Wheatstone Double-Mirror Stereoscope (in-office only)[14,15]		BO and BI amplitudes	Look-aways and BIM/BOP		
Eccentric circles (chiastopic and orthopic fusion)[14,15]			Fusion with BO and BI amplitudes	BO and BI amplitudes and look-aways	
Lifesaver Cards[d] (chiastopic and orthopic fusion)[14,15]				Fusion with BO and BI amplitudes	Look-aways and BIM/BOP (±1.50 D)

Abbreviations: BI, base in; BIM, base-in minus; BO, base out; BOP, base-out plus; D, diopters.

[a] Note that for the BIM/BOP test, the power of the flipper used increases with improved ability.

[b] Look-aways: Once fusion is achieved and held for between 5 and 10 seconds, the patient looks away at a relatively far distance (≥3 m) for approximately 5 seconds, and then looks back at the Lifesaver targets and attempts to regain fusion. This is repeated 5 to 10 times for each target separation.

[c] Sustained reading tasks requiring the patient to maintain clarity and fusion while alternating between reading for 2 minutes with either lenses or prism, followed by 2 minutes where the lens or prism is reversed (ie, from plus to minus, or from base in to base out, respectively). This procedure is used to challenge the adaptation component of the vergence response, and is typically performed for a period of 20 minutes.

[d] This test uses the Lifesaver card to stimulate both chiastopic (convergent) and orthopic (divergent) fusion.

		Never	(not very often) Infrequently	Sometimes	Fairly often	Always
1.	Do your eyes feel tired when reading or doing close work?			✓		
2.	Do your eyes feel uncomfortable when reading or doing close work?		✓			
3.	Do you have headaches when reading or doing close work?		✓			
4.	Do you feel sleepy when reading or doing close work?			✓		
5.	Do you lose concentration when reading or doing close work?		✓			
6.	Do you have trouble remembering what you have read?		✓			
7.	Do you have double vision when reading or doing close work?			✓		
8.	Do you see the words move, jump, swim or appear to float on the page when reading or doing close work?		✓			
9.	Do you feel like you read slowly?		✓			
10.	Do your eyes ever hurt when reading or doing close work?		✓			
11.	Do your eyes ever feel sore when reading or doing close work?		✓			
12.	Do you feel a "pulling" feeling around your eyes when reading or doing close work?			✓		
13.	Do you notice the words blurring or coming in and out of focus when reading or doing close work?			✓		
14.	Do you lose your place while reading or doing close work?		✓			
15.	Do you have to re-read the same line of words when reading?		✓			
		__ x 0	5 x 1	__ x 2	__ x 3	__ x 4

TOTAL SCORE __5__

Figure 1.20-2 Jed's Convergence Insufficiency Symptom Survey at the 3-month post–vision therapy progress evaluation.

		Never	(not very often) Infrequently	Sometimes	Fairly often	Always
1.	Do your eyes feel tired when reading or doing close work?			✓		
2.	Do your eyes feel uncomfortable when reading or doing close work?		✓			
3.	Do you have headaches when reading or doing close work?		✓			
4.	Do you feel sleepy when reading or doing close work?			✓		
5.	Do you lose concentration when reading or doing close work?		✓			
6.	Do you have trouble remembering what you have read?		✓			
7.	Do you have double vision when reading or doing close work?			✓		
8.	Do you see the words move, jump, swim or appear to float on the page when reading or doing close work?		✓			
9.	Do you feel like you read slowly?		✓			
10.	Do your eyes ever hurt when reading or doing close work?		✓			
11.	Do your eyes ever feel sore when reading or doing close work?		✓			
12.	Do you feel a "pulling" feeling around your eyes when reading or doing close work?			✓		
13.	Do you notice the words blurring or coming in and out of focus when reading or doing close work?				✓	
14.	Do you lose your place while reading or doing close work?		✓			
15.	Do you have to re-read the same line of words when reading?		✓			
		__ x 0	3 x 1	2 x 2	__ x 3	__ x 4

TOTAL SCORE __7__

Figure 1.20-3 Jed's Convergence Insufficiency Symptom Survey at the 6-month post–vision therapy progress evaluation.

clinical signs compared with performing either home-based pencil pushups, home-based computer vergence/accommodative therapy with pencil pushups, or office-based placebo therapy for the same duration in symptomatic children aged between 9 and 17 years.[11] Most of the children who were asymptomatic after a 12-week treatment program of office-based VT maintained their improvement (as assessed by clinical signs and symptoms) for at least 1 year after discontinuing treatment.[12] In a similar study on young adults, office-based vergence/accommodative therapy was the only treatment that produced clinically significant improvements in the near point of convergence, positive fusional vergence, and CISS scores.[13] Furthermore, the Convergence Insufficiency Treatment Study (CITS) compared home-based computer vergence/accommodative therapy with home-based, near target push-up therapy and home-based placebo treatment in symptomatic children aged between 9 and 17 years. While all 3 treatment groups had low and equivalent rates of success, problems with treatment compliance and follow-up between the treatment groups made interpretation of the results questionable.[14] In addition, the use of base-in prism was no more successful than placebo reading glasses in CI children.[1] However, in another study, base-in prism with progressive addition lenses has been shown to alleviate CI symptoms in presbyopic adults[15]—also see Chapter 1.24.

Although these studies demonstrated the most effective treatments for improving symptoms and clinical signs of CI, they were not designed to show the maximum possible improvement. Longer treatment durations (ie, more than 12 office visits) may have produced greater success. In addition, more home-based procedures, or longer periods of daily home-based therapy may also have provided greater success. It should be noted that the investigations cited earlier did not determine which procedures are most effective or whether other office-based treatment protocols could have proved more successful.

Finally, research investigations have noted that the vergence training increases convergence peak velocity, makes the movement of the 2 eyes more symmetrical, and reduces the number of saccades found within the early phase of the vergence response.[8,16] There is also evidence that VT may alter the response AC/A ratio.[17] In addition to the changes in eye movements, the amount of functional activity within the frontal areas of the brain, cerebellum, and brain stem also increase following CI treatment.[18] These neurologic changes are accompanied by improved functional connectivity within the brain, as well as metabolic levels in specific brain regions that are closer to binocularly normal subjects.[19]

CLINICAL PEARL

- Recent clinical trials have demonstrated that a program of office-based VT is the only treatment more effective than placebo for improving symptoms and clinical measurements of CI.

REFERENCES

1. Scheiman M, Cotter S, Rouse M, et al. Randomised clinical trial of the effectiveness of base-in prism reading glasses versus placebo reading glasses for symptomatic convergence insufficiency in children. *Br J Ophthalmol*. 2005;89:1318-1323.
2. Scheiman M, Wick B. *Clinical Management of Binocular Vision: Heterophoric, Accommodative and Eye Movement Disorders*. Philadelphia, PA: Lippincott Williams & Wilkins; 2013.
3. Griffin JR, Borsting EJ. *Binocular Anomalies: Theory, Testing & Therapy*. Santa Ana, CA; Optometric Extension Program Foundation; 2010.
4. Pang Y, Gabriel H, Frantz KA, Saeed F. A prospective study of different test targets for the near point of convergence. *Ophthal Physiol Opt*. 2010;30:298-303.
5. Rouse M, Borsting E, Mitchell GL, et al. Validity of the Convergence Insufficiency Symptom Survey: a confirmatory study. *Optom Vis Sci*. 2009;86:357-363.
6. Rouse MW, Borsting E, Hyman L, et al. Frequency of convergence insufficiency among fifth and sixth graders. *Optom Vis Sci*. 1999;76:643-649.
7. Porcar E, Martinez-Palomera A. Prevalence of general binocular dysfunctions in a population of university students. *Optom Vis Sci*. 1997;74:111-113.
8. Alvarez TL, Kim EH. Analysis of saccades and peak velocity to symmetrical convergence stimuli: binocularly normal controls compared to convergence insufficiency patients. *Invest Ophthalmol Vis Sci*. 2013;54:4122-4135.
9. Grisham JD, Bowman M, Owyang LA, et al. Vergence orthoptics: validity and persistence of the training effect. *Optom Vi Sci*. 1991;68:441-451.
10. Scheiman M, Cooper J, Mitchell GL, et al. A survey of treatment modalities for convergence insufficiency. *Optom Vis Sci*. 2002;79:151-157.

11. Convergence Insufficiency Treatment Trial (CITT) Study Group. Randomized clinical trial of treatments for symptomatic convergence insufficiency in children. *Arch Ophthalmol*. 2008;126:1336-1349.

12. Convergence Insufficiency Treatment Trial (CITT) Study Group. Long-term effectiveness of treatments for symptomatic convergence insufficiency in children. *Optom Vis Sci*. 2009:1096-1103.

13. Scheiman M, Mitchell GL, Cotter S, et al. A randomized clinical trial of vision therapy/orthoptics versus pencil pushups for the treatment of convergence insufficiency in young adults. *Optom Vis Sci*. 2005;82:583-595.

14. Pediatric Eye Disease Investigator Group. Home-based therapy for symptomatic convergence insufficiency in children: a randomized clinical trial. *Optom Vis Sci*. 2016;93:1457-1465.

15. Teitelbaum B, Pang Y, Krall J. Effectiveness of base in prism for presbyopes with convergence insufficiency. *Optom Vis Sci*. 2009;86:153-156.

16. Talasan H, Scheiman M, Li X, Alvarez TL. Disparity vergence responses before versus after repetitive vergence therapy in binocularly normal controls. *J Vis*. 2016;16(1):7, 1-19.

17. Singh NK, Mani R, Hussaindeen JR. Changes in stimulus and response AC/A ratio with vision therapy in convergence insufficiency. *J Optom*. 2017;10(3):169-175.

18. Alvarez TL, Vicci VR, Alkan Y, et al. Vision therapy in adults with convergence insufficiency: clinical and functional magnetic resonance imaging measures. *Optom Vis Sci*. 2010;87:E985-E1002.

19. Jaswal R, Gohel S, Biswal BB, Alvarez TL. Task-modulated coactivation of vergence neural substrates. *Brain Connect*. 2014;4:595-607.

1.21 Divergence Excess

Alejandro León and Sandra Milena Medrano

Carol, a 17-year-old female university student, reported that she had an eye turn since she was 4 years of age. Her aunt was the first person to notice the deviation, but it was considered intermittent at that time. When she was 8 years of age, her parents took her to the optometrist, because they noticed that her eye turned more frequently. At that time, she was prescribed glasses, patching (of each eye) for 5 hours per day and vision therapy (VT) including pencil push-ups and stereograms. She visited a different optometrist at 12 years of age who made the same recommendations.

Carol stated that when her eye starts to turn in, she tries to avoid double vision by doing pencil push-ups, although sometimes she would just close 1 eye. She also reported frontal headaches, photophobia, and that her eyes burn when she has to do near work (such as reading a newspaper or working on the computer). The same symptoms sometimes occur when she is watching television, and consequently she avoids both television and going to movie theaters.

Clinical Findings

Unaided distance VA	OD: logMAR −0.1 (20/15); OS: logMAR −0.1 (20/15); OU: logMAR −0.1 (20/15)
Unaided near VA	OD: logMAR 0.0 (20/20); OS: logMAR 0.0 (20/20); OU: logMAR 0.0 (20/20)
Distance cover test	40Δ alternating XT
Near cover test	30Δ alternating XT
Distance cover test after 45 min of sustained occlusion	36Δ alternating XT
Near cover test after 45 min of sustained occlusion	30Δ alternating XT
NPC	6 cm/9 cm
Extraocular muscle motility	Full OU
Retinoscopy	OD: Pl −0.50 × 180; OS: Pl −0.50 × 180
Subjective refraction	OD: Pl (logMAR −0.1[20/15]); OS: Pl (logMAR −0.1[20/15])
Cycloplegic retinoscopy	OD: +0.50 −0.50 × 180; OS: +0.25 −0.50 × 180
Distance vergence ranges	BI: x/15/12; BO: x/30/25
Near vergence range	BI: 10/20/15; BO: 25/50/38
NRA/PRA	+2.00/−2.00

AC/A (calculated)	9:1
AC/A ratio (gradient)	5:1
Stereopsis (Wirt circles)	400 s of arc
Accommodative lag (Nott retinoscopy)	OD +0.55 D; OS: +0.30 D
Worth 4-dot	Suppression OD at 6 m and 40 cm, although on occasion she reported simultaneous perception
Slit-lamp examination	Slight conjunctival injection; otherwise unremarkable OD and OS
Fundus examination	Unremarkable OD and OS with central and steady fixation in each eye

Abbreviations: AC/A, accommodative convergence to accommodative ratio; BI, base in; BO, base out; D, diopters; logMAR, logarithm of the minimum angle of resolution; NPC, near point of convergence; NRA, negative relative accommodation; OD, right eye; OS, left eye; OU, both eyes; Pl, plano; PRA, positive relative accommodation; VA, visual acuity; XT, exotropia.

Comments

Plano, single-vision photochromic lenses were ordered to help with photophobia. In addition, VT was recommended (both in-office therapy 30 minutes per week for 14 weeks, and home therapy 20 minutes per day was proposed). The in-office therapy consisted of the following:

1. Accommodative activities (eg, lens sorting, loose lens rock, binocular loose lens rock, binocular accommodative facility, and Hart chart distance-to-near accommodative rock).[1]
2. Antisuppresion and fusional vergence training (eg, Brock string in free space, Cheiroscope, variable and nonvariable anaglyphs and transanaglyphs, loose prism, vectograms, and stereograms).

After the VT had been completed, even though Carol reported that the diplopia was less frequent and that her eyes felt more comfortable during near work, she consulted an ophthalmologist, who performed extraocular muscle surgery. The precise details of the surgery are not available.

At a follow-up visit 6 months following the initial examination, Carol stated that not only were the photophobia and headaches still present, but she now noticed that her right eye turned upward. The new oculomotor findings were as follows:

Distance cover test	20Δ alternating XT, 3Δ right HT
Near cover test	12Δ alternating XT, 2Δ right HT
Distance vergence ranges	BI: x/25/20; BO: 14/30/25
Distance vertical ranges	RS 8/6; RI 10/6
Near vergence range (measured with 2 prism bars)	BI: 14/30/ 25; BO: 22/55/50
NRA/PRA	+3.00/−3.25
Stereopsis (Wirt circles)	32 s of arc
Accommodative lag (Nott retinoscopy)	OD: +0.17 D; OS: +0.65 D
Worth 4-dot	Flat fusion (4 lights) at both 6 and 0.4 m
Accommodative facility (±2.50 flipper at 33 cm)	OD: 15 cpm; OS: 15 cpm; OU: 15 cpm
Amplitude of accommodation (push-down)	OD: 9.00 D; OS: 9.60 D
Amplitude of accommodation (dynamic retinoscopy)	OD: 6.90 D; OS: 7.60 D
Afterimage test	Abnormal retinal correspondence (intermittently)

Abbreviations: BI, base in; BO, base out; D, diopters; HT, hypertropia; NRA, negative relative accommodation; OD, right eye; OS, left eye; OU, both eyes; PRA, positive relative accommodation; RI, right infraversion; RS, right supraversion; XT, exotropia.

Discussion

Divergence excess (DE) is a condition where the exodeviation is significantly greater at distance compared with near.[1] This disorder is relatively uncommon, and has been reported to occur in only 0.03% of the population.[2] Indeed, in a recently study, León et al[3] did not find any cases among a student population between 6 and 19 years of age in Colombia.

It has been suggested that the difference between the size of the deviation at distance and near should be at least 10Δ to be classified as DE.[4] Furthermore, Scheiman and Wick[1] observed that the main characteristic of DE is a larger exo deviation at distance compared with near, accompanied by a high accommodative convergence to accommodative (AC/A) ratio (greater than $6\Delta/D$). Accordingly, accommodation, and therefore accommodative vergence, will reduce the magnitude of the exodeviation at near. Nevertheless, in some cited DE cases, the AC/A ratio can be at an average level or even below average. For example, Cooper et al[5] observed that both the stimulus and response AC/A ratios were within the typical range for normal subjects in many cases of DE.

In this case, a prolonged occlusion test was used to confirm the presence of DE. One eye was patched for 45 minutes to achieve almost complete dissipation of slow fusional vergence. Nevertheless, the magnitude of the exodeviation at near did not change. The prolonged occlusion test is valuable for obtaining a more accurate measurement of the deviation. The sustained output of slow fusional vergence can prevent complete dissociation from being obtained. In addition, the patient showed intermittent strabismus at distance, as well as intermittent suppression. "Mixed" retinal correspondence was found. On occasion, Carol reported abnormal retinal correspondence with the after-image test, while at other times she said that the vertical and horizontal after-images overlapped (ie, normal retinal correspondence). Similar findings were also reported by Cooper and Medow,[4] although the underlying cause is unclear.

Patients with DE are often able to use disparity convergence to bring their eyes into alignment much of the time. Although both VT and extraocular muscle surgery reduced the size of the deviation, her symptoms persisted, albeit with reduced frequency. On occasions, multiple surgeries may be required for a heterotropia of this magnitude.[6] Unfortunately, a vertical deviation became apparent after the extraocular muscle surgery.

In summary, DE was diagnosed in this patient on the basis of a larger exodeviation at distance than near, a high AC/A ratio, no changes in the deviation at near after the prolonged occlusion test, and the presence of sensory changes (such as mixed retinal correspondence). While both VT and extraocular muscle surgery reduced the symptoms, a smaller exodeviation persisted, and we recommended additional VT to reduce her symptoms further.

CLINICAL PEARLS

- A prolonged occlusion test must be used to confirm DE.

- Patients with DE may still have a normal calculated AC/A ratio with anomalous retinal correspondence.

REFERENCES

1. Scheiman M, Wick B. *Clinical Management of Binocular Vision: Heterophoric, Accommodative, and Eye Movement Disorders.* Philadelphia, PA: Wolters Kluwer Health/Lippincott Williams & Wilkins; 2008.
2. American Optometric Association [Internet]. Optometric Clinical Practice Guidelines. St Louis, MO: AOA. Available from http://www.aoa.org/documents/optometrists/CPG-18.pdf.1998.Accessed March 7, 2017.
3. León Álvarez A, Medrano S, Márquez M, Nuñez S. Disfunciones no estrábicas de la visión binocular entre los 5 y los 19 años. *Ciencia & Tecnología para la Salud Visual y Ocular.* 2016;14(2):13-24.
4. Cooper J, Medow N. Major review: intermittent exotropia; basic and divergence excess type. *Binocul Vis Eye Muscle Surg* Q. 1993;8(3 suppl):187-216.
5. Cooper J, Ciuffreda KJ, Kruger PB. Stimulus and response AC/A ratios in intermittent exotropia of the divergence-excess type. *Br J Ophthalmol.* 1982;66(6):398-404.
6. Pineles SL, Ela-Dalman N, Zvansky AG, Yu F, Rosenbaum AL. Long-term results of the surgical management of intermittent exotropia. *J AAPOS.* 2010;14(4):298-304.

1.22 Clinical Use of Fixation Disparity

Sosena Tsz-Wei Tang

Ricky, a 47-year-old male office worker, presented for an eye examination. He had been struggling with close work for the past 2 months. Ricky wore single-vision spectacles through which his distance vision was clear, but he had to take them off to read small print. This was inconvenient as he attended a lot of meetings and needed to be able to see both distance presentations and read notes at a close distance. In addition, he used a desktop computer 40 cm away. When reading without his spectacles, his eyes felt like they were straining after 30 minutes. Also, the text became blurred, and he had to blink to clear it up. These symptoms improved if he took a short break from the computer. Ricky also reported frontal headaches at the end of the day. His general health was good, and he was not taking any medications. He had not undergone any other treatment on his eyes or been prescribed eye exercises in the past. His family, medical, and ocular histories were unremarkable.

Clinical Findings

Unaided distance VA	OD: 20/400; OS: 20/400; OU: 20/317
Unaided near (30 cm) VA	OD: N5 ($\approx$20/40); OS: N5 ($\approx$20/40); OU: N5 ($\approx$20/40)
Unaided cover test at near	20Δ exophoria, slow recovery
Ocular motility	Full OU
Near point of convergence	10 cm
Present Rx	OD: -3.50 -0.25×90 (20/20); OS: -4.00 sph (20/17)
Subjective Rx	OD: -3.75 -0.50×90 (20/17); OS: -4.00 sph (20/17)
Near add	ADD $+1.00$ OU (N5 at 25 to 40 cm; N6 at 40 cm)
Cover test (through subjective Rx)	Distance: 5Δ exophoria, moderate recovery Near: 15Δ exophoria, moderate recovery
Associated phoria measured with a near Mallett unit (Figure 1.22-1) through the subjective Rx (see Figures 1.22-1 and 1.22-2 and Discussion section)	Distance: 0Δ; Near (30 cm): 2Δ base-in OD and 1Δ base-in OS
Push-up amplitude of accommodation	OD: 6.0 D; OS: 6.0 D; OU: 7.0 D
Ocular health testing	Unremarkable OD and OS

Abbreviations: D, diopters; OD, right eye; OS, left eye; OU, both eyes; Rx, prescription; sph, sphere; VA, visual acuity.

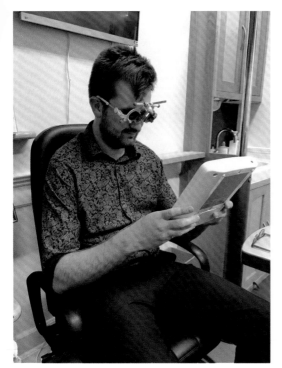

Figure 1.22-1   Use of the Mallett near vision unit to determine the associated phoria.

Comments

Ricky had become presbyopic, and benefited from a multifocal lens to improve his near vision. This form of correction will be helpful in business meetings. However, he had a significant oculomotor deviation at near, namely exophoria with exo fixation disparity. Correcting the fixation disparity (also termed uncompensated phoria) with a total of 3Δ base in at near may relieve his symptoms. Prescribing options included the following:

1. Progressive addition lenses (PALs) without prism for general use, for example, meetings, commuting, and daily life. In addition, a separate pair of single-vision reading spectacles with 1.5Δ base-in prism in each eye would be provided for prolonged near work.

2. Prism controlled bifocals, containing no prism in the distance portion and 1.5Δ base-in prism in the near segment for each eye.

3. Separate pairs of single-vision spectacles (1 for distance and 1 for near) with prism in the near pair only.

4. An occupational PAL containing the prism for intermediate and near work. This type of lens has only a minimal distance zone, and so he could keep his existing distance correction.

5. Progressive addition lenses containing a total of 3Δ base in for both distance and near.

The first option could be successful although somewhat inconvenient as Ricky would have to switch between the 2 pairs of glasses. The second option of prism controlled bifocals is likely to require a significant head tilt for a desktop computer user. This could result in significant neck discomfort unless the top of the segment was raised. This might interfere with general navigation. If Ricky was unhappy with the cosmetic appearance of a bifocal, the option of 2 pairs of single-vision lenses could be considered, although this would still be inconvenient for use in meetings. The occupational lens with prism could work for near reading and computer work but would still require a separate distance pair.

The fifth option contains prism for both distance and near viewing, even though the prism is not required at distance. This could induce symptoms during distance viewing, as he would have to diverge in order to overcome the prism.[1,2] His divergence ability could be tested by measuring fixation disparity through this amount of prism. If any additional fixation disparity is induced, then it would not be advisable to prescribe this option. However, if the patient insisted on a single pair of spectacles, then this option could be considered with caution.

Ricky decided to go with PALs (without prism) and single-vision reading glasses containing a total of 3Δ base-in prism. He was also advised to take regular breaks when using his computer or performing sustained near tasks. One week after collecting his new spectacles, he was asymptomatic and visually comfortable.

Discussion

Heterophoria describes the position of the 2 visual axes under dissociated conditions, that is, when fusion is interrupted. However, it

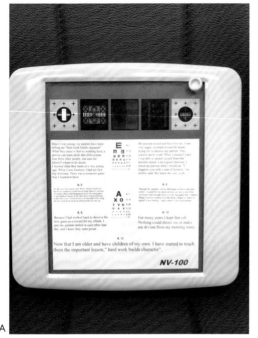
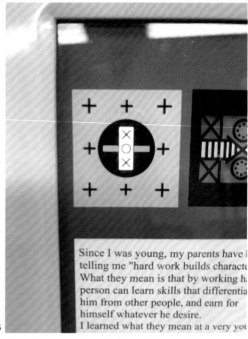

A   B

Figure 1.22-2   The near Mallett unit (A). The right hand figure (B) shows an enlarged view of the specific test used to measure the vertical associated phoria.

does not indicate whether the patient is compensating fully for their deviation by exerting the appropriate magnitude of fusional vergence when dissociation is removed. In contrast, fixation disparity reflects the position of the visual axes under associated conditions. This type of deviation is smaller than Panum's fusional area (typically around 6 to 10 minutes of arc at the fovea).[3]

A compensated heterophoria (where the patient is exerting the appropriate amount of disparity vergence) will generally be asymptomatic and requires no treatment. However, a heterophoria may become decompensated (and produce symptoms) due to factors such as a change in refractive error, increased visual demand, poor general health, accommodative stress, or a change in systemic medication. This case demonstrated a decompensated exophoria at near, exacerbated by the onset of presbyopia. The reduction in accommodation (and associated accommodative convergence) leads to increased exophoria. Signs of a decompensating heterophoria may include a slow recovery movement on cover test, an increase in the associated phoria, that is, prism to eliminate

the fixation disparity (also termed aligning prism),[4] reduced stereopsis, and decreased binocular VA. Interestingly, the likelihood of decompensation is not always proportional to the size of the heterophoria. Accordingly, measurement of heterophoria may not be essential.[5] On occasion, a decompensated heterophoria may be alleviated by simply taking regular work breaks or a change in working conditions, such as adopting a longer viewing distance or improving lighting conditions.

Fixation disparity can be a valuable tool for monitoring the effects of vision therapy or orthoptic exercises. Successful treatment should be accompanied by a reduction in the magnitude of this parameter. For those cases where vision therapy is less successful, or in the case of vertical deviations, prescribing the associated phoria may alleviate symptoms. Jenkins et al[6] observed that patients younger than 40 years of age who showed an associated phoria of at least 1Δ, or patients older than 40 years exhibiting an associated phoria of at least 2Δ were likely to be symptomatic (in the absence of prism). This suggests that these levels should be corrected in symptomatic patients.

One advantage of the Mallett near vision unit is that it demonstrates the position of each visual axis, that is, whether the decompensation is symmetrical between the 2 eyes. Indeed, Ricky's case required aligning prism of 2Δ and 1Δ base in in the right and left eyes, respectively. If decompensation occurs in only 1 eye, then the correcting prism is introduced before that eye. However, if the total associated phoria is greater than 2Δ, then the prism is usually split between the 2 lenses for increased patient comfort and improved cosmetic appearance. On occasion, spherical additions can also be used to correct decompensation, such as using additional minus power to stimulate accommodation (and accommodative convergence) in a pre-presbyopic, exophoric patient. The minimum amount of over-minus necessary to correct the associated phoria should be prescribed.[4]

The Mallett near vision unit , which includes a fixation disparity test, is a handheld device used to quantify the associated phoria (Figure 1.22-2). It should be held at the patient's habitual working distance. A binocular lock is provided as the 2 smaller circles are embedded within text in the original model. Other versions use a series of small crosses (as shown in the top right of Figure 1.22-2A). This is further enhanced by the "O X O" or "X O X" target. Adjacent to the central letter are 2 polarized green strips that are viewed dichoptically (1 for each eye) when viewing with a polarizing filter. Instructing the patient to fixate on the central letter within the fusion lock will improve the accuracy of the test.[7] While testing for horizontal deviations, the strips should appear to be directly above and below each other indicating no fixation disparity. However, if the polarized strips appear to be misaligned, then the patient is asked about the direction of misalignment, and whether 1 or both markers are in line with the center of the middle letter. This will indicate whether the fixation disparity is present in 1 eye or both eyes. Once ascertained, loose prisms are introduced (initially in 0.5Δ steps, and then in 1Δ steps) until the patient reports that the polarized strips are aligned with the center of the fusion lock. Vertical aligning prism is assessed with the target with horizontal markers on either side of the central lock (Figure 1.22-2B). It should be noted that the older units used an "O X O" configuration for the binocular portion of the target, rather than the newer "X O X." Some patients may report only 1 marker being present, which indicates suppression of that eye, or movement of the markers in cases of binocular instability. Rotation of the markers indicates cyclophoria.

Having good illumination during fixation disparity testing is important as poor lighting may result in the appearance of an uncompensated heterophoria at near.[8] In addition, some asymptomatic patients with fixation disparity either suppress 1 eye, or may avoid reading or performing other near vision tasks.[9] These individuals do not usually benefit from prism. Finally, it is important to exclude decompensation resulting from systemic or ocular disease. Appropriate referral may be necessary.

CLINICAL PEARLS

- Cases of decompensated heterophoria can be managed by prescribing the associated phoria (aligning prism), that is, the prism required to eliminate the fixation disparity.

- When measuring the associated phoria, it is important to use a target with a binocular fusion lock, as well as providing adequate lighting and precise instructions.

REFERENCES

1. Jenkins TC, Abd-Manan F, Pardhan S, Murgatroyd RN. Effect of fixation disparity on distance binocular visual acuity. *Ophthalmic Physiol Opt.* 1994;14(2):129-131.
2. Pickwell LD, Kaye NA, Jenkins TCA. Distance and near readings of associated phoria taken on 500 patients. *Ophthalmic Physiol Opt.* 1991;11(4):291-296.
3. Mallett RFJ. Techniques of investigation of binocular vision anomalies. In: Edwards K, Llewellyn R, eds. *Optometry.* 1st ed. London, UK: Butterworth & Co; 1988:238-269.
4. Evans BJ. *Pickwell's Binocular Vision Anomalies.* 4th ed. Oxford, UK: Elsevier Butterworth-Heinemann; 2004.

5. Rabbetts RB. *Bennett & Rabbetts' Clinical Visual Optics*. 3rd ed. Oxford, UK: Butterworth-Heinemann; 2000.

6. Jenkins TCA, Pickwell LD, Yekta AA. Criteria for decompensation in binocular vision. *Ophthalmic Physiol Opt*. 1989;9(2):121-151.

7. Karania R, Evans BJ. The Mallett fixation disparity test: influence of test instructions and relationship with symptoms. *Ophthalmic Physiol Opt*. 2006;26(5): 507-522.

8. Pickwell LD, Jenkins TC, Yetka AA. Effect of reading in low illumination on fixation disparity. *Am J Optom Physiol Opt*. July 1987;64(7):513-518.

9. Mallett, RFJ. Fixation disparity – its genesis and relation to asthenopia. *Ophthal Opt*. November 30, 1974;14:1659-1168.

1.23 Vision Therapy in an Adult With Congenital Nystagmus

Ira Strenger, Barry Tannen, and Kenneth J. Ciuffreda

Fred, a 25-year-old male patient, presented for evaluation and possible treatment of his congenital nystagmus. His chief visual complaints were loss of place and skipping of words while reading, impaired focusing, and eyestrain after reading for a short period of time, and a rightward head turn. He attributed all of these complaints to his nystagmus. In addition, he inquired about applying for an unrestricted New York State driver's license. The visual acuity (VA) requirement for licensure in the state is 20/40 in either eye, or both, with correction. He was concerned that his acuities might not be adequate to obtain a driver's license.

Fred was a photographer who used a graphics computer for several hours per day. There was no family history of nystagmus or albinism, and he appeared to have normal skin pigmentation. General medical history was unremarkable. Ocular history suggested that Fred's nystagmus was of a congenital, idiopathic nature. Treatment for the nystagmus was not recommended. In addition to the nystagmus, Fred had a constant, alternating esotropia that was treated concurrently and successfully, but that condition will not be discussed here. He had previously been prescribed spectacles, but did not wear them as he felt they did not improve his vision. Following successful vision therapy (VT), he was lost to follow-up.

Clinical Findings

Unaided distance VA (taken with a translucent occluder OD and OS to reduce the effect of the latent component on his nystagmus and resultant VA, both single letter and whole line)	OD: 20/70; OS: 20/60; OU: 20/60 No improvement with pinhole
Unaided near VA (taken with a translucent occluder OD and OS)	OD: 20/40; OS: 20/40; OU: 20/40
Pupil evaluation	PERRL; no RAPD
Confrontation visual fields	Full to finger counting OD and OS
Extraocular motility	Full OU slight V-eso pattern
Color vision (Ishihara)	All plates seen OD and OS
Previous Rx	Unavailable (not currently worn)
Dry retinoscopy	OD: +2.75 −0.75 × 180; OS: +3.00 −0.75 × 180
Wet retinoscopy (1 drop cyclopentolate OU)	OD: +5.75 −0.75 × 180; OD: +6.25 −0.75 × 180
Distance cover test	12Δ constant, alternating esotropia, with OS fixation preference

Near cover test	15Δ constant, alternating esotropia, with OS fixation preference (adding +3.00 D lenses over the dry retinoscopy did not affect the magnitude of the strabismus)
Worth 4-dot	OD suppression at all distances and room illuminations
Accommodative amplitude (minus lens technique)	OD: 4.75 D; OS: 4.75 D
Accommodative facility (±2.00 D)	0 cpm (difficulty with both plus and minus lenses)
Slit-lamp examination	Mild iris transillumination; otherwise unremarkable OD and OS
Dilated fundus examination	0.2/0.2 CD ratio; optic nerve head pink and distinct; foveal hypoplasia; hypopigmentation of the fundus; periphery intact OD and OS
Macular OCT (Figure 1.23-1)	No foveal pit OD and OS
Nystagmus (clinical estimate)	Variable amplitude, 3-5° horizontal right jerk nystagmus Frequency about 2.5 Hz (ie, 2.5 cycles per second) Null point about 15° to the left of primary gaze Noticeable rightward head turn Nystagmus dampened with convergence No oscillopsia reported

Abbreviations: CD, cup to disc; D, diopters; OCT, optical coherence tomography; OD, right eye; OS, left eye; OU, both eyes; PERRL, pupils equal, round, reactive to light; RAPD, relative afferent pupillary defect; Rx, prescription; VA, visual acuity.

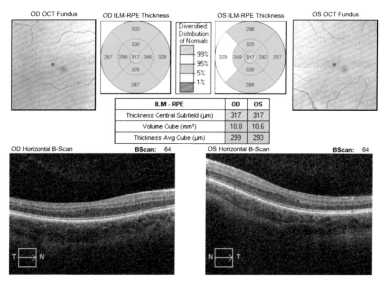

Figure 1.23-1   Macular optical coherence tomography showing foveal hypoplasia evident from the lack of foveal depression.

Discussion

Congenital nystagmus represents one of the least often discussed conditions of the clinical ophthalmic and oculomotor world, especially with respect to therapy to reduce the intensity of the condition (ie, nystagmus amplitude times velocity), to improve cosmesis and overall vision function (eg, VA, reading rate). Although congenital nystagmus is found in only ≈0.24% of the general population (≈1 in 400), its visual and psychological consequences can be considerable.[1] Thus, it is worthy of special consideration by the eye care practitioner.

Fortunately, there is a wide range of possible therapeutic interventions.[2,3] Most improve the cosmetic aspect reasonably well, typically with noticeable benefits to vision. The 3 most common approaches used by vision therapists and low vision optometrists to treat nystagmus include the following:

1. *Yoked prisms:* These are prisms with their bases in the same direction before each eye (eg, bases left). This simple solution works to reduce the frequently present head turn in nystagmus by shifting the patient's world toward the "null" position (ie, the lateral position of gaze where the nystagmus is most reduced). Thus, if the head turn is to the right, the null position is in left gaze, and the yoked prism bases (typically 10 to 15Δ in each eye) would be positioned to the right.

2. *Vision therapy:* This solution improves global oculomotor control. Nystagmus can be conceptualized as an extreme case of oculomotor dysfunction and treated accordingly. As with other patients having oculomotor dysfunction, one would train the fixation, saccadic, pursuit, vestibular and vergence oculomotor subsystems, first separately and then in combination. Start with relatively large, high-contrast targets, and gradually reduce the size and contrast to make the task progressively harder (ie, task loading). Once successful, the patient should perform the same tasks with distractors, such as audio noise, while conducting a conversation, walking down a crowded hallway, and so on. Vision therapy was used extensively in the present case.

3. *Contact lenses:* Either rigid or soft contact lenses can be used in lieu of spectacles, as they (a) create a less minified visual field (in myopes), which improves the fusional process; (b) produce a wider and relatively unobstructed field of view that assists the fusional process; and (c) perhaps most importantly, provide proprioceptive information to the brain via trigeminal nerve stimulation of the palpebral and bulbar conjunctiva regarding relative eye position and movement. The additional contact lens movement related to the nystagmus does not pose any unique problems related to corneal integrity.

There are other less common but excellent clinical techniques that have been used successfully in conjunction with those listed earlier.[1-3] These include the following:

1. *Visual feedback:* This technique has been employed in a variety of forms, including the use of (a) a flashed afterimage so that the patient can "visualize" their eye movements by seeing the correlated movement of the cortical afterimage. They then attempt to reduce movement of the afterimage, which indicates reduced nystagmus; and (b) a circular target comprised of a moiré pattern, which when rotated appears as a line that moves and is directionally correlated with the nystagmus. Again, the task is to try to reduce the movement of the line using volitional control, which the patient gradually learns to exert.

There have been 3 unique visual feedback techniques that Tannen and Ciuffreda of this case have developed over the past several years based on their experience with several hundred nystagmus patients.[1-4] These include the following:

(a) Have the patient gently touch their index finger to the lateral aspect of the upper eyelid to feel the nystagmus eye movements through the eyelid while fixating a target. Then they try to reduce the nystagmus intensity felt by the finger, as well as the palpebral and bulbar conjunctiva (thereby also incorporating proprioceptive feedback).

(b) The patient views a target consisting of a degraded, very low-contrast sinusoidal grating from a few feet away, so that they can just perceive the orientation of the grating (Figure 1.23-2). The patient then increases the viewing distance, until they first cannot perceive the orientation of the grating. At that point, the patient tries to use higher-level control strategies (eg, trying to hold the eye steady, trying to relax and look beyond the target, etc) to detect the target orientation. Once they have again identified the orientation, the process is repeated while gazing at gratings of different orientations, spatial frequencies, and test distances.

(c) Use direct visual feedback via the Visagraph reading eye movement system (Figure 1.23-3A and B). First, the eye movement goggles are aligned on the patient's eyes. The instrument mode is set for "measurement only." The patient performs a calibration by fixating small targets on the viewing screen positioned 57 cm away (so that 1 cm equals 1° when interpreting the recording). The targets are typically located at the center of the screen, as well as 5° to the left and right of center. The patient can now visualize a tracing of their nystagmus eye movements on the screen in real time (Figure 1.23-4A and B). The patient performs prescribed strategies to reduce the nystagmus movement observed on the screen. That is, they are instructed to try to make the jagged recording line straight. Before and after each 20 to 25 minute session, the nystagmus intensity is compared with the pre-therapy baseline value to assess for improvement. This eye-movement recording and related information can either be viewed grossly on the screen for any improvement or can be quantified and compared as shown in Table 1.23-1. Thus, the newly learned eye movement control ability is transferred to more naturalistic, free space viewing conditions.

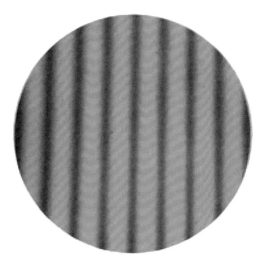

Figure 1.23-2   Low-contrast sine wave grating at the patient's contrast sensitivity threshold point.

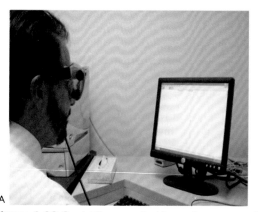

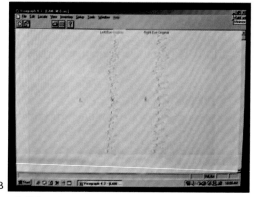

A   B

Figure 1.23-3   A, The set up for Visagraph nystagmus therapy. B, What the patient sees when wearing the Visagraph goggles. The patient fixates on the X, and the red (left eye) and blue (right eye) lines behind it are his recorded eye movements.

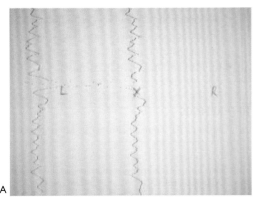 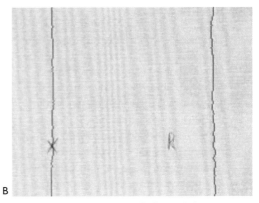

Figure 1.23-4   A, Recorded eye movements on the Visagraph at the beginning of therapy. B, Recorded eye movements on the Visagraph post-therapy.

Table 1.23-1	Pre- and Post-therapy Findings	
	Pre-therapy	**Post-therapy**
Nystagmus: amplitude/ frequency	3-5°/2.5 Hz	1°/1.5 Hz
Distance VA	20/60^{-2} OD/ OS/OU	20/40 OD/ OS/OU
Near VA	20/40 OD/ OS/OU	20/30 OD/ OS/OU

Abbreviations: OD, right eye; OS, left eye; OU, both eyes; VA, visual acuity.

These techniques were used extensively in the present case.

2. *Auditory-based feedback:* Tannen and Ciuffreda have been using auditory-based oculomotor feedback very successfully for nearly 3 decades. Essentially, the patient "hears" their nystagmus, and then tries to perform prescribed strategies to reduce the jerkiness of the tone, which is reflective of and correlated with their nystagmus eye movements. This technique involves the use of a recording system in which the eye-movement signal is transmitted to electronic circuitry that converts the incoming signal to a correlated tone/ pitch. For example, when the patient attempts to fixate a target, they would hear a tone of varying pitch reflecting their nystagmus intensity. The task would be to reduce the range of pitch variation, while concurrently either fixating or tracking the test target. For example, during either attempted pursuit or slow ramp of vergence, the patient tries to make the audible tone as smooth as possible. For vergence, they might hear a low tone indicating verging at far and a high tone indicating verging at near, with a desirable smooth auditory continuum between the 2 distances being the goal. One could also have the patient read, with the goal being reduced nystagmus and more efficient saccading from word to word (eg, a single saccade between each word with little or no nystagmus present). In addition, the patient attempts to reduce the jerkiness of the tone during steady fixation. This technique was used in the present case.

Most interestingly, Fred was able to reduce his jerk nystagmus amplitude for several seconds from a baseline of 3° to 5° to approximately 1° after only 2 sessions. After 10 sessions, he was able to dampen his nystagmus to 1° for 5 minutes or more. Visual acuity improved considerably to 20/40 (OD, OS, and OU) at distance, along with reduced asthenopia. Finally, the cosmetic improvement was marked, with his friends and relatives noticing both reduced nystagmus and head turn. Thus, there was a successful case outcome using a multimodal, therapeutic approach. The patient was also able to obtain a driver's license in New York State.

CLINICAL PEARLS

- The patient with nystagmus may present with a desire to improve vision function, often with a specific goal in mind (eg, obtaining a driver's license). Alternatively, they are frequently told by other doctors that "nothing can be done," and therefore are skeptical about the prospects for vision improvement. In either case, these patients can present a clinical challenge to the optometrist.

- Fortunately, there are several possible vision interventional approaches (eg, Visagraph-based visual feedback, oculomotor-based VT, contact lenses), which often have good outcomes in patients with nystagmus.

- A comprehensive vision rehabilitation approach can result in improved VA and other vision functions, enhanced quality of life, and improved cosmesis.

REFERENCES

1. Ciuffreda KJ, Tannen B, Rutner D. Multisensory feedback therapy for oculomotor dysfunction. In: Hung GK, Ciuffreda KJ, eds. *Models of the Visual System.* New York, NY: Kluwer Academic/Plenum Publishers; 2002:741-769.
2. Rutner D, Ciuffreda KJ. Visual feedback oculomotor training system for young children. *J Behav Optom.* 2002;13(4):91-98.
3. Ciuffreda MA, McCann AL, Gruning CF, Ciuffreda KJ. Multimodal treatment of congenital nystagmus: a case study. *J Behav Optom.* 2003;14(6):143-148.
4. Ciuffreda KJ, Tannen B. *Eye Movement Basics for the Clinician.* St. Louis, MO: Mosby; 1995:230-236.

1.24 Management of Convergence Insufficiency With Prism

Dashaini Retnasothie

William, a 56-year-old male, presented with a chief concern of double vision and asthenopic symptoms including headaches and eyestrain occurring several times a day. These symptoms began approximately 6 months ago, and were only noticed at intermediate and near distances (approximately 60 and 40 cm, respectively). William reported the diplopia to be horizontal and that it caused him to lose his place at the end of a line when reading. He noticed that his work efficiency (as a photographer doing many hours of editing at the computer per day) had declined significantly because of these symptoms. William was taking medication for high cholesterol and hypertension and had a family history of macular degeneration. He did not have any accompanying systemic signs or symptoms, such as changes in weight, appetite, or mood; gait or balance issues; or other visual disturbances.

Clinical Findings

Current distance Rx	OD: +2.00 −1.25 × 12 (20/20−)
	OS: +2.00 −0.50 × 25 (20/20−)
VAs through current intermediate/near Rx (PALs)	OD: +4.00 −1.25 × 12 (20/20− at 60 cm)
	OS: +4.00 −0.50 × 25 (20/20− at 60 cm)
	ADD: +1.00 OU (20/20− OD and OS at 40 cm)
Cover test	Distance: orthophoria;
	Near: 14Δ exophoria
Associated phoria (Wesson Card[1])	4Δ BI
Ocular motility	No restrictions or overactions OU
Near point of convergence	25 cm
Global stereopsis (Randot© test)	500 s of arc
Pupil evaluation	PERRL; no RAPD
Subjective refraction	OD: +2.00 −1.25 × 17 (20/20);
	OS: +2.00 −0.50 × 15 (20/20)
	ADD: +2.00 OU (20/20 OD and OS at 60 cm)
	ADD: +3.00 OU (20/20 OD and OS at 40 cm)
Near base-out vergence ranges	x/4/2
Convergence Insufficiency Symptom Survey (see Figure 1.24-1)	46

101

Intraocular pressure (GAT)	OD: 20 mm Hg OD; OS: 18 mm Hg at 11:00 AM
Slit-lamp examination	Unremarkable OD and OS
Fundus examination	Unremarkable OD and OS

Abbreviations: BI, base in; GAT, Goldmann applanation tonometry; OD, right eye; OS, left eye; OU, both eyes; PALs, progressive addition lenses; PERRL, pupils equal, round, reactive to light; RAPD, relative afferent pupillary defect; Rx, prescription; VA, visual acuity.

		Never	Infrequently	Sometimes	Fairly often	Always
1.	Do your eyes feel tired when reading or doing close work?	✓			✓	
2.	Do your eyes feel uncomfortable when reading or doing close work?	✓			✓	
3.	Do you have headaches when reading or doing close work?	✓			✓	
4.	Do you feel sleepy when reading or doing close work?	✓			✓	
5.	Do you lose concentration when reading or doing close work?		✓		✓	
6.	Do you have trouble remembering what you have read?		✓		✓	
7.	Do you have double vision when reading or doing close work?	✓			✓	
8.	Do you see the words move, jump, swim or appear to float on the page when reading or doing close work?	✓				✓
9.	Do you feel like you read slowly?		✓		✓	
10.	Do your eyes ever hurt when reading or doing close work?			✓	✓	
11.	Do your eyes ever feel sore when reading or doing close work?		✓		✓	
12.	Do you feel a "pulling" feeling around your eyes when reading or doing close work?	✓			✓	
13.	Do you notice the words blurring or coming in and out of focus when reading or doing close work?		✓		✓	
14.	Do you lose your place while reading or doing close work?		✓		✓	
15.	Do you have to re-read the same line of words when reading?		✓		✓	
To obtain score, total the number of "X"s in each column						
Multiply by the column value		x0	x1	x2	x3	x4
Sum 5 values						

Figure 1.24-1 William's responses on the Convergence Insufficiency Symptom Survey.[2] Blue checkmarks indicate responses at the initial examination (total = 46), and red checkmarks indicate responses at the 8-week follow-up (total = 9). The survey was administered using a blank form at each visit so the patient was unaware of their previous responses. Results are combined here for illustrative purposes.

Comments

Based on the case history and clinical findings, William was diagnosed with a decompensated exodeviation at near that presented as a classic case of convergence insufficiency (CI) (Table 1.24-1). While his near symptoms on the Convergence Insufficiency Symptom Survey (CISS)[2] were well substantiated by the large near exodeviation, receded near point of convergence, and reduced near positive fusional vergence, in view of the patient's age and recent onset of diplopia, it was important to look for any signs of underlying neurologic abnormality. Fortunately, both the case history and clinical findings did not indicate any neurologic signs or symptoms. Clinical testing showed that the magnitude of the deviation was equal in all angles of gaze when fixating with either eye (comitant). There was no evidence of an extraocular muscle paresis. It is likely that William always had near exophoria, but the magnitude had increased concurrent with the advent of presbyopia due to the loss of accommodative convergence. This would explain the recent onset of symptoms.[3]

Base-in (BI) prism correction and/or a vision therapy program designed to improve positive fusional vergence and sensorimotor fusion were presented as management options. William elected to be treated with

Table 1.24-1 Diagnostic Criteria for Convergence Insufficiency	
Convergence Insufficiency	Near exodeviation 4Δ more than distance
	Near point of convergence >6 cm
	Low positive fusional vergence at near (based on Sheard's criterion[4])

the prism correction only. To determine the amount of prism to prescribe, several different magnitudes were presented using Halberg clips over his glasses and trialed at the intermediate and near distances starting with 4Δ BI (his associated phoria determined using the Wesson card) and increasing in 2Δ steps. He reported significant improvement in comfort and clarity with 6Δ BI, and did not report any additional relief when presented with higher magnitudes of prism. Further details on determining the appropriate magnitude of prism is provided in the Discussion section. Ground prism was prescribed because the patient had thick, plastic frames and the prism magnitude was low. If cosmesis of the added prism was a concern, lens decentration could have been used because the lens power was relatively high. The following spectacle prescription was released to be made as an intermediate and near progressive addition lens (PAL) because this is where his symptoms were experienced (he had a separate pair of glasses for distance viewing):

Viewing Distance, cm	
60	OD: +4.00 −1.25 × 17; 3Δ BI; OS: +4.00 −0.50 × 15; 3Δ BI
40	ADD: +1.00 OU

Abbreviations: BI, base in; OD, right eye; OS, left eye; OU, both eyes.

At a follow-up visit 8 weeks after the initial examination, William reported excellent clarity, comfort, and resolution of diplopia with his new glasses. The CISS was readministered, and William's score improved from 46 to 9 (Figure 1.24-1). William was instructed to continue wearing his glasses, and to return for his yearly examination.

Discussion

Convergence insufficiency is a common binocular vision disorder that affects both children and adults. It is associated with a variety of symptoms during near viewing, including diplopia, blur, headaches, words moving on a page, and loss of place when reading.[2,4] The criteria for the diagnosis of CI are shown in Table 1.24-1. To quantify symptoms, the CISS, developed by the Convergence Insufficiency Treatment Trial (CITT) Study Group,[2,4] is valuable. A score of ≥16 for children[4] or ≥21[2] for adults is considered symptomatic. As shown in this case, this survey can also be useful for monitoring the effect of treatment.

Treatment options for patients with CI include simple monitoring, vision therapy (see Chapter 1.20), and/or prism correction. The effectiveness of BI prism was evaluated in a randomized clinical trial of CI patients aged between 9 and <18 years. The observed improvement in symptoms was equivalent in both of the groups, that is, those wearing prism correction and those in glasses without prism (the placebo group).[5] Teitelbaum et al[6] also evaluated the effect of BI prism in adults. While this study had limitations (such as a small sample size, use of a lens design not commercially available, and prescribing very low magnitudes of prism), presbyopic CI patients exhibited significantly greater improvement in symptoms when treated with prism, when compared with the group without prism in their glasses. These results give a preliminary indication that although equal to placebo treatment in children, BI prism may be more effective than placebo in adults. While more randomized clinical trials are needed, it does suggest that BI prism correction may be beneficial for adults with CI (like William).

To determine the amount of horizontal prism to prescribe, different magnitudes were presented in a trial frame while William viewed a computer screen at his habitual working distance. The magnitude was increased until the patient reported single, clear, and comfortable vision. The final prism magnitude to be prescribed was determined as the minimum necessary to eliminate the symptoms. William wore the trial prism for 20 minutes in the office to determine whether this was sufficient to eliminate symptoms with extended viewing. It was also made clear that changes to the magnitude could still be made as he tried the BI prism at home. A follow-up appointment was scheduled to evaluate whether such changes were necessary. Fresnel prism was recommended during this trial period to avoid the cost of grinding the prism in the event that a change needed to be made. It was noted that William did not like the quality of vision through the Fresnel prism and elected to have prism ground in right away. He was sufficiently symptomatic and was able to provide reliable subjective reports.

When examining a patient whose subjective reports are less reliable, or one who is not experiencing symptoms during the trial prism selection, there are other methods of determining the amount of prism to prescribe. For example, Sheard's criterion states that the fusional reserve should be at least twice the heterophoria. Based on this criterion, the equation "prism = ⅔ phoria − ⅓ compensating fusional vergence range" can be used to determine the required prism.[7] Alternatively, the amount of prism required to neutralize the fixation disparity (ie, the associated phoria) or the shape of their fixation disparity curve can be used.[8] Irrespective of the method adopted, using a trial frame to present the proposed amount of prism to the patient is highly recommended. This allows for minor changes once the starting point has been established by one of the methods described, that is, titrating the prism to determine the minimum amount to eliminate symptoms. It is important to emphasize that there is no single method to determine the amount of prism to prescribe. William had a specific task where he wished to achieve clear, comfortable, and single vision, so trying prism in a setting that simulated this as closely as possible was ideal. Had William encountered difficulty giving definitive subjective responses to the prism,

then an alternative method would have been attempted.

A challenge of using horizontal prism to alleviate symptoms of CI is that these patients require prism correction for near viewing only. If they view distance targets through the prism, this may cause symptoms including diplopia. Thus, BI prism can be added to a reading-only prescription or an intermediate-near bifocal or PAL, as was the case here. If the patient wears contact lenses, prescribing a pair of spectacles with prism may allow the patient to use them as needed for near viewing. Unfortunately, there are a limited number of commercially available spectacle lenses that allow for prism to be ground into the reading portion of the lens only (executive bifocals or in some cases a prism segment can be cemented in). Regular follow-up examinations are recommended in any case of prescribing prism to monitor for any necessary changes, especially in the event of prism adaptation.

A number of clinical trials have validated the effectiveness of vision therapy for managing CI,[9] and adults should be considered as good candidates for this form of treatment (see Chapter 1.20). However, if a patient is unable or unwilling to commit to the cost or time associated with vision therapy, BI prism can be an effective alternative treatment. Determining the ideal amount of prism to prescribe while preserving fusion at distance can require some trial and error. With patience, a successful outcome is possible, thereby allowing a patient to satisfy their visual requirements.

CLINICAL PEARL

- The Wesson card[1] is a quick method of quantifying fixation disparity. It is easy to administer and relatively inexpensive for the clinician to purchase. The amount of prism required to neutralize the patient's fixation disparity is a good starting point when prescribing both horizontal and/or vertical prisms.

REFERENCES

1. Wesson MD, Koenig R. A new clinical method for direct measurement of fixation disparity. *South J Optom.* 1982;1:48-52.
2. Rouse MW, Borsting EJ, Mitchell GL, et al. Convergence Insufficiency Treatment Trial Group.

Validity and reliability of the revised Convergence Insufficiency Symptom Survey in adults. *Ophthalmic Physiol Opt*. 2004;24(5):384-390.

3. Duke-Elder S. *System of Ophthalmology*. London, UK: Henry Kimpton; 1973.

4. Borsting EJ, Rouse MW, Mitchell GL, et al. Convergence Insufficiency Treatment Trial Group. Validity and reliability of the revised Convergence Insufficiency Symptom Survey in children aged 9 to 18 years. *Optom Vis Sci*. 2003:80(12):832-838.

5. Scheiman M, Cotter S, Rouse M, et al. Convergence Insufficiency Treatment Trial Study Group. Randomized clinical trial of the effectiveness of base-in prism reading glasses versus placebo reading glasses for symptomatic convergence insufficiency in children. *Br J Ophthalmol*. 2005;89(10):1318-1323.

6. Teitelbaum B, Pang Y, Krall J. Effectiveness of base in prism for presbyopes with convergence insufficiency. *Optom Vis Sci*. 2009;86(2):153-156.

7. Sheard C. Zones of ocular comfort. *Optom Vis Sci*. 1930;7(1):9-25.

8. Mallet RF. The investigation of heterophoria at near and a new fixation disparity technique. *Optician*. 1964;148:547-551.

9. Convergence Insufficiency Treatment Trial Study Group. A randomized clinical trial of treatments for symptomatic convergence insufficiency in children. *Arch Ophthalmol*. 2008;126(10):1336-1349.

1.25 Vertical Heterophoria

Paula Luke

Mike, a 30-year-old male, was referred to the eye clinic by a close friend. He was a student in the osteopathic medicine program and was having difficulty studying due to headaches and visual discomfort during sustained near work. The only relief he could obtain was by avoiding near tasks. He had received yearly eye examinations with unremarkable findings other than a correction for myopia. He had been prescribed blue overlays by a psychologist, which seemed to help for approximately 6 months, but he no longer felt any benefit from this treatment. Mike had a history of several concussions as a young child. He was not currently taking any medications. Family, medical, and ocular histories were unremarkable.

Clinical Findings

Habitual distance VA	OD: 20/15; OS: 20/15; OU: 20/15
Habitual near VA	OD: 20/20; OS: 20/20
Habitual Rx	OD: $-1.00 -0.75 \times 25$ OS: $-0.25 -1.00 \times 175$
Cover test	Distance: 2ΔRHP; near: 2Δ RHP, 2Δ XP (comitant in all diagnostic action fields)
Near point of convergence	15 cm/20 cm
Confrontation visual fields	Full to finger counting OD and OS
Pupil evaluation	PERRL; no RAPD
Subjective refraction	OD: $-1.00 -0.75 \times 25$ (20/15); OS: $-0.25 -1.00 \times 175$ (20/15)
Von Graefe	Distance: 2Δ right hyper; Near: 2Δ right hyper, 4Δ exo
NRA/PRA	+2.00/−2.50
Vertical associated phoria (Saladin Card)	1Δ base down OD

Abbreviations: NRA, negative relative accommodation; OD, right eye; OS, left eye; OU, both eyes; PERRL, pupils equal, round, reactive to light; PRA, positive relative accommodation; RAPD, relative afferent pupillary defect; RHP, right hyperphoria; Rx, prescription; VA, visual acuity; XP, exophoria.

Comments

The subjective refraction was prescribed with 0.5Δ base-down OD and 0.5Δ base-up OS. Mike was asked to return in 1 month to assess his symptoms. At this 1-month follow-up visit, Mike reported improved comfort in his reading. He was able to complete his homework and already noticed an improvement in school performance.

The following findings were recorded with the prescribed Rx and prism:

Cover test	Distance: ortho; near: 1Δ XP
Near point of convergence	5 cm/10 cm
Maddox rod at 6 m	1Δ right hyper
Modified Thorington (40 cm)	1Δ exo and 1Δ right hyper
6 m prism bar vergences	BI: x/4/2; BO: x/16/12
40 cm prism bar vergences	BI: x/12/10; BO: x/20/18

Abbreviations: BI, base in; BO, base out; XP, exophoria.

At a follow-up visit performed 6 months after the initial examination, Mike reported that he had passed his board exams in osteopathic medicine and was very happy with the prism Rx.

Discussion

A patient presenting with a history of visual discomfort while doing near work after a series of unremarkable eye examinations requires a careful assessment of vergence and accommodation. Given the report of multiple concussions as a child, there are a number of non-strabismic binocular dysfunctions associated with mild concussion that need to be ruled out (see Chapter 1.27). Convergence insufficiency, accommodative dysfunction, and saccadic dysfunction are the most common non-strabismic binocular vision disorders associated with traumatic brain injury.[1] While a small vertical heterophoria is not the most prevalent post-concussive vision disorder, it could still cause significant symptoms post-concussion.[2] Mike's vertical phoria was probably present at an early age, and the symptoms were exacerbated after the multiple concussions. The most common visual complaints following mild traumatic brain injury are blurred vision, diplopia, eye fatigue, words moving on a page, loss of place while reading, and difficulty sustaining attention.[1-4] Due to the elusive presentation of a vertical deviation and the presence of symptoms that overlap other conditions, a vertical deviation is often overlooked. Indeed, a psychologist suggested treatment with a blue filter, which did not offer any long-lasting benefit as the actual vision problem was the vertical oculomotor deviation.

Vertical heterophoria is present in approximately 20% of the general population. However, symptomatic vertical heterophoria is found in approximately 9% of the population.[5] Although the vertical heterophoria in the present case was small, Mike had difficulty compensating for the small vertical misalignment resulting in long-standing, nonprogressive visual discomfort. There is evidence that even a very small vertical deviation can cause significant symptoms after a concussion.[2]

Vertical heterophoria can be the result of a congenital hyperdeviation that is usually concomitant, a decompensated cranial nerve IV palsy or a newly acquired cranial nerve IV palsy.[6] It is important to determine the underlying cause of a vertical deviation, especially if it is associated with diplopia of sudden onset. Newly acquired cranial nerve IV palsies will be incomitant, but may become more concomitant over time. Mike had the symptoms for at least 3 years, did not report diplopia, and exhibited a concomitant deviation suggesting either a congenital vertical imbalance or a long-standing cranial nerve IV palsy. The likely cause for Mike's long-standing symptoms were related to his history of multiple concussions.

The treatment of choice for vertical heterophoria is prism.[5] Symptomatic patients with vertical deviations tend to respond well to prescribed prism with minimal or no adaptation. The prism may be ground into the glasses, prescribed as a Fresnel prism, or in the case of small amounts of vertical prism, prescribed in a contact lens.[7] Lower amounts of prism (<3Δ) do not need to be split between the 2 eyes. However, if all the vertical prism is ground into a single lens, it is recommended that it be in the base-up orientation to minimize visual distortions, which are present toward the prism base.[7]

Many methods are available to determine the appropriate amount of prism, including the associated phoria, the mid-point of the supra- and infra-vergence ranges, or a flip-prism technique.[5,7] In the flip-prism method, a 3Δ prism is introduced before 1 eye, first as base up, and then flipped to base down. The patient should report vertical diplopia with each flip of the prism. If no vertical phoria is present, then the separation of the double images will be equal for each prism orientation. However, if a vertical deviation is present, then the image displacement through the prisms will be unequal. Vertical prism is introduced into a trial frame in the direction necessary to reduce the larger displacement until the patient reports equal separation between base up and base down. The magnitude of prism required to equalize the image separation is the amount of prism recommended for trial. Alternatively, the midpoint of the vertical vergence ranges would work well in a patient with asymmetrical vertical vergences. The easiest and least complex method with a communicative patient having reliable subjective responses is to use the associated phoria, that is, the minimum amount of prism that eliminates the fixation disparity. Many computerized acuity charts have targets to determine the associated phoria with red/green glasses (Figure 1.25-1). It may also be measured at near with a Saladin or Wesson card. Prism is introduced until the patient reports precise vertical alignment. Vertical prism should be introduced in 0.50Δ steps. Mike gave reliable responses while testing the associated phoria indicating a value of 1Δ base-down OD with repeated testing.

Visual symptoms from a vertical phoria are typically alleviated with prism alone. If symptoms persist and horizontal vergence ranges remain reduced even after vertical prism

has been prescribed, vision therapy to improve the horizontal vergence ranges will often resolve the residual symptoms.[5] However, Mike gained relief from prism alone.

Symptomatic vertical heterophoria is a prevalent condition, occurring in approximately 9% of the general population. If a patient presents with long-standing visual symptoms and a history of normal eye examinations, then a vertical heterophoria should be considered. Patients with a history of concussion often benefit from very small refractive and prismatic corrections, as the size of the deviation is often unrelated to the severity of symptoms.[2] If there is any suspicion of a recent onset cranial nerve IV palsy or neurologic etiology, further assessment and management of the underlying cause are necessary (see Case 3.24).

CLINICAL PEARL

- Symptomatic vertical heterophoria occurs in approximately 9% in the general clinic population, and should be a differential diagnosis in any patient with a history of asthenopia.

REFERENCES

1. Capo-Aponte JE, Urosevich TG, Temme LA, Tarbett AK, Sanghera NK. Visual dysfunctions and symptoms during the subacute stage of blast-induced mild traumatic brain injury. *Mil Med.* 2012;177:804-813.
2. Rosner MS, Feinberg DL, Doble JE, Rosner AJ. Treatment of vertical heterophoria ameliorates persistent post-concussive symptoms: a retrospective analysis utilizing a multi-faceted assessment battery. *Brain Inj.* 2016;30(3):311-317.
3. Master CL, Scheiman M, Gallaway M, et al. Vision diagnoses are common after concussion in adolescents. *Clin Pediatr.* 2016;55(3):260-267.
4. Ciuffreda KJ, Kapoor N, Rutner D, Suchoff IB, Han ME, Craig S. Occurrence of oculomotor dysfunctions in acquired brain injury: a retrospective analysis. *Optometry.* 2007;78:155-161.
5. Scheiman M, Wick B. *Clinical Management of Binocular Vision.* Philadelphia, PA: Wolters Kluwer; 2013.
6. Richards BW, Jones FR Jr, Younge BR. Causes and prognosis in 4,278 cases of paralysis of the oculomotor trochlear, and abducens cranial nerves. *Am J Ophthalmol.* 1992;113:489-496; comment 1992; 114:777-778.
7. Cotter S. *Clinical Uses of Prism: A Spectrum of Applications.* St. Louis, MO: Mosby; 1995.

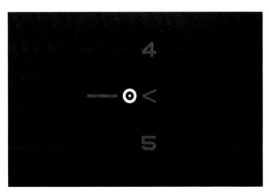

Figure 1.25-1   M&S system fixation disparity target.

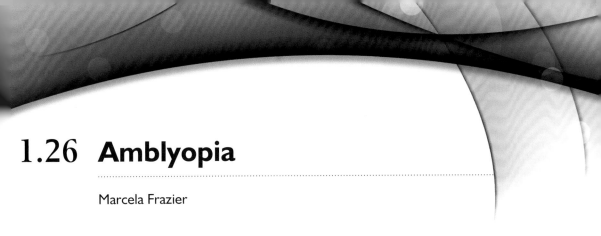

1.26 Amblyopia

Marcela Frazier

Daniel, a 4-year-old Hispanic male, presented for an eye examination. His mother stated that his right eye drifted in sometimes. She first noticed this when Daniel was 3 years old, but felt that it had worsened lately. Daniel had not previously had a comprehensive eye examination, but passed the pediatrician's vision screening every year. However, he failed a preschool vision screening this year. Family medical history was remarkable only for his mother being diagnosed with diabetes 2 years ago. His mother also reported that she had to wear an eye patch for a year when she was young due to amblyopia.

Daniel's medical history included high-functioning autism. He was very shy and did not make good eye contact. Otherwise, Daniel answered questions appropriately, and his mother stated that he was doing very well in school.

Clinical Findings

Distance VA (single-surrounded HOTV symbols using the EVA system)	OD: 20/200; OS: 20/80
Cover test	Distance: 20Δ constant RET; Near: 30Δ constant RET
Global stereopsis	None
MEM retinoscopy at 33 cm	1.25 D lead of accommodation OU (unstable)
Worth 4-dot test	Suppression of left eye at distance and near
Slit-lamp examination	Unremarkable OD and OS; no ptosis was observed
Intraocular pressure (Icare tonometer)	OD: 14 mm Hg; OS: 14 mm Hg at 10:33 AM
Cycloplegic retinoscopy (1 drop of 1% cyclopentolate and 1 drop of 2.5% phenylephrine OU)	OD: +5.25 sph; OS: +2.25 sph (BCVA was not obtained at this visit as Daniel was unreliable in his subjective responses after cycloplegia)
Fundus examination	Unremarkable

Abbreviations: BCVA, best corrected visual acuity; D, diopters; EVA, electronic visual acuity; MEM, monocular estimate method (retinoscopy); OD, right eye; OS, left eye; OU, both eyes; sph, sphere; RET, right esotropia; VA, visual acuity.

Comments

Daniel was diagnosed with hyperopia, anisometropia, and accommodative esotropia. He had a number of amblyopic risk factors. Glasses were prescribed with the following Rx: OD: +5.25 sph; OS: +2.25 sph. He was asked to return to the clinic in 2 months to evaluate the strabismus, adaptation to the glasses, and the need for additional amblyopia treatment.

Follow-up Visits

Date After the Initial Examination	VA (Single-Surrounded HOTV Symbols Using the EVA system)	Cover Test and Accommodation	Global Stereopsis	Other Actions or Recommended Treatment
2 months (with new Rx)	OD: 20/160; OS: 20/40	Ortho at distance; 6 Δ EP at near MEM retinoscopy OD +1.00; OS +0.50 Accommodative amplitude OD 8.3 D; OS 10 D (questionable reliability on amplitude measurement)	Nil	Continue wearing glasses full-time To return in 2 months.
4 months	OD: 20/160; OS: 20/40	Ortho at distance; Unreliable at near MEM retinoscopy OD +1.00; OS +0.50	Nil	Presented the choice of 6 h of daily patching vs daily atropine. The parents chose daily atropine. Started 1 drop of 1% atropine daily OS
6 months	OD: 20/125; OS: 20/40	Ortho at distance; Unreliable at near MEM retinoscopy OD +0.75; OS +3.00[a]	Nil	Continue atropine 1% 1 drop daily OS Mother told not to instill atropine 1 week before the next visit to obtain a more accurate CT result
8 months	OD: 20/80; OS: 20/40	Ortho at distance; 4Δ constant RXT at near MEM retinoscopy OD +1.00; OS +0.50 Atropine was stopped 1 week before this visit	Nil	Decrease atropine 1% OS from daily to 2 days per week
10 months	OD: 20/63; OS: 20/20	Ortho at distance; 4Δ constant RXT at near	Nil	Continue atropine 1% OS 2 days per week
12 months	OD: 20/40; OS: 20/20	Ortho at distance; Unreliable at near MEM retinoscopy OD fluctuating from +1.00 lag to −0.50 lead; OS +0.50	Nil	Continue atropine 1% OS 2 days per week Repeated cycloplegic retinoscopy: OD +5.25 sph; OS +2.00 sph

14 months	OD: 20/40; OS: 20/20	Ortho at distance; Unreliable at near due to cycloplegia OS	Nil	Continue atropine 1% OS 2 days per week
16 months	OD: 20/40; OS: 20/20	Ortho at distance; Unreliable at near	Nil	Visuoscopy and OCT of macula

Abbreviations: CT, computed tomography; D, diopters; EVA, electronic visual acuity; MEM, monocular estimate method (retinoscopy); OCT, optical coherence tomography; OD, right eye; OS, left eye; OU, both eyes; RXT, right exotropia; sph, sphere; VA, visual acuity.

[a] Mother forgot to stop atropine 4 days before the date of this appointment.

Comments

Due to the inability to obtain global stereopsis, plateauing of the visual acuity (VA) in the right eye and the poor reliability and inconsistency of the cover test at near, visuoscopy and optical coherence tomography (OCT) were performed. On visuoscopy, the right eye appeared to fixate eccentrically approximately 3Δ temporally and 1Δ inferiorly. However, obtaining an OCT image was challenging due to the unstable fixation of the right eye. The left eye fixated centrally. OCT images of each macula are shown in Figure 1.26-1.

Other Considerations

Daniel's mother reported that she had difficulty instilling the atropine drops initially. We recommended that she instill the drop while he was still asleep (early morning). Daniel also complained about blur at near, so we asked his teacher to provide slightly larger reading materials while he was undergoing treatment. After 14 months of treatment, he complained of photophobia while swimming, and we recommended either wearing sunglasses or switching to patching the left eye 2 hours per day. After trying patching for a couple of days, Daniel chose to go back to atropine, and wore tinted goggles while swimming.

In view of the large amount of anisometropia, the difference in the appearance of the right and left spectacle lenses may make the child self-conscious as he gets older. Contact lenses are a good alternative, especially as they will also relieve the differential vertical prism by decentration that occurs when he looks away from the optical center of the spectacle lenses. As the child matures, it is helpful to assess the amount of aniseikonia being generated by the anisometropia. Other tests of binocularity, suppression, and retinal correspondence, such as the Maddox rod, Bagolini striated lenses, and synoptophore testing may be helpful as the child gets older.

Discussion

Amblyopia is the most common cause of visual impairment in children, with a prevalence between 1% and 4 % in children younger than 6 years of age.[1,2] The main causes of amblyopia are uncorrected refractive error, strabismus,

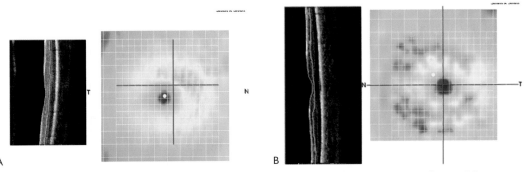

Figure 1.26-1   Optical coherence tomography of macula OD (A) and OS (B) shows eccentric fixation OD.
Abbreviations: OD, right eye; OS, left eye.

or a combination of strabismus and anisometropia. Recent population-based studies have shown uncorrected refractive error to be a more prevalent amblyogenic factor than strabismus in young children.[2] This may lead to the condition going undetected since parents are more likely to seek eye care for their children if they observe an eye turn, whereas uncorrected refractive error (especially hyperopia) may have no signs or symptoms in early childhood.

To maximize the visual outcome for children with amblyopia, early detection and treatment are very important. Children who fail vision screenings at primary care or preschool settings must receive a comprehensive eye examination that includes an appropriate assessment of ocular health, binocular vision testing, and cycloplegic retinoscopy. Single-surrounded Lea or HOTV symbols are recommended for VA testing to detect amblyopia in young children between 3 and 7 years of age.[3] If an amblyogenic refractive error is detected, then the appropriate optical correction should be worn until the VA stops improving. At that point, penalization or other amblyopia treatment can be initiated in addition to the glasses. In Daniel's case, the full amount of hyperopia was prescribed due to the presence of esotropia. The Pediatric Eye Disease Investigator Group (PEDIG)[4] has found that refractive correction with spectacles alone results in a clinically meaningful improvement in the VA of the amblyopic eye in most children.

Once VA improvement has maximized with optical correction alone, subsequent treatment options for unilateral amblyopia should include penalization of the "better" eye. Several PEDIG studies have shown that for the treatment of severe amblyopia (ie, VA between 20/100 and 20/400), 1 drop of 1% atropine per day is as effective as 6 hours of daily patching. For the treatment of moderate amblyopia (ie, VA between 20/40 and 20/80), 1 drop of 1% atropine given 2 nights per week is as effective as 2 hours of daily patching.[5]

Because the results of several amblyopia treatment studies have shown that penalization with patching versus atropine is equally effective, the choice of the modality of treatment falls on the family. Before making the decision whether to use patching or

atropine, the family should be informed about the common side effects of atropine, such as near blur, photophobia, stinging, and eye irritation, as well as about the less common side effects such as increased heart rate, restlessness, flushing, and irritability.

When treating children with anisometropic amblyopia, it is important to consider other differential diagnoses, or comorbidities, such as microtropia or unilateral optic nerve hypoplasia, especially in cases where the VA of the amblyopic eye reaches a plateau less than the normal value. In these cases, it is important to assess compliance with treatment, and to consider the possibility of subtle retinal, optic nerve, or gaze-control abnormalities. Birch et al[6] reported that the absence of stereoacuity may be associated either with a poor response to amblyopia treatment or unstable fixation. Accordingly, careful assessment of fixation is necessary. Children with a microtropia may have parafoveal eccentric fixation in their amblyopic eye.[7] This creates a challenge to binocularity when there is a "mismatch between the images of each eye."[6]

Most randomized-clinical trials investigating the treatment of amblyopia in children have demonstrated good results with monocular penalization. However, further evaluation of its effect on other near functions, such as accommodative facility, accommodative amplitude, stereopsis, and fusional suppression is necessary, especially for children with residual amblyopia and/or poor stereopsis. Binocular treatment modalities are being explored on adults in a laboratory setting, with excellent results.[8] Following on from these studies, the effect of binocular treatments for amblyopia in the clinical setting is currently being investigated.

CLINICAL PEARL

- Cycloplegic retinoscopy is required for the detection of amblyogenic refractive errors. Once these are detected, the appropriate optical correction should be worn until no further improvement in VA occurs between visits. Once VA improvement has maximized with optical correction alone, subsequent treatment options for unilateral amblyopia can be initiated.

REFERENCES

1. Friedman DA, Repka MX, Katz J, et al. Prevalence of amblyopia and strabismus in White and African-American children aged 6 through 71 months: The Baltimore Pediatric Eye Disease Study. *Ophthalmology*. 2009;116:2128-2134.
2. Multi-ethnic Pediatric Eye Disease Study Group. Prevalence of amblyopia and strabismus in African American and Hispanic children ages 6 to 72 months the multi-ethnic pediatric eye disease study. *Ophthalmology*. July 2008;115(7):1229-1236.
3. Holmes JM, Beck RW, Repka MX, et al. The Amblyopia Treatment Study visual acuity testing protocol. *Arch Ophthalmol*. 2001;119:1345-1353.
4. Writing Committee for the Pediatric Eye Disease Investigator Group. Optical treatment of strabismic and combined strabismic-anisometropic amblyopia. *Ophthalmology*. January 2012;119(1):150-158.
5. Repka MX, Cotter SA, Beck RW, et al. A randomized trial of atropine regimens for treatment of moderate amblyopia in children. *Ophthalmology*. November 2004;111(11):2076-2085.
6. Birch EE, Subramanian V, Weakley DR. Fixation instability in anisometropic children with reduced stereopsis. *J AAPOS*. June 2013;17(3):287-290.
7. Hardman Lea SJ, Snead MP, Loades J, Rubinstein MP. Microtropia versus bifoveal fixation in anisometropic amblyopia. *Eye (Lond)*. 1991;5:576-584.
8. Birch EE. Amblyopia and binocular vision. *Prog Retin Eye Res*. 2013;33:67-84.

1.27 Neuro-Optometric Rehabilitation of a Post-concussion Patient

Barry Tannen, Noah M. Tannen, and Kenneth J. Ciuffreda

Bill, a 20-year-old male student, presented for a vision therapy evaluation. He was referred by a medical concussion specialist based on a detailed case history, physical examination, and symptoms consistent with post-concussion. He had previously undergone a head computed tomography (CT) scan and brain magnetic resonance imaging (MRI), both of which were unremarkable. At the time of presentation, he had suffered 6 medically documented, sports-related concussions over the past 6 years; all of which occurred while playing hockey. The most recent incident occurred 4 months before the current vision evaluation. Bill reported that he had recovered fully from the first 5 concussions. His present symptoms included daily headaches and photosensitivity, especially in fluorescent illumination. Bill also experienced general asthenopia, intermittent horizontal diplopia at near, and loss of place while reading. This caused significant difficulties with reading comprehension, computer work, and completing class assignments. In fact, the symptoms became so severe that he was forced to take a 1 semester leave of absence during his junior year at college. This vision evaluation occurred in the summer between his second and third year of college. He was not taking any medications at the time of the vision examination.

Clinical Findings

Unaided distance VA	OD: $20/20^{-2}$; OS: $20/20^{-3}$
Near point of convergence	15 cm/25 cm (with diplopia)
Pupil evaluation	PERRL; no RAPD
Ocular motility	Full and comitant OD and OS
Subjective refraction	OD: Pl -0.50×105 (20/20); OS: Pl -0.75×72 (20/20)
Phoria (von Graefe)	Distance: orthophoria; Near: 5Δ exophoria
Near vergence ranges	BI: 8/16/12; BO: x/10/6
NRA/PRA	$+2.00/-1.50$
Accommodative facility (± 2.00 D)	OD: 12 cpm; OS: 12 cpm
Near vergence facility (12Δ BO/3Δ BI)	10 cpm (difficulty with BO)
Stereopsis (Wirt circles)	20 s of arc

Visagraph reading eye movement test	5th grade reading efficiency
Optokinetic drum	Disequilibrium (visual vertigo) reported peripherally in all directions of gaze

Abbreviations: BI, base in; BO, base out; D, diopters; NRA, negative relative accommodation; OD, right eye; OS, left eye; PERRL, pupils equal, round, reactive to light; PRA, positive relative accommodation; RAPD, relative afferent pupillary defect; VA, visual acuity.

Discussion

Bill was diagnosed with the following conditions: (a) bilateral, uncorrected astigmatism; (b) convergence insufficiency (based on the reduced near point of convergence and near vergence range findings); (c) fusional instability (based on relatively low BI and BO ranges at near); and (d) photosensitivity, especially under fluorescent illumination. These conditions are commonly found in the post-concussion (mTBI) population (Figure 1.27-1). Spectacles were prescribed to correct the astigmatism, having a bluish-purple tint (BPI Omega: his subjective preference) to alleviate the photosensitivity. He was also prescribed a regimen of vision therapy to treat the convergence insufficiency. This included 2 sessions per week of in-office, vision therapy (45 minutes each session) for 12 weeks. The goal was to improve accommodation, vergence, and versional eye movements, as well as higher-level visual-processing skills, selective and sustained attention (eg, computerized visual scanning and tachistoscope training) and visual–vestibular interaction (eg, walking

with a hand-held stereoscope[1,2]). Although accommodative deficits were not specifically found, accommodative training was integrated into the therapy program to help integrate vergence skills. Specifically, the vision therapy was divided into 3 phases, as described later, each with a specific goal.[3]

Phase 1: Visual Stabilization

This phase began with procedures to develop monocular, and then binocular, oculomotor, and accommodative ability. This therapy served to stabilize the vergence system at both distance and near. The goal was to improve/normalize the near horizontal vergence ranges, as well as accommodative amplitude and facility.

Phase 2: Binocular Visual Integration

In this phase, treatment emphasized binocular accommodative and oculomotor tasks, with an aim of improving vergence speed and accuracy. As this phase proceeded, more demanding tasks were added requiring the patient to respond to noncongruent (ie, unequal) vergence and accommodative demands, such as converging

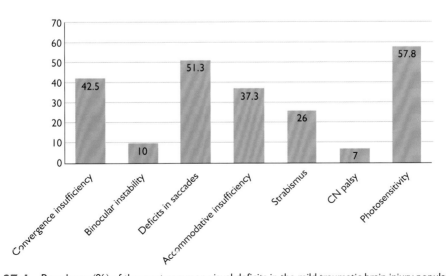

Figure 1.27-1   Prevalence (%) of the most common visual deficits in the mild traumatic brain injury population.

with plus lenses and diverging with minus lenses. This increasing difficulty was to ensure that the visual improvement could be maintained in more complex, naturalistic settings.

Phase 3: Visual Automaticity

This final phase refined visual skills, and increased response automaticity. Therefore, multisensory integration across modalities was incorporated. These techniques required integration of the vergence, accommodative, vestibular, tactile, and auditory systems, with the goal of increasing the speed, accuracy, and automaticity of visual and visuomotor responses. An example of such a procedure would be having the patient alternate between convergence and divergence by using prism flippers. The patient might walk toward and away from a 20/30 target on a wall while alternating between the convergence and divergence demands. In addition, they could time prism flips to a metronome in the background.

Outcomes

Bill manifested a wide range of vision improvements after completing the office-based vision therapy (Table 1.27-1). He reported wearing his tinted spectacles full-time, and visual symptoms were eliminated. Bill no longer experienced headaches or asthenopia while reading. He was able to read and study comfortably for longer periods of time (ie, 60 minutes vs 5 minutes). His visual efficiency based on the objective Visagraph results improved from the 5th to the 12th grade level. There was also a significant reduction in his photosensitivity and disequilibrium. Near point of convergence, horizontal vergence ranges, and dynamic vergence facility were all within the normal range, and most importantly, remained so at his 3-year follow-up vision examination (Table 1.27-1). No vision or other (eg, cognitive) therapy was performed during this 3-year follow-up period. Bill has

Table 1.27-1 Pre-/Post-vision Therapy Findings			
Test	**Pre-vision Therapy**	**Post-vision Therapy**	**Three-Year Post-vision Therapy**
Best-corrected visual acuity (Snellen)	OD 20/20 OS 20/20	OD 20/20 OS 20/20	OD 20/20 OS 20/20
Dry refractive error	OD plano −0.50 × 105 OS plano −0.75 × 072	OD plano −0.50 × 105 OS plano −0.75 × 072	OD −0.25 −0.50 × 100 OS −0.25 −0.50 × 70
Distance phoria (von Graefe)	Orthophoria	1Δ exophoria	Orthophoria
Near phoria (von Graefe)	5Δ exophoria	5Δ exophoria	7Δ exophoria
Near point of convergence (accommodative target)	15 cm/25 cm	5 cm/8 cm	5 cm/8 cm
Near vergence ranges (Δ)	BI 8/16/12 BO x/10/6	BI x/26/24 BO x/30/18	BI 14/26/20 BO 18/30/26
Vergence facility (3Δ BI/12Δ BO)	10 cpm	14 cpm	15 cpm
Accommodative facility (±2.00 D)	OD 12 cpm OS 12 cpm	OD 12 cpm OS 12 cpm	OD 13 cpm OS 14 cpm
Stereopsis (Wirt circles)	20 s	20 s	20 s
Visagraph reading eye movement test (Level 10)	5th grade level efficiency	12th grade level efficiency	Not performed

Abbreviations: BI, base in; BO, base out; D, diopters; OD, right eye; OS, left eye; Δ = prism diopter.

now successfully finished college and qualified as an accountant, an occupation that requires considerable sustained near work.

CLINICAL PEARLS

- Binocular vision problems occur with a high frequency in the mild traumatic brain injury population.

- These binocular vision problems can be remediated successfully with neuro-optometric rehabilitation.

REFERENCES

1. Ciuffreda KJ, Ludlam DP, Yadav NK, Thiagarajan P. Traumatic brain injury: visual consequences, diagnosis, and treatment. In: Yanoff M, ed., *Advances in Ophthalmology and Optometry*. Philadelphia, PA: Elsevier; 2016:307-333.
2. Ciuffreda KJ. Visual vertigo syndrome: clinical demonstration and diagnostic tool. *Clin Eye Vis Care*. 1999;11:41-42.
3. D'Angelo ML, Tannen B. The optometric care of vision problems after concussion: a clinical guide. *Optom Vis Perf*. 2015;3:298-306.

1.28 Intermittent Exotropia, Divergence Excess Type

Elaine C. Ramos and M. H. Esther Han

Elaine, a 6-year-old Asian female, was referred by her optometrist for the evaluation of a large intermittent exotropia. There was no report of double vision or headaches. Her mother was unsure when the eye turn first appeared and only noticed it occasionally. Elaine's medical and developmental histories were unremarkable. She was not taking any medications and had no known allergies. Elaine spoke limited English.

Clinical Findings

Present Rx	OD: $+1.00 -1.00 \times 10$ (20/20 at distance and near) OS: $+1.00 -1.00 \times 170$ (20/20 at distance and near)
Cover test (with present Rx)[a]	Distance: 25^Δ XP; near: 12^Δ XP
Near point of convergence	8 cm/13 cm with diplopia
Pupil evaluation	PERRL; no RAPD
Ocular motility	Full and comitant OU
Stereoacuity	Random dot stereograms 250 s; Wirt circles: 40 s
Dry retinoscopy	OD: $+1.00 -1.00 \times 10$; OS: $+0.50 -1.00 \times 170$
Subjective refraction	OD: $+1.00 -1.00 \times 10$ (20/20); OS: $+1.00 -1.00 \times 170$ (20/20)
Amplitude of accommodation (minus lens)	OD: 7.50 D; OS: 7.50 D
Binocular accommodative facility	0 cycles per minute (difficulty with minus)
Worth 4-dot	Flat fusion at 6 m, 3 m, and 0.40 m
Near phoria (modified Thorington through subjective Rx)	16^Δ exo
Distance vergence ranges (prism bar)	Base out: $x/6/0$; base in: $x/16/14$
Near vergence ranges	Base out: $x/18/14$; base in: $x/20/16$
Keystone visual skills (Keystoneview.com)	Distance: moderate exo posture Near: moderate exo posture
Clown vectogram ranges[1]	Base in: $x/11/3$; base out: $x/10/4$ Patient responded with normal responses, that is, reported floating and an ability to localize the image, and correctly indicated that the image became smaller and closer with base-out prism and became larger and moved further away with base-in prism (SILO)

118

Cycloplegic retinoscopy (1 drop 1% cyclopentolate OU)	OD: $+1.00 -1.00 \times 10$ OS: $+1.00 -1.00 \times 170$
Intraocular pressure (digital palpation)	Soft and symmetrical OD and OS
Slit-lamp examination	Unremarkable OD and OS
Fundus examination	Unremarkable OD and OS

Abbreviations: D, diopters; OD, right eye; OS, left eye; OU, both eyes; PERRL, pupils equal, round, reactive to light; RAPD, relative afferent pupillary defect; Rx, prescription.

[a] Intermittent alternating exotropia was noted only at the end of the evaluation after a prolonged (10 s) cover test at both distance and near.

Discussion

Intermittent exotropia of the divergence excess type (exodeviation greater at distance than near) has a higher incidence in females and within the Asian population.[2] Divergence excess is a variable type of ocular motor deviation. This was confirmed in the reports from Elaine's mother, the fluctuating magnitude observed either within the same visit or from visit to visit and Elaine's ability to maintain a phoric posture from 1 optometric vision-therapy session to the next. For example, at the initial evaluation, the tropia only became manifest at the end of the examination when Elaine was disassociated for a long period and probably became fatigued.

The parent's observations should be strongly considered when making a diagnosis of divergence excess exotropia in younger children, since the tropia may not be seen during the evaluation (as was the case for Elaine). This is also known as an exotropia of inattention, which a parent might notice more than the eye care professional during the course of the examination. Parents often report that the eye turns out when the child wakes up in the morning or right before bedtime. With this type of observation, a prolonged occlusion test is indicated to try and elicit the tropia. Finally, during the evaluation, prism bar ranges are preferred to in-phoropter testing in the younger pediatric population so that the eye movements can be observed.

Options for treatment include surgery, prisms, minus addition lenses, patching, botulinum toxin A injections, vision therapy, or simple observation.[3] At present, there is little evidence comparing these different treatment modalities, making it difficult to conclude which is the best management procedure. In addition, the natural history of the disorder is not well understood, so that its progression over time is unclear.[3] If a surgical treatment option is chosen for a larger magnitude strabismus, the parents should be informed that a high recurrence rate exists with frequent need for an additional surgical procedure within 10 to 15 years.[4] Although surgery may improve the cosmetic appearance, it may not improve binocularity or stereoacuity. Successful surgical outcomes are defined as deviations of less than 10Δ to 15Δ. Although Elaine's cover test findings ranged from 12Δ at near to 25Δ at distance, a surgical consultation was not indicated as these magnitudes were too close to what would normally be considered a successful surgical outcome.[4] A surgical referral can still be considered after a course of vision therapy in the younger patient, especially if the parents express cosmetic concerns due to the frequency of the eye turn.

Important factors when recommending vision therapy include patient's maturity and parent's motivation. However, they should not deter one from referring the very young patient for a vision therapy evaluation. There were several favorable prognostic factors in Elaine's case that suggested a good potential for vision therapy. She demonstrated a phoric posture most of the time, had random dot stereoacuity with flat fusion responses on the Worth 4-dot at all test distances and manifested a moderate angle of deviation. Another treatment modality to be considered for Elaine was additional minus power in her spectacles. However, this was not recommended since the amplitudes of accommodation were reduced for her age. In addition, a prismatic correction was not considered due to her age and level of maturity, along with her questionable subjective responses.

Table 1.28-1 Intermittent Exotropia Control Scale[5]

5 = Constant exotropia
4 = Exotropia >50% of the examination before dissociation
3 = Exotropia <50% of the examination before dissociation
2 = No exotropia unless dissociated, recovers in >5 s
1 = No exotropia unless dissociated, recovers in 1-5 s
0 = No exotropia unless dissociated, recovers in <1 s (phoria)

The aim of optometric vision therapy is to improve the patient's oculomotor/vergence control so the patient can demonstrate a greater frequency of phoria rather than tropia. Because the magnitude of the deviation is a poor indicator of severity, the intermittent exotropia control score (Table 1.28-1) provides a better tool to characterize the condition. This scale is applied for both distance and near fixation, yielding a total control score ranging from 0 to 10.[5] At the initial evaluation, Elaine had a control score of 2, which improved to 0 after successfully completing her therapy program.

Table 1.28-2 Summary of Vision Techniques Used in This Case[1,6]

Visual Efficiency Skill	Techniques	Therapy Considerations
Binocular	Brock String; Variable Vectograms; Computer Orthoptics VTS3 & VTS4; Lifesaver Cards; Cheiroscopic Tracing (Mirror and Correct-Eye Scope Stereoscopes); Aperture Rule; Stereoscope Cards (AN Series & EC Series Keystone Cards)	The goal was to shift from third-degree[a] (stereo) fusion to instrument (stereoscope)-based second-degree[b] (flat fusion) activities because this is more difficult for intermittent exotropes.
Anti-suppression	Monocular Fixation Binocular Field (MFBF); GTVT Chart & MFBF Perceptives (Bernell.com); Pola Mirror Walkaways; Split Quoit Walkaways & Alignment	Anti-suppression activities were emphasized before attempting higher level binocular activities.
Accommodation	Monocular Accommodative Rock (MAR) → Maximized to +2.00/−3.00 Binocular Accommodative Rock → Max to +/−1.50 with suppression check Base out with plus/base in with minus (BOP/BIM) with a max of +/−2.00 and using VTS3; 2 Variable Vectograms	
Oculomotor	Pegboard Rotator; Marsden Ball Looping; Beading a string	Activities were performed binocularly. While observing for ocular alignment, the patient would use her stereo/depth perception to complete the activity. For example, when the patient is asked to "loop" the Marsden ball, she could not touch the sides of the loop, which would require stereo.

[a] Third-degree fusion: When fused, the targets are perceived in 3 dimensions.

[b] Second-degree fusion: Identical targets that include a suppression check but are not perceived in 3 dimensions.

In Elaine's case, the goal of vision therapy was to decrease the frequency of her exotropia. In addition, she manifested a moderate accommodative insufficiency and a severe accommodative infacility. Elaine completed 17 sessions of in-office therapy, with re-evaluations scheduled after the 5th and 17th sessions. At the first re-evaluation (after 5 therapy sessions), Elaine was found to have exodeviations at distance and near of 25Δ and 12Δ, respectively. These decreased to 18Δ and 10Δ, respectively, at the second re-evaluation (after 17 therapy sessions). The therapy techniques used in this case are summarized in Table 1.28-2.

Patients with intermittent exotropia often display good stereoacuity and ocular alignment on presentation of a stereoscopic stimulus.[2] Therefore, therapy should begin with third degree (stereo) fusion targets, progressing later to second degree (flat fusion) images. It is common to begin with near targets, moving later to distance stimuli. Anti-suppression techniques should be incorporated to provide the patient with feedback as to when the eye is deviated. Patients with divergence excess can often converge to gain fusion as needed, and frequently exhibit normal convergence ranges.[3] Therefore, therapy should emphasize an improvement in the divergence ranges.

CLINICAL PEARLS

- When examining a divergence excess type exotropia, the clinician may not see the strabismus until the end of the examination.

- The parent's observations at home should be considered when diagnosing this type of exotropia in younger children.

- Prism bar ranges rather than vergence ranges in the phoropter should be utilized in the younger pediatric population so that the eye movements can be observed.

- Positive random dot stereopsis indicates that the exotropia is intermittent, and suggests a good prognosis for vision therapy depending on the magnitude of the tropia.

- A child's age should not preclude vision therapy being offered as a treatment option for intermittent exotropia. The child's maturity and the parent's motivation to comply with the recommendations are critical factors.

REFERENCES

1. Scheiman M, Wick B. *Clinical Management of Binocular Vision: Heterophoric, Accommodative, and Eye Movement Disorders*. 4th ed. Philadelphia, PA: Lippincott Willliams & Wilkins; 2014.
2. Nusz KJ, Mohney BG, Diehl NN. Female predominance in intermittent exotropia. *Am J Ophthalmol.* 2005;140(3):546-547.
3. Cooper J, Meadow N. Intermittent exotropia, basic and divergence excess type. *Binocul Vis Strabismus Q.* 1993;8:187-216.
4. Ekdawi NS, Nusz KJ, Diehl NN, Mohney BG. Postoperative outcomes in children with intermittent exotropia from a population-based cohort. *J AAPOS.* 2009;13(1):4-7.
5. Mohney BG, Holmes JM. An office-based scale for assessing control in intermittent exotropia. *Strabismus.* 2006;14(3):147-150.
6. Griffin JR, Grisham JD. *Binocular Anomalies: Diagnosis and Vision Therapy*. 4th ed. Amsterdam, The Netherlands: Butterworth-Heinemann; 2002.

1.29 Duane Retraction Syndrome

Rebecca Charlop and M. H. Esther Han

Rebecca, a 7-year-old South Asian female, presented with mild headaches and intermittent blur particularly at distance. Her mother noticed a mild head turn to the left when Rebecca was reading, and stated that she would typically cover 1 eye. Rebecca's mother was unsure which eye was covered. She also thought that Rebecca had poor peripheral vision. Rebecca would often bump into things and was very clumsy. Rebecca was in first grade and performing below average in reading, but at her grade level in math. She received occupational therapy twice a week in an attempt to improve her gross motor control. Rebecca had no significant health findings. She was not taking any medications and had no known allergies.

Clinical Findings

Unaided distance VA	OD: 20/20−; OS: 20/20−; OU: 20/20
Unaided near VA	OD: 20/20; OS: 20/20; OU: 20/20
Cover test (unaided)	Distance: ortho; near: 4Δ XP
Near point of convergence	46 cm/61 cm; OS turned out
Extraocular motility	OD: full
	OS: unable to abduct past the midline with mildly limited adduction and eyelid retraction (Duane retraction syndrome type I)
	A exo pattern (Figure 1.29-1)
Pursuit eye movements	Frequent losses of fixation OD and OS
Saccadic eye movements	20% undershoot in all gazes with unsteady fixation OD and OS
Stereoacuity	Wirt circles: 20 s
	Random dot stereograms: 250 s
Pupil evaluation	PERRL; no RAPD
Dry retinoscopy	OD: +0.25 −0.25 × 180; OS: +0.75 −0.50 × 180
Amplitude of accommodation (pull away)	OD: 14.00 D; OS: 14.00 D
Unaided distance phoria (Von Graefe)	1Δ exo
Unaided distance vergence ranges	Base-out: 10/14/2
	Base-in: x/6/2
Unaided near phoria (Von Graefe)	10Δ exo
Unaided near vergence ranges (unaided)	Base-out: x/6/8
	Base-in: x/20/16
Worth 4-dot	At 6 m: flat fusion
	At 3 m: flat fusion
	At 0.4 m: simultaneous perception (exo diplopia)

Slit-lamp examination	Unremarkable
Fundus examination	Unremarkable
Clown vectograms[1]	Base-out: $x/21/8$ Base-in: $x/16/6$ Patient responded with normal responses, that is, reported floating and an ability to localize the image. She correctly indicated that the image became smaller and closer with base-out prism and became larger and moved further away with base-in prism (SILO)
Keystone visual skills test (keystoneview.com)	Distance: ortho posture Near: exo posture

Abbreviations: D, diopters; OD, right eye; OS, left eye; OU, both eyes; PERRL, pupils equal, round, reactive to light; RAPD, relative afferent pupillary defect; VA, visual acuity; XP, exophoria.

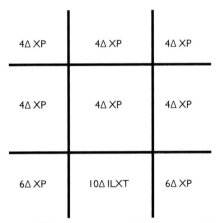

4Δ XP	4Δ XP	4Δ XP
4Δ XP	4Δ XP	4Δ XP
6Δ XP	10Δ ILXT	6Δ XP

Figure 1.29-1 Oculomotor balance at near (40 cm) in 9 cardinal gaze positions.

Abbreviations: ILXT, intermittent left exotropia; XP, exophoria.

Comments

Restricted eye movements, specifically mildly restricted adduction and an inability to abduct, could lead to diplopia, which would explain why Rebecca covered 1 eye when reading. The reported head turn is a strategy to minimize diplopia and/or discomfort. These symptoms and findings are characteristic of Duane retraction syndrome Type 1, as defined in the Discussion section.

Given the characteristics of this condition, an urgent neurologic referral was not considered necessary. Several treatment options exist to address alignment in primary gaze and elimination of an abnormal head posture. Yoked prisms can be prescribed to position the images in the unrestricted field of gaze, thereby alleviating the need for an anomalous head posture. Improving the efficiency of one or more of the extraocular muscles by surgical intervention can compensate for abnormal innervation.[2] Vision therapy will decrease the symptoms arising from tracking difficulties such as loss of place when reading. In addition, therapy will decrease her accommodative symptoms of headaches and blurred vision at distance. The latter treatment option was chosen for Rebecca so as to address a severe convergence insufficiency (particularly in downgaze), a moderate saccadic deficit, and a severe accommodative infacility (worse in the left eye). Rebecca completed 30 sessions of in-office therapy, with re-evaluations scheduled after the 10th and 20th sessions. After 10 sessions, her mother reported that Rebecca's reading had improved significantly, and on completing the program, she was reading at grade level. The therapy techniques used in this case are summarized in Table 1.29-1.

Even when formal therapy is not indicated, educational accommodations such as specific seating assignments in the classroom can be helpful. For example, Rebecca was advised to sit on the left side of the classroom to minimize the need for left gaze viewing, which would require her to abduct the left eye. Most patients develop suppression to eliminate diplopia in the affected direction of gaze, but may also exhibit an abnormal head posture for visual comfort.

Table 1.29-1 Summary of Vision Techniques Used in This Case. For More Information on These Procedures, See Scheiman and Wick[1]

Visual Efficiency Skill	Techniques	Therapy Considerations
Vergence	Brock string; variable vectograms; Computer Orthoptics VTS3; eccentric circles, Lifesaver cards; cheiroscopic tracing; aperture rule.	As there was greater OS suppression in left gaze, activities were initially placed to her right, and then moved toward the midline.
Anti-suppression	Monocular fixation binocular field (MFBF); GTVT Chart (Bernell.com).	Anti-suppression work with the left eye at near was emphasized before attempting higher level binocular activities.
Accommodation	Monocular accommodative rock up to +2.00/−4.00 Biocular rock: split Spirangle vectogram; red rock Binocular accommodative rock (with red/green stripe bar reader), up to ±2.00 with suppression check Base out with plus/base in with minus with a max of ±2.00 while using VTS3; 2 variable vectograms; 2 aperture rules.	Due to the severe accommodative infacility and intermittent left eye suppression, bi-ocular rock activities (which increase the accommodative stimulus in 1 eye while decreasing the stimulus in the fellow eye) were added to increase her flexibility between the eyes before attempting binocular accommodative activities.
Oculomotor	Near/far Hart chart; Wayne Saccadic Fixator; visual tracing; CPT visual search; CPT perceptual speed	Initially, all activities were done twice with the left eye, as the findings were worse in that eye.

Abbreviation: CPT, computer perceptual therapy; OS, left eye.

Discussion

Duane retraction syndrome is categorized as a neurologic strabismus, specifically a congenital cranial dysinnervational disorder.[3] The abnormalities within this disorder occur during development, and affect one or more cranial nerves leading to primary (absence of the nuclei) and/or secondary (abnormal nerve branch connections) dysinnervation. Duane retraction syndrome is nonprogressive, and can have sporadic or familial genetic inheritance patterns. The familial form will show an autosomal dominant inheritance pattern with significant clinical phenotypic variability.[3] Table 1.29-2 describes the genetic characteristics of the 2 phenotypes (which are distinct from Types I, II, III Duane retraction syndrome described in Table 1.29-2).

Duane retraction syndrome is a congenital disorder affecting the action of the lateral rectus muscle. While the unilateral condition is more prevalent, 15% to 20% of cases are bilateral.[3] During the fourth to eighth week of gestation, anomalies of the cranial nerve VI nuclei occur, which may be accompanied by aberrant innervation from cranial nerve III.[4] Characteristics of Duane retraction syndrome include limitation of abduction and/or adduction, as well as narrowing of the palpebral fissure and retraction of the globe on adduction. The narrowing of the palpebral fissure is due to the physical effect of the lids moving with the globe during retraction. This is the result of co-contraction of the lateral and medial recti, believed to be due to innervational abnormalities.[3,5,6] Along with eye movement deficits, these patients frequently manifest an abnormal head posture with the face turned toward the affected side (in 40% to 60% of cases), and can have atypical upward and downward eye movements when adducting the affected eye.[2,3] This

Table 1.29-2 Genetic Characteristics of the Specific Duane Retraction Syndrome I and II Phenotypes[3]

Phenotype	Clinical Characteristics	Genetic Characteristics
Duane retraction syndrome I (DURS1)	Unilateral or bilateral (15-20%) Limited abduction with normal or near normal adduction.	DURS1 gene located on chromosome 8 (8q13). A carboxypeptidase gene (CPAH) with 8 exons.
Duane retraction syndrome II (DURS2)	Almost always bilateral Limited adduction with normal or near normal abduction Associated with a variety of vertical deviations (superior oblique underaction and dissociated vertical deviation).	Autosomal dominant inheritance. CHN1 gene located on chromosome 2 (2q31). This gene is responsible for "neuronal path finding during the development of the abducens nerve and, to a lesser extent, the oculomotor nerve."

abnormal head posture allows for binocular vision, despite significant muscle restrictions. The unilateral condition is most common in females and more frequently affects the left eye.[3,7] Therefore, Duane retraction syndrome is clinically subdivided based on the gaze restriction, which differs from the specific gene phenotypes described in Table 1.29-2. The prevalence of types I (abduction deficit only), II (adduction deficit only), and III (both abduction and adduction deficits) are 78%, 7%, and 15%, respectively.

Before clinical testing, a careful case history should be performed, highlighting the ocular and medical histories as well as any past trauma. If the patient is symptomatic, the practitioner should determine when the symptoms first became manifest since Duane syndrome is a congenital condition. A careful examination of extraocular motility is critical for the diagnosis, along with careful observation of the patient's habitual head posture. One should look for narrowing of the palpebral fissure and retraction of the affected eye. It is important to determine whether the eye movement restrictions are due to Duane retraction syndrome or another motility disorder, such as a cranial nerve VI palsy. The latter condition is identified by the presence of esotropia in primary gaze and diplopia that is worse at distance compared with near. In Duane retraction syndrome, the patient may not be diplopic in the gaze of the affected eye due to the congenital and nonprogressive nature of the condition.

CLINICAL PEARLS

- Commonly, patients with Duane retraction syndrome will not exhibit a deviation in primary gaze, but will adopt an abnormal head posture.

- Careful observation of extraocular motility is critical for making the diagnosis, paying specific attention to globe retraction, and narrowing of the palpebral fissure on attempted adduction.

- Duane retraction syndrome is commonly unilateral and seen most frequently in the left eye of females.

- Because this is a congenital condition, the findings are typically stable and nonprogressive.

- Although clinical treatment may not be indicated, accommodations such as specifying classroom seating arrangements may be helpful for a school-aged patient with Duane retraction syndrome.

REFERENCES

1. Scheiman M, Wick B. *Clinical Management of Binocular Vision: Heterophoric, Accommodative, and Eye Movement Disorders*. 4th ed. Philadelphia, PA: Lippincott Willliams & Wilkins; 2014.
2. Kalevar A, Tone SO, Flanders M. Duane syndrome: clinical features and surgical management. *Can J Ophthalmol*. 2015;50(4):310-313.

3. Kekunnaya R, Sachdeva V. Chapter 83: Congenital cranial dysinnervation disorders. In: Lambert SR, Lyons CJ, eds. *Taylor and Hoyt's Pediatric Ophthalmology and Strabismus*. 5th ed. New York, NY: Elsevier; 2017:848-858.

4. Yuksel D, Orban de Xivry J-J, Lefevre P. Review of the major findings about Duane retraction syndrome (DRS) leading to an updated form of classification. *Vis Res*. 2010;50:2334-2347.

5. von Noorden GK, Campos EC. *Binocular Vision and Ocular Motility*. 6th ed. St. Louis, MO: Mosby; 2002.

6. Huber A. Electrophysiology of the retraction syndromes. *Br J Ophthalmol*. 1974;58:293-300.

7. DeRespinis PA, Caputo AR, Wagner RS, Guo S. Duane's retraction syndrome. *Surv Ophthalmol*. 1993;38(3):257-288.

1.30 **Pseudomyopia**

Reena A. Patel

Jennifer, a 12-year-old Caucasian female, presented with a chief concern of blurry distance vision. This started approximately 1 year ago and occurred intermittently, but most frequently on school days. The blur was not present in the morning, but would get progressively worse as the day went on. She reported clear vision when performing near tasks, but she did experience occasional headaches and eye strain after prolonged near work. Jennifer got her first pair of glasses when she was 8 years old and wore them full time. Her most recent eye examination was 2 years ago, when her glasses were last updated. She was in seventh grade and doing well in school. She had asthma, for which she used an albuterol inhaler as needed.

Clinical Findings

Unaided distance VA	OD: 20/40; OS: 20/40
Unaided near VA	OD: 20/20; OS: 20/20
Present Rx	OD: -1.00 sph (20/30); OS: -1.00 sph (20/30)
Cover test (aided):	Distance: ortho; near: 4Δ esophoria
Near point of convergence	To the nose
Confrontation visual fields	Full to finger counting OD and OS
Stereopsis	Random dot stereograms: 250 s Wirt circles: 40 s
Pupil evaluation	PERRL; no RAPD
Dry retinoscopy	OD: -2.50 sph; OS: -2.75 sph
Subjective refraction	OD: -2.25 sph (20/20); OS: -2.50 sph (20/20)
Near VA (with subjective Rx)	OD: 20/20; OS: 20/20
Amplitude of accommodation (push up)	OD: 15 D; OS: 15 D
NRA/PRA	$+1.00/-2.25$
MEM retinoscopy	OD: -0.50; OS: -0.75
Near vergence ranges	BI: $x/30/24$; BO: $x/40/34$
Intraocular pressure (GAT)	OD: 16 mm Hg; OS: 16 mm Hg at 10:00 AM
Cycloplegic retinoscopy (2 drops cyclopentolate [1%], 1 drop tropicamide [1%] OU)	OD: -1.00 sph; OS: -1.00 sph
Cycloplegic subjective refraction	OD: -1.00 sph (20/20); OS: -1.00 sph (20/20)

| Slit-lamp examination | Unremarkable OD and OS |
| Dilated fundus examination | Unremarkable OD and OS |

Abbreviations: D, diopters; GAT, Goldmann applanation tonometry; MEM, monocular estimate method (retinoscopy); NRA, negative relative accommodation; OD, right eye; OS, left eye; OU, both eyes; PERRL, pupils equal, round, reactive to light; PRA, positive relative accommodation; RAPD, relative afferent pupillary defect; Rx, prescription; sph, sphere; VA, visual acuity.

Discussion

A presenting complaint of blurred distance vision from a patient with myopia would most commonly indicate an increase in the myopic refractive error. However, this case highlights the importance of ruling out accommodative excess and pseudomyopia. The former refers to an excessive accommodative response during near work, while the latter is caused by excess accommodation during distance viewing after completing near work.

It should also be noted that the distance visual acuity (VA) measured through the current glasses (20/30 in each eye) would predict an increase in myopia of around 0.50 D,[1] which was significantly less than the increase found with non-cycloplegic retinoscopy and subjective refraction. In addition, unaided VAs of 20/40 were consistent with the −1.00 D cycloplegic refraction. These both provide an indication that the decreased distance VA was not produced by true myopia.

Patients with myopia will often accept more minus during the subjective refraction because the extra power makes the letters appear darker and therefore of higher contrast, but it is important to ensure that unnecessary minus power is not being prescribed. In this case, while additional myopia was found on dry retinoscopy, it was not present during the cycloplegic evaluation once Jennifer's accommodation was controlled. Accordingly, she was found to have pseudomyopia (ie, a failure to relax the accommodative response while viewing at distance) rather than true myopia, because the additional myopic prescription was only seen during non-cycloplegic testing.

Although not all cases of accommodative excess lead to pseudomyopia, the association between the 2 conditions should be understood. In Jennifer's case, a diagnosis of accommodative excess can be made based on (a) the lead of accommodation seen on monocular estimate method (MEM) retinoscopy, (b) a low negative relative accommodation (NRA) (reflecting difficulty relaxing accommodation), and (c) esophoria at near (likely due to excessive accommodative convergence[2]). This accommodative excess leads to an artificial increase of minus power in the distance prescription (pseudomyopia).

Scheiman et al[3] reported a 2.2% prevalence of accommodative excess in children. The excessive accommodative response during near tasks may lead to symptoms of headaches or eye strain during prolonged near work. In addition, the patient may have difficulty relaxing accommodation when looking into the distance after performing near work. This will lead to intermittent distance blur, as was seen here, whereas a true increase in myopia will be accompanied by constant distance blur. Differential diagnoses to consider include uncorrected refractive error, accommodative infacility, binocular vision disorders, and dry eye syndrome.

The treatment of pseudomyopia is aimed at reducing the accommodative response.[4] Treatment options include bifocals to decrease the accommodative demand and/or vision therapy to improve the accuracy of the accommodative response. An appropriate near prescription should provide normalized accommodative findings (typically a 0.50 D [±0.25] lag of accommodation and an NRA value between +1.50 and +2.50 D), which should eliminate the visual symptoms.[2] Because these patients have trouble relaxing accommodation, they may report some initial difficulty adapting to plus addition lenses. In addition to bifocals and/or vision therapy, patients should be advised to take frequent breaks when doing near work to reduce the accommodative response and prevent over accommodation. In this particular case, Jennifer's prescription was not changed, but she was asked to remove her glasses during prolonged near work, effectively giving her a +1.00 ADD at near.

CLINICAL PEARLS

- A cycloplegic examination may be important to obtain an accurate assessment of the refractive error, even in an older child with myopia.

- It is important to explain the findings and treatment recommendations clearly to the patients and their parents to ensure they understand why a simple increase in the prescription will not address the symptoms.

REFERENCES

1. Bennett AG, Rabbetts RB. *Clinical Visual Optics.* 2nd ed. London, UK: Butterworths; 1989.
2. Scheiman M, Wick B. *Clinical Management of Binocular Vision: Heterophoric, Accommodative, and Eye Movement Disorders.* 3rd ed. Philadelphia, PA: Lippincott Williams & Wilkins; 2008.
3. Scheiman M, Gallaway M, Coulter R, et al. Prevalence of vision and ocular disease conditions in a clinical pediatric population. *J Am Optom Assoc.* 1996;67:193-202.
4. American Optometric Association. *Optometric Clinical Practice Guideline. Care of the Patient with Myopia.* St. Louis, MO: American Optometric Association. http://www.aoa.org/documents/optometrists/CPG-15.pdf. 1997. Accessed June 1, 2017.

1.31 Comprehensive Color Vision Evaluation

Jason S. Ng

Ferris, a 31-year-old Caucasian male, presented for a comprehensive color vision evaluation. He reported failing an Ishihara test when he undertook a medical qualifying examination to enlist in the armed forces some years ago. Ferris now works in marketing at a university. He was surprised to be disqualified from the military, and often wondered about the severity of his color vision issue. Ferris had a comprehensive eye examination 1 month earlier and the findings were unremarkable. His unaided visual acuity (VA) was 20/20 in each eye at both distance and near and he did not wear a refractive correction. He did not perceive any difficulty with his color vision.

Color Vision Testing

Hardy Rand and Rittler Pseudo isochromatic Test (Richmond Products, Albuquerque, New Mexico—4th Edition)

Summary of results (see Figure 1.31-1)

Passed blue-yellow screening plates (2/2 correct)
Failed red-green screening plates (0/4 correct)
Diagnostic plates: Moderate deutan

Note that the degree of severity (medium) was based on the fact that the last plate missed was plate 17. The type of abnormality was determined from the total number of plates identified correctly in the protan and in the deutan columns (plates 11 through 20). The column with the greater number indicated the diagnostic type. In this case, a total of 3 and 9 plates were identified correctly in the protan and deutan columns, respectively. This indicated a deutan deficiency.

24 Plate Ishihara Test (1971)

Summary of results (see Table 1.31-1)

Failed red-green screening plates (1/15 correct).

Ferris read both diagnostic plates correctly. He was then asked whether the first or second numeral on plates 16 and 17 was more distinct or easier to see. For both plates, Ferris reported that the first numeral on each plate was easier to see. Accordingly, the diagnostic type and severity were assessed as a mild deutan deficiency.

Ishihara testing (binocularly) was repeated with a red trial lens before the right eye. All red-green screening plates were seen correctly with this additional lens.

Farnsworth D15 Test

Summary of results (see Figure 1.31-2)

First attempt: 0 major crossovers. Diagnosis: Mild defect. Note that the type cannot be established when no major crossovers (i.e., when 2 caps are positioned more than 3 places away) are present.

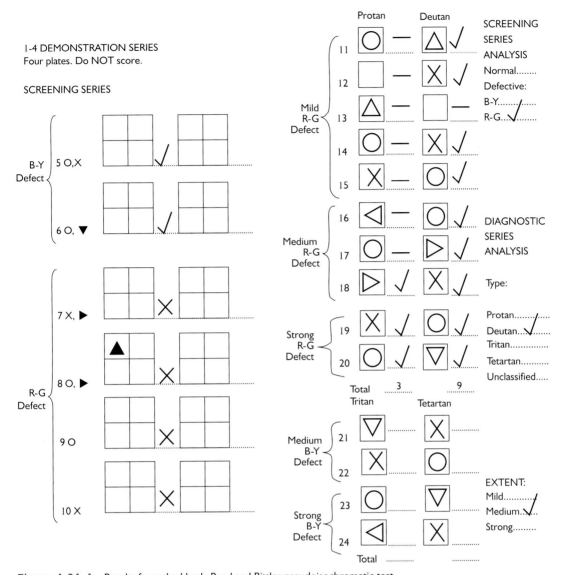

Figure 1.31-1 Results from the Hardy Rand and Rittler pseudoisochromatic test.

Second attempt: Identical result to the first attempt.

Lanthony D15 Test

Summary of results (see Figure 1.31-3)

First attempt: 8 major crossovers. Diagnosis: Deutan defect (severity cannot be established). Second attempt: 7 major crossovers (not illustrated here).

Anomaloscope

Summary of results

Range: 0-8 (normal range: 36-46);

Luminance: constant at 14; constant luminance settings are characteristic for color normals and patients with deutan deficiency;

Diagnosis: mild deutan defect (deuteranomaly).

Table 1.31-1	Results From the 24 Plate Ishihara Test (1971)	
Plate	Color Normal	CVD
1	(12)	12
2	8	(3)
3	29	(70)
4	5	(2)
5	3	(5)
6	15	(17)
7	74	(21)
8	6	(X)
9	45	(X)
10	5	(X)
11	7	(X)
12	16	(X)
13	73	(X)
14	X	(5)
15	X	45 "**43**"

Plate	Color Normal	P (Strong | Mild)	D (Strong | Mild)
16	(26)	6 | (2) 6	2 | 2 (6)
17	(42)	2 | (4) 2	4 | 4 (2)

Abbreviation: CVD, color vision deficiency.

Farnsworth-Munsell 100 Hue Test

Summary of results (see Figure 1.31-4)[1]

Total error score = 124

Upper limit of normal for patient's age = 106

Discussion

Patients often present for supplementary color vision testing when they have failed an earlier color vision test, perhaps at a school vision screening or during occupational testing. Deutan deficiencies are the most common red-green color vision deficiencies (CVDs), being present in up to 6% of males.[2] Deuteranomaly can be seen in 1 in 20 (5%) males. This CVD occurs because of a defect on the sex-linked X chromosome, which is typically transferred from the patient's maternal grandfather. Ferris was educated as to the likelihood of his passing the CVD onto his children. Assuming a future partner does not carry any CVD genes, any sons and daughters will have a 0% and 100% chance of becoming carriers of the CVD gene, respectively.

A deuteranomalous color vision deficiency occurs when the peak spectral sensitivity of the M cones is altered toward longer wavelengths. While the normal peak spectral sensitivity of M cones is approximately 530 nm, in deuteranomaly this peak may be shifted slightly (eg, to 532 nm) or to a greater degree (eg, to

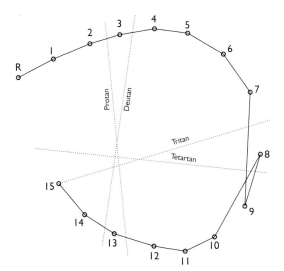

Figure 1.31-2   Results from the Farnsworth D15 test.

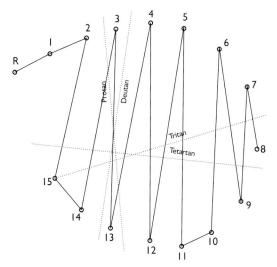

Figure 1.31-3   Results from the Lanthony D15 test.

556 nm—which is close to the peak spectral sensitivity of L cones).[3] The degree of deuteranomaly is consistent with the magnitude of the shift in peak spectral sensitivity.

Here, the Ishihara results show that the number of misses on the screening plates is a poor indicator of severity. Ferris missed every plate on the screening section except for the demonstration plate. Conversely, severe cases of CVD may not miss every screening plate. The test results of the diagnostic plates

were important in this case. Had an examiner simply recorded both diagnostic plates as correct, the opportunity to diagnose the type of CVD defect would have been lost. By asking the patient which of the 2 numerals were more obvious or easier to see, the determination of a diagnostic type was possible based on the Ishihara test alone. This same strategy can also be applied to the Hardy Rand and Rittler (HRR) test, especially when an equal number of protan and deutan diagnostic plates are identified. In this particular case, the diagnostic type was evident without this strategy. Because the HRR has more diagnostic plates than the Ishihara test, it is better at identifying both diagnostic type and severity.[4]

The screening book tests used here gave different degrees of severity for this CVD, with the Ishihara and HRR reporting a mild and moderate condition, respectively. Since there is no clear way to account for this difference, the results of the Farnsworth D15 test became critical. Having more than 1 major crossover generally constitutes a failure for the latter test. Some might support a more conservative criterion of no errors whatsoever to pass,[5] although even that demanding standard can be overcome by patients who attempt to subvert the test through practice.[6] A passing Farnsworth D15 finding with a failed book test is always interpreted as a mild CVD.[2] Finally, the Lanthony D15 results confirmed the diagnosis of a deutan defect. The Lanthony D15 results were expected to be worse than the Farnsworth D15, since the former uses desaturated (pastel-like) colors, and therefore is more demanding than the saturated Farnsworth D15 test.

The determination of CVD severity is more critical than diagnostic type. When comparing patients with protan and deutan deficiencies, although protans will have greater difficulty detecting red traffic signals or brake lights, there is no significant difference between the 2 groups for more general color-related tasks.[7] However, the severity of the CVD is directly proportional to patients' difficulty with colors.[7] Generally, patients with mild defects do not have significant issues with

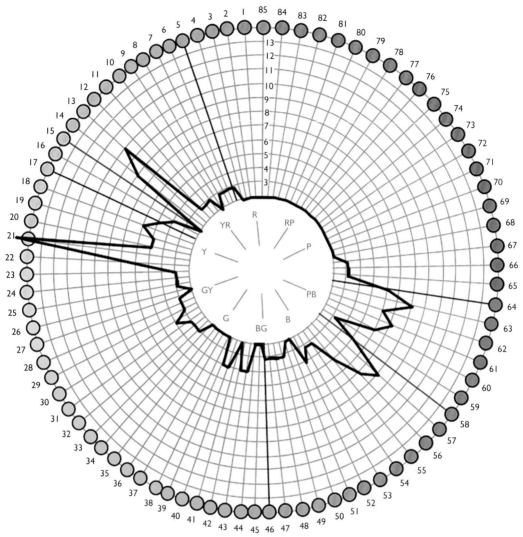

Figure 1.31-4   Results from the Farnsworth-Munsell 100 Hue test.

common color-related tasks, whereas patients with moderate- to severe-defects have greater problems with tasks, such as selecting color coordinated clothing, determining whether fruit is ripe, or when meat is cooked.

Anomaloscope testing was not critical in this case as differentiation between severe deuteranomaly and deuteranopia was not required. Similarly, the Farnsworth-Munsell 100 Hue test was not essential for the diagnosis, but was valuable when counseling the patient as to where in the color circle they should expect to have difficulties. The 100 Hue test is rarely valuable for diagnostic purposes, as even patients

with dichromacy may pass the test based on the age-related norms.[8]

Ferris had learned about the use of colored filters for CVDs, and expressed an interest in trying such a filter. He was informed about the limited utility of filters for managing CVDs.[9] In addition, he was questioned about any specific tasks he was having trouble with in his activities of daily living. As a demonstration, a red trial lens was introduced before 1 eye under binocular viewing conditions. Ferris was given time to walk around the clinic to experience the effects of the filter and have the Ishihara test repeated. It was explained that the red filter creates brightness differences in colors, thereby defeating the design of the Ishihara test. Using a colored filter for this type of test is generally considered cheating. Ferris was unable to identify any specific color-related tasks where he thought a filter may be useful. He was also disappointed by the limited effect of the filter, and decided not to pursue this treatment option any further at that time.

CLINICAL PEARLS

- Regardless of the number of misses, a color vision book test is never sufficient to diagnose fully a patient's color vision deficiency, and additional testing is indicated whenever such a failure occurs.

- Colored filters should never be used during color vision testing as they invalidate the test, and their use in the management of color vision deficiencies is patient and task specific.

REFERENCES

1. Verriest G, Van Laethem J, Uvijls A. A new assessment of the normal ranges of the Farnsworth-Munsell 100-hue test scores. *Am J Ophthalmol*. 1982;93:635-642.
2. Birch J. *Diagnosis of Defective Colour Vision*. 2nd ed. Oxford; Boston: Butterworth-Heinemann; 2001.
3. Simunovic MP. Colour vision deficiency. *Eye (Lond)*. 2010;24:747-755.
4. Cole BL, Lian KY, Lakkis C. The new Richmond HRR pseudoisochromatic test for colour vision is better than the Ishihara test. *Clin Exp Optom*. 2006;89:73-80.
5. Birch J. Pass rates for the Farnsworth D15 colour vision test. *Ophthalmic Phys Opt*. 2008;28:259-264.
6. Ng JS, Morton W. Case report: Invalidation of the Farnsworth D15 test in dichromacy secondary to practice. *Optom Vis Sci*. 2018;95:272-274.
7. Steward JM, Cole BL. What do color vision defectives say about everyday tasks? *Optom Vis Sci*. 1989; 66:288-295.
8. Birch J. Use of the Farnsworth-Munsell 100-Hue test in the examination of congenital colour vision defects. *Ophthalmic Physiol Opt*. 1989;9:156-162.
9. Swarbrick HA, Nguyen P, Nguyen T, Pham P. The ChromaGen contact lens system: colour vision test results and subjective responses. *Ophthalmic Physiol Opt*. 2001;21:182-196.

1.32 Color Vision Occupational Questions

Jason S. Ng

Christian, a 13-year-old Caucasian male, presented for a color vision evaluation. He had a comprehensive eye examination 3 months ago, and no abnormal findings were reported. Color vision testing was not performed at that time. Four years earlier, he underwent both a pseudoisochromatic plate and a Farnsworth D15 color vision test (see Figure 1.32-1), failing both evaluations. Christian had a family history of color vision deficiency (CVD) in his maternal grandfather. His parents were not known to have a CVD. Christian, currently a junior high school student, had an interest in becoming an aircraft pilot, and both he and his mother were wondering if the test results might have changed now that he was older. They did not think he should attempt to pursue a career in aviation if his color vision was severely affected. Beyond this consideration, the patient reported issues with identifying teammates in football games based on the color of their jersey, selecting color coordinated clothing, and identifying when he was sunburnt. Other than low hyperopia (+0.50 sph OU), his refractive findings were unremarkable.

Color Vision Testing

Hardy Rand and Rittler Pseudoisochromatic Test (Richmond Products, Albuquerque, New Mexico—4th Edition)
Summary of results (see Figure 1.32-2)

  2/2 blue-yellow screening plates correct

  1/4 red-green screening plates correct

  Diagnostic plates: strong protan

24 Plate Ishihara test (1971)
Summary of results (see Table 1.32-1)

  2/15 red-green screening plates correct

  Diagnostic plates: strong protan

Farnsworth D15
Summary of results (see Figure 1.32-1B)

  First attempt: 10 major crossovers

  Second attempt: 10 major crossovers (same errors)

  Diagnosis: severe protan defect

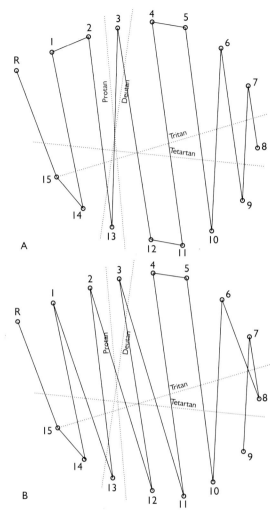

Figure 1.32-1 Results from the Farnsworth D15 test. The upper diagram (A) indicates the results taken 4 years ago (when he was 9 years old), while the lower diagram (B) shows the current findings.

Anomaloscope (Oculus, HMC)

Range of matches: 0-73 (ie, 73 units)

Luminance: decreasing with increasing red amount

Discussion

Given normal ocular health and visual acuity (VA), as well as the family history, the presumption was that Christian had a congenital CVD, since a logical genetic transmission existed. The maternal grandfather passed the color deficiency gene (on the X chromosome) to his daughter,

Christian's mother. As a carrier of the gene, the mother passed it on to her son. Christian had a 50% chance of receiving either the unaffected or the affected X chromosome from his mother. The Y chromosome is passed from the father, and no CVDs are carried on the Y chromosome.

Congenital CVDs are classified as either blue-yellow or red-green. A blue-yellow congenital deficiency, also known as a tritan deficiency, is relatively rare; the occurence being in 1 in 500 to 15 000 individuals.[1,2] Two types of red-green CVD exist, namely deutan and protan. Each of these types is classified as either dichromacy (ie, deuteranopia and protanopia) or anomalous trichromacy (ie, deuteranomaly or protanomaly). In dichromacy, 1 of the 3 cone photoreceptor types is either not functioning or absent. Protanopia and deuteranopia have equal prevalence, being found in approximately 1% of males and 0.02% of females.[2] In anomalous trichromacy, 1 of the 3 cone photoreceptor types is present and functioning, but is anomalous with a peak sensitivity shifted from away from the norm. Deuteranomaly and protanomaly have a prevalence of 5% and 1% of males, and 0.4% and 0.02% of females, respectively.

Both the Hardy Rand and Rittler (HRR) test and Ishihara tests are generally good at differentiating a deutan from a protan defect. The Farnsworth D15 is often used to confirm the type (deutan vs protan) and severity (mild vs moderate to severe) of the condition. The anomaloscope (the gold standard for color vision testing in a research setting) is the only instrument currently available that can distinguish reliably between patients with dichromacy and anomalous trichromacy.

Note that when performing the HRR color test, the degree of severity was determined by missing either plate 19 or 20. The type of abnormality is based on the total number of plates identified correctly in the protan and deutan columns (plates 11 through 20). The column with the greater number indicates the diagnostic type.

When scoring the D15 test, a major crossover is defined as 2 caps that are positioned more than 3 places away (eg, cap 14 is placed next to cap 1, a cap distance of 13). Figures 1.32-1A and 1.32-1B shows 8 and

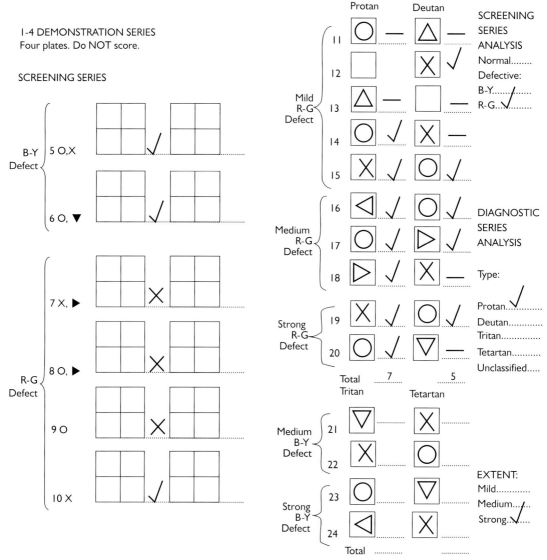

Figure 1.32-2   Results from the Richmond Hardy Rand and Rittler Pseudoisochromatic test, 4th ed.

10 major crossovers, respectively. Severity is scored based on the number of major crossovers. More than 1 major crossover is considered a failure, 2 to 5 major crossovers are considered a moderate defect, and greater than 5 major crossovers is a severe defect.[3] The type of abnormality is determined by identifying which of the marked axes (protan, deutan, or tritan) is most closely aligned with a line joining the major crossovers.

The anomaloscope is a color matching test where the observer varies a mixture of green and red light to match the appearance of a yellow-orange light. Patients with severe red-green color deficiency will perceive every color from green to red as matching the yellow-orange light. This is a range of 73 units on the anomaloscope scale since pure green is scored as 0 while pure red is scored as 73. Individuals with normal color vision will typically exhibit a small range (around 1 to 8 units) of colors that match the yellow-orange light.

In this case, the color vision tests were in agreement regarding the diagnostic type and severity. A pseudoisochromatic plate test and Farnsworth D15 would generally be enough

Table 1.32-1	Results From the 24 Plate Ishihara Test (1995)

Plate	Color Normal	CVD	
1	(12)	12	
2	8	(3)	
3	29	(70)	
4	5	(2)	
5	(3)	5	
6	15	(17)	
7	74	(21)	
8	6	(X)	
9	45	(X)	
10	5	(X)	
11	7	(X)	
12	16	(X)	
13	73	(X)	
14	X	(5)	
15	X	(45)	
		P (Strong | Mild)	D (Strong | Mild)
16	26	(6)| (2) 6	2 | 2 (6)
17	42 "8"	2 | (4) 2	4 | 4 (2)

Abbreviation: CVD, color vision deficiency.

to classify the type and severity in the case of a severe protan deficiency. Color vision tests typically agree on diagnostic type. Assessment of severity can be more variable, especially when the case involves a milder defect. In such situations, the optimal tests in order from the most to least reliable are the anomaloscope, Farnsworth D15, HRR, and Ishihara. However, an anomaloscope is rarely found in most optometric practices. Clinically, the important distinction regarding severity is whether the CVD is mild or severe. Historically, the Farnsworth D15 has been used to make such a differentiation. No clinical test is universally accepted as being able to separate moderate from severe CVDs. While this distinction may not be

critical, generally the more severe the defect the greater difficulty patients will have with color-related tasks, for example, selecting clothes, decorations or ripe produce, or distinguishing the colors of traffic lights.[4] Some investigators have suggested more than 5 major crossovers on a Farnsworth D15 test as a criterion for identifying severe defects.[3]

A second important determination from a color vision evaluation is the diagnostic type (ie, protan vs deutan). Interestingly, the *International Statistical Classification of Diseases and Related Health Problems (ICD-10)* system only differentiates between types, as there are no codes that distinguish between severity levels of CVD. Nevertheless, the degree of severity may be the most important aspect of a CVD for the clinician to communicate to the patient.

Similar to other congenital CVDs, protanopia is stable throughout life, and all other vision functions should be normal.[5] With age, acquired color vision defects can arise. These are generally asymmetric between the 2 eyes. Many ocular pathologies, such as cataracts, age-related macular degeneration, glaucoma and diabetic retinopathy, can lead to tritan defects. However, optic neuropathies commonly result in red-green deficiencies. Any acquired defects will be superimposed on an existing congenital color deficiency, and this may cause complex test results.

Patients with protanopia must be counseled that red lights will be harder to detect because they will appear dimmer than other colors. With protanopia, there are no L cones that have the highest sensitivity to long wavelength light. Indeed, patients with protan defects have slower reaction times to automobile brake lights and red traffic lights, as well as a higher rate of traffic accidents.[6] In addition, dark reds can be confused with black, while dark green may be confused with brown (which can be thought of as dark orange). In general, patients with protanopia will confuse shades of red, orange, yellow, and green. Blues and purples may be confused as well. More saturated colors are less likely to be confused.

In this case, Christian was counseled that a career in aviation would be difficult. Given a severe defect, he would not be able to pass any of the color vision tests needed to obtain an unrestricted aviation license. Christian could qualify for a restricted, private pilot's license that would limit his flying to daytime hours.

While this would allow recreational flying, it would rule out commercial flying.

Christian was reassured that his difficulties were consistent with the diagnosed CVD.[3] Overall, he was fully aware of his CVD, and had been educated by his mother since his maternal grandfather had the same condition. This made counseling much easier. Patients with CVD are not always fully educated about their condition, and can be in denial about the severity of diagnosis. Extra time should be spent counseling and providing additional resources.

CLINICAL PEARL

- Because congenital CVDs are nonprogressive, similar test results should be found on retesting.
  A patient who fails a color vison screening test should receive a comprehensive evaluation as early as possible, so that educational and occupational considerations can be discussed.

REFERENCES

1. Went LN, Pronk N. The genetics of tritan disturbances. *Hum Genet.* 1985;69:255-262.
2. Cole BL. Assessment of inherited colour vision defects in clinical practice. *Clin Exp Optom.* 2007;90: 157-175.
3. Birch J. Pass rates for the Farnsworth D15 colour vision test. *Ophthalmic Physiol Opt.* 2008;28:259-264.
4. Steward JM, Cole BL. What do color vision defectives say about everyday tasks? *Optom Vis Sci.* 1989;66:288-295.
5. Bailey JE. Color vision. Chapter 13. In: Eskridge JB, Amos JF, Barlett JD, eds. *Clinical Procedures in Optometry.* Philadelphia, PA: Lippincott; 1991: 99-120.
6. Cole BL. Protan colour vision deficiency and road accidents. *Clin Exp Optom.* 2002;85:246-253.

1.33 Hereditary Color Vision Deficiency in a Young Child

Jeff C. Rabin

Jimmy, a 4-year-old white male in good general health, was referred for a comprehensive color vision evaluation based on a positive family history of hereditary, red–green color vision deficiency. The patient's mother reported that her father had red–green color vision deficiency, and that her 2 older sons failed screening tests and were presumed to have color vision deficiencies as well. We sought to determine both the type and severity of color vision deficiency so as to be able to educate the patient, his parents, and the school about the nature of his condition. Jimmy's ocular and visual findings were otherwise unremarkable.

Color Vision Assessment

Cone Contrast Test

Normal red and blue cone results; significant decrease on the green cone test indicating hereditary deuteranomalous color vision deficiency OU (see Figure 1.33-1).

The Ishihara pseudo-isochromatic plate test was attempted, but Jimmy was unable to detect the demonstration number plate, which should have been visible for both normal and color deficient individuals. We attributed this to Jimmy's age and difficulty recognizing numbers, and attempted the ancillary plates in which the patient traces a colored line across the plate.

Unfortunately, Jimmy did not comprehend the task. Alternative tests that may have been more suitable include the Hardy Rand and Rittler (HRR) book test, which uses symbols rather than numbers, or a color naming test. However, Jimmy was more adept at recognizing letters, and greater diagnostic success was achieved with the cone contrast test (CCT; Innova Systems Inc., Burr Ridge, Illinois), a computer-based test that presents randomized, single-colored letters against a gray background (Figure 1.33-2). These targets stimulate only red-, green-, or blue-sensitive cones. The patient uses a mouse to select the letter seen from an adjacent matching display. An adaptive staircase adjusts cone contrast based on the patient's response to determine the red, green, and blue cone letter recognition thresholds. In this case, we had Jimmy callout the letters, and a clinician input his responses. Normally the test is conducted on each eye separately, but here the test was administered binocularly on 2 occasions to ensure repeatability. A passing score on each test ≥75 indicates that the patient does not have hereditary color deficiency. A score of 30 or less is indicates a moderately severe deficiency. As shown in Figure 1.33-1, Jimmy exhibited normal red and blue cone scores, but consistently failed the green cone CCT on 2 successive tests. This allowed us to identify both the type and severity of color vision deficiency. It is possible that his score may improve somewhat with increasing maturity and age.

Although we were unable to conduct any additional definitive tests on Jimmy due to his age, his elder brother, 9 years of age, was also deuteranomlous based on the Ishihara, CCT, D15 arrangement test, and the Oculus Heidelberger Multi-Color Anomaloscope. The latter test requires the patient match a red–green mixture to a yellow standard. The results for the elder brother are shown in

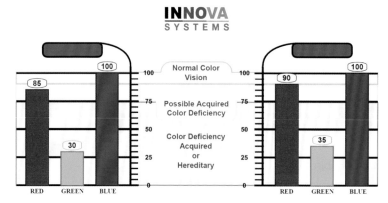

Figure 1.33-1   Cone contrast test results for Jimmy, age 4 years. The results definitively diagnose a green cone (deuteranomalous) color deficiency based on the selective decrease on the green cone contrast test.

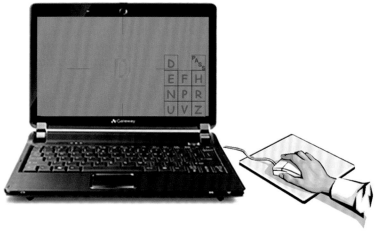

Figure 1.33-2   The cone contrast test display. A red, green, or blue cone specific letter appears briefly in the center of the display and the patient uses the mouse to select the letter seen.

Figure 1.33-3. Note that the matching range is quite wide, and the midpoint of the matching range is shifted toward green, confirming deuteranomalous color vision deficiency as found in his 2 brothers.

Discussion

Normal color vision is essential for accurate object detection, discrimination, and recognition.[1,2] Hereditary red-green color vision deficiency, which occurs in 8% of males and 0.5% of females, is an X-linked condition resulting in a shift of peak red or green cone absorption (protanomaly and deuteranomaly, respectively) or lack of either red (protanopia) or green (deuteranopia) cones.[3,4] The

importance of normal color vision has been identified for a variety of occupations requiring accurate hue discrimination in cue-limited settings, including transportation (aviation, railway, and driving), military settings, and law enforcement.[5-8] Hence, hereditary color vision deficiency is disqualifying for a number of occupations. Furthermore, acquired color vision deficiency may be an early sign of ocular, systemic or neurologic disease.

While pseudoisochromatic plate tests such as the Ishihara test are excellent for identifying the presence of a color vision deficiency, in this case we focused on tests that identified both the specific type and severity of the deficiency, including the CCT and the anomaloscope. With these tests, we were able to diagnose

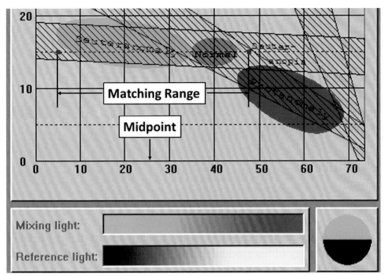

Figure 1.33-3   Oculus Heidelburg Multi-color Anomaloscope findings for the patient's elder brother. The matching range is wide with a midpoint shifted toward green.

severe deuteranomalous color vision deficiency in a patient who was only 4 years old. The family was counseled regarding the color vision deficiency, as well as its potential impact on school performance and future occupational implications. A letter was sent to the school describing the patient's color vision deficiency including illustrative depictions of how the patient sees the world in comparison with observers having normal color vision. The family greatly appreciated the extra effort to identify the specific color vision deficiency, and to convey this information to the patient's teachers and school.

CLINICAL PEARL

- In addition to standard color book tests, newer, computer-based tests can be used effectively in pediatric patients to diagnose both the type and severity of a hereditary color deficiency.

DISCLOSURE

The author has no financial interest in any of the instruments described in this report.

REFERENCES

1. De Valois RL, De Valois KK. A multi-stage color model. *Vis Res*. 1993;33:1053-1065.
2. Jacobs GH. Evolution of colour vision in mammals. *Philos Trans R Soc Lond B Biol Sci*. 2009;364:2957-2967.
3. Krill AE. Krill's hereditary retinal and choroidal diseases. In: Krill AR, Archer DB, eds. *Vol II: Clinical Characteristics..* New York, NY: Harper and Row; 1977: 335-390.
4. Pokorny J, Smith VC, Verriest G, eds. *Congenital and Acquired Color Defects*. New York, NY: Grune and Stratton; 1979.
5. Cole BL, Maddocks JD. Color vision testing by Farnsworth lantern and ability to identify approach-path signal colors. *Aviat Space Environ Med*. 2008; 79: 585-590.
6. Barbur J, Rodriguez-Carmona M, Evans S, Milburn N. *Minimum Color Vision Requirements for Professional Flight Crew, Part III: Recommendations for New Color Vision Standards*. DOT/FAA/AM-09/11, Final Report. Washington, DC: Office of Aerospace Medicine, 20591. ttp://www.faa.gov/library/reports/medical/oamtechreports/2000s/media/200911.pdf. June 2009. Accessed April 13, 2018.
7. Spaulding JAB, Cole BL, Mir FA. Advice for medical students and practitioners with colour vision deficiency: a website resource. *Clin Exp Optom*. 2010; 93:40-41.
8. Dain SJ, Casolin A, Long J, Hilmi MR. Color vision and the railways: Part 1. The Railway LED Lantern test. *Optom Vis Sci*. 2015;92:38-46.

1.34 Acquired Color Vision Deficiency

Jeff C. Rabin

Darin, a 65-year-old white male, was referred from a retinal specialist to our Visual Neurophysiology Service to ascertain the etiology of his gradual, painless loss of central vision over the past 15 years. Darin reported that he had recently stopped driving due to the severe loss of central vision. He also stated that his older brother had been diagnosed with a hereditary condition affecting cone function. He was otherwise in good general health, alert, and highly responsive during all clinical testing.

Clinical Findings

Best-corrected VA	OD: 20/400; OS: 20/150 (superior eccentric viewing in each eye)
Visual field (Humphrey 120 point screening)	OD: central field loss with a few discrete areas of mid-peripheral loss; OS: central field loss with loss in the superior and nasal fields, consistent with lower VA OS
Macular OCT	Thinning of all retinal layers OD and OS
Full-field, flash ERG	Normal dark and light-adapted amplitudes OD with borderline amplitudes OS under stimulus conditions involving cones with borderline cone implicit times OU to single flash and 30 Hz flicker
Multifocal ERG	Significantly decreased amplitudes centrally, with delayed latencies peripherally OD and OS, indicating cone and cone bipolar cell dysfunction
Slit-lamp examination	Unremarkable, OD and OS
Fundus examination (Figure 1.34-1—top figures)	OD: 0.6/0.6 CD ratio; healthy rim tissue with distinct disc margins; pigmentary changes in macular area; artery attenuation; periphery intact; OS: 0.65/0.65 CD ratio; healthy rim tissue with distinct disc margins; pigmentary changes in macular area; artery attenuation; periphery intact
Fundus autofluorescence (Figure 1.34-1—bottom figures)	OD: significant hypo-autofluorescence involving the fovea and macula; OS: central hyper-autofluorescence surrounded by a ring of hypo-autofluorescence
Color vision (cone contrast test, Figure 1.34-2)	OD and OS: significant decrease in red, green, and blue cone color contrast sensitivity

Abbreviations: CD, cup to disc; ERG, electroretinogram; OCT, optical coherence tomography; OD, right eye; OS, left eye; OU, both eyes; VA, visual acuity.

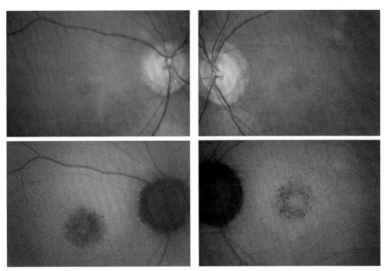

Figure 1.34-1 Standard retinal photography (top figures) and fundus autofluorescence (bottom figures) in a patient with cone dystrophy.

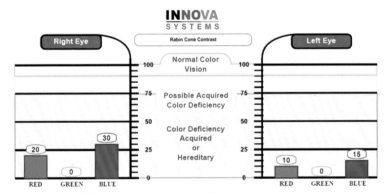

Figure 1.34-2 Red, green, and blue cone contrast test results.

Discussion

The significant decrease in red, green, and blue cone color contrast sensitivity is typical of cone dystrophy.[2] This, as well as the fundus appearance and multifocal electroretinogram (ERG), led us to diagnose Darin with a cone dystrophy. He was subsequently referred to our low vision service.

Acquired color vision deficiency (CVD) is often a sensitive early sign and/or symptom of vision-threatening ocular, systemic, and/or neurologic disease.[3-5] Accordingly, as primary care eye providers, sensitive color vision testing should be used to identify early disease. This case exemplified the significant loss of color vision in a patient with late-onset cone dystrophy, with severely impaired red, green, and blue cone function.

In comparison with the multifocal ERG (mfERG), which identifies cone and cone bipolar cell function from multiple focal sites, the full-field flash ERG reflects the overall rod only, rod and cone, or cone-only responses from the entire retina. Because both rods and cones exist in the central and peripheral retina, the flash ERG may show inconclusive diagnostic results for conditions such as cone or macular dystrophy and equally important Plaquenil toxicity, for which the mfERG is a highly recommended adjunctive test. In this case, the mfERG was grossly abnormal, which is consistent with a condition that primarily decreases cone function.

Tests that will assist in the diagnosis of acquired CVD include the Hardy Rand and Rittler (HRR) book test, which detects red, green, and blue CVD; the normal and desaturated D15 hue arrangement test; Farnsworth-Munsell (FM) 100 Hue test; Oculus Heidelberger Multi-color (HMC) anomaloscope; the cone contrast test (CCT); as well as several other new computer-based color vision tests. Short wavelength automated perimetry (SWAP) and color visual-evoked potentials offer additional approaches for detecting acquired CVD.[6,7] These tests will facilitate the detection of acquired CVD in various ocular diseases, including glaucoma, cone and macular dystrophies, optic neuritis and neuropathies, central serous retinopathy, as well as systemic diseases such as diabetes, multiple sclerosis, and other neurologic conditions.

CLINICAL PEARL

- Acquired color deficiency is a sensitive metric for detecting and monitoring ocular, systemic, and neurological disease.

REFERENCES

1. Rabin J, Gooch J, Ivan D. Rapid quantification of color vision: the cone contrast test. *Invest Ophthalmol Vis Sci*. 2011;52:816-820.
2. Pokorny J, Smith VC, Verriest G, eds. *Congenital and Acquired Color Defects*. New York, NY: Grune and Stratton; 1979.
3. Adams AJ, Rodic R, Husted R, Stamper R. Spectral sensitivity and color discrimination changes in glaucoma and glaucoma-suspect patients. *Invest Ophthalmol Vis Sci*. 1982;23:516-524.
4. Greenstein VC, Hood DC, Ritch R, Steinberger D, Carr RE. S (blue) cone pathway vulnerability in retinitis pigmentosa, diabetes and glaucoma. *Invest Ophthalmol Vis Sci*. 1989;30:1732-1737.
5. Rabin J. Quantification of color vision with cone contrast sensitivity. *Vis Neurosci*. 2004;21:483-485.
6. Johnson CA. Diagnostic value of short-wavelength automated perimetry. *Curr Opin Ophthalmol*. April 1996;7(2):54-58.
7. Rabin JC, Kryder AC, Lam D. Diagnosis of normal and abnormal color vision with cone-specific VEPs. *Transl Vis Sci Technol*. May 17, 2016;5(3):8. eCollection 2016.

1.35 Infant Hyperopia

Susan J. Leat

Lacey, an 11-month-old female, was brought in for a routine eye examination by her mother because her elder brother had glasses at 7 years of age, and her elder sister had an eye turn and wore glasses from 3 years of age. The mother thought that the sister's eye turn had corrected itself now. The mother had no current concerns with Lacey's vision. Lacey's general health was good, and she was meeting her developmental milestones. She was born at 39 weeks by Caesarian section, as she was in the breech position. Her birthweight was 7 pounds (3170 g). Her mother reported that Lacey was not taking any medications and had no allergies.

Family history included macular degeneration in the paternal grandmother and diabetes and hypertension in the maternal grandfather. The other grandparents had both had cataract surgery. Her father wore glasses for driving from 25 years of age, and her mother did not wear spectacles. So, they were surprised about the need for glasses in Lacey's older siblings.

Lacey was quite shy and turned her head away at the commencement of testing. No strabismus was noted during the case history. Toys were used to obtain her interest.

Clinical Findings

Ocular motility (with finger puppets)	Unrestricted
Hirschberg test	Non-strabismic
Unilateral cover test (thumb as occluder)	Non-strabismic
Jump near point of convergence	6 cm
Stereopsis (Lang I)	Pays attention to the car (550″)
Binocular VA (Teller acuity cards)	6.5 cpd (20/94) (Lacey was resistant to occlusion, but equally so with each eye)
Pupil evaluation	PERRL; no RAPD
Dry retinoscopy (Mohindra)	OD: +2.00 −0.75 × 180; OS: +2.25 −0.75 × 180
Gross external ocular health (penlight and 20 D lens)	No abnormalities detected OD and OS
Anterior chamber angles (penlight)	Open OD and OS

Abbreviations: D, diopters; OD, right eye; OS, left eye; PERRL, pupils equal, round, reactive to light; RAPD, relative afferent pupillary defect; VA, visual acuity.

At this point in the examination, Lacey's cooperation was decreasing, and she was getting tired, so a return appointment was recommended for a dilated fundus examination and cycloplegic refraction. At the end of the appointment, the mother mentioned that she may have seen an eye turn in Lacey, but it appeared very briefly. She was unsure of which eye was turning, but she thought that it may have occurred when Lacey was looking to her right. Since Lacey was returning for additional tests, it was suggested that the mother accustom her to having each eye occluded with the palm of her hand, so monocular acuity measurements could be attempted at the next visit.

Follow-up Visit (1 Week Following the Initial Examination)

Hirschberg test	Non-strabismic
Unilateral and alternating cover test (thumb as occluder)	Non-strabismic and orthophoric
Hirschberg and cover test in different directions of gaze	Non-strabismic
Unaided monocular VA (Teller acuity cards)	OD: 6.5 cpd (20/94); OS: 4.8 cpd (20/130)
Cycloplegic refraction (1 drop cyclopentolate 1% OU, with patient fixating the retinosocope)	OD: +2.75 −0.50 × 180; OS: +3.25 −0.50 × 180 (1.50 D subtracted from gross)
Media and fundus examination (direct ophthalmoscopy)	OD: media clear; macula clear with positive foveal reflex; OS: media clear; macula clear with positive foveal reflex;
Fundus examination (binocular indirect ophthalmoscopy)	OD: disc; healthy rim tissue with distinct disc margins, 0.3/0.3 CD ratio, temporal pigmentation. Normal vasculature. Periphery intact OS: disc; healthy rim tissue with distinct disc margins, 0.3/0.3 CD ratio, temporal pigmentation. Normal vasculature. Periphery intact

Abbreviations: CD, cup to disc; D, diopters; OD, right eye; OS, left eye; OU, both eyes; VA, visual acuity.

Discussion

Children of this age are difficult to examine. In many ways, younger infants are easier, as they are less active, shy, and can be strong-willed. Therefore, the clinician needs a number of different ways to assess vision. Start with tests that are less threatening, such as motility with a small toy or finger puppet (or multiple toys). With young children, many targets are needed to keep their attention. A guideline is 1 toy per look, or 1 toy for each side in the motility test. The Lang I test (Figure 1.35-1) gives an idea of the presence of gross stereopsis[1] (Bernell Optical, Mishawaka, Indiana). Note that the Lang II test is not valid as the position of the targets is easy to see monocularly (personal observation). For the unilateral cover test, place your fingers gently on the child's head and bring your thumb down to occlude the eye (Figure 1.35-2). This is less obstructing than an occluder, and the child will often tolerate it better. It is sometimes possible to do the alternating cover test this way as well. For near point of convergence testing, young children will usually stop looking at the target and refixate on your face once the target reaches approximately 15 cm away from the patient. However, this does not mean that convergence is reduced. The jump near point of convergence test overcomes this problem. Use a novel small target and bring it quickly from the side around 8 to 10 cm from the child's eyes. They will converge to see the new target. Demonstrating convergence (even the ability to converge and diverge along the midline) is useful to confirm the normal development of binocular vision. This is important at this age, especially if monocular acuities could not be measured, as at Lacey's first visit. Note also that the child was *equally* resistant to occlusion of either eye. More resistance to occlusion in 1 eye may be an indication of amblyopia in the non-occluded eye.

The visual acuities (VAs) were within the normal age range in this case.[2] To convert from cycles per degree (cpd) to Snellen acuity, use the following formula:

- Snellen denominator (in feet) = $20 \times 30/cpd$
- Snellen denominator (in meters) = $6 \times 30/cpd$

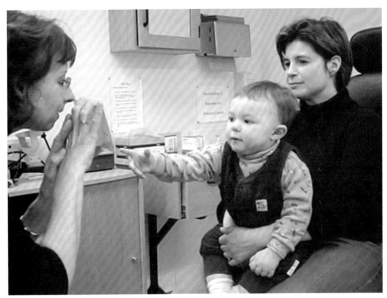

Figure 1.35-1 Lang stereotest.

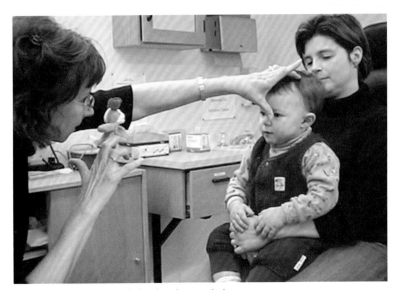

Figure 1.35-2 Unilateral cover test with the thumb as occluder.

An alternative, preferential looking test at this age is the Cardiff acuity cards (Good-Lite Co., Elgin, Illinois) or as an estimate, the Lea or Patti Paddles (Good-Lite Co. or Precision Vision, Woodstock, Illinois).

Undertaking a dry refraction gives useful information, even though at the first examination of a child, dilation with cycloplegia is becoming the standard of practice in many jurisdictions. The dry refraction can be used to decide which drug to use. If the refractive error is low and for a routine examination, tropicamide 1% gives good dilation and sufficient cycloplegia.[3] If there is a higher than average refractive error of any kind, strabismus, or a poor/uncertain/fluctuating result from the dry refraction, then cyclopentolate is indicated. For children with heavier skin/ocular pigmentation, when 1 drop of 1% cyclopentolate may be insufficient, a second drop of 1% tropicamide can increase the dilation and cycloplegia without added risk.[4] Atropine is rarely necessary and the author has not used it outside a hospital setting.

Although it may be possible to undertake the cycloplegic refraction on the same day, it is often better to have the child return for another visit. One unfavorable situation is when the drops are instilled, the child becomes tired and cannot cooperate with the further testing, and nothing is gained. However, this is a clinical decision on each occasion. Apart from the child's ability to cooperate, factors that may influence the decision to have the child return include the level of available financial coverage (eg, government programming, insurance or parental) and the clinical presentation and findings so far.

At the follow-up visit, both the cover test and Hirschberg test were repeated, because the mother mentioned concern of intermittent strabismus at the end of the first visit. Both tests can be undertaken in different directions of gaze if there is a concern. Parental observation of a strabismus in left or right gaze is often due to pseudo-strabismus caused by epicanthus. Having asked the parent to accustom the child to occlusion, monocular VAs could be measured and were found to be normal. Cyclopentolate was chosen for cycloplegia due to the slightly higher dry refraction for the child's age, the family history of spectacle wear and strabismus, and the mother's concern regarding strabismus. Dilated fundus examination can be undertaken before the refraction, as sufficient mydriasis occurs before full cycloplegia. Direct ophthalmoscopy gives a good view of the media (starting with high plus and decreasing the lens power) and macular area. Indirect ophthalmoscopy (binocular or monocular indirect ophthalmoscopes) or the direct ophthalmoscope in conjunction with the 20 D BIO lens to achieve a monocular indirect examination are used to gain a broader view of the fundus. The different quadrants of the periphery can be viewed by using toys to encourage the child to look in the different directions of gaze. A second person is often needed to hold the toys and obtain the child's attention. This could be the parent, while holding the child on their lap, or another family member, or staff person. At this age, retinoscopy is still undertaken with the child fixating the retinoscope light, as for the Mohindra technique, but the required correction factor will be larger. If full cycloplegia was obtained, then the full working distance correction of 2 D can be subtracted, but if it is thought that cycloplegia was incomplete then a value between the dry correction factor for a 0 to 2 year old child (0.75 D) and the full 2 D can be used. In this case, 1.5 D was subtracted from the retinoscopy findings. Cyclopentolate does not eliminate the accommodative response entirely.

For Lacey, there was no evidence of strabismus, and acuities were within normal limits. The hyperopia was higher than average and close to the level that might need correction in a child of this age.[5] There is still some chance that the hyperopia will emmetropize. Spectacles were not prescribed in this case, but Lacey will be seen again in 4 months, at which time it is hoped to see a reduction in hyperopia.

CLINICAL PEARLS

- Adapt your techniques, such as using the jump near point of convergence, and Hirschberg or cover test in different positions of gaze.

- Become expert at retinoscopy—you will have to prescribe based on the results.

- Use the direct ophthalmoscope to view the media and fovea/macular, and then switch to an indirect technique for the rest of the fundus examination.

- If good or complete results are not obtained on the first visit, have the child return on another day.

- When booking the appointment, always determine what is the best time of day for the child, which is when they are alert and neither hungry nor tired.

REFERENCES

1. Broadbent H, Westall C. An evaluation of techniques for measuring stereopsis in infants and young children. *Ophthal Physiol Opt.* 1990; 10:3-7.
2. Stereo Optical. *Teller Acuity Cards II Manual.* http://eiiwebassets.s3.amazonaws.com/s/sterooptical/pdf/other-manuals/TAC_II_manual.pdf. 2005. Accessed April 6, 2017.
3. Twelker JB, Mutti DO. Retinoscopy in infants using a near noncycloplegic technique, cycloplegia with Tropicamide 1% and cycloplegia with Cyclopentolate 1%. *Optom Vis Sci.* 2001;78:215-222.
4. Kleinstein RN, Mutti DO, Manny RE, Shin JA, Zadnik K. Cycloplegia in African-American children. *Optom Vis Sci.* 1999;76:102-107.
5. Leat SJ. To prescribe or not to prescribe. Guidelines for spectacle prescribing in infants and children. *Clin Exp Optom.* 2011;94:514-527.

1.36 High Refraction in Infancy

Susan J. Leat

Danny, a 6-month-old white male, was brought for his first routine examination, because his elder sister (who was 4 years old) was having her eyes examined. Their parents thought that they may as well have his eyes checked. The father had no concerns with Danny's vision and reported no eye turn. Danny's general health was good and he was meeting his developmental milestones. There were no complications with the pregnancy, and he was born at 40 weeks (birthweight = 10 lbs or 4.5 kg). His parents reported that Danny has had "pink eye a couple of times." The last occurrence was 2 months ago, subsequent to a cold. Antibiotic eye drops were instilled and it resolved within a few days.

The family history included macular degeneration in both the paternal grandfather and maternal grandmother. The father reported that he has astigmatism. The maternal grandfather had hypertension, had worn glasses since he was young and had an eye turn.

Clinical Findings

Ocular motility (with finger puppets)	Unrestricted
Hirschberg test	Non-strabismic
Near unilateral Cover test (thumb as occluder)	Non-strabismic
Unaided VA (Teller acuity cards)	OD: 3.2 cpd (20/190); OS: 3.2 cpd (20/190)
Dry retinoscopy (Mohindra)—see Figure 1.36-1	OD: +4.00 −2.00 × 180, OS: +3.00 −1.50 × 180
Dynamic retinoscopy (MEM in the vertical meridian). This was performed unaided, and these values represent the total error[1]	OD: +3.50; OS: +3.00
Pupil evaluation	PERRL/RAPD
Angles	Open by penlight
Gross external ocular health (penlight and 20 D lens)	OD and OS unremarkable

Abbreviations: D, diopters; MEM, monocular estimate method (retinoscopy); OD, right eye; OS, left eye; PERRL, pupils equal, round, reactive to light; RAPD, relative afferent pupillary defect; VA, visual acuity.

Danny was very cooperative so far, and so we continued with the cycloplegic refraction, which was indicated from the high refractive error. When the child is losing cooperation and becoming tired, it is frequently worthwhile to reschedule the cycloplegic and dilated fundus examination. This is especially true when a concern such as a high refractive error is found, as accurate results are particularly necessary. The worst scenario is that the child gets upset when the drops are instilled, and then is fussy and tired for the retinoscopy and ophthalmoscopy so that reliable results are not obtained and the cycloplegic examination has to be repeated later anyway. So 1 drop of 1% cyclopentolate was instilled OU.

152

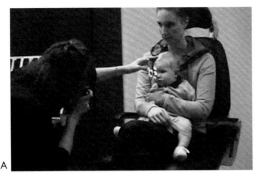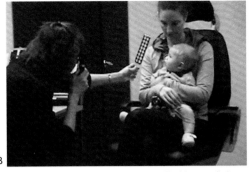

Figure 1.36-1   Mohindra retinoscopy. Note that this should be performed in complete darkness. Trial lenses (left figure) are less unsettling for a child than a lens bar (right figure). The child is less likely to be aware of them and push them away. The same technique at this age could be used for cycloplegic retinoscopy, but the correction factor would be 2 D (for wet refraction if a full dilation was obtained), rather than 0.75 D (for dry).

Internal Ocular Examination (After 20 Minutes)

Direct ophthalmoscopy	Media clear, fovea reflex present, macula clear OD and OS
Indirect ophthalmoscopy	OD: CD ratio 0.1, normal vasculature, periphery clear and no abnormalities detected. disc margins distinct, good color; OS: CD ratio 0.1, normal vasculature, periphery clear and no abnormalities detected. Disc margins distinct, good color
Cycloplegic refraction (30 min after instilling the drops, with Danny fixating the retinosocope)	OD: +6.00 −2.50 × 180; OS: +5.00 −1.50 × 180

Abbreviations: CD, cup to disc; OD, right eye; OS, left eye.

Management and Discussion

This infant has a high refractive error, which is close to the upper limit of the normal range for hyperopia.[2-5] According to Mayer et al,[3] the upper 95% limit of cycloplegic spherical equivalent is +4.4 D at 6 months. Mutti et al[4] found an upper limit of 4.3 D at 3 months and 3.1 D at 9 months (by my calculation), while Wen et al[5] reported an upper limit of 3.1 and 3.25 D in the right and left eyes, respectively, of non-Hispanic whites between 6 and 11 months of age. The mean spherical equivalent was 1.80 D, 1.36 to 2.16 D and 1.36 D in these studies, respectively. Danny's astigmatism was also high (outside the 95% range[5]) and close to the level that would be considered for prescribing.[2] We know that both of these refractive errors (hyperopia and astigmatism) are often high in the first year of life, and that emmetropization can occur for both parameters. We also know that without correction, a child with such a high level of hyperopia is at increased risk for esotropia, while visual acuity (VA) development may be arrested or slowed.[6,7] Uncorrected astigmatism may also result in poorer VA, and may negatively impact other visual functions later in life.[8,9] Weighed against this is the chance that emmetropization may still occur.

So which factors can aid in the decision of whether or not to prescribe spectacles? The first factor is the absolute level of hyperopia under cycloplegia. There is a 50% chance that emmetropization will occur with a hyperopic spherical equivalent 5 D or greater, and this decreases with higher levels of hyperopia.[10] High levels of ametropia seem to be beyond the "range" of the emmetropization process. The second factor is the level of VA. When this is poorer than the average or median value, there is a reduced chance of emmetropization. The third and fourth factors are the monocular estimate method (MEM) dynamic retinoscopy results and non-cycloplegic retinoscopy. When these are high, it indicates a less efficient or insufficient accommodation system, which may impact the development of VA. In Danny's case, the VA was lower than average (on the borderline of the normal range[11]), while the dry and MEM retinoscopy values were quite high. Another (and perhaps better) way to predict whether a child's refractive error will emmetropize is to monitor it over time. In conclusion, this child has high hyperopia that will require correction if emmetropization does not occur within 3 to 6 months. Therefore, a decision was made to review him in 4 months.

Follow-up Visit 4 Months Later (10 Months Old)

Ocular motility (with finger puppets)	Unrestricted
Hirschberg Test	Non-strabismic
Near unilateral Cover test (thumb as occluder)	Non-strabismic
Uncorrected VA (Teller acuity cards)	OD: 3.2 cpd (20/190); OS: 4.8 cpd (20/130)
Dry retinoscopy (Mohindra)	OD: +3.50 −1.50 × 180; OS: +3.00 −1.50 × 180
MEM retinoscopy (vertical meridian)	OD: +3.50; OS: +3.00
Pupil evaluation	PERRL/RAPD
Angles	Open by penlight

Abbreviations: MEM, monocular estimate method (retinoscopy); OD, right eye; OS, left eye; PERRL, pupils equal, round, reactive to light; RAPD, relative afferent pupillary defect; VA, visual acuity.

Cycloplegic refraction (1 drop of 1% cyclopentolate instilled OU, retinoscopy performed 30 minutes after instilling the drops, with Danny fixating the retinosocope):
OD: +5.50 −2.00 × 180: OS: +4.50 −1.00 × 180

Discussion

So how do we judge if this hyperopia is emmetropizing? Pennie et al[12] showed that individuals who emmetropize lose about half of their spherical equivalent (SE) refractive error in the first year. Given that the initial examination recorded a SE of +4.75 in the right eye (OD), one could expect a reduction in hyperopia of about 2.4 D, or 0.2 D per month over the first year. Since the second examination occurred 4 months later, this would predict (0.2 × 4) or 0.8 D less hyperopia. This makes the assumption that the emmetropization occurs steadily over the first year, which may not be the case.[12] However, it does give a guide regarding how much emmetropization would be hoped for. This child is not showing the predicted change in hyperopia (although the astigmatism has decreased). Visual acuity has improved by one level of the Teller cards in the left eye, but not in the right eye, so it remains at the lower borderline of normal. The MEM and dry retinoscopy are still higher than average.

Based on these findings (reduced rate of emmetropization, VA and levels of MEM and cycloplegic retinoscopy findings), it is appropriate to prescribe spectacles for Danny. He also exceeded the prescribing guideline for hyperopia of 3.5 D or more in the least hyperopic meridian.[2] In young infants and children who do not have any strabismus, a partial prescription is generally given. We do not want to interrupt the emmetropization process (if it is occurring) and most infants do not require the full correction, having accommodation that can overcome any uncorrected hyperopia. It has been shown that a partial correction does not significantly interfere with emmetropization.[7] So a prescription can be determined from the Atkinson protocol,[7] which was based on the refraction in plus cylinder format, namely:

- Sphere: prescribe 1 D less than the least hyperopic meridian
- Cylinder: prescribe half of the astigmatism, if it is >2.5 D

So the current findings are: OD: +5.50 −2.00 × 180; OS: +4.50 −1.00 × 180.

When transformed into plus cylinder format, this is: OD: +3.50 +2.00 × 90; OS: +3.50 +1.00 × 90.

Therefore, the prescription would be OD: +2.50 sph; OS: +2.50 sph, prescribed for full-time wear. While this is leaving a large amount of uncorrected hyperopia, we are aiming to leave the uncorrected portion as equal to, or slightly higher than, the "normal" amount of uncorrected refractive error for his age, which is about 1.75 D of hyperopia. The goal is to maintain either a normal or a slightly higher stimulus for emmetropization, because the rate of change in emmetropizing infants is proportional to the portion of the refractive error that remains uncorrected.

Often parents will wonder how they will get their 10-month-old child to wear glasses, but it is interesting to note how frequently a child with this amount of hyperopia will like wearing his or her glasses, and show improved alertness and interaction with his/her environment. This, of course, also indicates that they are benefiting from them. Parents are frequently concerned that wearing spectacles will make affect the child's eyes so that they will continue to need them. There is, however, no evidence that wearing a *partial* correction affects emmetropization,[7] and parents can be reassured about this.

With this reduced prescription, close follow-up is essential for the first few months. The accommodation system may have previously been quite inactive with this high uncorrected hyperopia and increased accommodative demand. Once the accommodation requirement is reduced by the spectacle correction, accommodation will become more active and may result in an accompanying esotropia. Careful counseling of the parent is important, with advice to return should they see any sign of an eye turn. The first follow-up appointment with the spectacles should be scheduled at about 6 weeks after prescribing, to allow time for the spectacles to be dispensed and for the child to adapt to wearing them. If the child does manifest an esotropia with the spectacles, then the prescription should be increased sufficiently to control the strabismus. The safest and textbook approach in such a case is to prescribe the full refractive error.

If emmetropization is seen over the following years, it may be possible to leave the hyperopic correction as it is, or even reduced to maintain a stimulus for emmetropization, keeping the uncorrected portion of hyperopia approximately equal to the average hyperopia for that age.[2] But if the hyperopia remains (which is more likely), it will be necessary to increase the prescription, so that the child remains corrected at the age-related guideline levels.[2] For example, if the refractive error remains constant, then by the time the child reaches 2 years of age, some of the astigmatism should be corrected. At this age, it is recommended to undercorrect the astigmatism by 1 D if it is either against-the-rule or with-the-rule, as in this case. Oblique astigmatism should be corrected at lower levels from a younger age, leaving a smaller amount undercorrected (see Leat[2] for details). At 4 years of age, it is recommended to undercorrect the hyperopia by 1.0 to 1.5 D, and to correct all of the astigmatism.

Follow-up

Danny was seen for follow-up 6 weeks after prescribing. He was still non-strabismic both with and without the spectacles. He showed good compliance, and his parents noted that he seemed more visually alert with them on. Corrected VA improved by 1 line when compared with his previous uncorrected VA.

CLINICAL PEARLS

- Consider VA, absolute levels of non-cycloplegic and cycloplegic refraction, and the accommodation response when deciding whether to prescribe spectacles.

- Monitor infants with high refractive errors over a 3- to 6-month period if unsure about prescribing. Parents will always appreciate that you are delaying prescribing spectacles, and it prepares them if you do have to prescribe.

- Correcting high levels of hyperopia can not only improve visual development, but also general development as well.

REFERENCES

1. Mutti DO, Mitchell GL, Jones LA, et al. Accommodation, acuity and their relationship to emmetropization in infants. *Optom Vis Sci*. 2009;86:666-676.
2. Leat SJ. To prescribe or not to prescribe. Guidelines for spectacle prescribing in infants and children. *Clin Exp Optom*. 2011;94:514-527.
3. Mayer DL, Hansen RM, Moore BD, Kim S, Fulton AB. Cycloplegic refractions in healthy children aged 1 through 48 months. *Arch Ophthalmol*. 2001;119:1625.
4. Mutti DO, Mitchell GL, Jones LA, et al. Axial growth and changes in lenticular and corneal power during emmetropization in infants. *Invest Ophthalmol Vis Sci*. 2005;46:3074-3080.
5. Wen G, Tarczy-Hornoch K, McKean-Cowdin R, et al.. Prevalence of myopia, hyperopia and astigmatism in non-Hispanic White and Asian children: multi-ethnic Pediatric Eye Disease Study. *Ophthalmology*. 2013;120:2109-2116.
6. Atkinson J, Braddick O, Robier B, et al. Two infant vision screening programmes: prediction and prevention of strabismus and amblyopia from photo- and videorefractive screening. *Eye*. 1996;10:189-198.
7. Atkinson J, Braddick O, Nardini M, Anker S. Infant hyperopia: detection, distribution, changes and correlates—outcomes from the Cambridge infant screening programs. *Optom Vis Sci*. 2007;84:84-96.
8. Gwiazda J, Bauer J, Thorn F, Held R. Meridional amblyopia does result from astigmatism in early childhood. *Clin Vis Sci*. 1986;1:145-152.
9. Harvey EM, Dobson V, Miller JM, Clifford-Donaldson CE. Changes in visual function following optical treatment of astigmatism-related amblyopia. *Vis Res*. 2008;48:773-787.
10. Mutti DO, Mitchell GL, Jones LA, et al. Accommodation, acuity, and their relationship to emmetropization in infants. *Optom Vis Sci*. 2009;86:666-676.
11. Stereo Optical. *Teller Acuity Cards II Manual*. http://eiiwebassets.s3.amazonaws.com/s/sterooptical/pdf/other-manuals/TAC_II_manual.pdf. 2005. Accessed April 6, 2017.
12. Pennie FC, Wood ICJ, Olsen C, White S, Charman WN. A longitudinal study of the biometric and refractive changes in full-term infants during the first year of life. *Vis Res*. 2001;41:2799-2810.

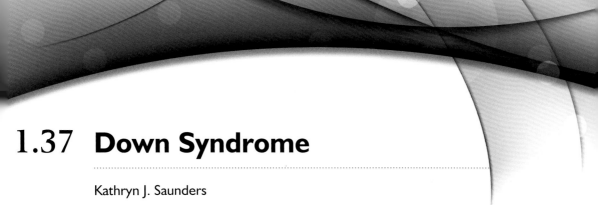

1.37 Down Syndrome

Kathryn J. Saunders

First Visit

Lucy, a 9-year-old girl with Down syndrome, attended for a routine eye examination. She had been seen in the hospital eye service since 3 years of age when she was diagnosed with strabismus and prescribed glasses to correct significant hyperopia. Her mother reported that her left eye used to turn in before she got glasses, but the eye turn is less noticeable when the spectacles are worn. At first, Lucy's compliance with glasses was poor due to problems with the fit, as well as getting used to the feel of the glasses on her face. Now, they are worn all the time, and Lucy looks for them as soon as she gets up in the morning, and only taking them off when she goes to bed. The hospital eye service prescribed patching of the right eye. Her mother reported that the vision in the left eye did get better, but it was never as good as the right eye. Lucy has now been discharged from the hospital service, and this was her first eye examination at the practice.

Lucy has been attending a mainstream school and had a full-time classroom assistant during the school day. Lucy liked to read and had been progressing well educationally. Her mother considered Lucy's vision to be good with her glasses on. She thought Lucy's glasses were getting a little small, and wanted a new frame that looked a little more grown-up.

Lucy's general medical health was good. She had good hearing. At birth she was noted to have a cardiac atrial-septal defect, which closed without treatment. She was no longer receiving specialist cardiac care. She had an underactive thyroid that was being monitored, but no medication was currently prescribed for this or any other conditions. She had no known allergies, although her mother reported that she used to get frequent coughs, colds, and other illness. However, she seemed more robust nowadays. Lucy used to get frequent blepharitis, but this was much improved and her mother reported that it is only comes back when Lucy has a cold or cough. She treated the condition by keeping the eyelids clean with cooled, boiled water.

Clinical Findings

Distance VA with current Rx[a] (crowded Sonksen LogMAR letter test @ 3 m)	OD: 0.35 logMAR (20/40); OS: 0.575 logMAR (20/70)
Near VA with current Rx[a] (crowded Sonksen LogMAR letter test @ 40 cm)	OU: 0.60 logMAR (20/80)
Current Rx	OD: +2.50 sph; OS: +3.00 sph The frame was in moderate condition but was too small. It was fitted with single vision CR39 lenses, which were mildly scratched.

Cover test with current Rx	Small Left Esotropia @ 6 m and 33 cm
	The eyes were cosmetically straight. Deviations were not measured with a prism bar.
Cover test unaided	Moderate Left Esotropia @ 6 m and 33 cm
Confrontation visual fields	Grossly full OU
Pupil evaluation	PERRL; no RAPD
Ocular movements	Grossly full; no incomitant deviation detected
Stereopsis	Not attempted (manifest strabismus present)
Accommodative function with current Rx (Ulster-Cardiff Accommodation CUBE @ 25 cm, see Figure 1.37-1A and B)	Significant lag (>1.00 D) OD and OS
Contrast sensitivity (Cardiff contrast test, with current Rx)	OU: 33. 3% contrast sensitivity—*this is below that expected for a younger child*
Retinoscopy (1 drop of 1% cyclopentolate OU)	OD: +2.50 sph; OS: +3.00 sph
Subjective refraction	Patient rejected any additional plus when viewing a distant target. A more detailed subjective examination could not be achieved.
Intraocular pressure (iCare tonometer)	OD: 11 mm Hg; OS: 11 mm Hg at 3:00 PM
Ocular health (binocular indirect ophthalmoscopy)	Healthy external eye media, fundi and discs, OU. Blue iris with Brushfield spots throughout OU

Abbreviations: D, diopters; logMAR, logarithm of the minimum angle of resolution; OD, right eye; OS, left eye; OU, both eyes; PERRL, pupils equal, round, reactive to light; RAPD, relative afferent pupillary defect; Rx, prescription; sph, sphere; VA, visual acuity.
[a] Both distance and near acuities were assessed using the matching card to identify letters. Cooperation was quite good, although Lucy was easily distracted and testing was not continuous.

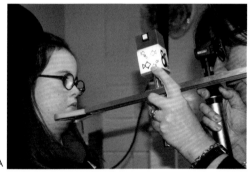 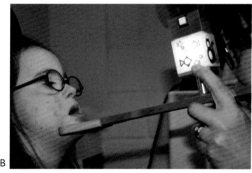

A   B

Figure 1.37-1   Lucy undergoing dynamic retinoscopy with her new bifocal spectacles. A, In this image Lucy is viewing the Ulster-Cardiff Accommodation Cube target at 25 cm through the distance portion of her new bifocals. The retinoscopist has to move back (>1.00 D) to achieve a neutral response, indicating a lag of accommodation. B, If the bifocals are addressing Lucy's accommodative deficit, when Lucy tips her chin up and views the target through her bifocals, the retinoscopist should achieve a neutral response when aligned with, or just slightly behind, the target position.

Comments

In view of Lucy's reduced near visual function (ie, significant accommodative lag and reduced near visual acuity [VA]), a bifocal correction was prescribed for full-time wear as follows:

OD: +2.50 sph; OS: +3.00 sph; ADD: +2.50 OU.

The chosen spectacle frame was adjusted to fit well on the bridge and behind the ears. A large, flat-top (D35) bifocal segment was fitted with the top of the segment positioned at the pupil center to optimize use. Trivex lenses were ordered. Lucy's mother was advised that poor focusing is a common finding in children with Down syndrome, and that bifocal wear has been shown to be a well-tolerated and successful method of improving near vision in this group. She was instructed that most children with Down syndrome appear to adapt very well to bifocals. However, during the first few days after getting the glasses, she was advised to monitor Lucy's mobility to ensure that she does not trip on stairs or the edges of the sidewalk.

The reduced vision in Lucy's left eye, as reported to her mother at previous hospital eye examinations, was confirmed. Her mother stated that this had been explained to her by the hospital orthoptist as being a consequence of the turn in Lucy's left eye. Although both patching and wearing glasses had improved the vision to some extent, Lucy's mother was aware that the vision remained poorer in this eye.

The right eye was the dominant, preferred eye. Lucy had better vision in this eye compared with the left, but the best-corrected VA in the right eye remained slightly below the level expected for a typical 9 year old. The level of contrast sensitivity in this eye was also below normal. These findings were discussed with Lucy's mother, and a brief written summary was provided for her to share with Lucy's teachers and others. This lay summary is included in Figure 1.37-2. This statement introduced the new bifocals and highlighted that Lucy had some visual limitations even when the glasses were worn. This letter also clarified that Lucy may benefit from sitting near the front of the class when whiteboard work is being presented, and care should be taken to ensure that educational material is of high contrast to ensure its visibility.

At a follow-up visit, 3 months after the initial examination, Lucy returned to evaluate how she was adapting to the new glasses and to assess her near vision through the bifocals. She was wearing them all day, and finding them helpful with school work. Both her teacher and

mother reported better attention and cooperation with school and homework. Lucy did not report any difficulty with steps, curbs, or other activities when wearing the bifocals. The following findings were observed:

Near VA with bifocal (crowded Sonksen logMAR letter test @ 40 cm)	0.20 logMAR OU *with matching letters, good co-operation*
Accommodative function with bifocal (Ulster-Cardiff Accommodation CUBE @ 25 cm)	Small lag (<1.00 D) OU
Accommodative function through distance portion of spectacles (Ulster-Cardiff Accommodation CUBE @ 25 cm)	Significant lag (>1.00 D) OU

Abbreviations: D, diopters; logMAR, logarithm of the minimum angle of resolution; OU, both eyes; VA, visual acuity.

Lucy was congratulated on doing so well with her new glasses and told that they are really helping her to see better. She was encouraged to keep wearing the glasses and to keep them in good condition. The improved near VA was explained to her mother, and a follow-up appointment was scheduled for 12 months time.

Discussion

In addition to slightly reduced best-corrected distance VA and contrast sensitivity, Lucy demonstrated another common visual problem found among children with Down syndrome.[1-4] She had a significant accommodative deficit (increased lag of accommodation), which reduced her near visual function. Unlike their typically developing peers, children with Down syndrome and other developmental disabilities often have reduced accommodative function.[2-5] Accommodative dysfunction has been reported in 55% to 85% of children with Down syndrome,[2-4] and 58% of children with cerebral palsy.[5] Recent research has

ULSTER UNIVERSITY OPTOMETRY CLINIC

VISUAL ASSESSMENT SUMMARY

NAME:　　LUCY　　　　　　　　　　　　DOB: 01.01.2008

Below is a brief summary of the findings from today's visual assessment;

Current glasses: Single vision　　OD+2.50sph　OS+3.00sph
New glasses: <u>Bifocal</u> glasses　　OD+2.50sph　OS+3.00sph　ADD +2.50 OU
These glasses should be used;　　All the time

Vision (with/~~without~~ glasses):　　Distance vision (@3m)　　OD 0.35 logMAR (6/12-)
　　　　　　　　　　　　　　　　　　　　　　　　　　　　　OS 0.575 logMAR (6/24+)

Focusing (with/~~without~~ glasses): using her old glasses Lucy has reduced focusing, she needs a bifocal to help with this.

Eye coordination: Lucy's left eye turns in (less when she wears her glasses) and she doesn't have 3D depth perception.

Contrast vision: Lucy has slightly reduced contrast sensitivity which means she finds faint, low contrast information harder to see than other children her age.

Lucy needs a pair of bifocals to help her see better far away and close up. Even with her glasses on her vision is slightly reduced compared to other children her age and she doesn't see faint (low contrast) information as easily. She should be allowed to sit near the front of the class for black/whiteboard work and may find copying from the board challenging. School- and homework should be high contrast and not too much presented at one time.

Children with Down syndrome are strong visual learners so it is important they have good eye care and, where appropriate, wear glasses to improve their vision. However, we know that most children with Down syndrome, even when they wear their glasses, don't see as well as other children. Simple strategies can make sure that visual difficulties aren't making learning and playing harder or less interesting for them*.

Material should be;

- **Larger**
- **Bolder** (use thick, dark pencils e.g. 6B or thick black pen; go over ruled lines on a page to make them more visible)
- **Less cluttered** (don't have lots of information or tasks on one page, cut and separate or cover parts of the page with black paper; remove unnecessary clutter/pattern from surfaces).

*The online <u>Ulster Vision Resources</u> contains information to support parents and others in working with children with a range of visual problems. Go to <u>http://biomed.science.ulster.ac.uk/research-institute/ulster-vision-resources</u> for more information and for examples of suitable print/picture sizes for children with different levels of vision.

Figure 1.37-2 Copy of the lay summary provided to Lucy's mother.

shown that in children with Down syndrome, while vergence eye movements are accurate and appropriate, these children often fail to use blur cues effectively to drive accommodative responses.[6,7] The use of bifocals is an effective and acceptable way of managing these cases.[8,9] Children with Down syndrome are frequently asymptomatic, even when significant deficits exist, and reduced function at near will compound underlying learning disabilities, as well as adversely impact educational and other outcomes.[3]

Objective measurement of accommodation is key to the detection and management of accommodative dysfunction in these children. Although reduced near VA may be indicative of an accommodative deficit, many children will perform quite well in a near VA assessment, even when a significantly decreased accommodative response (lag) is demonstrated with dynamic retinoscopy. This objective test is the optimal method to identify an accommodative deficit, which could be underestimated or missed entirely if only near VA is measured. A number of dynamic retinoscopy methods are available. Lucy cooperated well with the modified Nott method used in conjunction with the Ulster-Cardiff Accommodation Cube (see Figure 1.37-1). This cube encompasses research-derived, normative data so that practitioners can easily determine if the result lies within the normal range. It has also been shown to be both reliable and repeatable.[10,11] Alternative techniques include the monocular estimation method (MEM). However, a key advantage of Nott retinoscopy is that it does not require the use of supplementary lenses. These have been shown to interfere with the accommodative state during near viewing. In addition, not only do the supplementary lenses used during MEM retinoscopy change the magnitude of the accommodative response, but they can also be very distracting for young or intellectually challenged patients.

When considering the prescription of bifocals for a child with developmental disability, it is often good practice to prescribe single vision spectacles to correct any distance refractive error first, and check good compliance with this simpler format before progressing to bifocals. In this case, Lucy had been compliant with her full distance hyperopic correction for some time, and so the move to bifocals was straightforward. The use of a +2.50 D ADD is pragmatic, rather than evidence based. This addition has been used in research studies and appears to work well clinically.[8,12] An alternative method would be to measure how much supplementary plus power was required to reduce the accommodative lag at near to an acceptable level (eg, <1.00 D lag), and then prescribe an addition based on this value.[3] When testing a child who struggles to comply with lengthy test procedures, the use of the empirical +2.50 D addition may be preferable.

Once bifocals have been dispensed, future assessments should monitor the use of these lenses. Questions to be asked include: (a) Does the child actually use the bifocal segment when viewing detailed near objects? (b) What is the near VA through the near addition? (c) Is the accommodative response (as measured by dynamic retinoscopy) accurate when viewing a near target through the segment? (d) Is the accommodative response through the distance portion of the spectacles still reduced? Along with parental reports, the clinical answers to these questions will help the practitioner determine if the bifocal is having a positive impact.

Regarding the magnitude of the accommodative lag when the patient is viewing through the distance portion of the lens, it has been suggested that over time the bifocals may act as a positive treatment for the accommodative deficit.[12] If this is indeed the case, then it may be possible to go back to single vision lenses at some point in the future if accurate accommodation can be demonstrated through the distance portion of the spectacles. However, additional research is needed to determine whether bifocals can actually eliminate cases of accommodative dysfunction in Down syndrome, and if so, which patients are most likely to respond. Careful assessment of the accommodative response is critical before any change back to single vision lenses.

CLINICAL PEARLS

- Children with developmental disability are at increased risk for visual problems, and accommodative dysfunction is common and easily overlooked. All children with developmental disability should have an objective measure of accommodative function undertaken.

- Where an accommodative deficit is found, correct the distance refractive error. Then, when there is good compliance with single vision spectacle wear, reassess accommodative status through the distance correction. If an accommodative deficit remains, provide a near vision correction to optimize near visual function. Bifocals are well tolerated and negate the need for separate distance and near glasses, which can be easily misplaced or worn for the wrong purpose.

CONFLICT OF INTEREST

The author has a financial interest in the Ulster-Cardiff Accommodation Cube.

REFERENCES

1. John FM, Bromham NR, Woodhouse JM, Candy TR. Spatial vision deficits in infants and children with Down syndrome. *Invest Ophthalmol Vis Sci.* May 2004;45(5):1566-1572.
2. Woodhouse JM, Meades JS, Leat SJ, Saunders KJ. Reduced accommodation in children with Down syndrome. *Invest Ophthalmol Vis Sci.* 1993;34(7):2382-2387.
3. Nandakumar K, Leat SJ. Bifocals in children with Down syndrome (BiDS) – visual acuity, accommodation and early literacy skills. *Acta Ophthalmol.* September 2010;88(6):e196-204.
4. Anderson HA, Manny RE, Glasser A, Stuebing KK. Static and dynamic measurements of accommodation in individuals with Down syndrome. *Invest Ophthalmol Vis Sci.* 2011;52(1):310-317.
5. McClelland J, Parkes J, Hill N, Jackson AJ, Saunders KJ. Accommodative dysfunction in children with cerebral palsy: a population-based study. *Invest Ophthalmol Vis Sci.* 2006;47(5):1824-1830.
6. Doyle L, Saunders KJ, Little JA. Trying to see, failing to focus: near visual impairment in Down syndrome. *Sci Rep.* February 5, 2016;6:20444. doi: 10.1038/srep20444.
7. Doyle L, Saunders KJ, Little JA. Determining the relative contribution of retinal disparity and blur cues to ocular accommodation in Down syndrome. *Sci Rep.* January 10, 2017;7:39860.
8. Stewart RE, Margaret Woodhouse J, Trojanowska LD. In focus: the use of bifocal spectacles with children with Down's syndrome. *Ophthalmic Physiol Opt.* November 2005;25(6):514-522.
9. Adyanthaya R, Isenor S, Muthusamy B, Irsch K, Guyton DL. Children with Down syndrome benefit from bifocals as evidenced by increased compliance with spectacle wear. *J AAPOS.* October 2014;18(5):481-484. doi: 10.1016/j.jaapos.2014.07.158. Epub September 26, 2014.
10. McClelland J, Saunders K. Accommodative lag using dynamic retinoscopy: age norms for school-age children. *Optom Vis Sci.* 2004;81(12):929-933.
11. McClelland J, Saunders K. The repeatability and validity of dynamic retinoscopy in assessing the accommodative response. *Ophthalmic Physiol Opt.* 2003;23(3):243-250.
12. Al-Bagdady M, Stewart RE, Watts P, Murphy PJ, Woodhouse JM. Bifocals and Down's syndrome: correction or treatment? *Ophthalmic Physiol Opt.* July 2009;29(4):416-421.

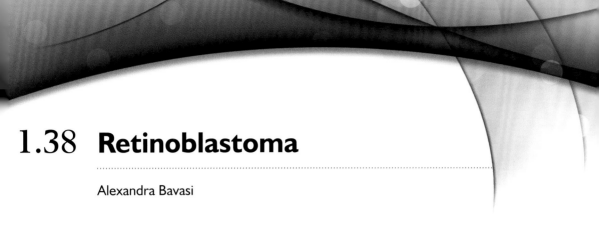

1.38 **Retinoblastoma**

Alexandra Bavasi

Gracie, a 2-year-old white female, presented following an urgent referral from her pediatrician a few hours earlier. Her mother had taken her to the pediatrician because she had noticed that Gracie's right pupil seemed larger than the left pupil, and that her right eye seemed to be pointing outward. She also stated that occasionally the right pupil seemed to "glow," or not look as black as the fellow pupil.

The pediatrician's notes confirmed a difference in pupil size, but he was unsure whether the difference was physiologic or pathologic. Neither direct ophthalmoscopy nor Bruckner testing had been performed, and there was no indication of leukocoria or a difference in the appearance of the red reflexes between the 2 eyes. Gracie's overall health was unremarkable. She was not taking any medications and had no known drug allergies. Family, medical, and ocular histories were also unremarkable.

Clinical Findings

Uncorrected distance VA (Pacific Acuity Test)	OD: oriented to a bright overhead light but unresponsive to hand motion; eye moved in nystagmoid searching pattern OS: 20/25 equivalent OU: 20/25 equivalent
Ocular alignment	Small right XT by gross observation; modified Krimsky indicated ≈15 prism diopters right XT
Pupil evaluation	Right pupil 1.5 mm larger than the left pupil in standard room illumination; + RAPD OD; right pupil had a subtle greyish appearance OD: abnormal direct and consensual responses to light OS: normal direct response to light; abnormal consensual response to light
Bruckner test	Inconclusive: the differences in red reflexes were difficult to assess due to pupil miosis
Ocular motility	Full OD and OS
Cover test	Patient unable to maintain fixation with her right eye
Direct ophthalmoscopy	OD: A large, white, vascular, retrolental mass was present. The tissue was multilobed, firm, and did not undulate. It formed a funnel shape that involuted posteriorly and appeared to fill the vitreal cavity. The optic nerve head was completely obscured by the mass. OS: Unremarkable
Intraocular pressure (digital palpation)	OD firmer than OS

Binocular indirect ophthalmoscopy	OD: Initially difficult to assess due to the anterior protrusion of the mass. By manipulating the condensing lens and working distance, the lesion could be visualized. It appeared to involve the entire retina. The tissue was whitish/yellowish in color, and overlying branch retinal vasculature could be visualized. Small, localized areas of white tissue were dispersed superficially on the multilobed mass. The tissue did not move on eye movement (Figure 1.38-1). OS: normal retinal architecture and optic nerve appearance

Abbreviations: OD, right eye; OS, left eye; OU, both eyes; RAPD, relative afferent pupillary defect; VA, visual acuity; XT, exotropia.

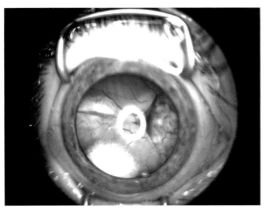

Figure 1.38-1 The funnel-like appearance of the multilobed tumor in the right eye can be seen through the dilated pupil.

Comments

Gracie was referred urgently to a pediatric ophthalmologist who confirmed the presence of a large retrolental mass consistent with a retinoblastoma in the right eye.[1] She was scheduled for an examination under anesthesia with an ocular oncologist, and magnetic resonance imaging (MRI) and B-scan ultrasonography were ordered to determine the extent of the mass and to rule out any involvement in the left eye.

The following week, Gracie presented for examination under general anesthesia. The following findings were noted:

Intraocular pressure (Tonopen)	OD: 35 mm Hg; OS: 16 mm Hg
Angle assessment	OD: shallow angles; OS: deep and quiet
Retinal appearance	OD: total bullous retinal detachment with retina in retrolental space; extensive subretinal fluid and whitish subretinal material; no obvious mass lesion OS: within normal limits
B-scan echography	OD: closed funnel appearance with dense subretinal debris. A few hyperreflective echoes consistent with exudate. No apparent solid mass, but no convection motion could be detected with dynamic viewing. OS: within normal limits
MRI of the brain and orbits with and without contrast (Figure 1.38-2)	Hyperintense mass occupying the majority of the right globe consistent with a retinoblastoma. No evidence of extra-orbital tumor extension. No evidence of abnormality in the left orbit, suprasellar cistern, pineal region, or elsewhere in the head.

Abbreviations: MRI, magnetic resonance imaging; OD, right eye; OS, left eye.

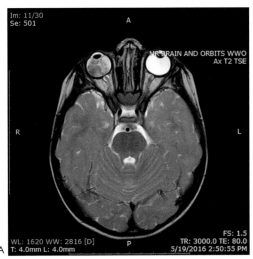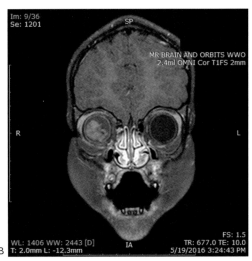

Figure 1.38-2 Axial T2 magnetic resonance imaging (MRI) (A) reveals multiple tumors within the right globe. Coronal T1 MRI with contrast and fat suppression (B) highlights dense tissue within the right globe.

Discussion

Although obvious abnormalities were found, the initial ocular oncologist's assessment produced diagnostic uncertainty. A unilateral, exudative, total retinal detachment with extensive subretinal material was observed in the right eye, but no clear mass lesion was present. A diagnosis of advanced Coats disease with total retinal detachment, rather than retinoblastoma, was considered. A second opinion was recommended before pursuing diagnostic and therapeutic enucleation of the right eye.

The following week, Gracie underwent another examination under general anesthesia at a different hospital under the oversight of retinoblastoma specialists, and her parents consented to immediate enucleation if retinoblastoma was confirmed. After extended ophthalmoscopy, B-scan echography, and MRI evaluation, the presence of retinoblastoma was confirmed, with a conglomeration of more than 10 tumors being found in the right eye.[2] Although each hospital used similar diagnostic testing, the specialists at the second hospital have evaluated many more cases of retinoblastoma annually, and their extensive experience may have assisted in the definitive diagnosis.

Enucleation of the right eye was carried out immediately. The optic nerve was cut as posteriorly as possible, because the second MRI showed possible anterior optic nerve involvement. A 20-mm orbital implant was inserted and anchored into place by suturing conjunctival tissue over the anterior aspect. A conformer, that is, a plastic shell that maintains the shape of the eye socket during healing, was placed over the implant, thereby saving space for the eventual prosthetic.[3] A temporary tarsorrhaphy was performed to keep the conformer in place and prevent accidental evulsion. The right globe was sent to pathology for evaluation.

The pathology report confirmed a dense retinoblastoma. Careful inspection revealed that cell abnormalities were consistent with early posterior extension of the tumor along the optic nerve. These findings confirmed the need for systemic chemotherapy to halt potential metastases.

After the orbit was dressed with a pressure patch, Gracie returned home to continue treatment at her local hospital. The pressure patch was removed 1 week later. The tarsorrhaphy sutures were removed 5 weeks later, and the conformer was replaced by a temporary prosthetic eye. This provided a cosmetic improvement while the eye socket continued to heal as she waited for her custom prosthetic fitting. Polycarbonate spectacles were prescribed to protect Gracie's healthy left eye.

Three weeks after enucleation, an implanted port was inserted 2 in below the Gracie's right clavicle, and 6 cycles of monthly chemotherapeutic infusions were initiated. MRI and B-scans during this time remained clear.

Eleven weeks post enucleation, Gracie was fitted for her first customized ocular prosthetic. Under general anesthesia, the temporary prosthetic was removed and a mold taken of her right eye socket. The hand-painted prosthetic was designed and inserted 2 days later.

Ocular prosthetics have their own complications, and Gracie frequently developed papillary conjunctivitis due to a mechanical reaction and hypersensitivity at the eyelid–prosthetic interface.[4] However, after a few months of treatment and modifications, the frequency of these episodes reduced.

Six months after the initial diagnosis, genetic testing was performed to search for mutations in the RB1 gene, which codes for a specific protein that acts as a tumor suppressor and controls how retinoblastoma cells grow and divide.[5] The results identified a single somatic RB1 mutation—del4→6—which resulted in a nonworking retinoblastoma protein in Gracie. No other somatic mutation was found on the RB1 gene. A somatic mutation indicates a change in any type of cell other than egg or sperm cells. Somatic mutations cannot be passed down to future generations. Additional changes outside the RB1 gene were found, suggesting the possibility of genomic instability, or chromothripsis, in the tumor. Analysis was unable to confirm or deny a germ line component of Gracie's retinoblastoma. Because of the uncertainty, it was estimated that she may have less than a 15% chance of carrying a second, unidentified mutation in her germ cells. This possibility indicates that her parents, siblings, and future children are at risk of carrying a mutation leading to retinoblastoma. Furthermore, Gracie is susceptible to developing retinoblastoma in her left eye, and potentially developing secondary cancers, such as sarcomas and melanomas.[5]

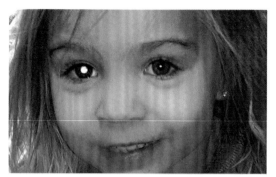

Figure 1.38-3   Gracie's appearance at 2 years of age. The "glow" in her right eye is clearly visible.

Gracie's parents and siblings presented for comprehensive eye examinations, and thankfully, each had normal ocular health. Gracie completed 6 months of chemotherapy, and her scans and blood work continued to be normal. Chemotherapy was discontinued.

Gracie's maintenance treatment plan will continue with monthly examinations under general anesthesia to assess the right eye socket, the retinal health of the left eye, B-scan ultrasounds, and MRI examinations to rule out the presence of metastases or contralateral involvement. These examinations and scans will continue until Gracie reaches 5 years of age, whereupon she will be monitored at 3-, and eventually 6-month intervals.

Although retinoblastoma is exceedingly rare, it reinforces the importance of accurately assessing and recognizing leukocoria, and to seek treatment immediately if it is suspected. Increased access to eye care for young children is critical, as is parental education. Figure 1.38-3 shows Gracie's appearance at 2 years of age. The camera flash reflects more intensely in her right pupil due to the yellowish/white color of the retinoblastoma mass. Tag lines, such as "know the glow," can be effective in educating parents, family, and friends to be aware of potential leukocoric abnormalities which can be observed in photographs (https://knowtheglow.org). When looking back at previous photographs taken of Gracie months before her diagnosis, her mother found many in which her right pupil "glowed."

CLINICAL PEARLS

- Do not underestimate the power of the direct ophthalmoscope, especially when examining children.

- When giving an alarming diagnosis, make yourself available to answer questions after the patient or parents have had time to process the initial shock.

- Examining pupillary function in children should never be skipped. If asymmetric pupillary responses or leukocoria are observed, then dilation is imperative.

REFERENCES

1. Aerts I, Lumbroso-LeRouic L, Gauthier-Villars M, Baisse H, Doz F, Desjardins L. Retinoblastoma. *Orphanet J Rare Dis*. 2006;1:31. doi:10.1186/1750-1172-1-31.
2. Balmer A, Zografos L, Munier F. Diagnosis and current management of retinoblastoma. *Oncogene*. 2006; 25(38):5341-5349. doi:10.1038/sj.onc.1209622.
3. Shields JA, Shields CL, DePotter P. Enucleation technique for children with retinoblastoma. *J Pediatr Ophthalmol Strabismus*. 1992;29(4):213-215.
4. Swann PG, Schmid KL. Giant papillary conjunctivitis associated with an ocular prosthesis. *Clin Exp Optom*. 2001;84:293-295.
5. Mallipatna A, Marino M, Singh AD. Genetics of retinoblastoma. *Asia-Pacific J Ophthalmol*. 2016;5: 260-264.

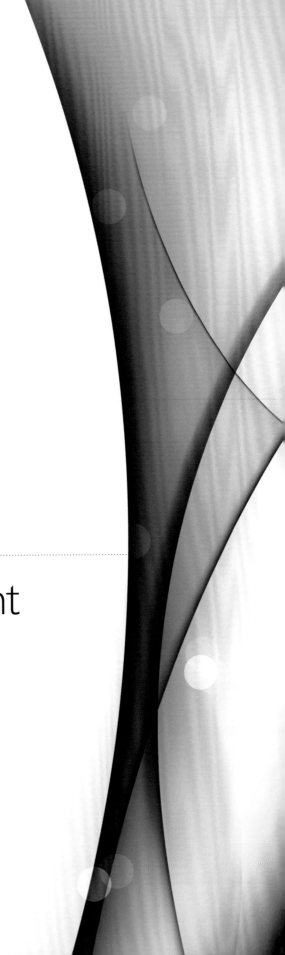

SECTION 2

Anterior Segment

Lead section editor: EUNICE MYUNG LEE

2.1 Use of Gas Permeable Versus Soft Contact Lenses

Lacey Haines

Jeffry, a 25-year-old male, presented for a contact lens fitting after receiving a comprehensive eye examination. The patient reported that he had tried soft contact lenses a few years ago but he did not continue wearing them because his distance vision with contact lenses was quite variable and not as good as through his glasses. He had heard that there were newer contact lens options available and was interested in trying them. He would prefer soft lens materials because he was under the impression that rigid lenses would be too uncomfortable and he would not be able to wear them for sports.

The patient worked as a real estate investor and was very active socially, especially with sporting activities, such as hockey, soccer, and golf. He was not taking any medications and there were no concerns with his general health. His comprehensive eye examination showed no ocular or visual problems.

Clinical Findings

Subjective refraction	OD: $+0.50 -4.50 \times 180$ $(20/20^{-2})$; OS: Pl -3.00×176 $(20/20^{-2})$
Slit-lamp examination	OD and OS: healthy lids, clear corneas, good tear break-up times
Horizontal visible iris diameter (HVID)	OD: 12.2 mm; OS: 12.3 mm (each slightly larger than average)
Pentacam corneal topography (Figure 2.1-1A and B)	OD and OS: high amounts of central corneal, regular astigmatism (4.4 D). Scans also showed regular astigmatism, elevation, and thickness patterns.

Abbreviations: D, diopters; OD, right eye; OS, left eye; Pl, plano.

The corneal topographies showed regular astigmatism, elevation, and thickness patterns, thereby ruling out the presence of corneal ectatic disorders such as keratoconus. It was determined that soft toric lenses would be appropriate. Due to the high cylinder component in this patient's refraction, he required extended range (XR) soft toric contact lenses. These are stock lenses available in powers outside the normal range and are not usually available in fitting sets because they are rarely used. These lenses are not completely custom so there is still some limitation of cylinder power and axis parameters. Because the patient's manifest refraction was available prior to the contact lens fitting appointment, the trial lenses were ordered in advance of the fitting visit based on the measured spectacle refraction vertexed to the corneal plane and availability of lens parameters. Extended range toric lenses were ordered with the following parameters for base curve, diameter, and power:
OD: $8.7/14.5/+0.50 -4.25 \times 180$
OS: $8.7/14.5/Pl -2.75 \times 175$

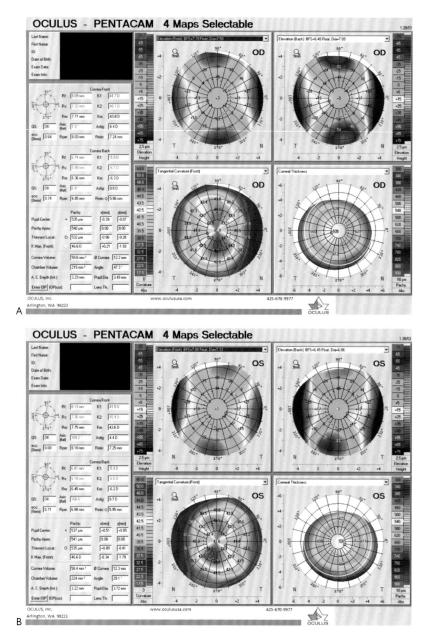

Figure 2.2-1   Pentacam corneal topography maps for the patient's right (A) and left (B) eyes demonstrate high amounts (4.4 D) of central corneal astigmatism in both eyes. The scans also show regular astigmatism, elevation, and thickness patterns.

After allowing the lenses to settle, the patient's visual acuities (VAs) were 20/25^{-2} OD and OS, and 20/20^{-3} OU. Over-refraction did not improve the patient's VA. Fit assessment showed lenses to have good centration and corneal coverage, and adequate movement on blinking and horizontal gaze on each eye. The right lens was stable and there was no rotation.

The left lens showed some mild rotation counterclockwise, but was still considered stable as it shifted only between the 5° and 10° marks after blinks.

Because Jeffry was satisfied with the initial comfort and vision of these lenses, he took them home after demonstrating proficiency in application, removal, lens care, and handling.

A follow-up appointment was scheduled for 1 week later.

One week later, Jeffry returned and reported that he was satisfied with the comfort of the lenses. However, he wanted to see if the vision could be improved. In particular, he found that vision fluctuated frequently and while he could tolerate the inconsistent vision for most activities, it was unacceptable for both sports and driving.

The lenses were assessed and while VA was OD 20/25^{+2}, OS 20/20^{-3}, it could not be improved with sphero-cylindrical over-refraction. Slit-lamp examination again showed good centration and movement, with good surface qualities, but both lenses now showed increased range of rotation between 5° and 15° counterclockwise and was deemed to be unstable. Because the lenses were clean and deposits were not an issue, this can be ruled out as a cause for the poor vision.

The lack of rotational stability, although relatively small, combined with the high amount of cylinder power was the most likely cause of unsatisfactory visual results.

These findings were discussed with the patient and it was determined that a scleral lens would be the best option to satisfy the patient's vision and comfort requirements. Given that the patient had a high refractive error, strong motivation for contact lens wear, and high expectations for visual outcomes, it was determined that a rigid gas-permeable (GP) lens would be the most appropriate. Since the patient wanted to wear contact lenses for sports, scleral lenses would be preferred over corneal GP lenses because of their better comfort and stability.

A scleral lens fitting was performed using diagnostic trial lenses and the following parameters were ordered:

Eye	Base Curve	Diameter	Power, sph[a]	Limbal Design	Periphery	Material
OD	8.40	15.2	+0.50	Extra limbal clearance	Toric: Standard × Flat 1	Boston XO
OS	8.40	15.2	+2.75	Extra limbal clearance	Toric: Standard × Flat 1	Boston XO

Abbreviations: OD, right eye; OS, left eye; sph, sphere.

[a] Note that despite the high amount of spectacle cylinder, only spherical powers were needed for the scleral lenses, because the patient's cornea is the main source for his astigmatism (Figure 2.1-1A and B) and GP lenses neutralize the majority of corneal cylinder.

The patient was to be scheduled for dispense of the scleral lenses once they arrived and the parameters were verified.

At the dispense visit, the scleral lenses were applied and assessed. The patient's vision was OD 20/20^{-1}, OS 20/20, with Pl sph over-refraction in each eye. Fit assessment showed good central corneal clearance of 200 micrometers, adequate limbal clearance, and good alignment of the scleral landing zones in each eye (Figure 2.1-2). Clearance values were estimated using an optic section with the slit-lamp biomicroscope and tear depth compared to lens center thickness. The patient stated that he was surprised by the initial good comfort and demonstrated only slight reflex tearing during the first 5 minutes of lens wear.

Because, fit, vision and comfort were all acceptable, the patient was trained on application and removal and the scleral lenses were dispensed. The patient was asked to return in 1 week for a progress check.

After wearing the scleral lenses for 1 week, Jeffry reported excellent vision and comfort. He had been able to wear the lenses for sports and driving, and they were preferable to wear compared to soft contact lenses or spectacles for being active because the vision was consistent. Jeffry admitted some difficulties with application and removal, but felt that he was improving each day.

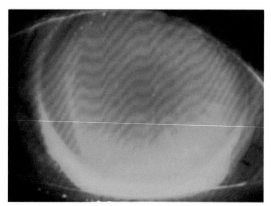

Figure 2.1-2   Sodium fluorescein pattern of the scleral lens demonstrating good central corneal clearance, adequate limbal clearance, and good alignment of the scleral landing zones.

Visual acuity through the scleral lenses was 20/20[+2] OD and OS, and did not improve with routine over-refraction. The fit showed slightly reduced (but still adequate) clearance of 175 micrometers in each eye. The limbal clearance and scleral landing zone alignments remained satisfactory.

No lens changes were required and the patient was asked to return 1 month later for a routine progress check.

Discussion

Nearly 94% of all new contact lens fits in Canada and the United States use soft lens materials, with the remaining 6% of fits involving rigid lens materials.[1] Although the development of new technologies has allowed soft lenses to satisfy a broader scope of patients, there is still an important need for GP lenses. It is well known that GP lenses provide superior visual correction over soft contact lenses.[2] However, some practitioners are still reluctant to choose this lens material because of the decreased initial comfort[3] and perceived complexity of fitting compared with soft lenses. Scleral lenses provide a good alternative in these cases, because they have good comfort and vision performance,[4] and product development continues to make the fitting process easier. The contact lens fitter can select from more efficient diagnostic strategies and improved lens designs. Furthermore, the large optical zone and excellent stability of scleral lens designs allow for the inclusion of more complex optical corrections,[4] such as high sphere and cylinder powers and multifocal optics. The stability of scleral lenses also makes them a great choice for playing sports, because they are less likely to become dislodged or trap debris in the post–lens tear layer.

When faced with reduced vision in an astigmatic soft lens wearer, it is important to rule out other causes, which may not be contact lens related. For example, if the VA with a toric soft lens was consistently reduced, corneal topography should be performed to rule out irregular cornea etiologies such as keratoconus. In addition, if the vision fluctuates throughout the day, lens dehydration should be ruled out by examining the surface quality of the soft lenses in situ with the slit-lamp biomicroscope and the patient's ocular health findings should be considered. In this case, the corneal topography, contact lens fit assessment, and ocular health findings demonstrated that the soft toric contact lens could not provide adequate and stable VA.

As with all contact lens fittings, the final lens design must be determined with a trial-wearing period with lens modification as required over several visits. Once lenses are finalized, the patient should be advised to maintain routine progress checks to avoid contact lens complications. It is generally recommended to follow-up with scleral lens wearers every 6 to 12 months in addition to annual comprehensive vision examinations.

CLINICAL PEARLS

- When refraction is available prior to the contact lens fitting, it is helpful to order diagnostic soft contact lenses in advance of the first visit, particularly when they are required in nonstandard and/or extended range parameters that would not be on hand, to provide optimal vision at the initial trial.

- Gas-permeable lens materials provide a superior alternative to soft lens materials in terms of their visual performance. This is especially apparent for higher and more complicated prescriptions.

- Scleral contact lenses may be an attractive GP lens choice for young and active patients, because they are more comfortable and stable when compared with smaller diameter rigid lens designs.

REFERENCES

1. Morgan PB, Woods CA, Ioannis GT, et al. International contact lens prescribing in 2016. *Contact Lens Spectr.* January 2017;32:30-35.

2. Michaud L, Barriault C, Dionne A, Karwatsky P. Empirical fitting of soft or rigid gas-permeable contact lenses for the correction of moderate to severe refractive astigmatism: a comparative study. *Optometry.* 2009;80:375-383.

3. Fonn D, Gauthier CA, Pritchard N. Patient preferences and comparative ocular responses to rigid and soft contact lenses. *Optom Vis Sci.* 1995;72(12):857-863.

4. Visser ES, Van der Linden BJ, Otten HM, Van der Lelij A, Visser R. Medical applications and outcomes of bitangential scleral lenses. *Optom Vis Sci.* 2013; 90(10):1078-1085.

2.2 Monovision Contact Lenses

Isabel Kazemi

Joseph, a 55-year-old Caucasian male who owned a small car dealership, presented for an annual eye examination with the following goals:

1. Joseph reported decreased distance vision with habitual contact lenses. There were no problems with near and computer vision.
2. Joseph was interested in laser vision correction.

His last eye examination was a decade ago. Joseph did not have any glasses, and wore his contact lenses overnight for 1 week before removing them to clean with multipurpose solution and disinfect overnight. He then wore them for another week, disposing lenses after 2 weeks of wear. He reported his contact lenses were comfortable. Ocular and health histories were unremarkable for the patient and his family.

Clinical Findings

Distance VA (through contact lenses)	OD: 20/70; OS: 20/60
Near VA (through contact lenses)	OD: 20/30; OS: 20/30
Contact lens parameters (2-week replacement)	Base curve 8.8 OD: −6.50 sph; OS: −7.50 sph
Spherical over-refraction	OD −2.00 (20/40); OS −1.50 (20/40)
Pupils	PERRL; no RAPD
Subjective refraction	OD −9.00 −1.00 × 110 (20/25); OS −10.50 −1.25 × 065 (20/25)
Near ADD	+2.00 OU (20/25)
Slit-lamp examination	1+ Superficial punctate keratitis, diffuse; otherwise unremarkable OU
Intraocular pressure (GAT)	OD 15 mm Hg, OS 15 mm Hg at 9:30 AM
Fundus examination	Unremarkable OU

Abbreviations: GAT, Goldmann applanation tonometry; OD, right eye; OS, left eye; OU, both eyes; PERRL, pupils equal, round, reactive to light; RAPD, relative afferent pupillary defect; sph, sphere; VA, visual acuity.

Comments

Joseph was an undercorrected presbyope, who wanted to see better at distance, but was seeing well at near. He was educated regarding the effect on his reading/near vision once distance vision was improved. This discussion had to occur prior to dilation to demonstrate this change to Joseph, due to the fact that he could not understand how his near would become worse (since he was not having any problems). After explaining presbyopia, Joseph was offered several options to correct his vision.[1]

1. Distance toric lenses with reading glasses (last choice because the patient wished to not wear glasses)

2. Multifocal toric contact lenses (can be a complicated fit, because both the astigmatic and multifocal component must be corrected)[2,3]

3. Gas-permeable (GP) or scleral multifocal contact lenses (with caution because the patient is a successful soft contact lens wearer)

4. Hybrid multifocal contact lenses (GP center for better acuity at distance and near with soft skirt for better comfort)

5. Monovision toric contact lenses[4]

Given Joseph's poor compliance and eye examination infrequency, it was felt that he may not return for frequent follow-up necessary for refitting into complicated contact lens designs. In addition, he was accustomed to decreased vision quality and could accept some blur (but should have good distance vision for driving). Additionally, due to his interest in vision corrective surgery, monovision would be the best choice because it could be replicated if he proceeded with refractive surgery. All the options were discussed with the patient, along with the best recommendation of monovision correction, which Joseph agreed to pursue.

Joseph's contact lens overwearing schedule was also discussed and the resulting superficial punctate keratitis that contributed to decreased best-corrected acuity. The importance of compliance and discontinuing extended wear was emphasized. He was offered daily disposable toric lenses for convenience and health. Joseph opted to adhere to a daily wear schedule utilizing 2-week replacement lenses.

Because Joseph was comfortable with his habitual silicone hydrogel brand, and it was available in astigmatic correction, he was refit into new toric contact lens powers. For refractive errors above +/−4.00 D, vertex distance in each meridian must be accounted for when prescribing contact lenses. For monovision, determine the distance contact lens prescription first, then calculate the "effective add" to the near eye for the initial

trial contact lenses. The near eye is typically the nondominant eye.

Initial contact lens Rx (based on lens parameter availability) with OD dominant:

OD: −8.50 −0.75 × 110 OS: −7.50 −0.75 × 070 (effective ADD +1.50 to +1.75)

The patient was retrained in application, removal, and lens care and was instructed to return for follow-up in 1 week wearing the contact lenses.

At the 1-week follow-up visit, his findings were as follows:

Spherical distance over-refraction	OD: Pl (20/20); OS: −1.75 (20/20)
Slit-lamp examination	Corneas clear with no SPK OD and OS

Abbreviations: OD, right eye; OS, left eye; Pl, plano; SPK, superficial punctate keratitis.

At this follow-up, Joseph was extremely happy with his vision at all distances. He desired to proceed with a surgical vision correction consultation. Due to his high refractive error, he was counseled that he may not qualify for refractive surgery.[5] If eligible, he would have to discontinue contact lens wear at least 2 to 3 weeks before any procedure and would need to wear glasses. Because he did not have any glasses, it would be necessary to order a pair for him to use.

The following spectacle options were offered:

1. Single vision distance correction (not ideal, because he would not be able to read or work at computer distance)

2. Bifocal lenses (possible, but may experience difficulty due to neck strain when having to view his computer through the near portion)

3. Progressive addition lenses

4. Monovision

Joseph was successful using monovision contact lens correction and he wanted to minimize the cost of glasses, because they would be for short-term use awaiting refractive surgery. Although monovision glasses are not commonly prescribed, in a case like this, it allows for consistent monovision status. The final glasses prescription was:

OD: −9.00 −1.00 × 110; OS: −8.50 −1.00 − 065 (effective ADD +2.00)

Discussion

For monovision contact lens (and occasional monovision glasses) correction, first determine the dominant eye, which is usually corrected for distance. There are several methods.[6]

- With both eyes open, place +1.50 trial lens over full distance correction in free space 1 eye at a time (or use retinoscopy +1.50 lens in the phoropter, if available). Ask the patient which degrades vision less. The dominant eye will be affected and the nondominant eye will notice little or no difference.

- Use a disposable camera, and ask the patient to pretend to take a photo—the eye the patient uses to sight through the viewfinder is likely the dominant eye.

- Hole in the hand/card test or pointing at an image. Sight a distance target through a small hole or point at a distance target. The eye that aligns with the target is the dominant eye.

- Handedness. Sometimes reported as being associated with eye dominance.

If the patient is uncomfortable with blur over either eye, he or she is likely not a good monovision candidate.

When considering monovision, the patient's age and appropriate add come into consideration. For patients requiring an ADD over +1.50 or +1.75, there is loss of intermediate vision (if a stronger add is prescribed for reading) or loss of near vision (if a lesser add is prescribed for intermediate vision). In general, prescribing an effective intermediate add works well for these patients, because most of close environment needs (computer, grocery store shelves, car dashboard) are viewed at an arm's length away. Additionally, a difference of 1.50 to 1.75 between the 2 eyes is usually well tolerated, while a larger difference

using higher effective adds may cause adaptation problems for patients, especially new to monovision.[7] Finally, patients can purchase over-the-counter +1.00 readers to use over their contact lenses for looking at very small print as needed.

Consult the appropriate Department of Motor Vehicles guidelines to ensure that the patient meets minimum driver's license vision requirements.

CLINICAL PEARLS

- When spherical over-refraction over contact lenses does not yield good VAs, suspect uncorrected astigmatism, amblyopia, pathology (anterior or posterior), or a combination of any of these. Just move on with the rest of your examination—by removing the contact lenses—to figure it out.

- Presbyopic patients with distance myopic changes require education as to what happens when their distance vision is corrected, creating a need for correction at near. Also, for pre-presbyopic patients, be cautious when making changes to a myopic shift and removing their slight effective add, which can push them into near vision problems.

- Presbyopic patients inquiring about laser vision correction—remember that their goal is to get rid of glasses. Therefore, a detailed discussion is warranted regarding expectations. Monovision is frequently recommended with trial monovision correction using contact lenses for at least 2 weeks, which is the time frame typically required to adapt to such modality.

- When refitting a patient to a different type of contact lens correction (single vision to toric or multifocal), consider what the patient is currently wearing. If the patient is happy with comfort and modality, adjust judiciously.

REFERENCES

1. Bedinhaus T. Contact lens options for people over 40. Verywell. January 8, 2017. https://www.verywell.com/contacts-for-people-over-40-3421627. Updated March 2018.
2. Potter R, Pal S, Stiegemeier MJ. Avoiding the soft multifocal failure. *Contact Lens Spectr*. March 1, 2016;31:22-25.
3. Davis R, Barry Eiden S, Sonsino J. Personalizing vision with custom soft lenses. *Contact Lens Spectr*. August 1, 2014;29:28-33.
4. Evans BJ. Monovision: a review. *Ophthalmic Physiol Opt*. September 27, 2007;5:417-439.
5. Den Beste BP. Where do you stand on these refractive surgery controversies? *Rev Optom*. October 15, 2014:30-36.
6. Glenn Hagele Dominant Eye Test, Council for Refractive Surgery Quality Assurance. January 1, 2013.
7. Sindt CW, Mataya Pietig M. Move over, monovision! *Rev Optom*. April 19, 2011.

2.3 Multifocal Gas Permeable Contact Lenses

Louis Frank

Fran, a 69-year-old female, complained of both a "glare and starburst effect" producing blur and "tunnel vision," which gave her a restricted field of view, while she was trying to read with her habitual, multifocal gas-permeable (GP) corneal contact lenses. Fran felt that it was necessary to turn her head to get adequate vision at near. She was visually comfortable, albeit cosmetically unhappy, when wearing her spectacles. The contact lenses were approximately 2 years old, and she had returned to her previous practitioner several times only to be told that the technology in multifocal contact lenses was limited and she needed to get used to her lenses. Fran also had primary open-angle glaucoma, for which she took 1 drop of 0.25% timolol maleate twice a day. Fran was seeking a second opinion on her contact lenses.

Clinical Findings

Present spectacle Rx	OD: -7.00 sph ($20/20^{-2}$); OS: $-5.25 -1.25 \times 016$ ($20/20^{-1}$); ADD: $+2.50$ OU ($20/30^+$)
Pupil evaluation	PERRL; no RAPD
Pupil diameter	OD and OS: 2.5 mm in bright light; OD and OS: 4.0 mm in dim light
Keratometry	OD: 42.30/43.50 at 075; OS: 43.00/43.90 at 090
Horizontal visible iris diameter	13 mm OD and OS
Vertical palpebral fissure	OD: 9 mm; OS: 8 mm
Manifest refraction	OD: -7.00 sph ($20/20^{-2}$); OS: $-5.50 -1.25 \times 016$ $20/20^{-1}$
Slit-lamp examination	Unremarkable OD and OS
Fundus examination	Unremarkable OD and OS

Abbreviations: OD, right eye; OS, left eye; OU, both eyes; PERRL, pupils equal, round, reactive to light; RAPD, relative afferent pupillary defect; Rx, prescription; sph, sphere.

Comments

The current GP multifocal lenses were as follows:

Overall diameter	OD: 9.8 mm; OS: 9.8 mm
Base curve	OD: 7.95 mm; OS: 7.85 mm
Power	OD: −7.00 sph ADD +2.00; OS: −5.50 sph ADD +2.00
Optic zone	OD: 7.1 mm; OS: 7.1 mm
Edge thickness	OD: 0.11 mm; OS: 0.11 mm
Color	Blue visibility tint OD and OS
Material	Boston ES OD and OS
Distance VA through contact lenses	OD: 20/20⁻¹; OS: 20/20⁻²
Distance over-refraction	OD: +0.50 (20/20); OS: +0.50 (20/20)
Near VA through contact lenses	OD: 20/25; OS: 20/20⁻²
Near over-refraction	OD: +0.50 (20/20); OS: +0.50 (20/20)

Abbreviations: OD, right eye; OS, left eye; sph, sphere; VA, visual acuity.

As assessment of the fit of the lenses showed appropriate alignment and movement, a new pair of multifocal GP corneal lenses having the same design was ordered with an increased optic zone diameter of 8.1 mm. The new prescription (Rx) was, OD: −6.50 sph; OS: −5.00 sph; ADD: +2.00 OU. On dispensing, Fran immediately reported elimination of the tunnel vision effect. This increased optic zone diameter, together with the lens power changes at both distance and near, resulted in a satisfied patient with excellent visual acuity (VA). With the new lenses, Fran was able to maintain between 12 and 15 hours of comfortable contact lens wear each day.

Discussion

Fran's blurred near vision was corrected by effectively providing additional plus power to the contact lenses. However, her primary complaint was related to the glare/starburst and tunnel vision effects when wearing the contact lenses. In considering the lens fits, the fluorescein patterns displayed central and secondary zone alignment between the contact lenses and the cornea, while the peripheral curves allowed good tear exchange. Edge lift was optimal in both lenses. The change in the optic zone diameter resolved her complaint.

Although technical expertise and clinical experience are required for the successful fitting of multifocal contact lenses, 1 must be cognizant of the basic design features of corneal GP lenses. Fran's multifocal GP design was characterized by front surface asphericity to reduce peripheral aberrations and back surface asphericity to provide the required add power. This particular lens was designed to be positioned superiorly on the cornea, with upper eyelid attachment, thereby causing the central optic zone to be displaced upward. This will limit the field of view, and can induce the tunnel vision effect seen in this case. Typically, the optic zone is designed to be approximately 1.5 to 2.0 mm smaller than the overall diameter of the contact lens. If the optic zone selected is too small, the apical fitting relationship to the cornea is flattened, the sagittal depth may be reduced, and most importantly the patient's pupil may lie within the transition zone between the central distance vision optic zone and the adjacent aspheric near zones, causing glare/starburst and limiting the field of view for near vision through the contact lens.

If a patient has significant astigmatism, a history of GP corneal contact lens wear, and/or has high visual demands or expectations, then GP bifocals may be the lens of choice as they provide excellent optics for both distance and near vision.[1] However, GP lenses require a full-time commitment by the patient. Patients desiring to wear contact lenses on an occasional basis must readjust to the comfort and awareness of the lenses after each interval without lens wear. If a patient has clinically significant residual astigmatism, then a toric lens design may be necessary for optimal distance vision. Such a lens may not be available in a bifocal design. Another potential obstacle to GP lenses may be multiple years of successful soft contact lens wear. Although a significant improvement in visual resolution may ensue, a long-term soft contact lens patient may be resistant to the initial discomfort/adaptation period, the greater awareness of movement, and the occasional foreign body discomfort that exists with GP contact lenses.

There are 3 categories of GP bifocal contact lenses, namely aspheric front and back surface lenses, concentric lenses, and alternating GP contact lenses. The first 2 types are characterized as simultaneous vision lenses, while the third category is described as translating lenses.[2] In corneal aspheric GP bifocal designs, the contact lens is generally a distance center design with a gradual transition to the maximum near Rx toward the periphery. Concentric GP bifocal contact lenses also usually have a distance center design, surrounded by a circular near Rx zone or zones. Contemporary aspheric and concentric GP bifocals are fit, where possible, superiorly on the cornea with upper eyelid attachment. The lenses make a mild excursion or translation from the distance center to the near add when looking downward to read. This translational eye movement is small; however, aspheric GP multifocal contact lenses are still categorized as simultaneous vision bifocal lenses.[3] Therefore, the position of the upper eyelid margin in relation to the superior limbus/cornea is important. To support a lid attachment fit, the upper eyelid should cover approximately 1.2 to 1.5 mm of the superior corneal surface when the patient is looking straight ahead. Even without a lid attachment fit, it is still possible to use aspheric and concentric GP designs but a significantly steeper base curve may be required for positional stability in the center of the cornea.

Translating GP contact lenses requires the lower eyelid be positioned at or just above the lower limbus in primary gaze. This allows the lower edge of the contact lens to rest on the eyelid margin. As the patient looks down to read, the lower eyelid pushes the lower edge of the contact lens upward, thereby moving the near segment of the translating bifocal contact lens in front of the pupil.

For patients electing soft contact lenses, several bifocal/multifocal lenses have been developed for presbyopia. Concentric or annular designs have a small central annular zone providing either distance or near correction, then are surrounded by a peripheral annulus generating the additional near or distance power, respectively. Aspheric soft multifocal designs use a gradual change of curvature along either the anterior, posterior, or both surfaces of the contact lens. The eccentricity, or rate of flattening, is significantly greater than found in single vision contact lenses, creating an increase in plus power from the center of the lens toward the periphery in a center distance design, or in minus power in a center near design. The quality of vision through aspheric soft contact lens designs can be slightly degraded due to spherical aberration. The highly motivated patient, with sufficient time to adapt to aspheric multifocal designs, can usually overcome an initial awareness of degraded imagery.[4] Aspheric soft multifocal contact lenses are better suited for the early and moderate presbyopes if the asphericity is placed on only 1 surface of the contact lens (usually the back surface). Aspheric soft multifocal lenses incorporating asphericity on both the front and back surface can allow the lens to generate as much as +3.00 diopter add power in some designs.[5]

Fitting bifocal contact lenses requires time, patience, and experience. However, the satisfaction, professional rewards and recognition, as well as the ability to develop a successful contact lens specialty practice make the challenge worthwhile.

CLINICAL PEARLS

- Present every suitable patient with the option of multifocal contact lenses.

- Ensure that your multifocal contact lens patient candidate is prepared to allow the necessary adaptation time as well as the multiple office visits required to achieve success.

- Determine whether your patient is best suited for a GP contact lens or a soft contact lens multifocal.

- Equip your practice with a sufficient number of both GP and soft multifocal contact lens designs to provide the optimal option for your patient.

REFERENCES

1. Bennett ES, Weissman BA. *Clinical Contact Lens Practice, Chapter 27 (Presbyopia)*. Philadelphia, PA: Lippincott Williams & Wilkins; 2005:531-548.
2. Toshida H, Takahashi K, Sado K, Kanai A, Murakami A. Bifocal contact lenses; history, types, characteristics, and actual state and problems, *Clin Ophthalmol.* December 2008;2(4):869-877.
3. Bennett ES. Innovations in gas permeable multifocal contact lenses. *Clin Optom.* 2010;2:85-90.
4. Benoit DP. Prescribing for presbyopia. What are you waiting for? *Contact Lens Spect.* October 2017;32:15.
5. Perez-Prados R, Pinero D, Perez-Cambrodi R, Madrid-Costa D. Soft multifocal simultaneous image contact lenses: a review. *Clin Exp Optom.* 2017;100:107-127.

2.4 Management of Keratoconus With Gas Permeable Contact Lenses

Beth Kinoshita

Theresa, a 23-year-old Caucasian female, presented with a chief concern of reduced vision over the past 2 years, particularly in her right eye. She did not use any refractive correction. The personal and family medical histories was unremarkable. Theresa denied any history of eye infection, injuries, or eye rubbing. There were no known ocular allergies.

Clinical Findings

Unaided distance VA	OD: 20/200 (PH 20/30^{-2}); OS: 20/200 (PH 20/30^{-2}); OU: 20/200
Pupil evaluation	PERRL; no RAPD
Keratometry (The Efron Grading Scale was used to grade the amount of distortion.[1])	OD: 51.00 × 47.00 @ 020; 2+ distortion OS: 50.00 × 45.00 @ 155; 2+ distortion
Medmont Corneal Topographer Simulated Keratometric Measurements (Figure 2.4-1)	OD: 52.20 @ 131/47.50 @ 041 OS: 49.50 @ 064/45.50 @ 154
Retinoscopy (scissor reflex was observed in each eye)	OD: +3.25 −3.25 × 105 OS: +4.25 −2.50 × 090
Subjective refraction	OD: +3.50 −3.25 × 105 (20/40) OS: +4.00 −3.50 × 080 (20/40)
Intraocular pressure (GAT)	OD: 12 mm Hg; OS 12 mm Hg at 2:36 PM
Slit-lamp examination	OD and OS: lids, lashes, lacrimal: clean; bulbar conjunctiva: white/quiet; palpebral conjunctiva: pink/healthy; cornea: trace striae, no scarring, no Fleischer ring; iris: flat/avascular; angles: 1:1 × 1:1 by Van Herick; anterior chamber: deep/quiet
Fundus examination	Unremarkable OU

Abbreviations: GAT, Goldmann applanation tonometry; OD, right eye; OS, left eye; OU, both eyes; PERRL, pupils equal, round, reactive to light; PH, pinhole; RAPD, relative afferent pupillary defect; VA, visual acuity.

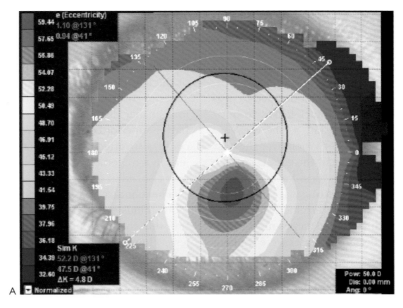

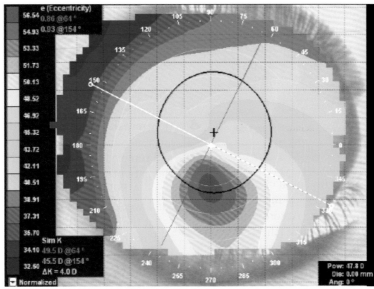

Figure 2.4-1 Axial maps showing inferior steepening with superior-nasal flattening in each eye. The black circle indicates the position of the pupil.

Comments

The topographic corneal maps (Figure 2.4-1) were consistent with a diagnosis of keratoconus with irregular astigmatism in each eye. Because corneal steepening coincided with the visual axis, this would explain the reduced visual acuity (VA).

Theresa was diagnosed with mild-to-moderate keratoconus with striae, and irregular astigmatism, which was worse in the right eye, thereby contributing to decreased best corrected VA through refraction. Inferior paracentral steepening with superior flattening was observed on corneal topography. Interestingly, compound hyperopic astigmatism is somewhat unusual in a patient with keratoconus.[2]

The patient was educated regarding this condition, including its incidence, progression, hypothesized etiology, and possible refractive treatment options. Spectacles were prescribed to achieve VA of 20/40, which was a marked improvement over her unaided vision. Alternative refractive options that were considered included gas-permeable (GP) (either corneal or scleral) contact lenses, customized soft contact lenses (SCL), and hybrid contact lenses, as well as corneal cross-linking and Intacs.

After discussion, the patient decided to proceed with corneal GP contact lenses to optimize distance and near vision, as she was very aware of the decline in her vision over the past 2 years. Both the position of the ectasia and the corneal eccentricity were ideal for an aspheric GP design. A diagnostic fitting was performed, with the initial lens determined from the keratometry reading in the steeper meridian.

The following diagnostic lenses were applied:

	OD	OS
Type	Aspheric KC lens	Aspheric KC lens
Base curve	52.00 D (6.49 mm)	50.00 D (6.75 mm)
Power	−10.00 D	−9.00 D
Overall diameter	9.6 mm	9.6 mm

Abbreviations: D, diopters; KC, keratoconus; OD, right eye; OS, left eye.

When positioned on the eye, both lenses decentered inferiorly with apical clearance. The lenses had unobstructed vertical movement with minimal superior edge lift. Accordingly, a lens with a 2.00 D flatter base curve (the next lens in the fitting set) was tried to improve centration, as steep lenses generally decenter inferiorly. Slight apical clearance with good centration was achieved in each eye. The over-refraction in each eye was +1.50 sph giving 20/20 acuity.

Lens order:

	OD	OS
Type	Aspheric KC lens	Aspheric KC lens
Base curve	50.00 D (6.75 mm)	48.00 D (7.03 mm)
Power	−7.50 D	−6.75 D
Overall diameter	9.6 mm	9.6 mm

Abbreviations: D, diopters; OD, right eye; OS, left eye.

Other options for improving the contact lens centration could have been to flatten the peripheral curve to allow for unobstructed vertical movement or to specify more eccentricity of the lens design to help align with the flatter superior cornea. The lens could also be ordered in a smaller diameter to interact less with the flatter superior cornea. The weight of the lens could also affect the centration. Ordering a lens in a material with a lower specific gravity may also aid in centration.

The contact lens prescription had much more minus power than the manifest refraction due to the steeper nature of the contact lens. However, these values are still relatively low, when compared with many cases of keratoconus. The patient was scheduled for a dispensing visit with training in application and removal.

At the dispensing visit, after the lenses were applied, Theresa exhibited immediate reflex tearing with moderate discomfort. However, once the lenses were allowed to settle, she reported improved comfort and good vision. Distance VA was 20/20 in each eye with a plano (Pl) sphere over-refraction. Slit-lamp examination revealed a well-centered lens with apical clearance and average edge lift OU. Application and removal were performed successfully, and the patient was instructed to build up wearing time. A follow-up appointment was scheduled for 1 week.

At the 1-week follow-up visit, both distance and near VAs were 20/20 in each eye with plano sphere over-refraction. No change in lens fitting was required. Theresa was scheduled for a 6-month progress examination and encouraged to continue with her current lens care cleaning products.

Discussion

Keratoconus is a disease that affects approximately 1 in 1800 people.[3] It is generally bilateral but sometimes presents asymmetrically.[2] The early, subclinical stage is best visualized with a corneal topographer where inferior corneal steepening with superior flattening is most commonly observed, although atypical presentations may occur. As this noninflammatory disease progresses, the corneal nerves become more prominent and the cornea

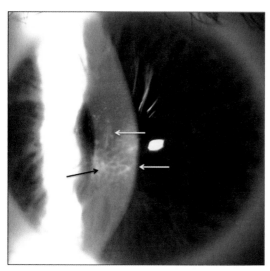

Figure 2.4-2 Advanced keratoconus with Vogt striae (white arrows) and corneal scarring (black arrow).

shows signs of thinning with Vogt striae (from the compression of Descemet membrane), a Fleischer ring (produced by iron deposition at the base of the corneal cone) and scarring (Figure 2.4-2).[2] Frequently, the most pronounced symptom is reduced best-corrected VA with spectacles and conventional soft contact lenses, although in the early stages of keratoconus, the patient may do well with these options. Late-stage findings include Munson's sign, that is, stretching of the lower lid on downgaze from the steep cornea, and Rizutti's sign, that is, the conical reflection of the nasal cornea when a light is shone onto the temporal limbus.

Keratoconus can be classified into 3 topographical morphologies. A nipple cone has a small diameter with a centered apex combined with a fairly regular peripheral cornea. The oval shape is the most common where the apex is located more inferiorly. This results in a steep inferior cornea with rapid superior flattening. The third type is keratoglobus, when 75% of the cornea is affected, and generally is considered the most challenging to fit with contact lenses.[2] Other, less common types of keratoconus include forme fruste keratoconus, which is a mild manifestation of keratoconus and posterior keratoconus, where the posterior cornea steepens more profoundly than the anterior cornea.

When making the diagnosis of keratoconus, other ectasias should be excluded. For example, pellucid marginal degeneration often exhibits a "kissing pigeons" topography (Figure 2.4-3). The inferior steepening is accompanied by corneal thinning in the inferior periphery. Generally, striae or corneal scarring are not associated with this condition. Terrien marginal degeneration shows stromal opacification in its early stages, with corneal thinning that starts superiorly and progresses circumferentially in the latter stages. Post-LASIK ectasia has topographic findings similar to keratoconus, but can be identified based on the history of refractive surgery.

The etiology of keratoconus is poorly understood despite extensive research into the condition. Hypotheses include the association of keratocyte apoptosis and keratoconus due to the higher presence of interleukin-1.[4] Interleukin-1 is also thought to be released by microtrauma to the cornea that may be exacerbated by contact lens wear, eye rubbing, or atopy.[5] The loss of keratocytes may lead to the release of degradative enzymes and the loss of stromal thickness.[4] Alternately, it may be associated with a decrease in the biochemical strength of the cornea due to decreased crosslinks within the stromal collagen fibers. This hypothesis has led to the use of collagen cross-linking in an attempt to stabilize and slow the progression of the disease. Vitamin B_2 (riboflavin) is applied to the cornea and exposed to ultraviolet A (370 nm) radiation to create covalent bonds between the stromal collagen fibers.[6] A recent investigation found stabilization of corneal curvature changes after this treatment.[7] However, the procedure is not recommended for corneas less than 400 micrometers thick, due to a higher likelihood of interaction with the endothelium. Generally speaking, cross-linking is recommended in eyes with progressive keratoconus.[6] The United States Food and Drug Administration (FDA) approved this procedure in April 2016. Current research suggests a stabilization of corneal curvature changes.[8]

There is also a genetic component to keratoconus. The estimated prevalence in first-degree relatives is between 15 and 67 times higher than in the general population.

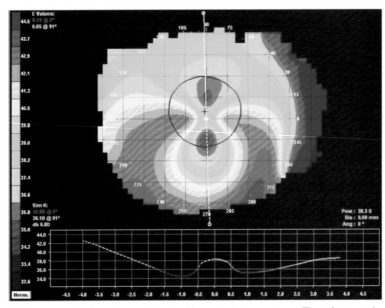

Figure 2.4-3   Axial topography of a patient with pellucid marginal degeneration. The inferior mid-peripheral steepening (red) surrounds a flatter central corneal curvature (blue).

A natural history study found no association between family history and the severity of the disease.[9]

Management of keratoconus with GP contact lenses has been shown to delay the need for surgical intervention in approximately 99% of cases.[10] Corneal GP contact lenses are used most commonly, although there is a resurgence in the use of other lens modalities, including hybrid, scleral, and custom SCL.

An aspheric corneal GP lens can achieve a higher rate of flattening so was chosen for Theresa due to her higher corneal eccentricity, which is common in keratoconus. This design can begin flattening from the center of the contact lens or have a spherical optical zone and then begin to flatten from the edge of the optical zone out to the periphery.

Theresa did well with corneal GP contact lenses. If this were not the case, a scleral lens would have been considered. In general, a starting point to consider a scleral lens is to determine the height difference along the meridian that has the largest elevation difference on an elevation topographical map. If that number is 350 micrometers or more, it is more likely that a scleral lens is more appropriate.[11] An appropriately fit scleral lens will vault the cornea and limbus and land on the sclera.

Generally, the visual complications of keratoconus are well managed with contact lenses. It seems likely that this condition will be diagnosed more frequently due to the greater prevalence of corneal topographers and other imaging devices, especially within refractive surgery centers. The contact lens management of keratoconus is considered the standard of care for mild- to moderate-forms of the ectasia. The lens creates a regular, anterior refractive surface, and allows the patient's tears to fill in the voids beneath the contact lens. The comfort and vision achieved with contact lenses can have a tremendous impact on the quality of life of patients with keratoconus.[12]

CLINICAL PEARLS

- In early forms of an ectasia, if there is only mild corneal distortion on keratometry and the manifest refraction yields good acuity, consider prescribing spectacles or an "off the rack" soft contact lens.

- When the retinoscopy reflex is scissoring or distorted and the refraction does not produce clear endpoints, consider performing keratometry or topography to screen for keratoconus prior to concluding the refraction. This will give you a good idea if there is high astigmatism or an ectasia contributing to the difficulty of the refraction.

- Many contact lens options are available specifically for keratoconus.

- When looking at the elevation topographical map, if there is more than 350 micrometers of corneal elevation difference along 1 meridian, consider fitting with a scleral contact lens.

- Corneal cross-linking is FDA approved for keratoconus that is documented as progressing.

REFERENCES

1. Efron N. *Contact Lens Complications*. 3rd ed. Philadelphia, PA: Saunders; June 19, 2012:5 pp.
2. Romero-Jimenez M, Santodomingo-Rubido J, Wolffsohn J. Keratoconus: a review. *Cont Lens Anterior Eye*. 2010;33:157-166.
3. Kennedy R, Bourne W, Dyer J. A 48-year clinical and epidemiologic study of keratoconus. *Am J Ophthalmol*. 1986;101(3):267-273.
4. Kim W-J, Rabinowitz Y, Meisler D, WIlson S. Keratocyte apoptosis associated with keratoconus. *Exp Eye Res*. 1999;69:475-481.
5. Wilson S, Mohan R, Mohan R, Ambrosio R, Hong J, Lee J. The corneal wound healing response: cytokine-mediated interaction of the epithelium, stroma, and inflammatory cells. *Prog Retinal Eye Res*. 2001;20(5):625-637.
6. Chan E, Snibson GR. Current status of corneal collagen cross-linking for keratoconus: a review. *Clin Exp Optom*. 2013;96:155-164.
7. Giacomin NT, Netto MV, Torricelli AA, et al. Corneal collagen cross-linking in advanced keratoconus: a 4-year follow-up study. *J Refract Surg*. 2016;32(7):6.
8. O'Brart D, Patel P, Lascaratos G, et al. Corneal cross-linking to halt the progression of keratoconus and corneal ectasia: seven-year follow-up. *Am J Ophthalmol*. 2015;160(6):10.
9. Szczotka-Flynn L, Slaughter M, McMahon T, et al. Disease severity and family history in keratoconus. *Br J Ophthalmol*. 2008;92:1108-1111.
10. Bilgin L, Yilmaz S, Araz B, Yuksel S, Sezen T. 30 years of contact lens prescribing for keratoconic patients in Turkey. *Cont Lens Anterior Eye*. 2009;32:16-21.
11. Zheng F, Caroline P, Kojima R, Kinoshita B, Andre M, Lampa M. Corneal elevation differences and the initial selection of therapeutic contact lens. Global Specialty Lens Symposium, Las Vegas, NV, 2015.
12. Wagner H, Barr J, Zadnik K. Collaborative Longitudinal Evaluation of Keratoconus (CLEK) Study: methods and findings to date. *Cont Lens Anterior Eye*. 2007; 30:223-232.

2.5 Contact Lens Noncompliance: Medico-legal

Barry A. Weissman

James, a 32-year-old Caucasian male, was referred by his local optometrist for specialty contact lens care. He had radial keratotomy (RK) performed in each eye 6 years ago. James reported that his unaided vision had been excellent in each eyes after the procedure, but over the past 12 to 18 months he had noted decreasing distance vision in both eyes, especially at night.

The optometrist's report documented a comprehensive eye examination performed 2 weeks earlier, including a dilated fundus evaluation, with no ocular or systemic health concerns apart from distorted and scarred corneas in each eye. Eight incision RK was seen in each eye with a few inclusion cysts. No staining, edema, infiltrates or neovascularization was noted. A new spectacle prescription had been provided as James did not have any glasses. However, it was recognized that this would be a challenging contact lens fitting, and it was suggested that he wait to fill the spectacle prescription pending contact lens care.

Clinical Findings

Unaided distance VA	OD: 20/80^{-1} (pinhole 20/25^{+1}); OS: 20/50^{-2} (pinhole 20/25^{+1})
Manual keratometry	OD: 40.39 × 38.00 @ 150; 2+ distortion; OS: 41.50 × 38.25 @ 170; 2+ distortion
Subjective refraction	OD: −0.50 −1.50 × 150 (20/50$^-$; pinhole 20/20) OS: +0.75 −2.00 × 122 (20/40$^-$; pinhole 20/20)

Abbreviations: OD, right eye; OS, left eye; VA, visual acuity.

Slit lamp and fundus evaluation confirmed findings of the referring optometrist.

Comments

James was diagnosed with distorted and scarred corneas secondary to RK with non-eroding inclusion cysts, and with resultant irregular astigmatism causing decreased visual acuity (VA) in each eye. It was recommended that James obtain a backup pair of spectacles, with the suggestion of polycarbonate lenses for eye protection. He was counseled regarding the persistent possible mechanical weakness of each cornea from the surgery that might potentiate any damage from trauma. Accordingly, eye protection was to be encouraged as much as possible, and particularly if James found himself in potentially hazardous situations. He was also counseled that spectacle vision would likely be variable and not as optimal as through gas-permeable (GP) contact lenses. A custom GP contact lens fitting was agreed on.

Over the course of 3 clinical evaluations, custom GP contact lenses were fitted and refined for each eye, having an overall diameter of 9.3 mm, a lens material with Dk of 100 and a base curve in reasonable alignment with the irregular corneas. On the third visit, the contact lenses appeared both mechanically and optically optimal (resulting in VA of 20/15^{-1} in each eye) and were dispensed. James was trained in appropriate contact lens application, removal, and care, and scheduled to return in 1 week for his first progress evaluation. He left the office apparently satisfied and appreciative of the care and improvement in vision.

Unfortunately, James failed to return for his follow-up evaluation. Several phone calls and voice messages were left for him (and documented in the record). Eventually, a letter was mailed to him asking him to make an appointment. He failed to respond to all communication.

Three months later, James telephoned the office requesting a replacement right lens. He reported loss of the lens while cleaning. This spare lens was dispensed in office following a professional evaluation that did not show any complications. He was advised to return in 2 weeks so that the continued adequacy of his contact lens prescription after a reasonable wearing time could be confirmed. It was documented in the record that he was advised that such care was not only necessary to prove his contact lenses were optimal, and if this was indeed the case, to allow for a finalized contact lens prescription in compliance with the US Fairness to Contact Lens Consumers Act. Unfortunately, he failed to keep his scheduled appointment, and again multiple telephone calls and voice mails were unsuccessful in getting him to return.

James next contacted the office by telephone 2 years later. He had lost the right contact lens (again). Although this was his chief and only complaint on the call, at the appointment to dispense the new lens, he also reported that both lenses were moving on his eyes more than he liked. Unaided and pinhole VA in the right eye were similar to that found at the previous evaluation. Aided vision (with the old contact lens) in the left eye was 20/20^{-}. Fluorescein evaluation suggested the left lens fit was now mildly steep, as well as loose in movement. On laboratory analysis, the left lens also was found to be warped. An undilated ocular examination suggested stability in all findings with the exception of his central keratometry readings, which

were each about 2 D flatter than previously measured, with a corresponding hyperopic shift in refractive error in each eye of about 2 D.

Impressions from this visit included continued non-eroding inclusion cysts and irregular astigmatism as well as a progressive hyperopic shift and corneal flattening due to corneal weakening; all of these changes were secondary to RK.[1] The following recommendations were provided:

1. A comprehensive eye examination with his previous optometrist including dilation and provision of emergency backup spectacle prescription (which the patient had never obtained).

2. Consultation with a corneal surgeon for consideration of cross-linking to assist corneal stability.[2]

3. A contact lens refit.

The initial portion of the refitting was performed immediately, and James was sent to the front desk so that new initial contact lenses could be ordered as well as to schedule the dispensing and other professional appointments as noted earlier.

At the end of the day, it was discovered that James had refused to order lenses or to make any of the recommended appointments for financial reasons. He did state that he would return within 2 weeks to follow through.

James next contacted the office about 9 months later by e-mail. He informed the office staff that he had no telephone and could only communicate in this manner. He requested a copy of the contact lens prescription determined 9 months earlier be sent to him by e-mail immediately. (These lenses had never been ordered, never dispensed, and never validated after wear in-office.) Otherwise, he demanded a refund of the charges for that professional examination. Several e-mails were sent to him explaining that this would not be good care, and that he should make an appointment for an in-office evaluation, as his corneas could have changed further in the intervening 9 months and a newer fitting might be more appropriate. In addition, he should have a general eye examination and a corneal specialist evaluation. However, he became more strident in tone and belligerent, eventually demanding the prescription without any professional care, quoting portions of the US Federal Fairness to Contact Lens Consumers Act.

The optometrist now took over the e-mail correspondence from the staff and again tried to explain the importance of professional care that was necessary for optimal results. James was also provided with a copy of the entire US 2004 Federal Fairness to Contact Lens Consumers Act, specifically pointing out that contact lens prescriptions are to be provided to patients only after the prescribing clinician has had the opportunity to ensure that such contact lenses are optimal on the eyes following some wear. It was explained that, due to the patient's (documented) corneal flattening as well as repetitive noncompliance, it was impossible to ensure that any contact lenses were adequate, let alone optimal, for his eyes at that time. Accordingly, there was no contact lens prescription to be forwarded. At this point, the patient became abusive to the optometrist and threatened legal action if the unfinalized contact lens prescription was not sent to him immediately and without further discussion.

After this communication, the optometrist took all of the records, including the complete e-mail exchange to legal counsel. After consideration, the lawyer advised that all actions appeared to have been totally appropriate. She advised that the patient be sent a "30-day letter" informing him that the office and/or optometrist would take care of any contact lens-related emergencies (which in her opinion did not include replacing lost contact lenses without further evaluation) for 30 days. Following that time interval, he would be responsible to transfer his contact lens and other ophthalmic care to another practitioner. Included in this letter was also an offer to provide a practitioner of his choice with a copy of the entire medical record. As the office had no valid mailing address for James, in lieu of a registered letter, the document was signed, scanned as an electronic file, and attached to an e-mail that was sent to the patient.

James has not contacted the office or optometrists since.

Discussion

Noncompliant patients can contribute to their own problems. This patient was also abusive and aggressive. Nevertheless, clinicians retain an obligation to teach, train, and advise what they believe, based on their best clinical judgment, to be in the patient's best interest. And when a patient choses an alternative path, that is also their right. It is the clinician's obligation to document the efforts that have been made to act in the patient's best interests. This will protect both the practitioner and the practice from any self-harm done by the noncompliant patient.

CLINICAL PEARLS

- As an eyecare practitioner, you must always act in what your knowledge, training, and experience leads you to believe is in the best interest of the patient. Rarely, this may be in conflict with the patient's desires. When such a conflict occurs, often the best course of action is to part ways with the patient. Although this will often be an amiable parting sometimes, as was seen here, it was less than friendly.

- Document every communication with the patient in the record, including all discussions, telephone calls, e-mails, text messages, and so on. That way you will be able to provide support for your clinical actions should that become necessary.

REFERENCES

1. Waring GO, Lynn MJ, McDonnell PJ. Results of the prospective evaluation of radial keratotomy (PERK) study 10 years after surgery. *Arch Ophthalmol.* October 1994;112(10):1298-308.
2. Elbaz U, Yeung SN, Ziai S, et al. Collagen crosslinking after radial keratotomy. *Cornea.* February 2014;33(2): 131-136.

2.6 Contact Lens Noncompliance: Therapeutic

Kathryn Deliso

Joey, a 20-year-old Caucasian male, presented with redness, itching, and an inability to wear his contact lenses for more than a few hours a day. He stated that a few hours after applying his contact lenses his vision seems blurry at both distance and near, which is temporarily relieved when he puts on a new pair of lenses the next day. As a college student, he reported that he is studying for midterm examinations and has been wearing his hydrogel contact lenses for "longer than he should- from about 7 AM to 10 PM." His current contact lenses were approximately 5 weeks old, and he generally disposed them when they felt uncomfortable or when they rip. He admitted it could be "several months." He cleaned the lenses with generic multipurpose solution and reported occasional overnight wear about 1 to 2 times per week. He did not have a pair of glasses with him but knew his prescription was around −4.50 in each eye.

Joey's last complete eye examination with a contact lens evaluation was about a year and a half ago with his hometown optometrist. Other than this recurring intolerance to his contact lenses, ocular history was reportedly unremarkable. He played rugby in college and occasionally took Advil for aches and injuries that occur on the field. He was otherwise in good health.

Clinical Findings

Aided distance VA (through contact lenses)	OD: 20/25−; OS: 20/30−2
Confrontation fields	Full to finger counting OD and OS
Pupil evaluation	PERRL/no RAPD
Slit-lamp examination	OD: lids/lashes: 1+ large papillae superior tarsal conjunctiva; conjunctiva: trace injection, loss of translucency; cornea: clear; iris: flat, no neovascularization; lens: clear OS: lids/lashes: 1+ large papillae superior tarsal conjunctiva; conjunctiva: trace injection, loss of translucency; cornea: clear; iris: flat, no neovascularization; lens: clear
Contact lens assessment	OD: full corneal coverage, 1-2 mm movement, small rip at 5 o'clock; OS: full corneal coverage, 1-2 mm movement, 1+ deposits

Abbreviations: OD, right eye; OS, left eye; PERRL, pupils equal, round, reactive to light; RAPD, relative afferent pupillary defect; VA, visual acuity.

Discussion

Joey presented with complaints of redness, itching, and contact lens intolerance. On further questioning, it became clear that he was overwearing his hydrogel contact lenses and wearing them as an extended/flexible wear contact lens. Slit-lamp evaluation revealed significant papillae on his

193

superior tarsal conjunctiva and loss of conjunctival translucency of both eyes, and he was diagnosed with giant papillary conjunctivitis (GPC) secondary to contact lenses (see Chapter 2.21). He was encouraged to discontinue contact lens wear until advised to resume, and he was prescribed loteprednol 0.5% to be used 4 times a day. At his 2-week follow-up, his symptoms had improved and the conjunctival papillae had decreased. It was recommended that he slowly resume contact lens wear starting with 4 hours per day up to a maximum of 12 hours per day after being refit with a daily disposable lens. He was told to reduce the loteprednol dosage to twice a day for 2 weeks. At his 1-month follow-up visit, he reported a significant improvement in lens tolerance and no irritation.

There were several issues of noncompliance in addition to the overwear of his contact lenses. Joey was not replacing his lenses according to the manufacturer's indication. As lenses are worn longer, they have the potential to buildup debris. To further exacerbate the condition of the lenses, Joey was using an unknown contact lens care system. It is important to prescribe a specific care system and to ensure the patient follows the instructions. It may be beneficial in office to have the patient actually demonstrate the steps taken each evening and morning. The importance of backup spectacles should also be emphasized. It is impossible for patients to discontinue lens wear if they have no available correction. This also discourages patients to give their eyes any break from contact lens wear in the morning and evening.

Giant papillary conjunctivitis is an inflammatory response that occurs secondary to mechanical stimuli of the tarsal conjunctiva. This can occur as a response to contact lenses, ocular prosthesis, or exposed sutures.[1] Giant papillary conjunctivitis has been observed with all types of contact lenses, but is most common with HEMA-based hydrogel contacts.[2] It can present after long-term contact lens wear or as soon as a few weeks after initiating contact lens wear. If unmanaged, it can be a cause for complete discontinuation of contact lens wear. Patients presenting with GPC generally have complaints of irritation or itching, conjunctival redness, mucus accumulation with subsequent blurred vision, and (if due to contact lens wear) excessive contact lens movement, discomfort,

and intolerance. On slit-lamp evaluation with lid eversion, there are papillae along the tarsal conjunctiva, variable conjunctival hyperemia, and mucus strands.[2] Conjunctival tarsal papillae increase in size as mechanical stimulation continues to occur. Eventually, papillae advance into a layered pattern of characteristic giant papillae (greater than 0.3 mm in diameter) with many being up to 1 mm in size.[1] Contact lenses may demonstrate excessive movement or superior decentration due to contact with the papillae on the tarsal plate. In severe cases, there may be severe hyperemia, copious mucus production, and papillary hypertrophy of the superior tarsal conjunctiva leading to loss of conjunctival translucency. Unless there is a unilateral exposed suture or foreign body, GPC is typically bilateral.

Although the diagnosis is usually straightforward, effective treatment of GPC can be a challenge, especially if the patient is not compliant. Initial treatment begins by removing the source of irritation by discontinuing all contact lens wear until there is sufficient resolution. Generally, contact lens wear can resume after improvement in symptoms and patients should be refit in a different lens type, material, and more frequent replacement schedule. If daily disposable lenses are not an option, patients are encouraged to decrease wear time, improve lens hygiene, and use hydrogen peroxide, and/or enzyme cleaning system. Cool compresses and chilled preservative-free artificial tears can also be recommended to improve symptoms. The frequency of follow-ups will vary with the severity of the condition. With proper treatment, approximately 80% of patients who develop GPC secondary to contact lenses can resume contact lens wear without discomfort.[3] Unfortunately, recurrence is common. In cases where GPC cannot be managed, refractive surgery options can be recommended to prevent recurrence.

CLINICAL PEARLS

- Patients presenting with GPC generally complain of irritation or itching, conjunctival redness, mucus accumulation with subsequent blurred vision, and (if due to contact lens wear) excessive contact lens movement, discomfort and intolerance.

- Palpebral conjunctiva evaluation with eyelid eversion reveals papillae along the tarsal conjunctiva, variable conjunctival hyperemia, and mucus strands.

- Effective treatment of GPC must involve removing the source of irritation and discontinuing all contact lens wear until symptoms have improved.

- Patient education regarding contact lens compliance is critical.

REFERENCES

1. Allansmith MR, Korb DR, Greiner JV, et al. Giant papillary conjunctivitis in contact lens wearers. *Am J Ophthalmol.* 1977;83(5):697-708.
2. Suchecki JK, Donshik P, Ehlers WH. Contact lens complications. *Ophthalmol Clin North Am.* September 2003;16(3):471-84.
3. Donshik P, Ballow M, Luistro A, Samartino L. Treatment of contact lens-induced giant papillary conjunctivitis. *CLAO J.* October–December 1984;10(4): 3466-3450.

2.7 Hordeolum

Padhmalatha Segu, Janet Garza, Marsha Thomas, and Bhagya Segu

Mario, a 36-year-old Hispanic male, presented for an emergency eye examination. He reported pain and discomfort in his left upper eyelid, which began 2 days ago. Mario reported that his upper left eyelid was swollen, painful, and tender to touch when he woke up. Associated symptoms included itching, watery discharge, and sensitivity to light. Mario denied any decrease in vision, diplopia, recent upper respiratory tract infection, fever or trauma. He reported a similar problem in the lower right eyelid 2 weeks ago. Mario stated the "bump" in his right eyelid was still present but no longer painful after it drained spontaneously. Mario's family ocular and medical histories were unremarkable. The only medication taken was a daily multivitamin. Mario has smoked 1 pack of cigarettes daily for the past 15 years. There were no allergies to medication, animals, or the environment.

Clinical Findings

Unaided Distance VA	OD 20/20; OS 20/20
Confrontation visual field	Full to finger counting OD and OS
Ocular motility	Unrestricted. No pain on eye movement OU
Pupil evaluation	PERRL; no RAPD
Intraocular pressure (NCT)	OD 16 mm Hg; OS 13 mm Hg at 2:00 PM
Preauricular nodes	Soft. No tenderness
Slit-lamp examination	OD: 1+ meibomian gland dysfunction; eyelid: 2-3 mm diameter, single nodular lower lid lesion not tender to palpation, no erythema; conjunctiva: pinguecula nasally; angles 4 × 4 by Van Herick estimation;
	OS: 1+ meibomian gland dysfunction; eyelid: 2-3 mm diameter, single nodular upper lid lesion with erythema and tenderness to palpation; conjunctiva: pinguecula nasally; angles 4 × 4 by Van Herick estimation
Tear breakup time	4-5 s OD and OS

Abbreviations: NCT, non-contact tonometry; OD, right eye; OS, left eye; OU, both eyes; PERRL, pupils equal, round, reactive to light; RAPD, relative afferent pupillary defect; VA, visual acuity.

Comments

Based on the clinical presentation and symptoms, diagnoses of an internal hordeolum in the left eye and a chalazion in the right eye were reached. These were treated with a combination of topical and oral antibiotics as well as supportive therapy. Mario was instructed to place warm compresses on his eyelids several times a day, to perform eyelid scrubs twice a day, use polysporin ointment OU at bedtime, and take oral doxycycline hyclate (100 mg) twice a day for 10 days. The latter was prescribed to help with the underlying meibomian gland dysfunction. The importance of lid hygiene was discussed, and premoistened lid scrub samples were dispensed. Proper lid hygiene and warm compresses will minimize potential future infections of the eyelid glands. Mario was instructed to return in 10 days or sooner if no improvement in symptoms was found.

At the 10-day follow-up, Mario reported an improvement in his symptoms, with resolution of pain and tenderness in the left eye. He reported using the warm compresses for a few days, but did not perform the lid scrubs. Mario did take the oral medication as prescribed, and used the topical medication at night with no reported side effects. The chalazion in the right eye persisted. He described his vision as being stable.

The following were his clinical findings at this visit:

Unaided distance VA	OD 20/20; OS 20/20
Slit-lamp examination	OD: trace to 1+ meibomian gland dysfunction; eyelid: 2 mm diameter, single nodular lower lid lesion not tender to palpation; conjunctiva: pinguecula nasally;
	OS: trace to 1+ meibomian gland dysfunction; eyelid: no lesion, internal hordeolum completely resolved; conjunctiva: pinguecula nasally
Tear breakup time	4 s OD and OS

Abbreviations: OD, right eye; OS, left eye; VA, visual acuity.

Comments

The internal hordeolum in the left eye had completely resolved. The chalazion in the right eye was still present. The need to maintain lid hygiene with warm compresses and lid scrubs daily was emphasized. To improve the quality of his tear film, non-preserved artificial tear

drops were prescribed (4 times daily in both eyes). Follow-up care was recommended until the chalazion in the right eye had resolved.

Discussion

A hordeolum is a painful mass originating from a bacterial infection of the glands located within the eyelid and/or lash follicle.[1] Individuals with inadequate lid hygiene are at risk for developing this lesion.[2] Patients with blepharitis, meibomian gland dysfunction, and acne rosacea may suffer from chronic eyelid infection and inflammation.[2] Clinical symptoms include a painful eyelid mass with associated swelling, which is tender to touch. The amount of pain is directly proportional to the amount of swelling.[2,3] Clinical signs include a localized swelling of recent onset, and erythema encompassing the infected gland.

An external hordeolum (commonly known as a stye[2,3]) is caused by an infection of the gland of Moll and/or Zeiss.[4] This type tends to point toward the infected gland along the eyelid margin in the form of a pustule.[4] An internal hordeolum is an infection that occurs within the sebaceous meibomian gland.[1,2,4] Here, diffuse eyelid edema may occur, and therefore it is important for the practitioner to examine the tarsal conjunctiva (including eyelid eversion) to localize the infected gland[4] (Figure 2.7-1). The development of a chalazion can occur in patients with a chronic internal hordeolum.[2]

Many cases are self-limiting, and these patients may not seek medical attention.[2] Typically, the condition resolves spontaneously within a few days or weeks following drainage of the abscess.[1-4] The main focus of treatment is to expedite recovery time and minimize symptoms. Warm compresses facilitate drainage of the infected gland.[3] The practitioner may consider epilation of any infected eyelash follicles to aid with abscess drainage.[2] Lid scrubs are beneficial to maintain lid hygiene and reduce the levels of bacteria. This should prevent reoccurrence of the hordeolum.[2] Artificial tears will stabilize the tear film, and wash away discharge as the hordeolum drains.

Staphylococcal bacteria are commonly associated with hordeola.[5] Therefore, oral and topical antibiotics are selected to target this

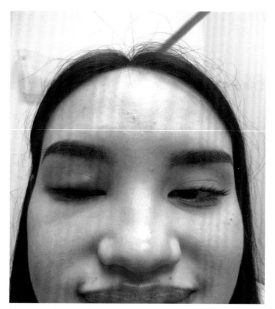

Figure 2.7-1   Example of an internal hordeolum.

infectious agent. Topical antibiotics minimize the risk of the infection spreading to the adjacent lash follicles, ocular surface, and skin.[2,4] Effective topical antibiotic ointments include bacitracin, erythromycin, and polysporin. Systemic antibiotics, such as medications from the penicillin, cephalosporin and/or tetracycline category are prescribed for an internal hordeolum, or when topical antibiotics are not effective.[2] The anti-inflammatory properties of doxycycline, when combined with antimicrobial effects, will treat the underlying meibomian gland dysfunction.[6]

As was seen here, patients with a hordeolum will present with a painful, tender "bump" on the eyelid. The management of Mario's case included supportive therapy, topical and systemic antibiotics. Swelling of the eyelid can be caused by a variety of conditions, including, but not limited to, blunt trauma, tumor, allergy, and infection.[4] Therefore, it is important for the practitioner to determine

the underlying source of the swelling, and to rule out any clinical signs associated with orbital malignancy such as loss of eyelid anatomy, madarosis, recurrent chalazia in the same location, ulceration of the skin, evidence of proptosis, or symptoms of diplopia.[7] The case history, clinical symptoms, and the clinical presentation will aid in the diagnosis of a hordeolum.

CLINICAL PEARLS

- Lid hygiene, including warm compresses, is an effective maintenance therapy option for meibomian gland dysfunction, the key predisposing cause for hordeola.

- During the ocular health examination, it is important for the practitioner to rule out underlying malignancies masquerading as hordeola.

- Early treatment of hordeolum may reduce the risk of chalazion formation.

- The amount of pain associated with a hordeolum is directly proportional to the amount of swelling.

REFERENCES

1. Carlisle RT, Digiovanni J. Differential diagnosis of the swollen red eyelid. *Am Fam Phys.* July 2015; 92(2):106-112.
2. Lindsley K, Nichols JJ, Dickersin K. Interventions for acute internal hordeolum. *Cochrane Database Syst Rev.* 2013;(4):CD007742.
3. Olson MD. The common stye. *J Sch Health.* February 1991;61(2):95-97.
4. Wald ER. Periorbital and orbital infections. *Infect Dis Clin North Am.* 2007;21(2):393-408, vi.
5. Lederman C, Miller M. Hordeola and chalazia. *Pediatr Rev.* 1999;20(8):283-284.
6. Duncan K, Jeng BH. Medical management of blepharitis. *Curr Opin Ophthalmol.* July 2015;26(4):289-294.
7. Gupta A, Stacey S, Amissah-Arthur KN. Eyelid lumps and lesions. *BMJ.* 2014;348:g3029.

2.8 Chalazia

Tamara Petrosyan

Anaya, a 38-year-old East Asian female, presented with a swelling on her upper left eyelid, which had been present for the past 4 weeks. Initially, the swelling was small, slightly red, and painful to touch, and eyelid was slightly swollen. Although the size of the lesion had been stable for a few weeks, the surrounding swelling had decreased, and it was no longer tender. She had had similar swellings previously in each eye, which had resolved without treatment. Anaya had visited her primary care physician 6 days ago who prescribed oral cephalexin (Keflex) 500 mg twice a day with no improvement. She denied any recent trauma or insect bites as well as any associated discharge, burning, itching, tearing, dryness, or pain on movement of either eye. All other visual, ocular, and medical histories were unremarkable.

Clinical Findings

Present Rx	OD: −0.75 sph (20/20); OS: −0.50 sph (20/20)
Pupil evaluation	PERRL; no RAPD
Confrontation visual fields	Full to finger counting OD and OS
Ocular motility	Full and comitant OD and OS
Slit-lamp examination	OD: eye lids: moderate capped meibomian glands; conjunctiva: small nasal pinguecula, otherwise white and quiet, no staining; cornea: clear, no staining; angle: 3 × 3; anterior chamber: deep and quiet, no cells and flare; lens: 2+ nuclear sclerosis; OS: eye lids: moderate capped meibomian glands, 4 mm horizontal × 3 mm vertical firm nodule on temporal left upper lid (Figure 2.8-1). No periorbital erythema or edema. No tenderness. Not warm to the touch. Surrounding eyelashes and tissue undisturbed with no feeder vessels or changes in pigmentation; conjunctiva: small nasal pinguecula, otherwise white and quiet, no staining; cornea: clear, no staining; angle: 3 × 3; anterior chamber: deep and quiet, no cells and flare. Lens: 2+ nuclear sclerosis.
Intraocular pressure (GAT)	OD: 17 mm Hg; OS: 16 mm Hg at 2:48 PM
Fundus examination	Unremarkable OD and OS

Abbreviations: GAT, Goldmann applanation tonometry; OD, right eye; OS, left eye; PERRL, pupils equal, round, reactive to light; RAPD, relative afferent pupillary defect; Rx, prescription; sph, sphere.

Comments

Anaya was diagnosed with a chalazion on the temporal aspect of her left upper eyelid, as well as blepharitis and dry eye disease in both eyes. Conservative therapy of warm compresses for 5 minutes followed by lid massage 3 to 4 times a day for 10 days of the left eye was recommended. She was asked to return in 10 days. In the event of no improvement after that time, either a

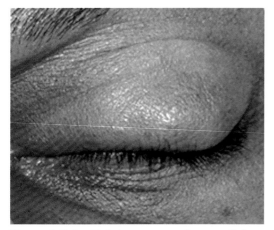

Figure 2.8-1   Chalazion on temporal aspect of left upper eyelid.

steroid injection or surgical removal of lesion would be considered. In addition, a warm compress mask was recommended followed by eyelid scrubs in both eyes twice daily. To treat the dry eye, artificial tears were prescribed for both eyes 4 times a day.

At the 10-day follow-up visit, Anaya reported good compliance with the treatment regimen and the lesion was reduced to 1 mm × 1 mm. It was much less bothersome to the patient. Although a small nodule was still present, she elected not to pursue further treatment. After discussing all treatment options, conservative therapy of warm compresses and lid massage 3 times a day was prescribed. Anaya was instructed to return if the lesion started to bother her, otherwise, she was scheduled for her yearly eye examination.

Discussion

Chalazia are the most common inflammatory lesions in the eyelids.[2] They are localized, chronic, lipogranulomatous inflammations caused by an obstruction of the sebaceous glands in the eyelid (meibomian and Zeiss).[3] The obstruction causes accumulation of secreted lipids in the stroma of the tarsal plate, triggering an immune reaction. The immune cells initially consist of neutrophils and later comprise lymphocytes, plasma cells, macrophages, mononuclear cells, eosinophils, and multinucleated giant cells.[2] In long-standing lesions, the capsular wall of the lipogranulomatous inflammation can become calcified.[3] This is in contrast to a hordeolum, which is typically warm and painful to the touch, and is caused by an infected sebaceous gland. Granulomatous inflammation can develop from a poorly resolved, infected hordeolum.[4]

A chalazion can affect individuals of all ages, race, and gender. Patients generally present with a persistent, painless nodule of the eyelid. Symptoms are usually restricted to poor cosmesis and local irritation. With larger lesions, mechanical ptosis, and reversible astigmatism due to corneal compression can arise.[4]

Depending on how advanced and bothersome the lesion is at the initial presentation, most practitioners will attempt conservative management first, as 25% to 50% of chalazia self-resolve over time.[5,6] These therapies, comprising a combination of frequent warm compresses, digital massage, and/or eyelid lid scrubs resolve between 40% and 80% of cases.[5,7] However, it is evident that this mode of treatment is not effective in all cases.

If conservative treatment is unsuccessful, the 2 most common interventions that follow are steroid injections and/or incision and removal of the inflammatory products.[8,9] Chalazia are inflammatory in nature, so the cells involved in formation are sensitive to steroids. The capsular wall poorly absorbs topically applied steroids, so the steroid is directly injected into the inflamed gland. The magnitude of the treatment effect will depend on the size, duration, and firmness of the lesion, with smaller, more recent onset, and softer lesions having a better treatment outcome. A 1-time steroid treatment, usually triamcinolone, injected transcutaneously or transconjunctivally, is effective between 60% and 84% of the time, with success rates increasing to 77% to 89% with 2 or more injections.[8-14] Using a transconjunctival approach is preferable as localized skin depigmentation, especially in darkly pigmented patients, is a common side effect. This is thought to be due to the inhibition of melanosome synthesis, impaired transfer of melanosome to the keratinocyte, or melanocyte ischemia.[15] Other possible side effects include increased intraocular pressure (IOP), atrophy of orbital and subcutaneous fat or accidental intraocular injection.[13]

Incision and drainage is a surgical treatment option for a recalcitrant chalazion (duration of more than 6 months), large lesions (larger than 11 mm in diameter) or where the capsular wall has calcified.[16] After administration of local anesthesia and eyelid eversion, the lesion is secured in a chalazion clamp and a scalpel is used to open the overlying conjunctiva. The granulomatous substance is then scooped out using a curette.[8] Depending on the size of the incision, cauterizing the wound or suturing may not be necessary. A single operation is effective in 79% to 87% of patients, with success rates increasing to 90% with 2 operations.[8,9] If the lesion is recurrent or the clinician is unclear of the diagnosis, the materials collected may be sent for pathologic analysis. This is particularly important when recurrences occur at the same location, as this may be a sign of a malignancy. In a study of 1060 cases where a lesion was diagnosed clinically as a chalazion, 68 (6.4%) were histopathologically shown to be misdiagnosed.[17] Sebaceous cell and basal cell carcinoma were the most commonly missed malignancies.[10,17-19]

Possible side effects resulting from incision and drainage surgery include discomfort, infection, bleeding and scarring or damage to lid structures. This procedure is also the most expensive treatment option. Recurrence of chalazion is common, even with the appropriate treatment. However, those patients whose lesions resolve completely are frequently lost to follow-up, so it is difficult to estimate the prevalence of recurrence. A 22% to 26% recurrence rate was reported after incision and drainage of chalazia. However, the use of thermal cautery did not impact the recurrence rate significantly.[20]

In Anaya's case, the oral antibiotic prescribed by her primary care physician was ineffective, because it was an inflammatory rather than an infectious lesion. Had any further treatment been considered necessary, incision and drainage would likely be preferred here as the patient had dark-pigmented skin. Steroid injection would therefore make her more prone to visible depigmentation.

CLINICAL PEARLS

- Chalazia are a localized, chronic, lipogranulomatous inflammation of the sebaceous glands that do not respond to antibiotic treatment.

- Depending on the symptoms and comfort of the patient, most practitioners will first attempt conservative management using frequent warm compresses, digital lesion massage, and/or eyelid lid scrubs.

- If conservative treatment fails, the 2 most common interventions that follow are steroid injections and/or incision and removal of the inflammatory products.

- In patients presenting with recurrent chalazia at the same location, one should suspect sebaceous cell carcinoma. Biopsy with histologic investigation is indicated.

REFERENCES

1. Kuiper J, Vislisel J, Oetting T. Chalazion: acute presentation and recurrence in a 4-year-old female. EyeRounds.org; available from http://EyeRounds.org/cases/193-Chalazion.htm. August 25, 2014. Accessed March 27, 2017.
2. Dhaliwal U, Arora VK, Singh N, Bhatia A. Cytopathology of chalazia. *Diagn Cytopathol.* 2004;31:118-122.
3. Ozdal PC, Codere F, Callejo S, Caissie AL, Burnier MN. Accuracy of clinical diagnosis of chalazion. *Eye.* 2004;18:135-138.
4. Sowka J, Kabat A. Options in Chalazia Management. *Rev Optom.* July 3, 2007;114(6). Retrieved from https://www.reviewofoptometry.com/article/options-in-chalazia-management-15417. Accessed 9 July, 2018.
5. Perry HD, Serniuk RA. Conservative treatment of chalazia. *Ophthalmology.* 1980;87(3):218-221.
6. Cottrell DG, Bosanquet RC, Fawcett IM. Chalazions: the frequency of spontaneous resolution. *Br Med J.* 1983;287:1595.
7. Garrett GW, Gillespie ME, Mannix BC. Adrenocorticosteroid injection vs. conservative therapy in the treatment of chalazia. *Am J Ophthalmol.* 1978; 85:818-821.
8. Goawalla A, Lee V. A prospective randomized treatment study comparing three treatment options for chalazia: triamcinolone acetonide injections, incision and curettage and treatment with hot compresses. *Clin Exp Ophthalmol.* 2007;35(8):706-712.
9. Simon GB, Rosen N, Rosner M, Spierer A. Triamcinolone acetonide injection versus incision and

curettage for primary chalazia: a prospective, random-ized study. *Am J Ophthalmol*. 2011;151:714-718.

10. Biuk D, Matic S, Barac J, Vukovic MJ, Biuk E, Matic M. Chalazion management-surgical treatment versus triamcinolon application. *Coll Antropol*. April 2013;37(suppl 1):247-250.

11. Watson AP, Austin DJ. Treatment of chalazions with injection steroid suspension. *Br J Ophthalmol*. 1984;68:833-835.

12. Ahmad S, Baig MA, Khan MA, Khan IU, Janjua TA. Intra-lesional corticosteroid injection vs surgical treatment of chalazia in pigmented patients. *J Coll Physicians Surg Pak*. 2006;16:42-44.

13. Vidaurri LJ, Pe'er J. Corticosteroid treatment of chalazia. *Ann Ophthalmol*. 1986;18:339-340.

14. Jacobs PM, Thaller VT, Wong D. Intralesional cortico-steroid therapy of chalazia: a comparison vs. incision and curettage. *Br J Ophthalmol*. 1984;68:836-837.

15. Kligman AM, Willis I. A new formula for depigmenting human skin. *Arch Dermatol*. 1975;111:40-48.

16. Dhaliwal U, Bhatia A. A rationale for therapeutic decision-making in chalazia. *Orbit*. December 2005;24(4):227-230.

17. Ozdal PC, Codère F, Callejo S, Caissie AL, Burnier MN. Accuracy of the clinical diagnosis of chalazion. *Eye (Lond)*. February 2004;18(2):135-138.

18. Tesluk, G. Eyelid lesions: incidence and comparison of benign and malignant lesions. *Ann Ophthalmol*. 1985;17:704-707.

19. Costea CF, Petraru D, Dumitrescu G, Sava A. Sebaceous carcinoma of the eyelid: anatomoclinical data. *Rom J Morphol Embryol*. 2013;54(3):665-668.

20. Sendrowski DP, Maher JF. Thermal cautery after chalazion surgery and its effect on recurrence rates. *Optom Vis Sci*. November 2000;77(11):605-607.

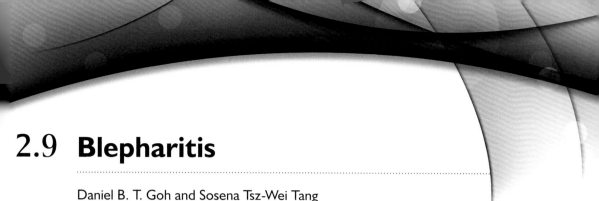

2.9 Blepharitis

Daniel B. T. Goh and Sosena Tsz-Wei Tang

Anna, a 49-year-old female teaching assistant, experienced soreness and burning in both eyes since undergoing laser refractive surgery 7 years ago. These symptoms were present throughout each day and were mild to moderate in intensity but occasionally severe. Her vision was variable and she reported ghost images when looking at digital readouts on audio-visual equipment (especially at night), light sensitivity, and inability to read for more than 10 minutes without significant discomfort. She had experienced long-standing floaters in both eyes for more than 30 years, but no photopsia. Anna indicated that she had been unhappy with her vision immediately after the bilateral LASIK procedure, as there was a residual spectacle prescription. There had also been an increase in the postoperative prescription over the following 18 months. She recalled that she had been about a 7.00 D myope preoperatively, and had worn soft monthly disposable contact lenses as she disliked her appearance in spectacles and their weight. Despite preferring contact lens wear, she had problems with comfort after around 3 to 4 hours wear and she "occasionally" used over-the-counter drops (no specific details were available). She had not worn spectacles or contact lenses since the LASIK surgery. She reported that her general health was good. Her family history was unremarkable.

Clinical findings

Unaided VA	OD: 20/200; OS 20/80 (with ghost images); OU: 20/40^{-2}
Pupil evaluation	PERRL; no RAPD
Subjective refraction	OD: −0.50 −2.75 × 170 (20/40); OS: −0.50 −1.00 × 175 (20/30); ADD: +1.75 OU (20/20)
Slit-lamp examination (all grading is on a scale from 0 to 4)	OD: lid redness: 2.0; lid roughness: 1.0; discharge: serous 1; meibomian glands: Grade 3; marginal tear strip: 0.1 mm (irregular); lower volume temporally; bulbar conjunctiva: 2.0 conjunctival folds; limbal redness: 0.5; cornea: staining area 5 type 1; extent 2.5 depth 1; LASIK flap margins visible; anterior chamber: deep and quiet, no cells/flare;
	OS: lid redness 2.5; lid roughness: 0.5; discharge: clear serous 1; meibomian glands: Grade 3; marginal tear strip: 0.1 mm (irregular), lower volume temporally; bulbar conjunctiva: 1.5 conjunctival folds; limbal redness: 0.5; cornea: staining area 5 type 1; extent 2.5 depth 1; LASIK flap margins visible; anterior chamber: deep and quiet, no cells/flare
Tear breakup time	OD: 2 s; OS 2 s
Intraocular pressure (Goldmann)	OD: 16 mm Hg; OS: 16 mm Hg at 11:15 AM

Fundus examination	Unremarkable OD and OS
Topography	No ectasia OD and OS

Abbreviations: OD, right eye; OS, left eye; OU, both eyes; PERRL, pupils equal, round, reactive to light; RAPD, relative afferent pupillary defect; VA, visual acuity.

Comments

Anna was diagnosed with posterior blepharitis, meibomian gland dysfunction, and post-laser refractive surgery dry eye. Differential diagnoses included allergy, dermatoconjunctivitis medicamentosa, parasitic infection, herpes (simplex or zoster), meibomian gland carcinoma, exposure keratopathy, and lagophthalmos.[1]

Recommendations for this case included the following:

1. Regular lid hygiene, that is, lid cleansing with commercially available lid wipes, twice a day (preferably after hot compresses).

2. Hot compresses using a commercially available hot compress bag twice a day for 3 weeks then once a day ongoing, each time to be followed by gentle lid massage with finger or lid massager.

3. Avoidance of eye liner and mascara.

4. Omega eye capsules (Omega-3 oil capsules with Vitamin D3) 4 times a day.

5. Flaxseed oil capsules (1000 mg) twice a day (at breakfast and at evening meal).

6. Artificial tears, that is, 0.1% sodium hyaluronate combined with 2% dexpanthenol, 4 times a day or more often as required.

7. Unmedicated lubricant ointment at bedtime.

8. Conscious full blinks at least every 20 minutes, especially when engaged in concentrated activities such as reading or computer work.

Anna had been miserable since having LASIK, experiencing discomforting dry eyes and a poor visual outcome. She was now very motivated to improve her ocular comfort. Anna was advised that the blepharitis may be contributing to her symptoms, but was reassured that the management plan should provide some relief. She was also told that chronic dry eye sometimes occurs following LASIK, and that both the quantity and quality of her tear film were inadequate to promote visual clarity and ocular comfort. She was informed that creating the flap during the LASIK procedure had damaged the corneal nerves. These can recover over time or may remain abnormal.[2] Anna was asked to return in 8 weeks for follow-up.

The findings from the 8-week follow-up visit are as follows:

Subjective refraction (repeated as the ocular surface was compromised at the first visit)	OD: −0.50 −2.75 × 170 (20/40⁺³); OS: −0.50 −1.00 × 175 (20/30⁺²); OU: 20/30⁺²
Slit-lamp examination (all grading is on a scale from 0 to 4)	OD: discharge: nil; meibomian glands: Grade 1; marginal tear strip: 0.15 mm, more regular; bulbar conjunctiva: 0.5; limbal redness: 0.5; cornea: staining area 5 type 1, extent 0.5 depth 1, flap margins visible; anterior chamber: deep and quiet, no cells/flare; OS: discharge: nil; meibomian glands: Grade 1; marginal tear strip: 0.15 mm, more regular; bulbar conjunctiva: 1.0; limbal redness: 0.5; cornea: staining area 5 type 1, extent 0.5 depth 1, flap margins visible; anterior chamber: deep and quiet, no cells/flare
Tear breakup time	OD: 6 s; OS 6 s

Abbreviations: OD, right eye; OS, left eye; OU, both eyes.

Anna was very motivated to carry out the treatment plan and experienced no difficulties with it. She was much happier and after 8 weeks both eyes were much more comfortable. Examination revealed significantly less meibomian gland blockage in each eye with an increased tear breakup times/tear meniscus height, and a definite reduction in inferior punctate staining. She could see much more clearly at both distance and near with her newly dispensed spectacles and felt these suited her cosmetically. Anna did report some initial disorientation but was adapting. She understood that the treatment plan would have to be executed long term to maintain relief and prevent the symptoms returning. A follow-up appointment was scheduled for 6 months. She was told to come back earlier if her symptoms worsened.

Discussion

Transient symptoms of dry eyes are common following LASIK, usually lasting less than 6 months, but a small proportion of individuals with preexisting issues, such as lid disease and reduced tear quality, experience chronic problems.[2] The presentation will be similar to blepharitis and dry eyes.

Dry eye and blepharitis are presented together in this case. After LASIK, dry eye may occur due to the disruption of normal corneal innervation when the flap is created. This action interrupts the relationship between the ocular surface and the lacrimal secretions causing disruption to the tear film. This may also unmask or exaggerate preexisting ocular surface disease.[3]

Blepharitis is a common inflammation of the eye lid margins that can present as an acute or chronic condition with reoccurring episodes. Blepharitis can be due to allergy or infection, which might be bacterial (eg, staphyloccocus), viral (eg, herpes simplex) or may also be caused by demodicosis (demodex mite).[1] It can also be classified based on the position of the affected eye lid margin. Anterior blepharitis presents with bilateral lid margin hyperaemia, crusts or collerettes at the base of the lashes and lid margin swelling. It is often associated with bacterial infection or seborrhea.

Some patients may exhibit eye lash loss, whitening, or trichiasis. The lids may show unevenness due to ulceration. In chronic cases such as the present case, typical symptoms are nonspecific general irritation and lid stickiness on awakening. Posterior blepharitis (meibomian gland dysfunction) will show plugging of the meibomian glands ducts, reoccurring lid cysts (eg, chalazia), foamy tears, conjunctival hyperemia, and inferior corneal staining/vascularization. Patients can present with blepharitis in either or both locations.[1]

The acute form often has a sudden onset, with moderate discomfort or pain and occurs concurrent with an infection elsewhere such as a cold. It is usually unilateral and can be associated with conjunctivitis or keratitis. Signs may include more dramatic swelling of lid margins and redness.[1]

Treatment should aim to reduce dry eye symptoms using topical, preferably preservative-free, artificial tears to substitute for the compromised postsurgical tear film.[4] Underlying meibomian gland dysfunction should be treated to minimize discomfort.[1] Commercially available, reusable eye masks that can be heated in a microwave oven and used as a warm compress are a suitable intervention to maintain long-term improvement.[2,5] Optimal lid hygiene should include warm compresses for 5 to 10 minutes followed by lid massage to remove blocked matter from the glands, lid scrubs to clear the debris and excessive bacteria and toxins from the lid margins, and tear supplementing eye drops or ointment. Lid scrubs can be either commercially available preparations (available as a solution or presoaked pad) or made from a solution of 1 part baby shampoo to 10 parts warm water.[1]

Additional hygiene measures, such as frequent face and scalp cleaning should be recommended for seborrheic cases. This should be performed 2 to 3 times a day for at least 1 to 2 weeks, and then maintained on a daily basis. Makeup behind the eye lash line should also be avoided as this may block the meibomian glands.[1]

Oral re-esterified Omega-3 capsules improve tear osmolarity, tear breakup time, and many of the symptoms associated with dry eye.[6] Oral flaxseed oil capsules reduce ocular surface inflammation and improve symptoms in patients with serious dry eye disease.[7] A combination of these treatments (lid wipes, artificial tears, and nutritional supplements) produces significant improvement in comfort.[8] In addition, inferior punctate corneal staining caused by neurotrophically reduced or incomplete blinking can be alleviated by blink exercises.[9]

If the condition is not improved by these initial therapies, pharmacologic treatment may be employed. Some patients benefit from oral tetracyclines for posterior blepharitis such as oxytetracycline, minocycline, or doxycycline. Two to three months of low-dose antibiotic treatment may be needed.[10] Short-term treatment of 2 to 4 weeks of topical steroids, such as prednisolone or flouromethalone,[1,11,12] or the insertion of punctal plugs[13] may also be beneficial. For stubborn cases, topical cyclosporine 0.05% and autologous serum may be required.[14,15]

The long-term management of blepharitis can be tedious for patients. As commonly occurs, Anna was very motivated for the first 4 weeks of treatment, but her adherence decreased even as symptoms improved. We advise patients to use phone alerts or to incorporate the management into their daily routine, but appreciate that this can be difficult. For follow-up care, we advise patients to find out what level of intervention works for them as symptoms and signs improve.

CLINICAL PEARLS

- Dry eye and blepharitis are very common and adequate eye lid hygiene is often overlooked.

- The eyelids and ocular surface should be in optimal condition before any elective procedure (such as refractive surgery) that might exacerbate dry eye type symptoms is performed.

REFERENCES

1. The College of Optometrists Clinical Management Guidelines: Dry eye and blepharitis. www.college-optometrists.org. 2016. Accessed April 26, 2017.
2. Shtein RM. Post LASIK dry eye. *Expert Rev Ophthalmol*. 2011;6(5):575-582.
3. Nettune GR. Post LASIK tear dysfunction and dysesthesia. *Ocul Surf*. 2010;8(3):135-145.
4. Pflugfelder SC, Solomon A, Stern ME. The diagnosis and management of dry eye: a twenty-five year review. *Cornea*. 2000;19(5):644-649.
5. Bilkhu PS, Naroo SA, Wolffsohn JS. Randomised masked clinical trial of the MDDRx eyebag for the treatment of meibomian gland dysfunction-related evaporative dry eye. *Br J Ophthalmol*. 2014;98(12): 1707-1711.
6. Epitropoulos AT, et al. Effect of oral re-esterified Omega-3 nutritional supplementation on dry eyes. *Cornea*. 2016;35(9):1185-1191.
7. Pinheiro MN Jr, dos Santos PM, dos Santos RC, Barros Jde N, Passos LF, Cardoso Neto J. Oral flaxseed oil in the treatment for dry eye Sjögren's syndrome patients. *Arg Bras Oftalmol*. 2007;70(4):649-655.
8. Korb DR, Blackie CA, Finnemore VM, Douglass T. Effect of using a combination of lid wipes, eye drops, and Omega-3 supplements on Meibomian gland functionality in patients with lipid deficient/evaporative dry eye. *Cornea*. 2015;34(4):407-412.
9. McMonnies CW. How blink anomalies can contribute to post-LASIK neurotophic epitheliopathy. *Optom Vis Sci*. 2015;92(9):241-247.
10. Doughty MJ. On the prescribing of oral doxycycline or minocycline by UK optometrists as part of management of chronic meibomian gland dysfunction (MGD). *Cont Lens Anterior Eye*. 2016;39(1):2-8.
11. The College of Optometrists Optometrists' Formulary. www.college-optometrists.org. 2016. Accessed May 1, 2017.
12. Pflugfleder SC, Maskin SL, Anderson B, et al. A randomised double masked, placebo controlled, multicentre comparison of loteprednol etabonate ophthalmic suspension, 0.5%, and placebo treatment of keratoconjunctivitis sicca in patients with delayed tear clearance. *Am J Ophthalmol*. 2004;138(3):444-457.
13. Yang HY, Toda I, Sakai C, Yoshida A, Tsubota K. Punctal plugs for treatment of post-LASIK dry eye. *Jpn J Ophthalmol*. 2012;56:208-213.
14. Salib GM, McDanald B, Smolek M. Safety and efficacy of cyclosporine 0.05% drops versus unpreserved artificial tears in dry-eye patients having laser in situ keratomileusis. *J Cataract Refract Surg*. 2006;32:772-778.
15. Alio J, Rodriguez AE, WrobeDudzinska DW. Eye platelet-rich plasma in the treatment of ocular surface disorders. *Curr Opin Ophthalmol*. 2015;26:325-332.

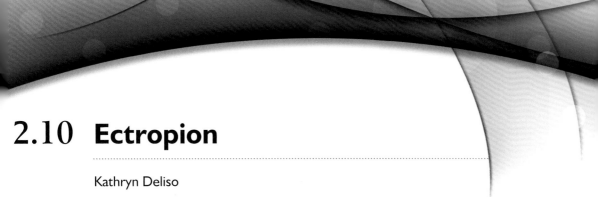

2.10 Ectropion

Kathryn Deliso

Maurice, a 74-year-old Caucasian male, presented with a watery, irritated left eye. He reported that this had been an ongoing issue for the past few years, but had been bothering him more recently. He now had to carry tissues all the time to wipe away the tears. Maurice had a positive history of dry eye, and while he had found improvement in the past by using warm compresses and generic artificial tears, now they only provided very temporary relief.

Maurice indicated that over the past year, the vision in his right eye had declined at both distance and near. He also noticed that glare bothered him significantly while driving at night. He had tried wearing his wife's "night driving" yellow glasses over his prescription bifocals, and this did seem to help a little.

Maurice's last eye examination was 1 year ago, when he was told that he had a cataract in his right eye. He had cataract surgery on his left eye approximately 2 years ago without any complications. Maurice was in good health and took lisinopril (20 mg/d) for hypertension and simvastatin (40 mg/d) for high cholesterol.

Clinical Findings

Present Rx	OD: $-0.50 -1.25 \times 092$ (20/50⁻; pinhole: 20/40⁻²); OS: $+0.25 -0.25 \times 180$ (20/20⁻²) ADD: +2.50 OU
Pupil evaluation	PERRL; no RAPD
Confrontation visual fields	Full to finger counting OD and OS
Keratometry	OD: 44.50/43.50 at 006; OS: 44.50/44.00 at 013
Subjective refraction	OD: $-1.00 -1.00 \times 090$ (20/40); OS: Pl -0.25×180 (20/20⁻²); ADD: +2.50 OU (OD: 20/30⁻²; OS: 20/20⁻²)
Intraocular pressure (GAT)	OD: 16 mm Hg; OS: 15 mm Hg at 1:55 PM
Slit-lamp examination	OD: lids/lashes: dermatochalasis, trace blepharitis; conjunctiva: trace injection; cornea: arcus; lens: 2+ nuclear sclerosis, 1+ anterior capsular cataract; OS: lids/lashes: dermatochalasis, trace blepharitis, lower punctal and medial ectropion (Figure 2.10-1); conjunctiva: trace injection, early inferior palpebral keratinization; cornea: arcus, trace staining inferiorly; lens: posterior chamber IOL, trace posterior capsule opacification
Fundus examination	Unremarkable with the exception of early epiretinal membrane OD Unremarkable OS

Abbreviations: GAT, Goldmann applanation tonometry; IOL, intraocular lens; OD, right eye; OS, left eye; OU, both eyes; PERRL, pupils equal, round, reactive to light; Pl, plano; RAPD, relative afferent pupillary defect; Rx, prescription.

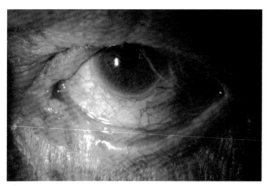

Figure 2.10-1 Lower punctal and medial ectropion OS.

Abbreviation: OS, left eye.
Photo credit: Raymond Chew, OD, FAAO

Table 2.10-1 Orbicularis Tone Classified With the Eyelid Snap Test. Based on These Results, Maurice Was Diagnosed With Involutional Ectropion

Grading	Time for Eyelid to Reposition Against the Globe
Grade 0	Less than 2 s
Grade I	2-3 s
Grade II	4-5 s
Grade III	Greater than 5 s
Grade IV	Does not return to position against the globe

Comments

The lower lid distraction test was used to assess eyelid laxity. This measures the separation between the lower lid and the globe when the lid is pulled away from the eye. A normal finding is between 2 and 3 mm. If there is more than 6 mm of separation between the eyelid and the globe, then significant laxity is present.[1] In Maurice's case, a finding of 5.5 mm was found in the left eye and 3 mm in the right eye.

In addition, the snap test was used to assess the tone of the orbicularis muscle. Here, the lower eyelid is everted down and away from the orbit and the response is noted as the examiner releases the lid. In the presence of normal eyelid muscle tone, the eyelid will return to its proper position against the globe in 1 to 2 seconds, with or without a blink. A positive snap test occurs when the eyelid fails to snap against the globe, and there is visible lower lid laxity. Results can be classified further based on the time taken for the eyelid to return to apposition with the orbit (Table 2.10-1[2]). In this case, a finding of 6 seconds (Grade III) was observed.

Discussion

A 74-year-old presenting with symptoms of epiphora and ocular irritation should lead the practitioner to evaluate eyelid position. Ectropion is a common clinical presentation among the elderly as eyelid laxity increases with age. Although decreased vision does not typically occur with ectropion unless significant corneal exposure has occurred, it may be a possible causative factor if significant keratitis occurs. However, Maurice had decreased vision in the fellow eye, which was attributed to an early epiretinal membrane and nuclear sclerotic cataract leading to a small myopic shift in refractive error.

When the lower eyelid margin turns outward away from the globe, the ectropion can be classified as involutional, cicatricial, paralytic, mechanical or congenital.[1,2] Involutional ectropion is the most common type, and generally occurs due to acquired horizontal laxity of the eyelid and canthal tendons (lateral, medial), thereby causing the eyelid to turn outward. This is frequently associated with significant loss of orbicularis muscle tone and tarsoligamentous elasticity, leading to abnormal snapback and lid distraction test findings. Cicatricial ectropion results from an insult to the integrity of the eyelid structure following surgery, trauma, chronic dermatitis, thermal or chemical exposure or burns. These may lead to vertical tightening of the eyelid skin. Paralytic ectropion is generally associated with an ipsilateral facial nerve palsy, which can lead to significant exposure keratoconjunctivitis. Mechanical ectropion occurs when there is a physical structure (such as a mass, large chalazion or fibroma) or swelling causing the eyelid to turn outward. Congenital ectropion (the least common etiology) occurs most frequently in Down syndrome.[2] This often presents with vertical tightening of the skin, similar to cicatricial ectropion, and may require surgical management by tightening the lateral canthal tendon.

Patients with ectropion may complain of excessive tearing, redness, irritation, foreign body sensation, itching, and discharge. Symptoms can range from mild to severe depending on the degree of corneal exposure and sensitivity. The conjunctiva is typically injected and as the tarsal conjunctiva becomes exposed, thickening, inflammation, and keratinization may be observed. In addition, staining may be present inferiorly. The practitioner should enquire about a history of facial burns, trauma, surgery or palsy. Recognition of possible malignant or space-occupying lesions is essential as the differential diagnosis of ectropion includes eyelid malignancy, retraction secondary to proptosis, and neurologic dysfunction.

If significant corneal exposure occurs, it is imperative to provide adequate corneal coverage to prevent persistent corneal epithelial defects, ulceration, or perforation. The surgical management of involutional ectropion involves horizontal tightening and shortening of the eyelid, both medially and laterally if there is severe laxity.[3]

Conservative treatment may be adequate if the patient is unsure about, or does not yet require surgery. Topical lubrication with high viscosity or preservative-free artificial tears should be recommended, as well as the use of a lubricating ointment at bedtime, with or without eyelid taping. In the case of a paralytic ectropion, temporary relief can be achieved by applying adhesive tape from the lower lid to above the outer canthus. Patients with significant epiphora should be encouraged to wipe the tears upward and inward toward their nose rather than down or out, as the latter can lead to increased lid laxity. Moisture chamber goggles may also be recommended for patients with corneal exposure, and follow-up visits should be scheduled to monitor corneal staining in these patients. Maurice was prescribed preservative-free artificial tears for use 4 times a day in the right eye and a lubricating ointment at bedtime. He was also referred for an oculoplastic consultation. The possibility of cataract surgery on his right eye was also discussed. The prognosis of ectropion is generally good if it is addressed early, but may vary depending on the underlying etiology. Generally, surgical correction is curative in the absence of paretic or cicatricial involvement.

CLINICAL PEARLS

- Ectropion can present with epiphora, chronic redness, irritation, and discharge.

- Eyelid laxity can be categorized using the snap test. If the eyelid does not return to its proper position opposed against the globe within 1 to 2 seconds, with or without a blink, the patient has some degree of eyelid laxity that can lead to corneal exposure.

- Conservative management is achieved with higher viscosity or preservative-free artificial tears and ointment applied at night.

- For patients deferring or declining surgical intervention for ectropion, it is imperative to provide corneal coverage to prevent persistent corneal epithelial defects, ulceration, or perforation.

REFERENCES

1. Kanski JJ, Bowling B. *Kanski's Clinical Ophthalmology: A Systematic Approach.* 7th ed. Amsterdam, the Netherlands: Elsevier; 2011:45-46.
2. Piskiniene R. Eyelid malposition: lower lid entropion and ectropion. *Medicina (Kaunas).* 2006;42(11): 881-884.
3. Freitag SK, Lee NG. Eyelid malpositions: entropion and ectropion. *Facial Surg.* 2014;12:221-232.

2.11 Blepharospasm

Nadine M. Furtado and Andre Stanberry

Patricia, a 67-year-old Caucasian female, presented with complaints of severe photophobia in each eye for the past 6 months. The symptoms first occurred suddenly while she was driving at night. Although there was no specific instigating factor, the initial onset did occur at a particularly stressful time in her life. The photophobia increased in frequency and severity over the following few weeks, with episodes so severe that she had to keep her eyes closed for extended periods of time, opening them only intermittently as needed. She stopped driving shortly thereafter.

Approximately 2 months ago, Patricia started experiencing episodes of what she described as uncontrollable excessive blinking and squeezing of her eyes. In addition, over the past month, she had been having neck muscle spasms and noted that her head tended to fall forward onto her chest, which resulted in her having to hold her head up with her arm. This awkward head posture caused significant pain in her neck and across her shoulders.

Patricia's ocular history was unremarkable. Her medical history was positive for iron deficiency anemia, which she treated with daily ferrous sulfate tablets. She also took daily vitamin C tablets to help with iron absorption. For pain management, she used acetaminophen as needed. She denied any environmental or medication allergies. She had never smoked and did not drink alcohol. Her family history included a maternal aunt diagnosed with dystonia in her 30s.

Clinical Findings

Habitual Rx	OD: $-0.75 -2.00 \times 085$ (20/20); OS: $-1.00 -1.50 \times 082$ (20/20); ADD: +2.25 OU (OD: 20/20; OS: 20/20)
Pupil evaluation	PERRL; no RAPD
Ocular motility	Full in all gazes OD and OS
Confrontation visual field	Full to finger counting OD and OS
Cranial nerve testing	CNII through CNXII were normal
Color vision testing	Normal OU with desaturated D-15 test
Gross examination	Frequent bilateral spastic movements of orbicularis oculi Occasional uncontrollable head and neck movements
Slit-lamp examination	Trace nuclear sclerosis OD and OS; all else unremarkable OD and OS
Intraocular pressure (GAT)	OD: 16 mm Hg; OS: 17 mm Hg at 11:15 AM
Fundus examination	OD: CD 0.35/0.35; optic nerves well perfused with intact neural retinal rims; macula: flat and intact OS: CD 0.35/0.35; optic nerves well perfused with intact neural retinal rims; macula: early epiretinal membrane causing mild distortion to fovea and perimacular regions Peripheral retinal examination was unremarkable OD and OS, however, views were fleeting in certain quadrants due to frequent blinking

Goldmann visual field testing	No neurologic defects OD and OS
Electrodiagnostic evaluation	Full field ERG showed no signs of cone or rod pathway abnormalities
Magnetic resonance imaging	Large dural-based meningioma of the left cerebellar hemisphere (determined to be noncontributory to symptoms)

Abbreviations: CD, cup to disc; ERG, electroretinogram; GAT, Goldmann applanation tonometry; OD, right eye; OS, left eye; OU, both eyes; PERRL, pupils equal, round, reactive to light; RAPD, relative afferent pupillary defect; Rx, prescription.

Comments

Patricia was diagnosed with severe blepharospasm with photophobia. The neurologic testing was ordered to rule out other potential diagnoses. In addition, due to the limited views with binocular indirect funduscopy and the inability to attain optical coherence tomography (OCT) scans as a result of the severe blepharospasm, an electrodiagnostic evaluation was carried out.

Discussion

Benign essential blepharospasm (BEB) is a primary focal dystonia characterized by involuntary and excessive muscle contractions of the orbicularis oculi muscles, as well as the corrugator and procerus muscles in the upper face. The blink rate becomes more frequent, forceful, and enduring as the condition progresses. In addition, patients with BEB often experience spasms of the lower facial and neck muscles (Meige syndrome) and photophobia due to trigeminal hyperexcitability. Although visual acuity (VA) is usually normal, patients can become functionally blind, which leads to social impairment. The age of onset is usually in the sixth decade of life, with women being affected more than men.[1,2]

Benign essential blepharospasm is believed to result from a combination of predisposing genetic factors and environmental influences.[3] Approximately one-third of patients report a family history of dystonia or movement disorder.[2] Potential influences include stress, ocular surface disease, and a history of head trauma.[3] Eyelid spasms are absent during sleep, and may reduce in frequency when the individual engages in specific sensory activities, such as humming or singing.[3] Animal models implicate dysfunction in the basal ganglia

response to cerebellar activity, which causes aberrant neuroplasticity resulting in trigeminal hyperexcitability and spastic lid closure.[3,4]

A comprehensive case history is important in making an accurate diagnosis, and to differentiate BEB from secondary blepharospasm that can occur in association with certain neurodegenerative diseases, movement disorders, and other ocular conditions. Assessment for associated abnormal facial muscle contractions or rigid neck movements should be done to rule out Meige syndrome and extrapyramidal disease, respectively. A neurologic examination with neuroimaging should also be conducted to assess for potential underlying neurologic etiology. In addition, reflex blepharospasm due to ocular irritation and lid myokemia are differential diagnoses that must be excluded. If the orbicularis oculi spasms remain unilateral, then the diagnosis is hemifacial spasm. Medication history should also be reviewed as certain drugs have been shown to induce blepharospasm, including antipsychotics, dopamine-stimulating drugs, sympathomimetics, and nasal decongestants.

At the onset of BEB, patients often experience only mild twitching of their eyelids, which may initially be unilateral. As the condition progresses, the muscle spasms increase in frequency and intensity in a synchronous and symmetrical manner; during very severe episodes, patients may report an inability to keep their eyelids opened. In addition, patients may experience photophobia and ocular surface discomfort related to dry eyes.[2]

Various oral medical treatments have been proposed to treat BEB, but their efficacy has been limited. Botulinum toxin is currently the most commonly used treatment; injection into the orbicularis muscle weakens the contractions and usually provides temporary relief for most patients.[5] However, treatment typically needs to be administered every 3 to 4 months as the effects wear off and the muscle regains its functional ability. In addition, patients should be made aware of possible side effects, including transient ptosis and diplopia.[6] In severe cases, where patients are unresponsive to botulinum toxin treatment, surgical options can be pursued; an eyelid myectomy can be performed to excise the orbicularis oculi, corrugator supercilii, and/or procerus muscles, depending on the severity of the blepharospasm.

CLINICAL PEARL

- Benign essential blepharospasm is a diagnosis of exclusion. Ancillary testing, including a complete neurologic assessment, should be conducted to rule out secondary blepharospasm due to an alternative underlying cause.

REFERENCES

1. Hallett M, Evinger C, Jankovic J, Stacy M. Update on blephrospasm: report from the BEBRF International Workshop. *Neurology.* 2008;71:1275-1282.
2. Ben Simon GJ, McCann JD. Benign essential blepharospasm. *Int Ophthalmol Clin.* 2005;45(3):49-75.
3. Evinger C. Benign essential blepharospasm is a disorder of neuroplasticity: lessons from animal models. *J Neuroophthalmol.* 2015;35:374-381.
4. Kranz G, Shamim EA, Lin PT, Kranz GS, Voller B, Hallett M. Blepharospasm and the modulation of cortical excitability in the primary and secondary motor areas. *Neurology.* 2009;73:2031-2036.
5. Simpson DM, Hallett, M, Ashman EJ, et al. Practice guideline update summary: botulinum neurotoxin for the treatment of blepharospasm, cervical dystonia, adult spasticity, and headache. *Neurology.* 2016;86(18): 1818-1826.
6. Czyz CN, Burns JA, Petrie TP, Watkins JR, Cahill KV, Foster JA. Long-term botulinum toxin treatment of benign essential blepharospasm, hemifacial spasm, and Meige syndrome. *Am J Ophthalmol.* 2013;156:173-177.

2.12 Dacryocystitis

Anna K. Bedwell

Avani, a 23-year-old Indian female, presented for an urgent care visit due to swelling and tenderness around her right eye. This had begun 2 days earlier. She graded the discomfort as 4 out of 10. She reported watering and a thick, yellow discharge from the right eye.

She was last seen at the clinic 9 months ago for a comprehensive contact lens examination. The records indicated that she was wearing monthly disposable contact lenses. She reported wearing her lenses an average of 14 hours per day, and did not sleep in them. She used a generic, multipurpose, contact lens solution. Ocular history indicated that 2 years ago, Avani experienced a red right eye and she had been told it was due to her over-wearing her contact lenses. This was treated with an antibiotic/steroid combination drop and resolved fully. Medical history was positive for seasonal allergies for which she took loratadine (Claritin) as needed.

Clinical Findings

Current contact lens Rx	OD: −2.00 sph (20/20⁻); OS: −2.00 sph (20/20)
Pupil evaluation	PERRL; no RAPD
Extraocular motility	Full and smooth OD and OS. No pain or diplopia
Confrontation visual fields	Full to finger counting OD and OS
Slit-lamp examination	OD: moderate lower lid edema and erythema localized nasally (see Figure 2.12-1). Mucopurulent discharge through the punctum observed on palpation. Moderate tear film debris. Cornea and conjunctiva clear; OS: unremarkable
Intraocular pressure (GAT)	OD 10 mm Hg, OS 10 mm Hg at 10:02 AM
Fundus examination	Unremarkable OD and OS

Abbreviations: GAT, Goldmann applanation tonometry; OD, right eye; OS, left eye; PERRL, pupils equal, round, reactive to light; RAPD, relative afferent pupillary defect; Rx, prescription; sph, sphere.

Comments

Avani was diagnosed with acute dacryocystitis. She was prescribed oral cephalexin 500 mg twice a day, 1 drop of moxifloxacin 0.5% 4 times a day in the right eye and advised to use warm compresses with digital massage 4 times a day. Avani was instructed to follow this treatment regimen for the next 7 days. She was told to discontinue contact lens wear until the condition had resolved.

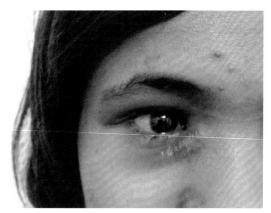

Figure 2.12-1   Photo of the patient's right eye showing edema and erythema localized to the nasal aspect of the lower eyelid.

At the follow-up visit 3 days later, Avani felt much better and had noticed that the swelling and tenderness had nearly resolved. She was compliant with the previous instructions and taking the cephalexin and moxifloxacin as directed.

Distance VA (through current spectacles)	OD: 20/20; OS: 20/20
Slit-lamp examination	OD: 75% reduction in edema compared with the previous visit, no erythema; mild tear film debris with a thick tear meniscus. Cornea and conjunctiva clear; OS: unremarkable.

Abbreviations: OD, right eye; OS, left eye; VA, visual acuity.

Discussion

Avani presented with painful edema and erythema localized over the right lacrimal sac consistent with a diagnosis of acute dacryocystitis. Differentials to consider are other ocular soft tissue infections, such as preseptal cellulitis, canaliculitis, and orbital cellulitis. At the 1-week follow-up visit, the infection had fully resolved. However, the patient still complained of persistent epiphora. A Jones Test 1 was performed by instilling sodium fluorescein dye in the right eye. Because this did not pass through her nose, it indicated obstruction was present as this is a negative test result. The left side was patent. Avani was referred to an oculoplastics specialist who performed a dacryocystorhinostomy.

Dacryocystitis is generally attributable to a nasolacrimal duct obstruction causing a secondary infection. It is most commonly seen in adults older than 40 years, with a high preponderance for postmenopausal females.[1] This is due to a narrow nasolacrimal fossa and middle nasolacrimal duct caused by osteoporotic changes in the older female population.[1] It can also develop in infants with congenital nasal lacrimal duct obstruction.[2] This patient was in her early 20s and so did not fit into the typical demographics for dacryocystitis. The diagnosis was made based on the signs and symptoms alone.

Secondary development of preseptal cellulitis or conjunctivitis is common.[3] Although progression to orbital cellulitis is a rare but serious, sight-threatening concern, any ocular soft tissue infection with proptosis, limited ocular motility, fever or pupillary defect should be referred promptly for intravenous antibiotic therapy.

Dacryocystitis can be categorized as either acute or chronic. The acute form presents as lacrimal sac distention with painful inflammation localized medially in the lower eyelid of short duration.[4] In contrast, chronic dacryocystitis exhibits significantly less inflammation. Individuals with the chronic form may report symptoms of swelling or discharge lasting over 2 weeks.[4]

Management of dacryocystitis in adults includes a 7- to 10-day course of broad spectrum oral and topical antibiotics with warm compresses to the inner canthal area. Topical therapy alone is inadequate.[3] Pain management can be provided as needed. Although the infecting organism varies, it is most commonly Gram-positive bacteria.[4] Thus, cephalosporins and amoxicillin/clavulanic acid are good oral treatment options. Irrigation or surgery should be deferred until the infection has resolved. Persistent epiphora or chronic dacryocystitis can then be managed with dacryocystorhinostomy. This creates an anastomosis between the lacrimal sac and the nasal cavity. An endoscopic approach is more commonly used nowadays, rather than the traditional, external dacryocystorhinostomy as it does not leave an external scar. Both techniques offer equally high success rates.[5]

CLINICAL PEARL

- Patients may not fit the classic age, race, or gender profile for a disease. Use the history, symptoms, and signs to reach the proper diagnosis.

REFERENCES

1. Babar TF, Masud MZ, Saeed N. An analysis of patients with chronic dacryocystitis. *J Postgrad Med Inst.* 2004;18(3):424-431.
2. Kapadia MK, Freitag SK, Woog JJ. Evaluation and management of congenital nasolacrimal duct obstruction. *Otolaryngol Clin North Am.* 2006;39(5):959-977.
3. Pinar-Sueiro S, Sota M, Lerchundi TX, et al. Dacryocystitis: systematic approach to diagnosis and therapy. *Curr Infect Dis Rep.* 2012;14:137-146.
4. Mills DM, Bodman MG, Meyer DR, Morton AD; ASOPRS Dacryocystitis Study Group. The microbiologic spectrum of dacryocystitis: a national study of acute versus chronic infection. *Ophthal Plast Reconstr Surg.* 1993;9(1):38-41.
5. Farzampour S, Fayazzadeh E, Mikaniki E. Endonasal laser-assisted microscopic dacryocystorhinostomy: surgical technique and follow-up results. *Am J Otolaryngol Head Neck.* 2010;31(2):84-90.

2.13 Dry Eye Disease

Tracy Doll

George, a 43-year-old Caucasian male pharmacist, was referred for a dry eye workup based on his concerns of persistent ocular irritation during his primary eye examination. His main concern was contact lens intolerance for the past 5 years. He had been experiencing excessive blinking, burning, and irritation on a daily basis, which became worse toward the end of his computer-intensive workday. He could not tolerate wearing contact lenses anymore and his primary goal was to be able to wear them on the weekend for skiing and fishing.

George had tried both temporary intra-canalicular punctal plugs and topical cyclosporine ophthalmic emulsion 0.05% (Restasis) for 6 months without success. He was using non-preserved lipid-enhanced artificial tears 6 times a day, as well as consuming a teaspoon (5 mL) of ground flaxseed for Omega-3 support. He reported being told by a previous provider that he should "blink more frequently."

Medical history was significant for gout, which was successfully treated with allopurinol, and infrequent eczema for which he was not receiving treatment. George suspected he may have mild rosacea based on his "rosy cheeks," but had no formal diagnosis. He denied any autoimmune conditions, muscle aches, or excessive thirst. Family, ocular, and medical histories were unremarkable.

Clinical Findings

Habitual distance VA	OD: 20/15; OS: 20/20
Ocular motility	Full range of motion OD and OS
Confrontation visual fields	Full to finger counting OD and OS
Pupil evaluation	PERRL; no RAPD
Slit-lamp examination	Lids (upper and lower): scalloped and telangiectasia with line of Marx staining (lissamine green) intermittently over upper and lower meibomian glands; low tear meniscus with mild tear debris; diffuse, mild conjunctival injection and mild diffuse lissamine green punctate staining; no follicles or papillae; trace inferior punctate corneal staining with lissamine green OD and OS
Meibomian gland expression (upper and lower lids)	Yellow and clear secretions, no toothpaste-like white secretions OD and OS
Standardized SPEED dry eye questionnaire (SPEED Q; Figure 2.13-1)	16 (range 0-28; 10 and greater is indicative of dry eye)
Lipid layer thickness (LLT) by white light interferometry (Figure 2.13-2)	OD: 56 nm average, indicating borderline-low lipid layer of the tear film on the ocular surface; OS: 72 nm average, indicating borderline-low lipid layer of the tear film on the ocular surface.

Partial blink rate (Figure 2.13-2)	OD: 0/7, demonstrating complete blinking; OS: 0/4, demonstrating complete blinking
Dynamic meibography imaging (Figure 2.13-2)	OD: Grade 1 gland drop-out of the lower eyelid, Grade 1 duct dilation upper and lower eyelid; OS: Grade 1 duct dilation upper and lower eyelid
Non-invasive tear breakup time by keratograph (NIKBUT) (Figure 2.13-3)	OD: 2.68 s first break, this is reduced OS: 1.72 s first break, this is reduced.
Korb-Blackie lid seal test for nocturnal lagophthalmos	Complete eyelid closure OD and OS
InflammaDry test (Figure 2.13-4)	Mildly (faint pink) positive at 10 min OD and OS
Meibomian glands yielding liquid secretion score (MGYLS)	OD: 4 clear secreting glands, indicating moderate meibomian gland dysfunction (OD > OS) OS: 9 clear secreting glands, indicating moderate meibomian gland dysfunction (OD > OS)

Abbreviations: OD, right eye; OS, left eye; PERRL, pupils equal, round, reactive to light; RAPD, relative afferent pupillary defect; VA, visual acuity.

Patient Name: _____   ☐ RIGHT EYE

Date: _____   ☐ LEFT EYE

DRY EYE QUESTIONNAIRE - SPEED

Please answer the following questions by checking the box that best represents your answer. Select only one answer per question.

1. Report the type of SYMPTOMS you experience and when they occur:

SYMPTOMS	AT THIS VISIT		WITHIN PAST 72 HRS		WITHIN PAST 3 MONTHS	
	YES	NO	YES	NO	YES	NO
Dryness, Grittiness or Scratchiness						
Soreness or Irritation						
Burning or Watering						
Eye Fatigue						

2. Report the FREQUENCY of your symptoms using the rating list below:

SYMPTOMS	0	1	2	3
Dryness, Grittiness or Scratchiness				
Soreness or Irritation				
Burning or Watering				
Eye Fatigue				

0 = Never   1 = Sometimes   2 = Often   3 = Constant

3. Report the SEVERITY of your symptoms using the rating list below:

SYMPTOMS	0	1	2	3	4
Dryness, Grittiness or Scratchiness					
Soreness or Irritation					
Burning or Watering					
Eye Fatigue					

0 = No problems
1 = Tolerable – not perfect but not uncomfortable
2 = Uncomfortable – irritating but does not interfere with my day
3 = Bothersome – irritating and interferes with my day
4 = Intolerable – unable to perform my daily tasks

4. Do you use eye drops for lubrication? ☐ YES ☐ NO If yes, how often? _____

Figure 2.13-1 Standardized Patient Evaluation of Eye Dryness (SPEED) Questionnaire.

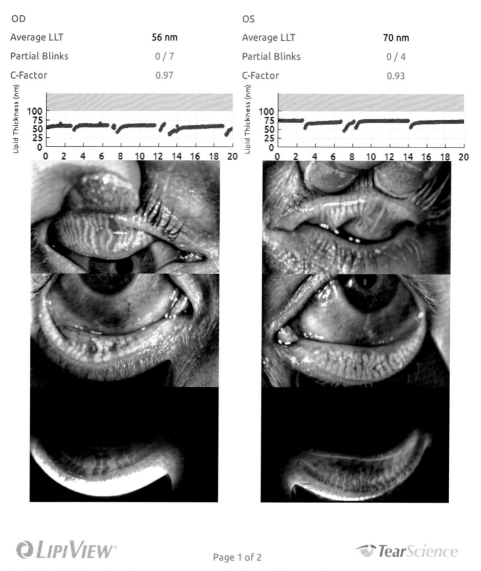

OD		OS	
Average LLT	56 nm	Average LLT	70 nm
Partial Blinks	0 / 7	Partial Blinks	0 / 4
C-Factor	0.97	C-Factor	0.93

Figure 2.13-2   LipiView II baseline summary report: lipid layer thickness, blink analysis and meibography.

Comments

Based on the borderline Korb meibomian gland evaluator and lipid layer thickness findings, with the appearance of the eyelids and cornea, George was diagnosed with meibomian gland dysfunction (MGD), with a probable inflammatory dry eye component. He received therapy over a 4-month time period, as outlined in Table 2.13-1, including anti-inflammatory eyelid home regimen, LipiFlow Vectored Thermal Pulse therapy, and a lifitegrast 5% (Xiidra) regimen. Table 2.13-2 compares the baseline and 4-month treatment findings.

George was able to achieve his goal of returning to contact lens wear with scleral contact lenses within 6 months of the initial appointment. Scleral contact lenses were recommended for their ability to create a moisture chamber for the cornea.

Discussion

Dry eye diagnostic and treatment techniques have expanded rapidly since the release of the DEWS I Report in 2007[1] the DEWS II Report in 2017.[2] This case illustrates how the use of classic primary care techniques and newer

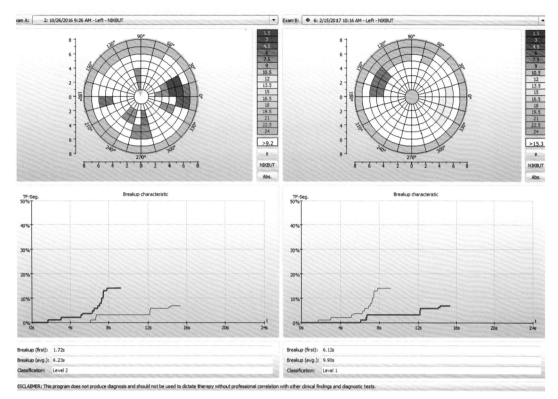

Figure 2.13-3   Serial noninvasive tear breakup time with oculus keratograph 5M OD (top) and OS (bottom).
Abbreviations: OD, right eye; OS, left eye.

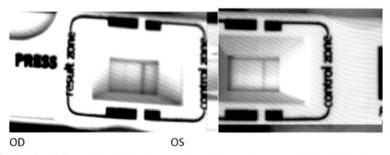

OD   OS

Figure 2.13-4   Baseline InflammaDry testing for matrix metalloproteinase-9, positive at 10 minutes.

advanced technologies can be combined to give the practitioner a more complete picture of the causes underlying ocular surface dryness. It is now understood that ocular surface dryness is chronic and progressive whether the cause is evaporative, inflammatory or a combination of the 2.[1,2]

A newer diagnostic technique that can be easily added to the biomicroscope routine to assess the function of the meibomian glands is the meibomian glands yielding liquid secretion (MGLYS) score obtained with the Korb Meibomian Gland Evaluator (MGE). This instrument simulates a complete blink, which is the stimulus needed to express the meibomian glands to release meibum onto the lid margin.[3] The quantity of functional meibomian glands can be combined with examination of forcefully expressed meibum. Low functional MGLYS scores and turbid quality indicate MGD. The Korb MGE is a simple addition for primary care dry eye evaluation, as it requires very little time

Table 2.13-1	Treatment Protocol
Time Period	**Treatment Protocol**
Month 1	Initiate eyelid cleaning home regimen: lid scrubs twice a day, fish oil-based Omega-3 fatty acid dry eye supplement 2 capsules daily[a] Continue: flaxseed 5 mL daily, lipid-enhanced artificial tears 4 times a day
Month 2	In-office LipiFlow Vectored Thermal Pulse therapy OU Continue: lid scrubs, lipid-enhanced artificial tears 4 times a day, dry eye supplement 2 capsules daily Initiate Iifitegrast (Xiidra) twice a day 1 week post-LipiFlow
Month 5	Continue: lifitegrast twice a day, lid scrubs twice a day, dry eye supplement 2 capsules daily, lipid-enhanced artificial tears 4 times a day Refer for scleral contact lens fitting
Months 6-7	Scleral contact lens fit and dispense

Abbreviation: OU, both eyes.

[a] It should be noted that after the initial home therapy regimen prescribed at the first visit, including lid scrubs and a fish-oil based Omega-3 fatty acid, George felt no significant relief over baseline at month 2. Home therapy was not enough to help George's symptoms and in-office treatment was initiated.

Table 2.13-2	Comparison of Findings at Baseline and After 4 Months of Treatment		
Finding	**Baseline**	**After 4 Months of Therapy**[a]	**Normative Values**
SPEED Q	17 OD and OS	11 OD and OS	>10 is indicative of significant dry eye
Meibomian glands yielding liquid secretion score	Functional glands: OD: 4; OS: 9	Functional glands: OD: 10; OS: 11	10 glands are normal <6 correlated with dry eye symptoms
Noninvasive tear breakup time (by keratograph) first break	OD: 2.68 s; OS: 1.72 s	OD: 4.59 s; OS: 6.12 s	<10 s is indicative of dry eye
Lipid layer thickness (average)	OD 56 nm; OS: 72 nm	OD: 67 nm; OS: 55 nm	<60 nm correlated with dry eye symptoms
InflammaDry	Mild positive (light pink test line) at 10 min OD and OS	Negative (no test line visible) at 10 min OD and OS	Any visible test line, even intermittent or faint, is considered positive for the presence of MMP-9 on the ocular surface

Abbreviations: MMP-9, matrix metalloproteinase-9; OD, right eye; OS, left eye.

[a] At the contact lens fitting appointments (6-7 months into therapy), no signs of punctate keratitis were seen, which had been observed at month 4.

to complete the measurement (under 1 minute for both lower eyelids) and is compatible with slit-lamp biomicroscopy.

For advanced diagnostics, an additional measurement of meibomian gland functionality is lipid layer thickness (LLT). Interferometry (with the LipiView II) quantifies the thickness of the lipid layer of the tear film on the ocular surface. A finding of less than 60 nm has been shown to correlate with dry eye symptoms.[4]

Tear breakup time has been classically measured utilizing sodium fluorescein dye techniques. The advent of computer software combined with infrared technology (such as in the Oculus Keratography 5M), allows for a noninvasive measurement of the tear breakup time to the millisecond. This can be compared over time to demonstrate any improvement, as shown in George's case (Figure 2.13-3). In the absence of equipment for assessment of the noninvasive tear breakup time, classic sodium fluorescein dye should still be used.

The in-office medical laboratory test, InflammaDry (by RPS Diagnostics) detects the presence of the inflammatory marker, matrix metalloproteinase-9 (MMP-9), on the ocular surface.[5] This test confirms that inflammation is present and this finding can be demonstrated to the patient (Figure 2.13-4). This can be helpful for monitoring inflammation and assigning chronic anti-inflammatory therapy, including lifitegrast (Xiidra) or topical cyclosporine (Restasis).

LipiFlow vectored thermal pulsation therapy is a US Food and Drug Administration (FDA)-approved treatment for MGD. This has been shown to be a safe and effective treatment for expressing blocked glands and thereby improving patient symptoms.[6]

The impact of complete lid closure is crucial in a dry eye evaluation. While George demonstrated complete blinks on the blink analysis (LipiView II), it is a common phenomenon that computer users experience a high rate of incomplete blinks, which may also be accompanied by reduced blink frequency. This leads to tear film instability.[7] Reminding patients to take breaks every 10 to 15 minutes while viewing a digital screen can help combat occupational dryness. Blink analysis may also help to explain a mismatch between normal MGYLS scores and a low LLT. If a patient does not blink adequately, readily available meibum may not be transferred to the tear film. Doctors without blink analysis software can detect infrequent blinking during conversation and also note incomplete lid closure with biomicroscopy. On occasion, incomplete lid closure can also occur at night. The Korb-Blackie lid seal test, utilizing a transilluminator on closed eyelids, can be useful to rule out nocturnal lagophthalmos and morning dryness.[8]

This combined inflammatory and evaporative dry eye case illustrates the breadth of options available to ocular surface dryness patients. Primary care evaluation techniques, such as the MGE, biomicroscopy, and lid closure evaluations can help guide the modern practitioner. Other advanced options are available for those seeking ocular surface dryness referral-based resources. The combination of a clean ocular surface, meibomian gland therapy, and oral and topical anti-inflammatory agents provided George with improved comfort and a return to contact lens wear.

CLINICAL PEARLS

- Contact lens intolerance, a history of skin problems, and occupational computer use are each potential signs of dry eye disease.

- Home therapy without in-office treatment is often insufficient to help patients with significant dry eye symptoms. A combination of home therapy, in-office treatments, and topical anti-inflammatory pharmaceuticals can be far more successful.

REFERENCES

1. The definition and classification of dry eye disease: report of the Definition and Classification Subcommittee of the International Dry Eye WorkShop (2007). *Ocul Surf.* April 2007;5(2):75-92.
2. Bron AJ, De Paiva CS, Chauhan SK, et al. TFOS DEWS II pathophysiology report. *Ocul Surf.* July 2017;15(3):438-510.
3. Korb DR, Blackie CA. Meibomian gland diagnostic expressibility: correlation with dry eye symptoms and gland location. *Cornea.* December 2008;27(10): 1142-1147.

4. Eom Y, Lee JS, Kang SY, Kim HM, Song JS. Correlation between quantitative measurements of tear film lipid layer thickness and meibomian gland loss in patients with obstructive meibomian gland dysfunction and normal controls. *Am J Ophthalmol*. June 2013;155(6):1104-1110.

5. Chotikavanich S, de Paiva CS, Li de Q, et al. Production and activity of matrix metalloproteinase-9 on the ocular surface increase in dysfunctional tear syndrome. *Invest Ophthalmol Vis Sci*. July 2009;50(7):3203-3209.

6. Blackie CA, Carlson AN, Korb DR. Treatment for meibomian gland dysfunction and dry eye symptoms with a single-dose vectored thermal pulsation: a review. *Curr Opin Ophthalmol*. July 2015;26(4):306-313.

7. Hirota M, Uozato H, Kawamorita T, Shibata Y, Yamamoto S. Effect of incomplete blinking on tear film stability. *Optom Vis Sci*. 2013;90(7):650-657.

8. Blackie CA, Korb DR. A novel lid seal evaluation: the Korb Blackie light test. *Eye Contact Lens*. March 2015;41(2):98-100.

2.14 Dry Eye Disease Associated With Secondary Sjögren Syndrome

Jillian F. Ziemanski

Mary, a 67-year-old Caucasian female, was referred regarding severe dry eye disease associated with secondary Sjögren syndrome and systemic lupus erythematosus. She reported progressive, constant, and severe dryness of both eyes despite current treatment alternating with artificial tears and lubricant eye gel 6 times per day. This was in addition to the past treatment with intermittent cyclosporine (Restasis), Omega-3 fatty acids, and punctal plugs. She denied any other relevant ocular history. She was first diagnosed with both systemic lupus erythematosus and secondary Sjögren syndrome 16 years ago. Her medical history was otherwise unremarkable.

Clinical Findings

Ocular Surface Disease Index (OSDI) symptom survey	89.5 (range from 0 to 100; values $\geq$33 reflect severe disease[1])
Habitual VA	OD: 20/25^{-2}; OS: 20/25^{-1}
Tear osmolarity	OD: 379 milliosmoles/L; OS: 359 milliosmoles/L (mOsms/L)
Matrix metalloproteinase 9 (MMP-9) testing	OD: negative; OS: negative
Lipid layer thickness	OD: 88 nm; OS: 77 nm
Dynamic meibography imaging (Figure 2.14-1)	Right lower lid: 50% dropout Left lower lid: 30% dropout
Slit-lamp examination	OU: eyelids: margins mildly edematous with moderate posterior lid margin hyperemia, moderate lid wiper epitheliopathy, significant reduction in meibomian gland expression with digital pressure; cornea: scattered anterior stromal scars, moderate superficial punctate epitheliopathy inferiorly; tear film: moderate cellular debris
Tear breakup time	2 s OD and OS
Phenol red thread test (wetting in 15 s)	OD: 12 mm; OS 14 mm

Abbreviations: OD, right eye; OS, left eye; OU, both eyes; VA, visual acuity.

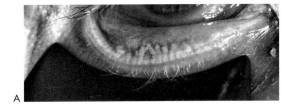

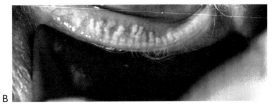

Figure 2.14-1 Meibography images of the right lower (top image) and left lower (bottom image) lids taken by the LipiView II.

Comments

Mary was diagnosed with combined-etiology dry eye disease (both aqueous-deficient and evaporative) (see Chapter 2.13) associated with meibomian gland dysfunction and secondary Sjögren syndrome. A multifaceted treatment plan was established to manage her dry eye disease. She was advised to resume oral Omega-3 fatty acid supplements (2 g/d), to invest in moisture-chamber spectacles particularly for outdoor use, and to begin warm compresses for 10 minutes twice daily. Cyclosporine ophthalmic emulsion (Restasis) was prescribed twice per day together with loteprednol etabonate (Lotemax) 3 times per day for 6 weeks, then twice per day for 1 week, then once per day for 1 week. Artificial tears and lubricating gel were continued, alternating every 2 hours. If her signs and symptoms did not improve significantly after 3 months of therapy, then an amniotic membrane graft would be considered.

Mary was seen 10 days after starting loteprednol to ensure no IOP increase resulted from the topical steroid. After 3 months of treatment, no significant relief was apparent. Therefore, an amniotic membrane graft was used in each eye (provided at separate visits). The grafts dissolved within 5 days, and the bandage contact lenses were removed without incident. Mary noted an immediate improvement in overall dryness and ocular irritation. Cyclosporine was reinitiated but later switched to lifitegrast.

Thirteen months after the initial consultation, Mary's dry eye was well managed with lifitegrast as the primary therapeutic agent, supplemented by Omega-3 fatty acids, moisture-chamber spectacles, warm compresses, lubricating gel, and artificial tears. Her Ocular Surface Disease Index (OSDI) had improved to 31 (a moderate value), though this was complicated by visual symptoms from recently developed posterior subcapsular cataracts. The cataract development was presumed to be secondary to oral prednisone, which had been prescribed by her rheumatologist 2 months earlier. Best-corrected visual acuity (VA) had reduced to OD: 20/40; OS: 20/30, prompting a referral for cataract surgery. She was to maintain her current dry eye therapy with acute episodes to be reassessed.

Discussion

Sjögren syndrome is an autoimmune exocrinopathy that often leads to severe and debilitating dry eye disease. Approximately 2 to 4 million people in the United States are afflicted with the condition, with 9 times more females than males.[2] It is most common in individuals between 40 and 55 years of age, although it is becoming more prevalent in younger subjects. Sjögren syndrome can occur primarily as an isolated autoimmune condition, or secondarily in association with other autoimmune conditions, such as rheumatoid arthritis or systemic lupus erythematosus. It is estimated that 60% of Sjögren syndrome cases are secondary to other autoimmune conditions.[2,3]

The underlying pathogenesis of Sjögren syndrome is poorly understood. The prevailing theory is that a predisposed individual has multiple genetic polymorphisms, which ultimately accumulate to make her more susceptible to an environmental trigger. The most recognized factor is exposure to particular viral or bacterial microbes that are structurally similar to other molecules naturally present in the human body. Once sensitized to these microbial antigens, predisposed individuals begin an immune response against their own tissues that contain structurally similar antigens.[3] Hormonal changes have also been implicated in the disease pathogenesis. Sjögren disease is common in peri- and postmenopausal women, when estrogen levels are known to decline. Since estrogen is considered protective of exocrine glands, reduced estrogen levels may make the lacrimal and salivary glands vulnerable to apoptotic death and subsequent immune insult.[3]

Patients with Sjögren syndrome are most likely to present with dry eye symptoms. Associated complaints may include burning, stinging, grittiness, soreness, itching, photosensitivity, glare, or blurred vision. Dry eye associated with Sjögren syndrome almost always results from a deficiency in aqueous tear production, but is also commonly associated with meibomian gland dysfunction. Ocular surface inflammation is frequently, but not ubiquitously, present. Due to the severity of dry eye disease, these patients are more likely to experience recurrent corneal erosions, corneal ulceration, and, rarely, corneal perforation necessitating transplantation.[2,3]

Clinical evaluation of Sjögren syndrome patients should go beyond a routine eye examination and be tailored to their presenting complaints. Problem-focused dry eye evaluations should document severity so that changes in the response to treatment or the natural progression of the disease can be recorded. Testing should include tear osmolarity, tear MMP-9 detection, tear film imaging, meibography, slit-lamp examination, fluorescein staining, lissamine green staining, meibomian gland expression, and tear production testing (eg, Schirmer or phenol red thread test).

Sjögren syndrome is a systemic disease that is capable of immune attack of nearly all body systems. The second most common manifestation is xerostomia, or dry mouth. Patients may also experience dryness of other surfaces, such as the skin, nasal passages, throat, and vagina. Up to half of all Sjögren syndrome patients develop extraglandular manifestations, primarily affecting the articular, pulmonary, or neurologic systems[4,5] but also extending into hematologic, gastrointestinal, and dermatologic systems, among others.[2] Notably, up to 10% of patients with Sjögren syndrome develop life-threatening neoplastic conditions, such as non-Hodgkin's B-cell lymphoma.[4,6]

Given that Sjögren syndrome is a systemic autoimmune condition, a thorough review of systems should be completed for every dry eye patient. The disease should be considered in patients who report dry mouth symptoms or swelling of their salivary glands. Patients who demonstrate severe ocular surface signs, such as a Schirmer test finding without anesthesia ≤5 mm/5 min or significant corneal staining, especially when their disease is recalcitrant to standard treatment, should be evaluated for Sjögren syndrome.[3]

Anti-SSA (anti-Ro), anti-SSB (anti-La), rheumatoid factor (RF), and antinuclear antibodies (ANA) are the classic autoantibodies associated with Sjögren syndrome. However, these antibodies have come under scrutiny due to concerns that they may be late-stage markers, thereby lacking the sensitivity needed to detect early Sjögren syndrome.[3] Animal studies have revealed 3 additional autoantibodies toward novel proteins in early disease: salivary protein-1, carbonic anhydrase 6, and parotid secretory protein.[7,8]

Just as with other forms of dry eye disease, milder presentations of Sjögren syndrome may be managed with artificial tear supplementation, warm compresses, lid hygiene, and moisture-chamber spectacles. Oral Omega-3 fatty acid supplementation is a potential anti-inflammatory treatment option for mild-to-moderate cases.[9] With moderate signs and symptoms, punctal plugs or topical treatment with corticosteroids, cyclosporine, or lifitegrast may be indicated. For more severe presentations, treatment may include autologous serum tears, amniotic membrane graft placement, and/or scleral contact lenses.[9] These patients are often best managed with a combination of these treatment options to provide a multifactorial defense against autoimmune dry eye disease.

In this case, aggressive dry eye treatment was initiated with a corticosteroid due to its rapid onset of action, while simultaneously initiating the slower-acting cyclosporine. The patient was switched to lifitegrast due to its differing mechanism of action. Amniotic membrane graft placement was also used, for its anti-inflammatory, anti-scarring, and anti-angiogenic effects,[10] which is generally reserved for severe cases of dry eye. Although not considered a long-term treatment option, amniotic membrane graft placement may be particularly helpful in reducing ocular surface inflammation, allowing the attenuated condition to be managed with topical therapeutics.

Treating Sjögren syndrome systemically with immunomodulary medications or other disease-modifying anti-rheumatic drugs provides little or no benefit for the ocular surface condition.[3] For recalcitrant cases of dry eye disease associated with Sjögren syndrome, a rheumatologic evaluation may be indicated, although successful treatment of the ocular surface is more likely to be attained by a combination of palliative measures and topical therapeutic interventions.

CLINICAL PEARLS

- A targeted review of systems emphasizing dry mouth, swollen salivary glands, and joint pain can raise suspicion for undiagnosed Sjögren syndrome. Initiating the appropriate systemic workup will assist with the diagnosis of the condition.

- While specialty diagnostic equipment will expand one's ability to assess the etiology of dry eye disease, a thorough examination can still be obtained with a competent ocular surface biomicroscopic examination. This should include fluorescein staining assessment of the cornea, lissamine green staining assessment of the lid and conjunctiva, and either phenol red thread or Schirmer testing. The meibomian gland structure can be evaluated by transillumination, and meibomian gland function assessed by digital expression. These tests can differentiate between aqueous- and lipid-deficient subtypes.

- A targeted and systematic dry eye evaluation allows more accurate identification of the underlying etiology in order to tailor a more specific treatment plan.

- Dry eye disease associated with Sjögren syndrome can be slow to respond to therapy. A well-devised, multifactorial treatment plan is likely to demonstrate slow and steady improvement over time. Patience from both the patient and the practitioner is paramount.

REFERENCES

1. Miller KL, Walt JG, Mink DR, et al. Minimal clinically important difference for the ocular surface disease index. *Arch Ophthalmol.* 2010;128(1):94-101.
2. Kassan S, Moutsopoulos HM. Clinical manifestations and early diagnosis of Sjogren syndrome. *Arch Intern Med.* 2004;164:1275-1284.
3. Foulks GN, Bunya VY, Hammitt K, et al. Improving diagnosis and outcomes of Sjogren's disease through targeting dry eye patients: a continuing medical education enduring material. *Ocular Surf.* 2015;13(4S):S1-S33.
4. Voulgarelis M, Tzioufas AG, Moutsopoulos HM. Mortality in Sjogren's syndrome. *Clin Exp Rheumatol.* 2008;26(5)(suppl 51):S66-S71.
5. Ramos-Casals M, Brito-Zeron P, Solans R, et al. Systemic involvement in primary Sjogren's syndrome evaluated by the EULAR-SS disease activity index: analysis of 921 Spanish patients (GEAS-SS Registry). *Rheumatology.* 2014;53:321-331.
6. Manganelli P, Fietta P, Quaini F. Hematologic manifestations of primary Sjogren's syndrome. *Clin Exp Rheumatol.* 2006;24:438-448.
7. Shen L, Suresh L, Lindemann M, et al. Novel autoantibodies in Sjogren's syndrome. *Clin Immunol.* 2012;145:251-255.
8. Pertovaara M, Bootorabi F, Kuuslahti M, et al. Novel CA autoantibodies and renal manifestations in patients with pSS. *Rheumatology.* 2011;1453-1457.
9. Management and therapy of dry eye disease: report of the management and therapy subcommittee of the International Dry Eye Workshop. 2007;5(2):163-178.
10. Cheng AMS, Zhao D, Chen R, et al. Accelerated restoration of ocular surface health in dry eye disease by self-retained cryopreserved amniotic membrane. *Ocular Surf.* 2016;14(1):56-63.

2.15 Preseptal Cellulitis

Phillip T. Yuhas

Elaine, a 25-year-old Asian female, presented with a swollen, painful left eye. She reported that her symptoms had been worsening since they began 1 week ago, and graded them as an 8 on a 0 to10 scale. She also noticed recently a clear or white discharge in the affected eye. She initially thought that these symptoms were associated with her rigid gas-permeable (GP) contact lenses, but the eye pain and swelling continued after she discontinued lens wear, 3 days earlier. The patient practiced good contact lens hygiene and denied any photophobia, diplopia, painful eye movements, or fever.

A review of systems revealed anxiety, depression, and menstrual headaches. The patient denied using tobacco or recreational drugs, and there was no history of facial or ocular trauma. Her ocular history was positive only for mild refractive error. Current medications included duloxetine and acetaminophen. No allergies were reported. The patient was oriented to time, place, and person. Her mood and affect were normal.

Clinical Findings

Blood pressure	105/68 mm Hg RAS at 2:10 PM
Body mass index	24.1 kg/m² (normal female range: 18.5-29.9 kg/m²)
Aided distance VA	OD 20/30⁺; OS 20/25⁺
Motility	Full OU, without pain or diplopia
Pupil reactions	PERRL; no RAPD
Intraocular pressure (GAT)	OD 11 mm Hg; OS 11 mm Hg at 2:20 PM
Gross evaluation of the ocular adnexa	OD: unremarkable; OS: 2+ edema and erythema without vesicles of upper and lower eyelid. No proptosis.
Preauricular nodes	Right: unremarkable; Left: palpable
Slit-lamp examination	OD: unremarkable; OS: lid margins and cilia: inspissated meibomiam gland upper lid, 2+ scurf; bulbar conjunctiva: normal; palpebral conjunctiva: 1+ erythema, 1+ papillae; cornea: clear; tear film: uneven; sclera: normal; anterior segment: deep and quiet
Fundus examination	Unremarkable OD and OS

Abbreviations: GAT, Goldmann applanation tonometry; OD, right eye; OS, left eye; OU, both eyes; PERRL, pupils equal, round, reactive to light; RAPD, relative afferent pupillary defect; VA, visual acuity.

Comments

The differential diagnosis list for this patient included allergic dermatitis, viral conjunctivitis with secondary eyelid swelling, orbital cellulitis, and preseptal cellulitis. The clinical findings of unilateral eyelid erythema, edema, and tenderness without the presence of proptosis, pain with eye movement, restricted ocular motility, ocular itch, and follicular conjunctivitis led to the diagnosis of preseptal cellulitis. The infection most likely began as an internal hordeolum in the inspissated meibomian gland and subsequently spread to the surrounding soft tissue. She began oral antibiotic therapy in the form of 1 amoxicillin-clavulanate 875/175 mg capsule twice a day for 10 days. She was instructed to return for a follow-up appointment in 2 days, but sooner if she experienced diplopia, vision loss, or fever.

At follow-up, the patient reported that her symptoms had improved dramatically after starting antibiotic therapy. Visual acuity and extraocular muscle function remained normal. Anterior segment evaluation revealed trace erythema and edema in the left eyelid. An internal hordeolum was seen when the left upper lid was everted. The conjunctiva, sclera, and cornea were unremarkable. The patient was instructed to continue amoxicillin-clavulanate as directed and to initiate warm compresses and lid scrubs. She was also counseled to return after completing the course of antibiotics if her symptoms did not resolve completely. No additional visit was required.

Discussion

Preseptal cellulitis is a localized infection in the soft tissue of the eyelids. This adnexal disease often begins as a contained infection in a specific structure of the eyelid or head that expands into the surrounding soft tissue and skin. Thus, ethmoid sinusitis, hordeolum, dacryocystitis, impetigo, upper respiratory infection, otitis media, conjunctivitis, and blepharitis are all predisposing factors for the development of preseptal cellulitis.[1] A break in the skin over the eyelid from trauma, an insect bite, or a foreign body may also expose the soft tissue of the eyelid to infection.[1] The

orbital septum, a thin barrier of connective tissue connecting the tarsal plate to the periosteum at the orbital margin, prohibits infectious expansion posteriorly into the orbit. Although a wide range of fungal and bacterial pathogens have been implicated in preseptal cellulitis cases, Staphylococcus aureus is the most common etiological pathogen.[2] The prevalence of methicillin-resistant Staphylococcus aureus (MRSA) is increasing, and this dangerous bacterium must be addressed in recalcitrant preseptal cellulitis cases.[3]

Preseptal cellulitis is a common condition that affects males and females at equal rates.[2] The peak incidence occurs in children between 1 week and 5 years of age.[4,5] Young adults are more commonly affected than the middle-aged or older individuals, and the mean age having the highest prevalence is between 19.1 and 34.2 years.[2] The disease occurs most commonly during spring and typically occurs unilaterally without any predilection for the right or left eye.[2]

The clinical presentation of preseptal cellulitis is distinct. Slowly developing erythema and edema in the eyelids are the 2 most common clinical signs.[6] Less common signs may include fever, chemosis, ocular discharge with epiphora, ptosis, and a palpable preauricular node.[1,6] Otherwise, the health of the globe is unremarkable, with normal VAs, extraocular muscle function without proptosis, and intraocular pressure.[6] Warmth and tenderness of the area are the 2 most common symptoms associated with preseptal cellulitis.[6] The average duration of symptoms is approximately 4 days.[7]

Common differential diagnoses for preseptal cellulitis include viral conjunctivitis or ocular allergy with eyelid involvement. Unlike preseptal cellulitis, viral conjunctivitis with eyelid involvement typically presents with conjunctival follicles, conjunctival hyperemia, or skin vesicles. Allergic conjunctivitis with eyelid involvement often presents bilaterally with significant ocular itching, but preseptal cellulitis is more commonly unilateral with mild ocular itching, if present at all. Due to its vision- and life-threatening sequelae, orbital cellulitis is the most important differential diagnosis of preseptal cellulitis. Unlike preseptal cellulitis, orbital cellulitis will present with decreased VA, restricted extraocular muscle function, ophthalmoplegia, or proptosis. Patients presenting with either these signs, or those of preseptal cellulitis with the additional symptoms of drowsiness, vomiting, or severe headaches should be referred immediately to an oculoplastic surgery department or emergency department for potential advanced orbital imaging and surgical intervention to rule out orbital cellulitis and/or treatment.

The initial treatment of preseptal cellulitis should include aggressive oral antibiotic therapy to prevent the infection from spreading into the orbit. For uncomplicated cases, amoxicillin-clavulanate or a cephalosporin are adequate first-line treatments.[5] In the case of a patient with penicillin allergy, a macrolide or fluoroquinolone is an appropriate substitute. Trimethoprim-sulfamethoxazole (TMP-SMX) or clindamycin are efficacious against MRSA and should be used in cases where its presence is suspected, such as hospital in-patients, or previous failure with oral antibiotic therapy.[8,9] The first follow-up visit should be no more than 24 to 48 hours after the initial diagnosis, with subsequent appointments every 2 to 7 days until the condition resolves.

The outcome of appropriate treatment for preseptal cellulitis is usually excellent.[2,7] Less commonly, subsequent complications can include cicatricial entropion, lid abscess, and lagophthalmos.[5]

CLINICAL PEARLS

- Preseptral cellulitis is an infection of the soft tissue of the eyelids that lies anterior to the orbital septum. It presents as diffuse eyelid erythema and edema.

- A broad-spectrum antiobiotic such as amoxillin-clavulanate is a strong first-line medication in the management of preseptal cellulitis. In cases where MRSA is the suspected infectious agent, trimethoprim-sulfamethoxazole should be considered.

- Additional signs and symptoms including decreased VA, restricted extraocular muscle function, ophthalmoplegia, proptosis, drowsiness, vomiting, and severe headache could indicate that the infection has moved retrograde into the orbit, resulting in vision- and life-threatening orbital cellulitis.

REFERENCES

1. Chaudhry IA, Shamsi FA, Elzaridi E, Al-Rashed W, Al-Amri A, Arat YO. Inpatient preseptal cellulitis: experience from a tertiary eye care centre. *Br J Ophthalmol.* 2008;92:1337-1341.
2. Bagheri A, Tavakoli M, Aletaha M, Salour H, Ghaderpanah M. Orbital and preseptal cellulitis: a 10-year survey of hospitalized patients in a tertiary eye hospital in Iran. *Int Ophthalmol.* 2012;32:361-367.
3. Mera RM, Suaya JA, Amrine-Madsen H, et al. Increasing role of *Staphylococcus aureus* and community-acquired methicillin-resistant *Staphylococcus aureus* infections in the United States: a 10-year trend of replacement and expansion. *Microb Drug Resist.* 2011;17:321-328.
4. Jackson K, Baker SR. Periorbital cellulitis. *Head Neck Surg.* 1987;9:227-234.
5. Brugha RE, Abrahamson E. Ambulatory intravenous antibiotic therapy for children with preseptal cellulitis. *Pediatr Emerg Care.* 2012;28:226-228.
6. Rao VA, Hans R, Mehra AK. Pre-septal cellulitis–varied clinical presentations. *Indian J Ophthalmol.* 1996;44:225-227.
7. Pandian DG, Babu RK, Chaitra A, Anjali A, Rao VA, Srinivasan R. Nine years' review on preseptal and orbital cellulitis and emergence of community-acquired methicillin-resistant *Staphylococus aureus* in a tertiary hospital in India. *Indian J Ophthalmol.* 2011;59:431-435.
8. Frei CR, Miller ML, Lewis JS II, et al. Trimethoprim-sulfamethoxazole or clindamycin for community-associated MRSA (CA-MRSA) skin infections. *J Am Board Fam Med.* 2010;23:714-719.
9. Miller LG, Daum RS, Creech CB, et al. Clindamycin versus trimethoprim-sulfamethoxazole for uncomplicated skin infections. *N Engl J Med.* 2015;372:1093-1103.

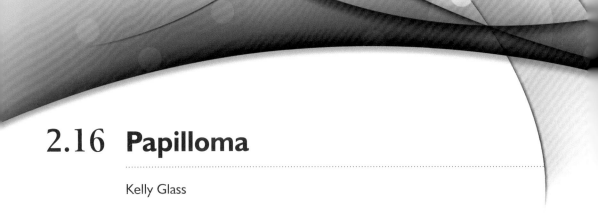

2.16 Papilloma

Kelly Glass

Trent, a 78-year-old male, presented for a general eye examination. He reported dry, irritated eyes and fluctuations in vision throughout the day, affecting the left eye more than the right. This had been occurring for several years, but it had become significantly worse over the past 3 months. In addition, he stated that the lesion on his left upper lid was bothersome. A growth had been present for at least a decade with no noticeable changes in size, shape or color, and it was diagnosed as an eyelid papilloma several years ago. He used artificial tears in both eyes as needed, which provided only minimal relief. His ocular history was positive for bilateral cataract surgery 1 year ago. Trent was prescribed ipratropium bromide and albuterol (Combivent), terazosin and hydrochlorothiazide for chronic obstructive pulmonary disease and hypertension. He used a continuous positive airway pressure (CPAP) machine at night.

Clinical Findings

Unaided distance VA	OD: 20/20; OS: 20/25 (pinhole 20/20)
Present Rx	OD: +0.75 sph (20/20); OS: +1.25 sph (20/20); ADD: +2.25 OU (20/20)
Confrontation visual fields	Full to finger counting OD and OS
Pupil evaluation	PERRL; no RAPD
Subjective refraction	OD: +1.00 −1.00 × 085 (20/20); OS: Pl −0.50 × 095 (20/20)
Intraocular pressure (GAT)	OD: 13 mm Hg; OS: 11 mm Hg at 10:30 AM
Slit-lamp examination	OD: 2+ meibomitis, TBUT 5 s, low tear meniscus (−) SPK OS: 2+ meibomitis, TBUT 5 s, low tear meniscus (−) SPK, nonpigmented squamous papilloma on superior temporal margin measuring 5.5 mm × 3 mm, no lashes missing, small vessels throughout but no feeder vessel, no bleeding, crusting or ulceration
Fundus examination	Unremarkable OD and OS

Abbreviations: GAT, Goldmann applanation tonometry; OD, right eye; OS, left eye; OU, both eyes; PERRL, pupils equal, round, reactive to light; Pl, plano; RAPD, relative afferent pupillary defect; Rx, prescription; sph, sphere; SPK, superficial punctate keratitis; TBUT, tear breakup time; VA, visual acuity.

Comments

Trent was diagnosed with a squamous papilloma in the left upper eyelid and dry eye syndrome in both eyes (Figure 2.16-1). He was provided with samples of artificial tears to be used 4 times a day in each eye and advised to perform warm compresses twice a day for 10 minutes. A moist heat eye compress was recommended for use at night to deflect air seeping from the CPAP machine

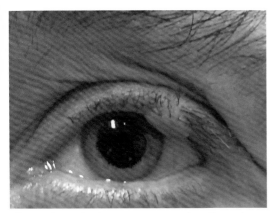

Figure 2.16-1 Large nonpigmented papilloma along left upper eyelid margin.

(see Chapter 2.30). At his request, Trent was referred to an oculoplastics specialist for removal and biopsy of the lid lesion. He was to return in 3 months for a dry eye checkup.

Trent opted to return to the primary eye care provider for removal of the lid lesion. The risks, benefits, alternative procedures, and potential complications were explained to him and consent was reviewed and signed. Approximately 80% of the lesion was removed and it was decided to not go any deeper due to larger vasculature beneath the lesion and greater bleeding possibility. Trent tolerated the procedure well and was instructed to use erythromycin ointment 3 times a day until the tube ran out. He was very satisfied with the outcome immediately after the procedure but was educated more of the bump could be removed at a 5-week follow-up visit.

At the 5-week follow-up visit, the patient reported, "It is worlds better without that big, old knot on my lid that was getting in my way and in my vision." On evaluation, the nonpigmented papilloma was 80% to 90% reduced with only a slight remaining smooth elevation. Lashes were growing superior to the lesion. The biopsy result could not be obtained.

Discussion

Squamous papilloma is a general term referring to a benign sessile or pedunculated proliferation of epithelial tissue. It may occur as a single growth or multiple mulberry-like lesions. On careful examination, one may observe a central

core of vascular tissue within each lesion, which provides a blood supply to the proliferating epithelium. Typically, the surface is covered by hyperkeratotic and acanthotic epithelium. Eyelid papilloma most commonly develops in middle-aged or elderly patients.[1]

Squamous papilloma may also contain varying amounts of pigmentation. Symptoms are generally restricted to cosmetic concern. In rare instances, a large lesion may generate ocular discomfort or lid dysfunction. Squamous papilloma may have a myriad of etiologies, but typically they emerge as a gradual senescent skin change. Squamous papilloma may, on rare cases, constitute precancerous lesions. Accordingly, malignant transformation should remain a consideration.[2]

The case history should include questions regarding chronicity, tenderness, discharge, and growth of the lesion. Additional pertinent factors to consider are a history of skin cancer, sun exposure, immunosuppression, and fair skin type.[3] Slit-lamp examination should include an evaluation of the appearance of the lesion and adjacent skin's surface. The clinician should look for common characteristics of malignant lesions including ulceration with irregular pigment, pearly edges, bleeding or crusting, and the loss of normal eyelid architecture. A significant number of malignant eyelid tumors are misdiagnosed, particularly by nondermatologists.[3] The typical management involves photodocumentation, periodic observation, and patient education.[4] When in doubt, any suspicious lesion should be sent for biopsy.[2] Trent's lid neoplasm, although large in size, exhibited no change in size, shape, color, or border over several years. The presence of eyelashes in the papilloma was a fortuitous sign, lowering suspicion of malignancy. The eyelid architecture remained unchanged and no discharge occurred near the neoplasm site; however, the lid growth did alter the left upper eyelid margin causing more noticeable dry eye symptoms in the affected eye.

When necessary, papilloma are often removed via electrocautery and surgical curettage. The electric current produces iatrogenic necrosis resulting in regression of the lesion, usually within about a week. Without local anesthesia, electrocautery and curettage can be a painful experience for the patient. Scarring is a common displeasing result of these procedures.[5] Laser ablation is also available for removal of these lesions.

CLINICAL PEARLS

- Never assume that a previous practitioner has asked whether the patient would like to have the papilloma removed.

- Consider lid architecture alterations secondary to a squamous papilloma in addition to potential malignant transformation.

REFERENCES

1. Sindt C. Don't overlook the eyelids: what a thorough exam can reveal. *Rev Optom.* 2015;152(3):44-50.
2. Kersten RC, Ewing-Chow D, Kulwin DR, Gallon M. Accuracy of clinical diagnosis of cutaneous eyelid lesions. *Ophthalmology.* 1997;104:479-484.
3. Lober CW, Fenske NA. Basal cell, squamous cell, and sebaceous gland carcinomas of the periorbital region. *J Am Acad Dermatol.* 1991;25(4):685-690.
4. Kasenchak J, Notz D. Eyelid lesions: diagnosis and treatment. *Rev Ophthalmol.* April 2016:71-75.
5. Kabat A, Sowka JW. Kill 'em with chemicals: in most states, ODs can safely and effectively cauterize benign skin lesions with dichloroacetic acid. *Rev Optom.* 2014;151:72-75.

2.17 Molluscum Contagiosum

Bhagya Segu and Padhmalatha Segu

Maria, a 51-year-old Hispanic female, clinic for the removal of a suspected molloscum contagiosum lesion from her right upper eyelid. Maria's ocular history indicated that she had a similar lesion removed from her right lower eyelid 6 months earlier. Subsequent biopsy of that lesion confirmed the diagnosis of molloscum contagiosum. Maria reported that the current lesion developed 1 month after the removal of the earlier lesion. Maria's medical history indicated that she has had osteoarthritis for 5 years, and had bladder surgery and a hysterectomy 7 years ago. There was no history of blood transfusions or a compromised immune system. She had no known drug or seasonal allergies. Current medications include naproxen (Naprosyn) for joint pain. Her family ocular and medical history were unremarkable. Maria was employed as a housekeeper and she denied coming into contact with anyone having a similar lesion. She did not report any history of alcohol consumption, smoking, or steroid use. She tested negative for the human immunodeficiency virus (HIV) after the removal of the first molluscum contagiosum lesion.

Clinical Findings

Aided distance VA	OD: 20/20; OS: 20/20^{-2}
Pupil evaluation	PERRL; no RAPD
Ocular motility	Full range of motion with no restrictions OU
Confrontation visual field	Full to finger counting OD and OS
Intraocular pressure (NCT)	OD: 9 mm Hg; OS: 9 mm Hg at 9:00 AM
Slit-lamp examination	OD: 4 mm horizontal × 2.5 mm vertical flesh colored, dome shaped eyelid lesion with umbilicated center on temporal aspect of upper eyelid; several smaller papillomas along upper and lower eyelid margins. Mild flaking and crusting of skin along upper lid margin. All other findings unremarkable. OS: no flesh colored lesions having umbilicated center; few scattered eyelid papillomas. All other findings unremarkable.
Fundus examination	Unremarkable OD and OS

Abbreviations: NCT, noncontact tonometry; OD, right eye; OS, left eye; OU, both eyes; PERRL, pupils equal, round, reactive to light; RAPD, relative afferent pupillary defect; VA, visual acuity.

Comments

A tentative diagnosis of molloscum contagiosum was based on the clinical appearance of the lesion on the temporal aspect of the right upper eyelid. With Maria's informed consent, the suspected molloscum contagiosum lesion and 2 smaller papillomas were removed from the right eyelid using a local anesthetic followed by excision and cautery and sent to pathology for analysis. Maria was prescribed polysporin ophthalmic ointment twice a day for 5 days for use on her right eyelid, as well as recommended to apply cold compresses over her right eye. She was advised to take acetaminophen (Tylenol) for any postoperative pain. Maria was educated on the contagious nature of molloscum contagiosum, and to avoid direct contact or manipulation of any similar lesions. In addition, Maria was educated on maintaining proper hygiene such as frequent hand washing, no towel sharing, discarding previously used eye makeup, and wearing gloves during work to prevent transmission of the virus. The biopsy was positive for molloscum contagiosum bodies, and the diagnosis was confirmed with Maria at her subsequent follow-up appointment.

Discussion

Molluscum contagiosum is a benign, self-limiting disease of the skin caused by a DNA poxvirus. After an incubation period of 2 weeks to 6 months, the molloscum contagiosum virus undergoes DNA replication resulting in the formation of a flesh-colored, dome-shaped, umbilicated lesion with an average diameter of 2 to 6 mm (Figure 2.17-1).[1] Molloscum contagiosum lesions can be located anywhere on the body depending on the mode of transmission.[2-4] The condition resolves spontaneously within 6 to 12 months without scarring in patients with normal immune systems.[1] However, immunocompromised individuals may have persistent atypical presentation.[5,6] Molloscum contagiosum virus is contracted by direct or indirect contact with an infected individual and is prevalent in young children, sexually active adults, and individuals with compromised immune systems.[1,5]

Ocular manifestations of molloscum contagiosum lesions typically occur along the eyelid margin and rarely the cornea or conjunctiva. If virus particles are shed into the tear film, a toxic follicular keratoconjunctivitis may develop.[7] If the viral conjunctivitis becomes chronic, it may result in conjunctival scarring, corneal scarring, conjunctival chemosis, pannus formation, epiphora, photophobia, and blurred vision.[2,8,9] Eyelid lesions have also been documented to cause contact dermatitis, eczema in surrounding tissue, pruritus, irritation, and pain.[1,2,8]

Nonsurgical management includes palliative therapy such as artificial tears and cold compresses for patients with a superficial keratoconjunctivitis. Topical application of agents such as imiquimod (Aldara), silver nitrate paste, trichloroacetic acid, salicylic acid, cantharidin, tretinoin (Retin-A) potassium hydroxide, and cidofovir cream (Vistide) may also be administered to treat active molloscum contagiosum. The various methods for surgical management include curettage, cryotherapy, electrocautery, electrodessication, and excision of the lesion.[8]

Patients with an atypical presentation such as numerous (>30), large lesions (>1 cm in diameter) with frequent recurrences should be questioned about their immune status and tested for immunosuppressive diseases such as HIV.[5] Patients taking immunosuppressive medications such as prednisone and methotrexate may suffer from widespread molloscum contagiosum lesions. Prior to the availability of highly active antiretroviral therapy (HAART), patients who were seropositive for HIV and had molloscum contagiosum would exhibit a lower CD4 count. In the era of immune reconstitution for treatment of HIV, patients may have isolated molloscum contagiosum lesions without widespread disease, thereby indicating an appropriate T-cell response to the antiretroviral therapy.[10]

Regardless of the method of treatment, all patients must be educated about proper hygiene to prevent the spread of this condition. Infected patients should be counseled on avoiding swimming pools, community baths, contact sports, and sharing towels. Furthermore, the

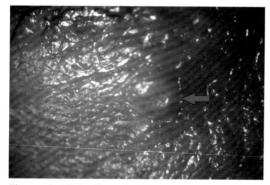

Figure 2.17-1 Example of a molluscum contagiosum lesion located on the right lower eyelid.

patient should avoid direct contact with their lesions, expressing the contents, or shaving the lesion.

CLINICAL PEARLS

- Patients with an atypical presentation, such as numerous (>30), large lesions (>1 cm in diameter) with frequent recurrences, should be questioned about their immune status and tested for immunosuppressive diseases.

- Due to the contagious nature of molloscum contagiosum, patients must be educated about proper hygiene and avoidance of lesion manipulation to prevent the spread of this condition.

- Molloscum contagiosum lesion(s) on the eyelid may result in a follicular keratoconjunctivitis if virus particles are shed into the tear film.

- Molloscum contagiosum spontaneously resolves within 6 to 12 months without scarring in patients with normal immune systems although topical or surgical management may be implemented in symptomatic patients.

REFERENCES

1. Hansen D, Diven DG. Molluscum contagiosum. *Dermatol Online J*. 2003;9(2):2.
2. Husar K, Skerlev M. Molluscum contagiosum from infancy to maturity. *Clin Dermatol*. March-April 2002;20(2):170-172.
3. Smith KJ, Skelton H. Molluscum contagiosum: recent advances in pathogenic mechanisms, and new therapies. *Am J Clin Dermatol*. 2002;3:535-545.
4. Fornatora ML, Reich RF, Gray RG, Freedman PD. Intraoral molluscum contagiosum: a report of a case and a review of the literature. *Oral Surg Oral Med Oral Pathol Oral Radiol Endod*. 2000;92:318-320.
5. Birthistle K, Carrington D. Molluscum contagiosum virus. *J Infect*. 1997;34:21-28. doi:10.1016/S0163-4453(97)80005-9.
6. Robinson MR, Udell IJ, Garber PF, Perry HD, Streeten BW. Molluscum contagioscum of the eyelids in patients with acquired immunodeficiency syndrome. *Ophthalmology*. 1992;99:1745-1747.
7. Ingraham HJ, Schoenleber DB. Epibulbar molluscum contagiosum. *Am J Ophthalmol*. March 1998; 125(3):394-396.
8. Molluscum Contagiosum. *Handbook of Ocular Disease Management*. October 4, 2003.
9. Charteris DG, Bonshek RE, Tullo AB. Ophthalmic molluscum contagiosum: clinical and immunopathological features. *Br J Ophthalmol*. 1995;79:476.
10. Albini T, Rao N. Molluscum contagiosum in an immune reconstituted AIDS patient. *Br J Ophthalmol*. 2003;87:1427-1428.

2.18 Adult Inclusion Conjunctivitis

Kaira Kwong

Janice, a 37-year-old Asian female, presented with redness in both eyes. She had been diagnosed with epidemic keratoconjunctivitis (EKC) in her right eye 1 month earlier. Despite treatment with povidone-iodine solution (Betadine), the symptoms of redness, itchiness, and early morning mucous discharge in the right eye were still present with minimal improvement. Now she had similar symptoms in her left eye for the past 4 days.

Her medical history was positive for recurring candida vaginosis with vaginal discharge over the past 3 days. She reported switching dating partners 6 months ago. She was otherwise healthy with no systemic conditions.

Clinical Findings

Present Rx	OD: −3.25 −2.00 × 180 (20/25, no improvement with pinhole); OS: −3.75 −1.75 × 180 (20/25, no improvement with pinhole)
Pupil evaluation	PERRL; no RAPD
Ocular motility	Full and comitant OU
Confrontation visual field	Full to finger counting OD and OS
Slit-lamp examination	OD: lids/lashes: clear; conjunctiva: diffuse conjunctival hyperemia, grade 2 follicles, and papillae, mild mucopurulent discharge, 1 temporal bulbar follicle; cornea: diffuse superior punctate keratitis, no infiltrates; anterior chamber: deep and quiet, no cells/flare; OS: lids/lashes: clear; conjunctiva: diffuse conjunctival hyperemia, grade 2 follicles, and papillae, mild mucopurulent discharge; cornea: diffuse superior punctate keratitis, no infiltrates; anterior chamber: deep and quiet, no cells/flare
Intraocular pressure (GAT)	OD: 18 mm Hg; OS: 18 mm Hg at 10:18 AM
Fundus examination	Unremarkable OD and OS
Ancillary tests	No preauricular nodes

Abbreviations: GAT, Goldmann applanation tonometry; OD, right eye; OS, left eye; OU, both eyes; PERRL, pupils equal, round, reactive to light; RAPD, relative afferent pupillary defect; Rx, prescription.

Comments

The clinical findings of mixed tarsal follicles and papillae in both eyes, a bulbar conjunctival follicle OS and chronic red eyes despite previous treatment with povidone-iodine led to the working diagnosis of adult inclusion conjunctivitis. A tarsal conjunctival scrape was obtained. Erythromycin ophthalmic ointment was prescribed 4 times a day OU while waiting for the results of the culture. Janice was asked to abstain from sexual activity and return in 1 week.

At the 1-week follow-up visit, Janice's clinical findings remained stable. Her conjunctival culture was positive for chlamydia trachomatis. She was started on a single dose of 1 g oral azithromycin. A referral was provided for a visit with her gynecologist for comanagement of her vaginosis, as well as treatment for her sexual partner.

Discussion

Adult inclusion conjunctivitis, also known as Chlamydial conjunctivitis, is a sexually transmitted disease caused by an obligate, intracellular, Gram-negative bacterium, Chlamydia trachomatis serotypes D-K.[1] Chlamydiae are unique in that they can behave as both bacteria (containing both DNA, RNA, and a cell wall) and viruses (only growing intracellularly). Therefore, the clinical presentation can mimic both bacterial and viral conjunctivitis, characterized by a mixed papillary and follicular tarsal conjunctival response, a bulbar follicular conjunctival response, mucopurulent discharge, and conjunctival hyperemia. Corneal involvement may occur in the form of superior punctate keratitis, subepithelial infiltrates and pannus. The presentation is typically unilateral, but bilateral cases may present. Swollen preauricular nodes can be observed on the ipsilateral side of the involved eye. As there is an overlap between the signs and symptoms of viral conjunctivitis and adult inclusion conjunctivitis, Janice was originally diagnosed with an EKC. Individuals who present with recurrent, chronic red eyes with a marked follicular response and failure to respond to conventional topical antibiotic treatment should be suspected of having adult inclusion conjunctivitis. This diagnosis is supported by concomitant vaginal discharge or chronic vaginitis in women. Men will often be asymptomatic systemically.

Diagnosis is typically made clinically based on patient presentation. The clinical diagnosis can be confirmed by a conjunctival culture and serum levels of immunoglobulin IgG. Basophilic, intracytoplasmic epithelial inclusion bodies are revealed in Giemsa staining of the conjunctival scrapings, hence the name inclusion conjunctivitis.

The patient and their sexual partners should be treated concurrently with systemic antibiotics to prevent reinfection, and also evaluated for other sexually transmitted diseases.[2] The most common antibiotics prescribed for adult inclusion conjunctivitis are azithromycin 1 g orally in a single dose or doxycycline 100 mg orally twice a day for 7 days.[3] Alternatives include tetracycline 500 mg orally 4 times a day for 7 days, erythromycin 500 mg orally 4 times a day for 7 days or ofloxacin 200 to 400 g orally twice a day for 7 days. Topical antibiotics have not been proven to be an effective mode of treatment.

Janice was comanaged with her gynecologist and returned 2 weeks later. Her ocular symptoms had improved significantly. She no longer had symptoms of ocular discharge, redness, tearing or burning. Her gynecologist tested her serum IgG levels and continued her and her partner on a repeated dose of 1 g oral azithromycin. It is not unusual for patients to require multiple treatments to eradicate this disease completely. After 1 month, all ocular and vaginal symptoms had resolved, and her serum IgG levels were normal. She was discharged to follow-up for her annual eye examination in 6-months' time.

According to the US Centers for Disease Control and Prevention (CDC), chlamydia is among the most common notifiable diseases in the United States.[4] The World Health Organization (WHO) reported that it is also the world's leading infectious cause of blindness.[5] An untreated, chronic ocular chlamydial infection can lead to inflammation and scarring of the conjunctival tissue, trichiasis, entropion, corneal opacity, and blindness. Systemically, undiagnosed chlamydia can lead to pelvic inflammatory disease, infertility, and neonatal infection. Multiple treatments may be necessary for the complete eradication of the disease. Accordingly, early diagnosis and adequate follow-up care is paramount for overall treatment success.

CLINICAL PEARLS

- Adult inclusion conjunctivitis is a sexually transmitted disease caused by a Gram-negative bacterium, Chlamydia trachomatis, serotypes D-K.

- Chlamydiae behave as both a bacteria and virus, causing the clinical presentation to resemble both of these types of conjunctivitis.

- Clinical signs of chlamydial conjunctivitis can include a mixed papillary and follicular tarsal response, a bulbar follicular response, mucopurulent discharge, conjunctival hyperemia, and corneal involvement.

- Adult inclusion conjunctivitis is treated with systemic antibiotics.

- Sexual partners must be treated concurrently to avoid reinfection.

REFERENCES

1. *Conjunctivitis Preferred Practice Pattern – 2013*. San Francisco, CA: American Academy of Ophthalmology. https://www.aao.org/preferred-practice-pattern/conjunctivitis-ppp--2013. October 2013. Accessed February 16, 2017.
2. *External Disease and Cornea*. San Francisco, CA: American Academy of Ophthalmology; 2009.
3. Malamos P, Georgala I, Rallis K, et al. Evaluation of single-dose azithromycin versus standard azithromycin/doxycycline treatment and clinical assessment of regression course in patients with adult inclusion conjunctivitis. *Curr Eye Res*. December 2013;38(12):1198-1206.
4. *Chlamydia. 2015 Sexually Transmitted Diseases Surveillance*. Atlanta, GA: Centers for Disease Control and Prevention. https://www.cdc.gov/std/stats15/chlamydia.htm. Last reviewed October 17, 2016. Accessed February 16, 2017.
5. *WHO Guidelines for the Treatment of Chlamydial Trachomatis*. Geneva, Switzerland: World Health Organization; WHO Press. http://apps.who.int/iris/bitstream/10665/246165/1/9789241549714-eng.pdf.s. Accessed March 1, 2017.

2.19 Epidemic Keratoconjunctivitis

Navjit Kaur Sanghera

Sarah, a 15-year-old African American female, presented with a sudden red, painful, blurry, watery, swollen, and photophobic right eye. She reported that the symptoms began 5 days ago with slight discomfort and foreign body sensation and had since become worse. Sarah had gone to the local emergency department 2 days ago and was given an antibiotic ointment, but reported no improvement. She stated she was recovering from an upper respiratory infection with a temperature as high as 101.7°, approximately 1 week ago. No other family members had the condition, although her boyfriend also had red eyes. Her most recent eye examination was 10 months earlier and she had never worn glasses. Her past medical, surgical, and allergy histories were unremarkable.

Clinical Findings

Unaided distance VA	OD: 20/20⁻; OS: 20/20⁻
Pupil evaluation	PERRL; no RAPD
Ocular motility	Full range of motion OU
Confrontation visual fields	Full to finger counting OD and OS
Intraocular pressure (GAT)	OD: 15 mm Hg; OS: 14 mm Hg at 12:30 PM
Slit-lamp examination	OD: adnexa: clear; lid/lashes: (+) edema upper/lower lids; conjunctiva: diffuse 2+ hyperemia; follicles; petechial hemorrhages; (+) pseudomembrane with temporal symblepharon lower lid; sclera: 1+ diffuse injection; cornea: trace SPK; anterior chamber: deep and quiet; angle, iris, lens: unremarkable;
	OS: adnexa: clear; lid/lashes: clear; conjunctiva: diffuse 2+ hyperemia; follicles; petechial hemorrhages; cclera: 1+ diffuse injection; cornea: trace SPK; anterior chamber: deep and quiet; angle, iris, lens: unremarkable
Fundus examination	Unremarkable OD and OS
Supplementary testing	Right palpable preauricular lymph node. Patient reported tender to touch;
	Left preauricular lymph node unremarkable

Abbreviations: GAT, Goldmann applanation tonometry; OD, right eye; OS, left eye; OU, both eyes; PERRL, pupils equal, round, reactive to light; RAPD, relative afferent pupillary defect; VA, visual acuity.

Comments

Sarah was diagnosed with epidemic keratoconjunctivis (EKC), which is a common, but serious ocular surface infection caused by adenovirus disease.[1] Although there are many laboratory tests such as cell culture in combination with immunofluorescence staining, serologic methods, antigen detection, polymerase chain reaction,[1] and the noninvasive RPS Adeno Detector, which can confirm the diagnosis within 10 minutes in office, these are rarely used or necessary. There

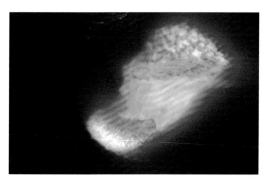

Figure 2.19-1   Pseudomembrane formation in the right inferior conjunctiva.

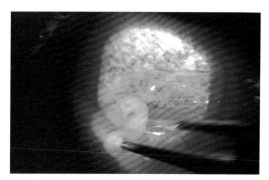

Figure 2.19-2   Removal of pseudomembrane with jeweler's forceps.

are no known treatments for these viral infections and management is usually palliative with cool compresses, artificial tears, and vasoconstrictors. Due to the presence of the pseudomembrane (Figure 2.19-1), which can prolong recovery, it was decided to perform a membrane peel. The initial attempts to use a wet, cotton-tipped applicator to roll the membrane were not successful so jeweler's forceps were used (Figure 2.19-2). Based on the amount of difficulty and resultant bleeding, it was determined there was symblepharon formation in the fornices. Due to the adhesive properties of the membrane, the patient was given proparacaine every 5 minutes for comfort and phenylephrine to increase vasoconstriction and decrease bleeding. The patient was also given gatifloxacin (Zymar) pre- and post-procedure for antibiotic coverage due to increased risk of bacterial infection post peel. There were no complications.

Due to the removal of the membrane and bleeding during the procedure, the patient was prescribed 1 drop of tobramycin/dexamethasone (Tobradex) every 3 hours OD and tobramycin/dexamethasone ointment 4 times per day OD for comfort, reduction of membrane response and antibacterial coverage. Although conjunctival findings are usually self-limiting within 2 to 4 weeks, the patient remains infectious during this time. Sarah was advised to limit close personal contact, wash hands frequently, wipe down all surfaces such as doorknobs and counter tops, and to wash all personal items such as linens, pillows, and towels in hot water. She was also advised to educate her boyfriend regarding her diagnosis for further prevention

of exposure to others. She was asked to return in 2 days for a follow-up visit.

Sarah missed her 2-day follow-up visit and instead returned in 2 weeks. She was instilling tobramycin/dexamethasone drops during the day, albeit only twice a day, and she used the tobramycin/dexamethasone ointment at night. She reported using artificial tears throughout the day and cold compresses as needed. Her symptoms were improving, but she now reported slight blur in her right eye. Clinical findings were as follows:

Unaided distance VA	OD: 20/25; OS: 20/20
Slit-lamp examination	OD: presence of pseudomembrane, resolved lid edema and conjunctival chemosis, diffuse injection, follicles (Figure 2.19-3), 1(+) SEIs central cornea OS: (−) pseudomembrane

Abbreviations: OD, right eye; OS, left eye; SEIs, subepithelial infiltrates; VA, visual acuity.

All other clinical findings remained unchanged. The cause of the decreased vision in the right eye was the presence of the corneal central subepithelial infiltrates. The pseudomembrane, which had reformed, was removed easily with a wet cotton-tipped applicator. No complications were noted. Since Sarah's symptoms had improved, she was instructed to taper her tobramycin/dexamethasone drops to once daily for 1 week and then to stop. She was

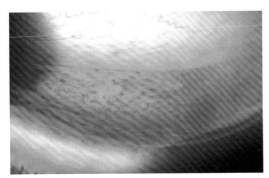

Figure 2.19-3 Visible follicles of the right eye at the 2-week follow-up.

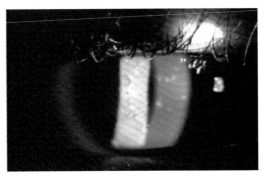

Figure 2.19-4 Presence of central scattered subepithelial infiltrates in the right eye.

also instructed to discontinue the tobramycin/dexamethasone ointment, but to continue her artificial tears throughout the day. Sarah was reminded of the infectious nature of her condition and to continue taking precautions. She was asked to return in 2 weeks.

Sarah missed her 2-week follow-up appointment, but instead returned in 7 weeks after the initial presentation. She had discontinued all medications by this time and reported feeling much better, although she stated that vision in her right eye was still blurry. Clinical findings were as follows:

Unaided distance VA	OD: 20/30; OS: 20/20⁻
Slit-lamp examination	OD: (+) central scattered subepithelial infiltrates (Figure 2.19-4); OS: mild conjunctival redness

Abbreviations: OD, right eye; OS, left eye; VA, visual acuity.

All other clinical findings remained unchanged.

At this point, the EKC was following its natural course and the presence of multiple subepithelial infiltrates was not uncommon. Sarah was educated on the reduction in visual acuity (VA) secondary to her corneal findings and their slow resolution (few weeks to months and in some cases years). In the meantime, she was asked to return in 1 month to monitor resolution with possible refraction at that visit.

Discussion

A patient who initially presents with marked foreign body sensation, photophobia, profuse tearing, and hyperemic eyes should always be considered for a viral conjunctivitis. Although there are many possible causes for a red eye, unilateral followed by bilateral involvement, profuse watery discharge, history of a recent upper respiratory infection, and a palpable preauricular node, help to rule out allergic or bacterial conjunctivitis. The initial presentation of a viral conjunctivitis is usually unilateral with the second eye becoming less severely involved approximately 5 to 10 days later. In Sarah's case, the right eye was affected 5 days prior to her first visit with less involvement of the left eye at the initial presentation. The VA OU was stable when compared with her last eye examination 10 months earlier. In the early stages of the disease, VA is typically unaffected, but this can change if the cornea becomes involved. The stages of EKC-related keratitis are outlined in Table 2.19-1. The patient's presentation of multifocal subepithelial infiltrates at the 2-week appointment supports the diagnosis of EKC, as their presence is considered pathognomonic for the disease.[1]

Conjunctival redness is common along with edema of the lids, caruncle, and conjunctiva. The incubation period is typically 2 to 14 days after inoculation when follicles begin to develop, typically inferiorly. During this time, the patient is asymptomatic and may spread the virus inadvertently.[1] The patient may remain infectious for 10 to 14 days after the onset of symptoms, which tend to last between 7 and

Table 2.19-1   Stages of Keratitis in Epidemic Keratoconjunctivitis[2]

Stage 1 (days 2-5)	Fine, diffuse punctate epithelial keratitis
Stage 2 (days 4-8)	Focal white subepithelial opacities Cornea stains with rose bengal
Stage 3 (days 6-12)	Coarse granular infiltrates
Stage 4 (as early as 2 wk)	Classic subepithelial infiltrates that do not stain Infiltrates may persist for weeks to months to years and can cause permanent scars

21 days. The fellow eye is involved in more than 50% of the cases (usually within 7 days of onset), although the signs and symptoms are typically less severe in the second eye.

Pseudomembranes can form in one-third of cases[3] often making the follicles very difficult to see. This was true in Sarah's case, as a pseudomembrane was present in the right eye (Figure 2.19-1) with subtler underlying follicles. The follicles were clearly visible in her left eye on lower lid eversion as there was no pseudomembrane. Commonly present in EKC, the pseudomembrane is composed of fibrin and leukocytes, and in prolonged cases fibroblasts and collagen deposits. If left untreated, the presence of a pseudomembrane containing high amounts of viral load can delay recovery and lead to possible conjunctival scarring, symblepharon formation, and patient discomfort.

The use of steroids when no pseudomembrane is present may be controversial due to the masking of patient symptoms, stimulation of viral replication, and prolonged viral shedding. If a steroid is considered absolutely necessary, a mild steroid should be considered such as fluorometholone (FML Forte) or loteprednol etabonate (Lotemax) and tapered after 2 weeks. In the later stages of the condition, a steroid can be used for the subepithelial infiltrates if there is significant vision loss or prolonged/severe symptoms, but it should be tapered very slowly

to decrease recurrence of the infiltrates. Topical ganciclovir ophthalmic gel 0.15% has shown efficacy against adenovirus and can shorten the recovery time.[4] Cidofovir reduces the viral replication cycle and can also be effective as a prophylactic agent.[5] Antiviral medications such as trifluridine (Viroptic) are ineffective against the adenovirus because adenovirus does not encode any of the enzymes that are commonly inactivated by trifluridine. Though off-label, povidone-iodine (Betadine) solution (5%) will provide an immediate reduction in patient symptoms and decreased formation of pseudomembranes and subepithelial infiltrates. Although this treatment was not applied in Sarah's case, it is commonly performed and the process is highlighted as follows[1]:

- Instill 1 drop of 0.5% proparacaine
- Instill 1 to 2 drops of topical non steroidal anti-inflammatory drug (NSAID)
- Instill 4 to 5 drops of povidone-iodine 5% ophthalmic prep solution
- The patient should roll his/her eyes for full exposure
- Swab lid margin(s) with cotton-tipped applicator with lids closed
- Wait for 60 seconds
- Lavage ocular tissues with sterile saline irrigation solution
- Prescribe loteprednol etabonate 4 times a day for 4 to 5 days

Epidemic keratoconjunctivis is one of the most serious forms of adenoviral infections and the infectious agent can survive on nonporous surfaces such as tonometer tips for approximately 34 days.[4] In the eye care practitioner's office, all clinical surfaces and ophthalmic instruments should be disinfected immediately. The US Centers for Disease Control and Prevention (CDC) recommends that "semicritical items" that have come in contact with mucous membrane tissue or non-intact skin should be wiped clean and disinfected for 5 to 10 minutes with either 3% hydrogen peroxide, 5000 ppm chlorine, 70% ethyl alcohol or 70% isopropyl alcohol, then rinsed in tap water and air dried before use. Most manufacturers of medical devices also include at least 1 validated cleaning and disinfection or sterilization protocol for their devices for reference. For instrumentation that has come into contact with blood, sterilization is recommended by first properly cleaning and disinfecting the instrument, then placing in peel pouches and autoclaved.[1]

Consideration should also be given to more detrimental differential diagnoses such as pharyngoconjunctival fever (which is common in children, although high fever and corneal involvement is rare) and acute hemorrhagic conjunctivitis (often associated with a large subconjunctival hemorrhage). Any underlying conditions that have the potential to lead to viral conjunctivitis should be managed accordingly.

CLINICAL PEARLS

- Keep all equipment, instruments, and chair areas clean to avoid staff and patient contamination.

- Advise the patient to use his or her own washcloths, towels, pillows, and utensils. Recommend the patient wash all fabric items regularly for at least 2 weeks.

- Advise the patient to wash hands regularly or wear plastic gloves when at home for at least 2 weeks. Having the practitioner wear gloves during the examination will emphasize their importance.

- Reserve steroids for severe cases as infiltrates usually resolve independently of treatment. Topical NSAIDS are another option prior to steroids. If steroids are used, perform a slow taper as the condition resolves.

- Patients should be educated that symptoms will worsen before they get better.

REFERENCES

1. Pihos AM. Epidemic keratoconjunctivitis: a review of current concepts in management. *J Optom.* 2013;6(2):69-74. doi:10.1016/j.optom.2012.08.003.
2. Piccolo M, Victor M. Viral infectious diseases. *Ocular Therapeutics Handbook: A Clinical Manual.* Philadelphia, PA: Wolters Kluwer/Lippincott Williams & Wilkins; 2011:311-17.
3. Bagheri N, Wajda BN, Calvo CM, Durrani AK, Friedberg MA, Rapuano CJ. *The Wills Eye Manual: Office and Emergency Room Diagnosis and Treatment of Eye Disease.* Philadelphia, PA: Wolters Kluwer Health/Lippincott Williams & Wilkins; 2017:14-38.
4. Heiberger MH, Madonna RJ, Nehmad L. *Emergency Care in the Optometric Setting.* New York: McGraw-Hill; 2004.
5. Hillenkamp J, Reinhard T, Ross RS, et al. The effects of cidofovir 1% with and without cyclosporin a 1% as a topical treatment of acute adenoviral keratoconjunctivitis: a controlled clinical pilot study. *Ophthalmology.* May 2002;109(5):845-850.

2.20 Vernal Keratoconjunctivitis

Kaira Kwong

Olivia, a 12-year-old white female, was referred for a "corneal ulcer" in the right eye. She was complaining of sharp, needle-like pain, photosensitivity, mucoid discharge and blurry vision OD for 2 days. She had a history of allergic conjunctivitis and intense itching OD that started a month ago. Olivia reported frequent scratching of her eyes. Her medical history was significant for asthma and seasonal allergies. This visit took place in the autumn. She was not taking any systemic medication or eye drops.

Clinical Findings

Distance VA (through habitual Rx)	OD: 20/100 (pinhole 20/60); OS: 20/30 (pinhole 20/25)
Pupil evaluation	PERRL; no RAPD
Ocular motility	Full and comitant OU
Confrontation visual fields	Full to finger counting OD and OS
Subjective refraction	OD: −4.75 sph (20/100); OS: −4.75 sph (20/20)
Slit-lamp examination	OD: lids/lashes: erythematous with a reactive ptosis; conjunctiva: hyperemia, giant cobblestone papillae superior > inferior palpebral conjunctiva OD >> OS with thick, ropy mucoid debris in between papillae (Figure 2.20-1); cornea: ulcer superiorly extending to central cornea with top lesion 6 mm vertical × 4 mm horizontal connected to lower lesion 3 mm × 3 mm on visual axis (Figure 2.20-2); diffuse superior punctate keratitis 360°, stromal haze 360° and obscurity of pupil; anterior chamber: deep and quiet to the extent seen; iris: clear; angle: 3 × 3.
	OS: lids/lashes: clear; conjunctiva: hyperemia, giant cobblestone papillae superior > inferior palpebral conjunctiva OD >> OS; cornea: clear; anterior chamber: deep and quiet to the extent seen; iris: clear; angle: 3 × 3.
Intraocular pressure (GAT)	OD: 16 mm Hg; OS: 16 mm Hg at 10:15 AM
Fundus examination	Unremarkable OD and OS

Abbreviations: GAT, Goldmann applanation tonometry; OD, right eye; OS, left eye; OU, both eyes; PERRL, pupils equal, round, reactive to light; RAPD, relative afferent pupillary defect; Rx, prescription; sph, sphere; VA, visual acuity.

Discussion

Olivia presented with conjunctival vernal keratoconjunctivitis (VKC). She had pathognomonic giant cobblestone papillae on her superior tarsal conjunctiva, that was evident on lid eversion, with ropy mucoid debris between the papillae (Figure 2.20-1), a shield ulcer (Figure 2.20-2), and ptosis OD. Her left eye had a milder presentation of chronic allergic conjunctivitis.

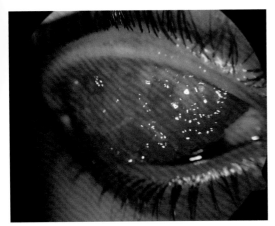

Figure 2.20-1   Cobblestone papillae OD.
Abbreviation: OD, right eye.

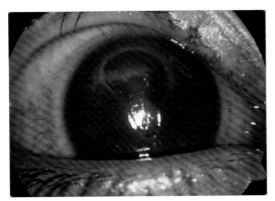

Figure 2.20-2   Shield ulcer OD.
Abbreviation: OD, right eye.

Vernal keratoconjunctivitis is a severe, sight-threatening ocular disease that occurs predominantly in school-age children (5 to 15 years of age).[1] The condition has a 3 to 4 times predilection for males rather than females in patients younger than 20 years. This disease typically lasts between 4 and 10 years and resolves after puberty.[2] Vernal keratoconjunctivitis is found throughout the world with a wide range of racial and geographic variation, and is most prevalent in warm Mediterranean countries.[1] Although vernal implies that it occurs in the spring, the disease commonly occurs throughout the year. In Olivia's case, the condition was long-standing and the development of a shield ulcer caused her to present in the autumn.

Patients typically present with intense itching, discharge, blepharospasm, photophobia, tearing, and redness. They often have a systemic history of allergic rhinitis or asthma. There are 3 distinct types of VKC, namely tarsal, limbal, and mixed presentations.[3] The tarsal form of the disease is characterized by giant, cobblestone papillae, greater than 1 mm in diameter, on the upper tarsal plate. Mucous accumulation can be observed between the papillae. The limbal form of VKC is characterized by Horner–Trantas dots, which are gelatinous, light-gray limbal infiltrates containing epithelial cell debris and degenerated eosinophils.[3] Mixed VKC, as the name suggests, is simply a combination of these 2 entities. Olivia presented with the tarsal form of VKC.

Corneal involvement can vary between mild (punctate epithelial keratitis) and severe (macroerosions and sterile ulcers). A shield ulcer is seen in approximately 3% to 11% of VKC patients, and is the main cause of permanent visual reduction.[1] Shield ulcers are oval-shaped, sterile, epithelial defects with an intact Bowman membrane that are usually located on the upper half of the visual axis. In more chronic cases, they can have an overlying fibrin or mucous plaque that may need to be removed surgically. Superficial corneal neovascularization may be a manifestation of VKC, and its presence suggests active palpebral disease. In the resolved stages of the disease, pseudogerontoxon lesions can be found in the peripheral cornea. These are gray–white lipid deposits that appear similar to arcus senilis (also known as generontoxon) and is caused by the waxing and waning corneal damage from VKC.[4]

Vernal keratoconjunctivitis is both an IgE- and non-IgE-mediated ocular allergy. It was previously thought to be caused by an IgE-mediated response only from mast cell release. However, this theory did not explain the varied inflammatory response, and why episodes did not always coincide with environmental factors.[1] It is now believed that CD4[+] Th2 lymphocytes also play an important role in the development of VKC by increasing the expression of co-stimulatory molecules, cytokines, chemokines, and interleukins. This cascade promotes mast cell degranulation, the release of histamines and triggers a type I and type IV hypersensitivity reaction.[5] Giant papillae are caused by epithelial thickening and fibroblast formation. Damage to the cornea is caused by metalloproteinases, neurotoxins, eosinophils, and eosinophil-derived basic proteins.[1] This cycle of chronic inflammation causes tissue remodeling changes and the clinical signs of VKC.[1,6]

In young patients, VKC will generally resolve upon reaching puberty. However, it can be debilitating if severe or treated inappropriately. Potential consequences may be corneal scarring, glaucoma from prolonged steroid use and blindness. The mainstay of treatment for VKC is medical treatment in a stepwise sequence depending on the level of disease (Table 2.20-1).[6]

The first line of treatment is environmental modification and to remove the offending agents triggering the immune response. For mild cases, cool compresses, artificial tears, topical antihistamines (levocabastine 0.05%, emadastine 0.05%) and mast cell stabilizers (sodium cromoglycate 2% to 4%, lodoxamide 1%) are successful. Note that olopatadine 0.1%, a dual-acting mast cell stabilizer and antihistamine, has been shown to be more effective compared to either mast cell stabilizer or antihistamines alone.[1,6]

For moderate cases, topical corticosteroids, such as prednisolone, fluorometholone, and dexamethasone are added to the treatment regimen. However, one must monitor for glaucoma, cataract, and opportunistic infections during steroid use. Loteprednol is a good alternative to prednisolone as it has less effect on the intraocular pressure and is equally efficacious.[7]

Severe cases of VKC can be treated with the addition of immunomodulating agents, such as cyclosporine A and tacrolimus. They have the ability to inhibit T-cell activation, and have been shown to be safe and effective to use in children.[1] Surgical treatment is rarely required unless a corneal plaque develops. Giant papillae can be removed with excision and mitomycin-C. Amniotic membranes can be effective for refractory cases.[8]

Olivia was started on prednisolone acetate 1% 4 times daily OD, moxifloxacin (Vigamox) 4 times daily OD for infection prophylaxis, cyclopentolate 1% 3 times daily for pain and olopatadine (Patanol) twice daily OU to control her underlying inflammatory condition. Her pediatrician was consulted, and prescribed sodium montelukast (Singulair) to control her asthma and allergies. She was also sent for immunology testing. At a 2-week follow-up visit, visual acuity (VA) in the right eye had improved slightly to 20/50 with pinhole. Her left eye had a best-corrected VA of 20/20, and showed an improved papillary response. An amniotic membrane lens was inserted at this visit OD due to the slow resolution of the corneal shield ulcer. This was removed 1 week later, whereupon the epithelial defect resolved with a remaining anterior stromal scar. Figure 2.20-3 shows the appearance of

Table 2.20-1	Sequential Treatment of Vernal Keratoconjunctivitis Based on Severity of Disease	
Severity	**Clinical Signs**	**Treatment**
Mild	Small papillae No corneal involvement	Environmental modifications Cool compresses Artificial tears Antihistamines Mast cell stabilizers
Moderate	Cobblestone papillae Mucoid debris Corneal neovascularization	Topical steroids
Severe	Cobblestone papillae Corneal macroerosions Shield ulcer Persistent inflammation	Immunomodulatory agents

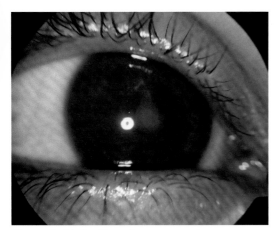

Figure 2.20-3   Corneal appearance after amniotic membrane lens removal.

her cornea 2 days after removal of the amniotic membrane lens.

At the 2-month follow-up visit, the following findings were observed:

Pupil evaluation	PERRL; no RAPD
Ocular motility	Full and comitant OU
Confrontations	Full to finger counting OD and OS
Refraction	OD: −4.75 sph (20/25); −4.75 sph (20/20)
Slit-lamp examination	OD: lids/lashes: clear; conjunctiva: clear with no papillae; cornea: dumbbell-shaped scar affecting visual axis with no epithelial defect; anterior chamber: deep and quiet to extent seen; OS: lids/lashes: clear; conjunctiva: clear with no papillae; cornea: clear; anterior chamber: deep and quiet to extent seen
Intraocular pressure (GAT)	OD: 15 mm Hg; OS: 15 mm Hg at 9:30 AM

Abbreviations: GAT, Goldmann applanation tonometry; OD, right eye; OS, left eye; OU, both eyes; PERRL, pupils equal, round, reactive to light; RAPD, relative afferent pupillary defect; sph, sphere.

Olivia was followed on an annual basis after this examination. She was advised to return sooner if her symptoms recurred, to use olopatadine (Patanol) twice daily as necessary should she experience symptoms of ocular allergies, to refrain from eye rubbing and to follow-up on a regular basis with her pediatrician for control of her systemic allergies and asthma.

CLINICAL PEARLS

- Vernal keratoconjunctivitis is a sight-threatening disease that occurs predominantly in school-aged children and typically resolves after puberty.

- Vernal keratoconjunctivitis occurs predominantly in males.

- Vernal keratoconjunctivitis is often associated with a systemic history of allergic rhinitis, asthma or atopy. As such, it is seasonally recurring.

- Clinical signs of VKC include giant, cobblestone papillae in the upper tarsal plate, Horner–Tranta's dots and corneal involvement (punctate epithelial keratitis, macroerosions, shield ulcers).

- Treatment of VKC may include environmental modifications, topical antihistamines, and mast-cell stabilizers, topical steroids and immunomodulating agents.

REFERENCES

1. Vichyanon P, Pacharn P, Pleyer U, Leonardi U. A vernal keratoconjunctivitis. A severe allergic eye disease with remodeling changes. *Pediatr Allergy Immunol.* 2014;25:314-322.
2. Leonardi A. Vernal keratoconjunctivitis: pathogenesis and treatment. *Prog Retin Eye Res.* 2002;21: 319-339.
3. Leonardi A, Bogacka E, Fauquer JL, et al. Ocular allergy: recognizing and diagnosing hypersensitivity disorders of the ocular surface. *Allergy.* 2012;67:1327-1337.
4. Jeng BH, Whitcher JP, Margolis TP. Pseudogerontoxon. *Clin Exp Ophthalmol.* August 2004;32(4):433-434.
5. Kumar S. Vernal keratoconjunctivitis: a major review. *Acta Ophthalmologica.* 2009;87(2):133-137.

6. Kraus C. *Vernal keratoconjunctivitis*. San Francisco, CA: American Academy of Ophthalmology. https://www.aao.org/pediatric-center-detail/vernal-keratoconjunctivitis-5. April 28, 2016. Accessed March 12, 2017.

7. Oner V, Turkcu FM, Tas M, et al. Topical loteprednol etabonate 0.5% for treatment of vernal keratoconjuncitivits: efficacy and safety. *Jpn J Ophthalmol*. 2012;56:312-318.

8. Guo P, Kheirkhah A, Zhou WW, Qin L, Shen XL. Surgical resection and amniotic membrane transplantation for treatment of refractory giant papillae in vernal keratoconjunctivitis. *Cornea*. June 2013;32(6):816-820.

2.21 Giant Papillary Conjunctivitis

Rebekah Montes, Lucy E. Kehinde, Susana C. Moreno, and Naomi Chun

Bekah, a 24-year-old Hispanic female, presented with intermittent blurred vision at distance and significant itching after removing her contact lenses. This began 2 months ago. The contact lenses were biweekly, soft silicone hydrogel lenses, which were worn approximately 12 hours every day. Bekah reported that she often changed lenses only every 4 weeks and napped for about 30 minutes in her lenses about twice a week. With a fresh pair of lenses, she experienced improvement of her symptoms but only for a day or 2. She used a branded multipurpose solution daily and denied any water exposure to her lenses. She reported that after removal, she rubbed each lens on both sides with the cleaning solution, and replaced the solution in the case on a daily basis. She also replaced the contact lens case every 2 to 3 months.

Associated symptoms included redness and burning, which was worse toward the end of the day. She used artificial tears (brand unknown) once or twice a day, although this did not provide any relief. Bekah denied any discharge of mucus, crusting, pain or photophobia. Her past medical history was positive for corneal infections secondary to contact lens overwear, perennial allergies, and a family history of atopy and hypertension. Current medications included over-the-counter oral antihistamines as needed, a nasal steroid spray once daily for nasal symptoms associated with perennial allergies, and ibuprofen for occasional headaches. No known drug allergies were reported. Bekah drank alcohol socially, but did not report any use of tobacco or narcotics.

Clinical Findings

Aided distance VA (through contact lenses)	OD: −2.00 sph (20/15); OS: −2.00 sph (20/15)
Pupil evaluation	PERRL; no RAPD
Slit-lamp examination	OD: lids/lashes: clean and clear; cornea: 1+ inferior superficial punctate keratitis; conjunctiva: 3+ papillae at margin of the tarsal plate extending from nasal to temporal aspects with 1+ injection; anterior chamber: dark and quiet; lens: clear; angle: 4 × 4; OS: lids/lashes: clean and clear; cornea: 1+ inferior superficial punctate keratitis; conjunctiva: 3+ papillae at margin of the tarsal plate extending from nasal to temporal aspects with 1+ injection; anterior chamber: dark and quiet; lens: clear; angle: 4 × 4
Intraocular pressure (NCT)	OD: 15 mm Hg; OS: 15 mm Hg at 1:02 PM

Abbreviations: NCT, noncontact tonometry; OD, right eye; OS, left eye; PERRL, pupils equal, round, reactive to light; RAPD, relative afferent pupillary defect; sph, sphere; VA, visual acuity.

Comments

Bekah was diagnosed with giant papillary conjunctivitis (GPC) (see Chapter 2.6). She was instructed to discontinue contact lens wear immediately, and to return for a follow-up examination in 1 week. She was prescribed loteprednol 0.5% ophthalmic suspension to be used 4 times a day in both eyes, along with olopatadine hydrochloride ophthalmic solution (Pataday) once daily. A lipid-enhanced lubricant was provided, to be used 2 to 3 times a day for ocular dryness. She was also recommended to use an overnight gel at bedtime.

At the follow-up visit, 1 week after the initial examination, Bekah reported a significant improvement in her symptoms, good compliance with the prescribed drops, and had not worn her contact lenses for the past week. Findings at that time were as follows:

Aided distance VA (through glasses)	OD: 20/15; OS: 20/15
Slit-lamp examination	OD: lids/lashes: clean and clear; cornea: clear and healthy; conjunctiva: 2+ papillae at margin of the tarsal plate extending from nasal to temporal aspects with trace injection; OS: lids/lashes: clean and clear; cornea: clear and healthy; conjunctiva: 2+ papillae at margin of the tarsal plate extending from nasal to temporal aspects with trace injection.
Intraocular pressure (NCT)	OD: 15 mm Hg; OS 15 mm Hg at 2:02 PM

Abbreviations: NCT, noncontact tonometry; OD, right eye; OS, left eye; VA, visual acuity.

The final impression of this case was resolving GPC. Loteprednol was tapered to twice a day for 1 week, followed by once a day for 1 more week, and discontinued thereafter. Bekah was prescribed olopatadine for long-term maintenance therapy. After resolution of the acute event, she was advised to return for fitting with daily disposable lenses. She was also educated on the proper care of her contact lenses and instructed not to sleep in them.

Discussion

Giant papillary conjunctivitis, also known as contact lens–induced papillary conjunctivitis, is a condition resulting from an immunoglobulin E-mediated hypersensitivity reaction in conjunction with mechanical injury to the palpebral conjunctiva.[1] It has been postulated that eyelid movement over a foreign object is responsible for the formation of papillae along the superior tarsal conjunctiva.[1] Giant papillary conjunctivitis is commonly associated with extended wear of silicone hydrogel and hydrogel contact lenses, while less often seen in rigid gas-permeable lens wear.[1,2] Biofilms on a contact lens may influence the development of GPC as they collect deposits onto the surface of the lens, which may elicit an immune response of the conjunctiva.[3] Higher water content contact lenses are especially prone to accumulating protein deposits, which lead to an immunologic response from the conjunctiva. Additional causes of GPC include an extruding scleral buckle, sutures, filtering blebs, ocular prosthetics, elevated corneal scars, and corneal foreign bodies.[3,4]

Symptoms of GPC include foreign body sensation, mucus discharge, blurred vision, contact lens awareness, and itching after the removal of the lenses.[1,2] The hallmark findings are large papillae along the superior tarsal edge of the palpebral conjunctiva (Figures 2.21-1 and 2.21-2).[1-3] Using fluorescein sodium dye can further help highlight the areas with papillae (Figure 2.21-3). It is important to evert the upper lid to evaluate the conjunctiva thoroughly in these cases.[3] Most patients will also have a history of seasonal or perennial allergies.[2,3]

A grading scale has been proposed that separates the superior tarsal conjunctiva into 5 zones, thereby delineating the extent of papillae into a local or general presentation, as shown in Figure 2.21-4.[3,5] Local responses are limited to

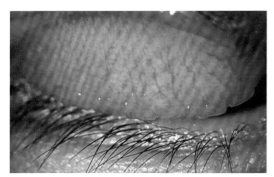

Figure 2.21-1 Example of large papillae on superior conjunctiva.

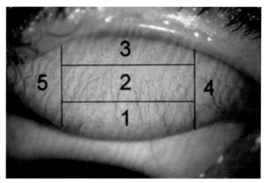

Figure 2.21-4 Grading zones for giant papillary conjunctivitis.[3,5]

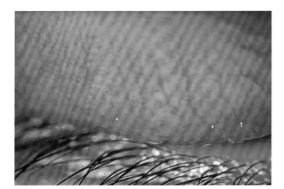

Figure 2.21-2 Magnified view of large papillae from Figure 2.21-1.

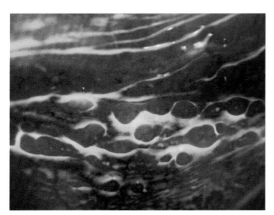

Figure 2.21-3 Example of inferior papillae with fluorescein staining.

and edge shape.[3] However, a general response is believed to result from an immunologic reaction.[3]

The primary focus in the management of GPC is to remove the offending agent.[1-3] The initial treatment includes the temporary discontinuation of contact lens wear for 1 to 3 weeks, followed by refitting into daily disposable lenses.[1-3] In moderate cases, topical steroids such as loteprednol or fluorometEhalone may be used to treat the associated inflammation in conjunction with antihistamine/mast cell stabilizers.[6,7] Evaluation of intraocular pressure is important at all follow-up visits to check for an adverse response to the steroid.[1,2] In more severe cases, the off-label use of tacrolimus may provide relief.[8]

The prognosis for GPC is generally good, and most patients may continue wearing lenses after the initial acute event. Antihistamine/mast cell stabilizers may be used for long-term maintenance therapy. As in this case, patients may also present with associated dry eye, and care should include the use of artificial tears throughout the day, as well as lubricating ointments at nighttime for patients with nocturnal lagophthalmos. Management of the meibomian glands with lipid-based artificial tears should also be implemented, as the majority of contact patients exhibit meibomian gland pathology.[9]

Patient education should focus on proper lens care, such as not sleeping in their lenses, avoiding lens exposure to water, and decreasing wear time when possible.[13] In the event that a patient is unable to use daily disposable contact

zones 2 or 3 while a more general response can be found in zones 1 to 3.[5] However, papillae may form in all zones.[5] A local response may be caused by mechanical irritation, and relevant factors include the modulus of elasticity of the contact lens, as well as its peripheral fit lenses, switching to a hydrogen peroxide-based disinfecting solution may also be useful with reusable lenses.[1] All patients should have a backup pair of glasses when not wearing their contact lenses, or in the event that they need to discontinue wear for a period of time. There is a significant likelihood of recurrence, especially if the patient does not adhere to the long-term maintenance therapy.

CLINICAL PEARLS

- Always evert the superior eyelid to assess the palpebral conjunctiva in patients reporting itching or lens awareness with contact lens use.

- Consider switching to a daily disposable modality to lessen the symptoms associated with GPC.

- Using a mast cell stabilizer/antihistamine combination drop will help maintain the patient's symptoms long term.

- Do not hesitate to recommend additional allergy remedies; that is, intranasal steroids, over-the-counter allergy medications, etc., for patients reporting systemic allergy symptoms.

REFERENCES

1. Onofrey BD, Skorin, L Jr, Holdeman NR. *Ocular Therapeutics Handbook: A Clinical Manual*. 3rd ed. Philadelphia, PA: Wolters Kluwer/Lippincott Williams & Wilkins; 2011.
2. Ehlers JP, Shah CP. *The Wills Eye Manual: Office and Emergency Room Diagnosis and Treatment of Eye Disease*. Philadelphia, PA: Lippincott Williams & Wilkins; 2008.
3. Strapleton F, Stretton S, Papas E, Sknotisky C, Sweeny DF. Silicone hydrogel contact lenses and the ocular surface. *Ocul Surf*. 2006;4(1):24-43.
4. Dunn JP Jr, Weissman BA, Mondino BJ, Arnold AC. Giant papillary conjunctivitis associated with elevated corneal deposits. *Cornea*. October 1990;9(4):357-358.
5. Skotnitsky CC, Naduvilath TJ, Sweeney DF, Sankaridura PR. Two presentations of contact lens-induced papillary conjunctivitis (CLPC) in hydrogel lens wear: local and general. *Optom Vis Sci*. 2006;83(1):27-36.
6. The Loteprednol Etabonate Giant Papillary Conjunctivitis Study Group. A double-masked, placebo-controlled evaluation of the efficacy and safety of loteprednol etabonate in the treatment of giant papillary conjunctivitis. *Am J Opthalmol*. 1997;123:455-464.
7. Khurana S, Sharma N, Agarwal T, et al. Comparison of olopatadine and fluorometholone in contact lens-induced papillary conjunctivitis. *Eye Contact Lens*. July 2010;36(4):210-214.
8. Diao H, She Z, Cao D, Wang Z, Lin Z. Comparison of tacrolimus in mild-to-moderate contact lens-induced papillary conjunctivitis. *Adv Therapy*. 2012;29(7):645-653.
9. Arita R, Fukuoka S, Morishige N. Meibomian gland dysfunction and contact lens discomfort. *Eye Contact Lens*. 2017;43(1):17-22.

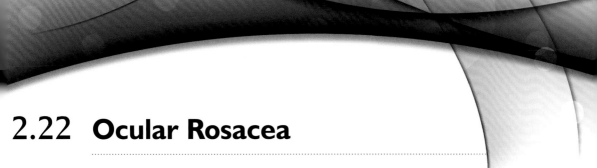

2.22 Ocular Rosacea

Nadine M. Furtado and Andre Stanberry

Mary, a 59-year-old Caucasian female, complained of difficulty reading at near. She reported that her eyes became fatigued after reading for 15 minutes and that she experienced intermittent blurred vision even while wearing her reading glasses. In addition, she reported bilateral ocular redness, which was worse in the morning, as well as tearing and mild itching. These symptoms had been present for the past few months, but she felt as though they were getting progressively worse. She denied any symptoms of photophobia, discharge, or pain.

Mary had undergone a bilateral laser peripheral iridotomy 2 years ago for anatomically narrow angles. She was not using any ocular medications or lubricants. Her medical history was positive for dyslipidemia, which was being treated with simvastatin. She denied any environmental allergies or allergies to medications.

Clinical Findings

Current Rx	OD: +1.00 −0.75 × 090 (20/20); OS: +0.75 −0.50 × 095 (20/20) ADD: +2.00 OU (OD: 20/25; OS: 20/25)
Pupil evaluation	PERRL; no RAPD
Confrontation visual fields	Full to finger counting OD and OS
Subjective refraction	OD: +1.50 −0.75 × 090 (20/20); OS: +1.25 −0.75 × 095 (20/20); ADD: +2.00 OU (OU: 20/20)
Slit-lamp examination	OD and OS: mild telangiectasia of lid margins; inspissated meibomian glands—moderate pressure to the glands revealed turbid expression; oily tear film; mild bulbar conjunctival hyperemia and moderate punctate epithelial erosions on inferior cornea; trace nuclear sclerosis; patent laser peripheral iridotomy superiorly
Intraocular pressure (GAT)	OD: 12 mm Hg; OS: 12 mm Hg at 1:20 PM
Fundus examination	Unremarkable OD and OS
Gross examination	Erythema of cheeks and nose with an area of pronounced telangiectasia on right cheek; pustules visible on both cheeks

Abbreviations: GAT, Goldmann applanation tonometry; OD, right eye; OS, left eye; OU, both eyes; PERRL, pupils equal, round, reactive to light; RAPD, relative afferent pupillary defect; Rx, prescription.

Comments

Mary was diagnosed with ocular rosacea and commenced a course of treatment including oral doxycycline 100 mg daily and 0.5% loteprednol etabonate ophthalmic suspension (Lotemax) in both eyes 4 times a day. In addition, she was advised to use warm compresses for 10 minutes followed by lid massage every day and to use preservative-free artificial tears at least 4 times a day in both eyes. An updated spectacle prescription was also provided.

Mary returned for a follow-up visit 1 month later reporting an improvement in her symptoms. Facial erythema was reduced and the skin pustules showed signs of improvement. Anterior segment examination revealed an improvement in the quality of the meibomian gland secretions and reduced conjunctival hyperemia (Figure 2.22-1).

Discussion

Rosacea is a chronic inflammatory skin disorder, which primarily affects the centrofacial area. The pathophysiology is not completely understood, but it is a multifactorial disease related to dysregulation in the innate and adaptive immune systems.[1,2] The ROSacea COnsensus (ROSCO) panel, an international group of dermatologists and ophthalmologists, has proposed a global, phenotype-based approach to addressing the diagnosis and classification of this condition. This system of assessment is based on 2 features being independently diagnostic for rosacea, namely (a) the presence of persistent, centrofacial erythema, which is accompanied by periods of exacerbation; and (b) phymatous changes.[3] Other characteristics, such as flushing, transient centrofacial erythema, inflammatory papules and pustules,

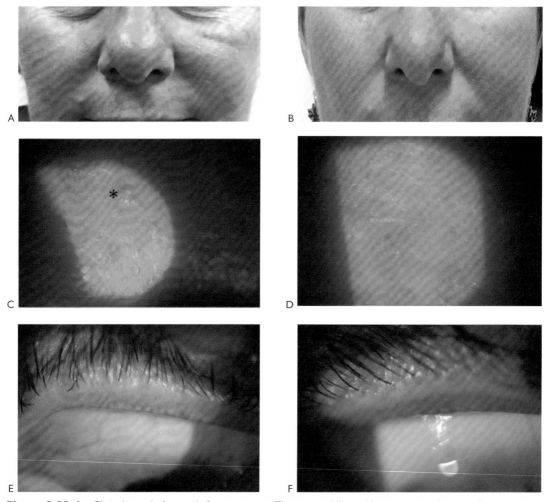

Figure 2.22-1   Clinical signs before and after treatment. The top, middle, and bottom pairs of images demonstrate improvement in facial erythema, resolution of pustules on the cheek (indicated by the asterisk), and improved meibomian gland secretions, respectively.

telangiectasia and ocular manifestations were considered to be major features of rosacea but none, in and of themselves, are sufficient to make a diagnosis.

There are varying reports on the prevalence of rosacea, but it is estimated to affect 10% to 20% of the population.[1] Although some sources report that rosacea is more prevalent in fair-skinned individuals, this may be the result of a reporting bias due to a lack of diversity in the populations being studied.[4] The onset of signs and symptoms of rosacea usually occurs between the third and fifth decades of life. Although rosacea is a chronic inflammatory disorder, there are certain triggers that can exacerbate the condition. Specifically, ultraviolet radiation, exposure to heat, stress, caffeine intake, alcohol consumption, spicy food, and smoking are all considered known triggers of rosacea.[1] In addition, certain microorganisms, such as *Demodex folliculorum*, *Demodex brevis*, *Helicobacter pylori*, and *Staphylococcus epidermidis*, may play a potential role in aggravating the disease.[4]

Although rosacea is primarily a dermatologic condition, between 58% and 72% of affected patients will have ocular involvement, with more than half of them being symptomatic.[4] Ocular symptoms include redness, tearing, burning, itching, foreign body sensation, and eyelid swelling. In more severe cases, patients may be symptomatic for photophobia and pain. Depending on the extent of corneal involvement, patients may also report blurred vision. Clinical signs of ocular rosacea include eyelid erythema and telangiectasia. Blepharitis and meibomian gland dysfunction are often present, with individuals frequently reporting a history of recurrent hordeola or chalazia. Conjunctival tissue frequently becomes inflamed, usually manifesting as interpalpebral bulbar hyperemia and conjunctivochalasis. Corneal sequela can also occur, ranging from punctate epithelial erosions and peripheral stromal infiltrates to recurrent corneal erosions, edema, and neovascularization. As the disease advances, infiltrates can progress and possibly lead to stromal ulceration and even corneal perforation. There are often abnormalities in the tear film and tear production, which result in a reduced tear breakup time and a hyperosmolar ocular surface. The latter results in increased concentrations of interleukin-1α and matrix metalloproteinase-9 (MMP-9), a pro-inflammatory cytokine and an extracellular matrix degrading enzyme, respectively, which further reduce tear volume and exacerbate symptoms of dry eye.

There is no known cure for ocular rosacea, so treatment and management are focused on reducing the symptoms experienced by patients. Given that the disease is exacerbated by exposure to certain conditions, patients diagnosed with ocular rosacea should be counseled to avoid these triggers. Localized treatment is appropriate for mild ocular rosacea, including the use of warm compresses for 10 minutes with digital massage and eyelid scrubs. Lubricating drops and ointments should be used to address ocular surface dryness, with preservative-free formulations being recommended if frequent instillation is required. In addition, nutritional oral supplementation with omega-3 fatty acids has been shown to be beneficial in treating blepharitis and meibomian gland dysfunction by reducing inflammation and should be suggested as part of the treatment unless otherwise contraindicated.[4]

Moderate to severe cases of ocular rosacea should be treated with systemic antibiotics, which are prescribed for their anti-inflammatory characteristics and ability to inhibit MMP-9. Tetracyclines are the most effective treatment, with doxycycline being most commonly prescribed because it has few side effects.[5] Azithromycin is an alternative oral treatment, which can be used for individuals who cannot tolerate doxycycline.[6] Topical cyclosporine and punctal occlusion can also be valuable treatment modalities to address the chronic ocular surface dryness and symptoms related to ocular rosacea.[7] Surgical management is indicated in advanced cases to prevent or treat complications. For example, corneal thinning, the most common advanced complication, can be addressed with the use of tissue adhesives, amniotic membrane transplants, or conjunctival flaps, whereas corneal opacification or perforation are managed with lamellar or penetrating keratoplasty.[4]

CLINICAL PEARLS

- Always assess facial skin for signs of rosacea in patients being diagnosed with meibomian gland dysfunction and/or ocular surface disease.

- Although more easily observed in fair-skinned people, rosacea can also be present in darker-skinned individuals. Careful assessment is needed to appreciate rosacea in these patients as the clinical presentation is much more subtle.

REFERENCES

1. Tan J, Berg M. Rosacea: current state of epidemiology. *J Am Acad Dermatol.* 2013;69:S27-S35.
2. Steinhoff M, Schuber J, Leyden JJ. New insights into rosacea pathophysiology: a review of recent findings. *J Am Acad Dermatol.* 2013;69:S15-S26.
3. Tan J, Almeida LM, Bewley A, et al. Updating the diagnosis, classification and assessment of rosacea: recommendations from global ROSacea Consensus (ROSCO) panel. *Br J Dermatol.* 2017;176:431-438.
4. Vieira AC, Mannis MJ. Ocular rosacea: common and commonly missed. *J Am Acad Dermatol.* 2013; 69:S36-S41.
5. Sobolewska B, Doycheva D, Deuter C, Pfeffer I, Schaller M, Zierhut M. Treatment of ocular rosacea with once-daily low-dose doxycycline. *Cornea.* 2014;33:257-260.
6. Akhyani M, Ehsani AH, Ghiasi M, Jafari AK. Comparison of efficacy of azithromycin vs. doxycycline in the treatment of rosacea: a randomized open clinical trial. *In J Dermatol.* 2008;47(3):284-288.
7. Arman A, Demirseren DD, Takmaz T. Treatment of ocular rosacea: comparative study of topical cyclosporine and oral doxycycline. *Int J Ophthalmol.* 2015;8(3):544-549.

2.23 Childhood Ocular Rosacea

A. Mika Moy and Michelle Chun

Julie, an 18 year-old multiethnic (Persian and Caucasian) female, presented with intermittent red, irritated eyes. This problem first began when she was 8 years of age. She had never sought professional care for this complaint, but felt that the redness was getting worse. Julie reported particular difficulty when outdoors or in windy conditions. She also felt that her face flushed easily, and her cheeks were often rosy. Julie denied any past ocular surgery or trauma and had no history of contact lens wear. She stated that her father had chronic eye redness as well. Her medical history was positive for polycystic ovarian syndrome for which she was taking levonorgestrel and ethinyl estradiol (Aubra) to regulate her menstrual cycle. She was not taking any other medications or recreational drugs and denied tobacco use.

Clinical Findings

Unaided distance VA	OD: 20/20; OS: 20/20
Pupil evaluation	PERRL; no RAPD
Slit-lamp examination	OD: mild blepharitis, small hordeolum of upper right eye lid (Figure 2.23-1 A). Meibomian glands somewhat stagnant on expression with slightly turbid secretions. Grade 1-2+ hyperemia (greater inferiorly than superiorly) of palpebral and bulbar conjunctiva, corneal neovascularization 360° extending 2.5 mm inferiorly and 1 mm superiorly toward central cornea (Figure 2.23-2). Trace positive fluorescein staining near leading edge of the inferior vessels, and trace negative staining between that and limbus indicating some corneal edema (Figure 2.23-3). Cornea between blood vessels appeared relatively clear. No anterior chamber reaction;
	OS: mild blepharitis (Figure 2.23-1 B). Meibomian glands somewhat stagnant on expression with slightly turbid secretions. Grade 1-2+ hyperemia (greater inferiorly than superiorly) of palpebral and bulbar conjunctiva, corneal neovascularization 360° extending 2.5 mm inferiorly and 1 mm superiorly toward central cornea. Cornea between blood vessels appeared relatively clear. No anterior chamber reaction
Intraocular pressure (GAT)	OD: 14 mm Hg; OS: 14 mm Hg at 4:00 PM
Fundus examination	Unremarkable OD and OS

Abbreviations: GAT, Goldmann applanation tonometry; OD, right eye; OS, left eye; PERRL, pupils equal, round, reactive to light; RAPD, relative afferent pupillary defect; VA, visual acuity.

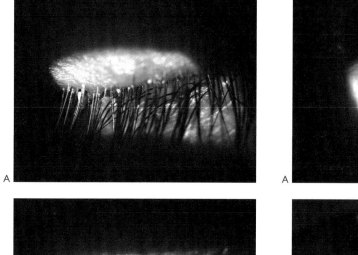

Figure 2.23-1   A, Right upper lid showing scurf and small hordeolum. B, Left upper lid showing scurf.

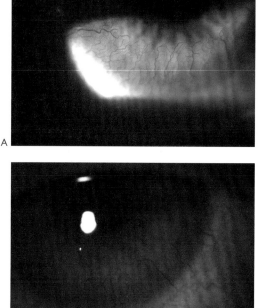

Figure 2.23-2   Extensive corneal neovascularization of the (A) right eye and (B) left eye.

Comments

Julie was given a tentative diagnosis of staphylococcal marginal keratitis and was prescribed moxifloxacin (Vigamox) ophthalmic solution 4 times a day OU to provide broad spectrum coverage. Although simply gram-positive coverage may have been sufficient, the diagnosis was tentative and therefore broad spectrum coverage was desired. To rule out a systemic infectious etiology, the following laboratory blood work was ordered: complete blood count (CBC) with differential, Lyme titer, T-SPOT for tuberculosis, fluorescent treponemal antibody absorption (FTA-ABS), and rapid plasma reagin (RPR) for syphilis. Julie was asked to perform lid scrubs and warm compresses twice a day and to return in 1 week for a follow-up care.

At the 1-week follow-up visit, Julie reported her symptoms had improved. Anterior segment evaluation revealed stable findings with a slight improvement in corneal staining.

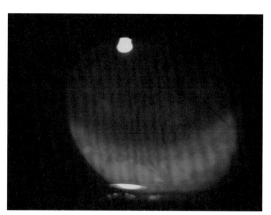

Figure 2.23-3   Sodium fluorescein staining of the right eye showing slight positive and negative staining.

The central cornea seemed clearer, which allowed for visualization of edema between the neovascular blood vessels and areas of fibrosis that had not been observed 1 week earlier. All laboratory tests were within normal limits. A new working diagnosis of ocular rosacea was established.

Julie was advised to discontinue moxifloxacin and commence loteprednol etabonate 0.2% (Alrex) ophthalmic suspension 4 times per day in each eye in view of the negative bloodwork results. Azithromycin (AzaSite) ophthalmic solution was added as a lid scrub twice a day to improve the appearance of the lid margin. She was instructed to first clean with the commercially available lid scrub to clear the scurf and then rub the base of her eyelashes again with the azithromycin. Doxycycline 100 mg tablets were prescribed twice a day. Julie was advised of all side effects of the prescribed medications, and she confirmed verbally that she was neither pregnant nor was she at risk for becoming pregnant. She was advised to return in 2 weeks for a follow-up appointment.

At the follow-up appointment 3 weeks after the initial diagnosis, Julie reported no further episodes of redness or irritation since starting the medical therapy. Anterior segment evaluation revealed improved blepharitis, resolution of the small hordeolum on the right eye and that the bulbar and palpebral conjunctiva hyperemia had resolved. The corneal neovascularization had started to fade and ghosting of vessels was apparent. Intraocular pressures remained stable.

With the improving signs and symptoms, Julie was advised to continue lid hygiene with warm compresses and the dual lid scrub regimen. Doxycycline was reduced to 100 mg once per day, with the intent to reduce it to 50 mg once a day, with continued improvement. Loteprednol was tapered to 3 times per day in each eye. She was asked to return in a further 2 weeks.

At the follow-up appointment 5 weeks after the initial diagnosis, Julie reported continued improvement of symptoms and that she could not "remember when (her) eyes have felt so good." Her visual acuity (VA) was stable at 20/20 in each eye. Slit-lamp biomicroscopy revealed the absence of scurf on the lashes, hyperemia or conjunctival injection. There was continued ghosting of corneal blood vessels.

Julie was advised to taper the loteprednol to twice a day for 1 week, then once a day for 1 week, and then discontinue. Azithromycin was discontinued, although she was encouraged to continue warm compresses and over-the-counter lid scrubs twice a day, and the chronic nature of the condition was explained. The doxycycline tablets were tapered to 50 mg once per day for 60 days.

Julie was asked to return for an anterior segment evaluation in 2 months, and at that time a lower dose of doxycycline would have been considered. Unfortunately, she was lost to follow-up and has not returned to the clinic.

Discussion

Rosacea is a chronic inflammatory skin condition with variable levels of severity that involves vasomotor instability with flare-ups and periods of remission.[1] There are 4 subtypes of rosacea, namely erythematotelangiectatic, which causes flushing and persistent redness, papillopustular, which causes the more classic acne appearance, phymatous or a thickening of the skin most commonly associated with the nose and ocular rosacea, which causes lid margin thickening, and meibomian gland dysfunction leading to corneal neovascularization.[2] Rosacea typically occurs in adults between the age of 30 and 50 years with no gender predilection. In rare cases, it can occur in childhood.[1]

Rosacea affects over 45 million people worldwide and 16 million American adults.[2] Although more commonly present in people with fair complexions,[3] 4% of rosacea patients are of African, Hispanic, and Asian descent.[4]

The pathophysiology of rosacea is unclear as there are no histological or serological markers.[5] Some environmental factors have been found to exacerbate the condition including wind, hot and spicy foods, alcohol, sunlight, extreme temperature, anxiety, stress, anger, embarrassment, and exercise. One theory is that these environmental factors, such as sunlight, can damage both the blood vessels and connective tissue within the skin. This theory is supported by the distribution of erythema and telangiectatic vessels on areas of the face that are less protected from the sun. These chronically dilated vessels may leak inflammatory material initiating a cascade that results in papule and pustule formation.[6]

A more recent theory is that the clinical features of rosacea are caused by a hypersensitivity reaction to microorganisms.[1,3] The demodex mite is commonly found on the skin and has been observed in significantly higher quantities in patients with papulopustular rosacea compared with age-matched controls.[3,7] The patient may exhibit a hypersensitivity reaction to the microbes that live on the demodex mite, rather than the arachnid itself.[3] There may also be a genetic component, as 40% of rosacea patients report that at least 1 family member also suffers from the disease.[8]

Ocular rosacea can be diagnosed with the presence of 1 or more of the following signs: interpalpebral conjunctival hyperemia, telangiectasia of the conjunctiva and lid margin, or lid and periocular erythema. The patient may also experience foreign body sensation, burning or stinging, dryness, itching, light sensitivity, or blurred vision.[5] Recurrent chalazia or hordeola are also common. It may be difficult to distinguish between meibomian gland dysfunction and ocular rosacea without concurrent dermatologic rosacea signs. The severity of symptoms and difficulty in controlling signs can help the clinician make that distinction. Ocular rosacea affects both genders equally and the incidence ranges from 6% to 72%.[4]

Corneal manifestations may occur in up to 33% of patients with rosacea, most commonly affecting the inferior cornea.[2] Ocular rosacea is found in 58% of patients with dermatologic rosacea; however, approximately 20% of adults with rosacea have ocular symptoms that precede any dermatologic findings.[5,7]

The prevalence of childhood rosacea is unknown. However, it is likely that there is an underreporting of cases due to a lack of diagnostic criteria. Retrospective evaluation of 20 children between the age of 1 and 15 years with a diagnosis of cutaneous, ocular or oculocutaneous rosacea showed that the clinical features in children are similar to those found in adults, other than no phymatous changes were observed in the younger age group.[1] The authors proposed a classification system for childhood rosacea similar to that of the adult condition. However, they proposed that 2 primary features must be present to diagnose childhood rosacea as opposed to 1 criteria in adult rosacea. Interestingly, using these criteria, Julie would not have been diagnosed with rosacea as a child when her ocular symptoms first began.

The treatment of rosacea depends on the severity of the symptoms. If the patient is aware of sensitivity to a specific trigger, then clearly this should be avoided. Topical agents that are commonly employed include metronidazole, sodium sulfacetamide, azelaic acid, benzoyl peroxide, and antibiotic ointments such as erythromycin and clindamycin.[9] Systemic antibiotics are also indicated for ocular rosacea and include tetracyclines and macrolides.

Second-generation tetracyclines (eg, minocycline and doxycycline) have fewer side effects and are effective in treating inflammatory disease due to their anti-inflammatory properties.[10] The sub-antimicrobial dose of doxycycline, that is, the maximum dose that achieves plasma concentrations consistently below those required for an antimicrobial effect, although maximizing its anti-inflammatory properties is well established.[11] A 20 mg-dose of doxycycline administered twice a day showed an effective inflammatory reduction without producing any detectable effect on microbial counts.[12] This indicates that patients can be left on low-dose doxycycline without fear of developing bacterial resistance.

Macrolide antibiotics are also useful when treating rosacea. For example, erythromycin is as effective as tetracyclines in resolving inflammatory lesions and improving symptoms. Azithromycin is a newer macrolide that penetrates tissues quickly, has an affinity for inflammatory tissues, maintains prolonged tissue levels, and allows for less frequent dosing. Azithromycin can also be used safely in pregnant women as the placenta provides an effective barrier to the fetus.[6] The recommended dose of azithromycin in rosacea is 500 mg 3 times per week and then tapered to a single dose of 500 mg, once a week.[6] Unfortunately, macrolides have been associated with increased bacterial resistance.[6]

There is disagreement regarding the appropriate maintenance therapy using oral medications in rosacea. It is important to balance a good patient outcome while avoiding bacterial resistance. Other factors such as the cost of medicine and possible side effects must also be considered. Recurrence is common after the cessation of systemic therapy. It has been reported that 25% of patients had a relapse within 1 month of discontinuing therapy, while 55% and 70% showed recurrence 6 months and 1 to 4 years after stopping the medication, respectively.[12] Some suggest therapy should be maintained for a few months followed by gradual tapering, while others recommend the long-term use of oral antibiotics for at least 1 year, with prompt intervention of mild occurrences.[13]

CLINICAL PEARLS

- Childhood rosacea is a rare entity that is more likely than adult rosacea to present with ocular symptoms first.

- Prescribing tetracyclines in children is contraindicated, therefore secondary antibiotics such as macrolides should be considered.

- Untreated ocular rosacea can lead to permanent vision loss.

REFERENCES

1. Chamaillard M, Mortemousque B, Boralevi F, et al. Cutaneous and ocular signs of childhood rosacea. *Arch Dermatol.* 2008;144(2):167-171.

2. Vieira ACC, Höfling-Lima AL, Mannis MJ. Ocular rosacea: a review. *Arq Bras Oftalmol.* 2012;75(5):363-369.

3. Crawford GH, Pelle MT, James WD. Rosacea: I. Etiology, pathogenesis, and subtype classification. *J Am Acad Dermatol.* 2004;51(3):327-341.

4. Geria AN, Culp B, Scheinfeld NS. Rosacea: a review. *Kosmet Medizin.* 2008;29(6):303-308.

5. Wilkin J, Dahl M, Detmar M, et al. Standard grading system for rosacea: report of the National Rosacea Society Expert Committee on the Classification and Staging of Rosacea. *J Am Acad Dermatol.* 2004; 50(6):907-912.

6. Akhyani M, Ehsani AH, Ghiasi M, Jafari AK. Comparison of efficacy of azithromycin vs. doxycycline in the treatment of rosacea: a randomized open clinical trial. *Int J Dermatol.* 2008;47(3):284-288.

7. Nazir SA, Murphy S, Siatkowski RM, Chodosh J, Siatkowski RL. Ocular rosacea in childhood. *Am J Ophthalmol.* 2004;137(1):138-144.

8. Kroshinsky D, Glick SA. Pediatric rosacea. *Dermatol Ther.* 2006;19(4):196-201.

9. Pelle MT, Crawford GH, James WD. Rosacea: II. Therapy. *J Am Acad Dermatol.* 2004;51(4):499-514.

10. Valentín S, Morales A, Sánchez JL, Rivera A. Safety and efficacy of doxycycline in the treatment of rosacea. *Clin Cosmet Investig Dermatol.* 2009;2:129-140.

11. Sloan B, Scheinfeld N. The use and safety of doxycycline hyclate and other second-generation tetracyclines. *Expert Opin Drug Saf.* 2008;7(5):571-577.

12. Bikowski JB. Subantimicrobial dose doxycycline for acne and rosacea. *Skinmed.* 2003;2(4):234-245.

13. Voils SA, Evans ME, Lane MT, Schosser RH, Rapp RP. Use of macrolides and tetracyclines for chronic inflammatory diseases. *Ann Pharmacother.* 2005;39(1):86-94.

2.24 Phlyctenule

A. Mika Moy

Paul, a 20-year old East Indian male, presented with a complaint of redness, slight photophobia, itch, and watery discharge in each eye that had started 2 days ago. He was otherwise in good health and was not taking any medications. He had no known systemic or drug allergies. There was no significant family ocular or medical history.

Paul stated that this type of red eye had occurred "several times" in the past and that he wanted a prescription for topical antibiotics, because these had previously provided relief. Regarding the current episode, he stated that the right eye became red first, followed by the left. Paul felt that the symptoms were getting worse. He had returned from a trip to India 1 month ago.

Clinical Findings

Unaided distance VA	OD: 20/20; OS: 20/20
Pupil evaluation	PERRL; no RAPD
Slit-lamp examination	OD: 1+ blepharitis with a few capped meibomian glands; trace, mixed papillary and follicular reaction (Figure 2.24-1) with mild hyperemia of the inferior palpebral conjunctiva (Figure 2.24-2A); 1+ sectoral conjunctival hyperemia nasally and temporally surrounding multiple raised, circular areas along the limbus approximately 0.2-2 mm in size (Figure 2.24-3); the lesions stain with sodium fluorescein; cornea and anterior chamber are unremarkable;
	OS: 1+ blepharitis with a few capped meibomian glands (Figure 2.24-2B); 1+ sectoral conjunctival hyperemia at 4:00 surrounding multiple raised lesions along the limbus approximately 0.2-0.5 mm in size; the lesions stain with sodium fluorescein; cornea and anterior chamber are unremarkable
Intraocular pressure (GAT)	OD: 13 mm Hg; OS: 13 mm Hg at 11:00 AM
Fundus examination	Unremarkable OD, OS

Abbreviations: GAT, Goldmann applanation tonometry; OD, right eye; OS, left eye; PERRL, pupils equal, round, reactive to light; RAPD, relative afferent pupillary defect; VA, visual acuity.

Comments

Paul was diagnosed with phlyctenular conjunctivitis and blepharitis. He was educated on the likelihood of recurrence, and the difference between this condition and bacterial conjunctivitis. He was prescribed tobramycin 0.3%/dexamethasone 0.1% ophthalmic suspension to use 4 times a day in each eye. Paul was instructed to perform warm compresses and lid scrubs twice a day in each eye to treat the blepharitis.

The patient reported returning from a trip to India 1 month ago. Because Paul had recently returned from a tuberculosis (TB)-endemic area, even though he denied any symptoms of TB,

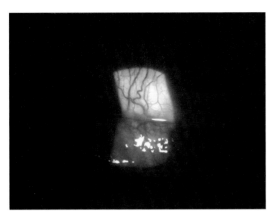

Figure 2.24-1 Inferior palpebral conjunctiva OD showing epiphora, and trace follicular reaction.

Abbreviation: OD, right eye.

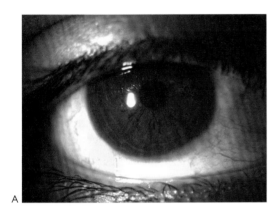

A

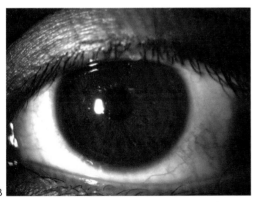

B

Figure 2.24-2 A, Low magnification view of OD. Note sectoral redness from 2:00 to 4:00 and 7:00 to 10:00. B, Low magnification view of OS. Note sectoral redness from 3:30 to 5:00. Note also capped meibomian gland in view centrally on the upper eyelid.

Abbreviations: OD, right eye; OS, left eye.

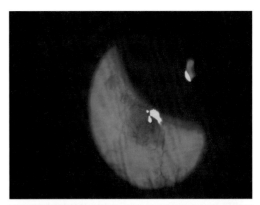

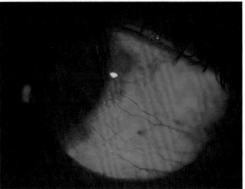

Figure 2.24-3 Right eye nasally and temporally showing circular, elevated areas that pick up sodium fluorescein staining. Lesions vary in size from 0.2 to 2 mm in diameter.

such as cough, chest pain, fever, decrease in appetite, night sweats, weakness or fatigue, a T-SPOT (Interferon Gamma Release Assays or IGRA) blood test was ordered to rule out TB. He was asked to return in 1 week.

At the 1-week follow-up visit, all conjunctival staining had resolved, and Paul reported that his symptoms had ended 2 to 3 days after taking the topical antibiotic/steroid suspension. His TB test was negative and the intraocular pressure measurements were similar to those recorded the previous week.

Discussion

Phlyctenular keratoconjunctivitis (PKC) is a hypersensitivity (Type IV) reaction to bacterial antigens, with staphylococcus being one of the most common organisms. The phlyctenules are composed of macrophages and T-lymphocytes with no microorganisms present.[1] Therefore, this is an allergic rather than an infectious reaction and the patient must first be sensitized to the antigen and have a subsequent re-exposure.

Previously, when TB was more prevalent, it was associated with phlyctenules. Patients would be re-exposed to the TB bacillus either from their own body or others (eg, through coughing). Because TB is encountered much less frequently in the United States currently, the likelihood of a sensitized individual coming into contact with that antigen is remote, unless they have recently traveled to a TB endemic area such as sub-Saharan Africa, China, India, or Russia.[2] Indeed, today, even patients with active TB have a low rate of phlyctenules.[3]

Interferon Gamma Release Assays screen for TB by measuring how strongly the immune system (specifically, interferon gamma) reacts to TB bacteria.[4] These tests have the further benefit of not requiring 2 patient visits, as is the case for the more common purified protein derivative (PPD) test. Other antigens associated with PKC include chlamydia, coccidioides, candida, herpes simplex virus, and parasites.

Treatment for phlyctenules must include a topical steroid to reduce the inflammatory response. Reduction of the antigen is also key in the treatment, so efforts must be made to identify the responsible antigen. In the United States nowadays, this is most likely to be staphylococcus. An antibiotic–steroid combination drug was selected to help reduce both the bacterial load of the ocular surface and the inflammatory response. Patients with recurrent cases where extended topical steroid use is a concern or who are known steroid responders can be managed successfully with topical cyclosporin A.[5]

Phlyctenules that only affect the conjunctiva tend to be associated with mild symptoms. However, PKC can also affect the cornea, and although this is rarer, it will produce more severe symptoms. These lesions tend to move across the cornea, leaving areas of scarring in their wake. Both the cause and treatment are the same regardless of affecting the conjunctiva or the cornea.

CLINICAL PEARLS

- Phlyctenules are caused by a type IV hypersensitivity reaction to a microbial antigen. Although there was a strong association with TB in the past, in the United States currently, the rates of TB have declined to the point where a staphylococcus origin is much more likely. Chlamydia, herpes simplex virus, and parasites can also be causative agents.

- Treatment of PKC includes a topical steroid to address the phlyctenule as well as reducing the offending antigen when possible. In recalcitrant cases, topical cyclosporin A has been shown to be effective.

REFERENCES

1. Abu el-Asrar AE. Phenotypic characteristics of inflammatory cells in phlyctenular eye disease. *Doc Ophthalmol.* 1989;70:353-362.
2. WHO. *Global Tuberculosis Report.* Geneva, Switzerland: World Health Organization; 2015.
3. Biswas JBS. Ocular morbidity in patients with active systemic tuberculosis. *Int Ophthalmol.* 1995-1996; 19(5):293-298.
4. Zwelling AE. Interferon-gamma release assays for tuberculosis screening of healthcare workers: a systematic review. *Thorax.* 2012;67:62-70.
5. Doan SE. Topical cyclosporine A in severe steroid-dependent childhood phlyctenular keratoconjunctivitis. *Am J Ophthalmol.* 2006;14:62-66.

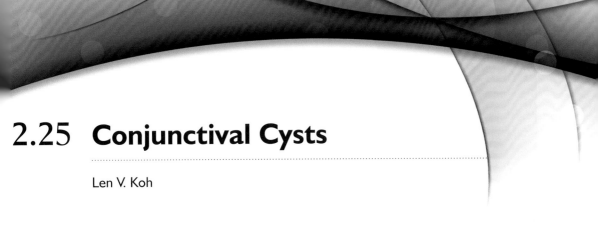

2.25 Conjunctival Cysts

Len V. Koh

Clara, a 26-year-old white female, complained of a watery left eye, which started 4 days ago. In addition, she observed a cyst on her conjunctiva this morning. This was the first occurrence, and there was no prior history of ocular trauma. Clara used over-the-counter artificial tears 4 times a day for dry eye. Her last physical and eye examinations were 3 months ago. Clara's review of systems was unremarkable and she had no known drug allergies. She was not a smoker and took birth control pills.

Clinical Findings

Present Rx	OD: −2.25 −0.50 × 180 (20/20); OS: −2.75 −0.50 × 180 (20/20)
Ocular motility	Full OD and OS
Confrontation visual fields	Full to finger counting OD and OS
Pupil evaluation	PERRL; no RAPD
Slit-lamp examination	OD: unremarkable OD; OS: 4 mm ellipsoid cysts in the superior temporal conjunctiva OS (Figure 2.25-1 A), all other findings unremarkable
Intraocular pressure (GAT)	OD: 16 mm Hg; OS: 16 mm Hg at 10:23 AM
Fundus examination	Unremarkable OD and OS

Abbreviations: GAT, Goldmann applanation tonometry; OD, right eye; OS, left eye; PERRL, pupils equal, round, reactive to light; RAPD, relative afferent pupillary defect; sph, sphere; Rx, prescription.

Comments

The conjunctival cysts were lanced with a 27-gauge sterile needle after administration of 1 drop of proparacaine. Moxifloxacin ophthalmic drops were prescribed 4 times a day left eye for 1 week. Clara was asked to return for follow-up in a few days, or sooner if needed. Anterior segment photography (Keratograph 5M, Oculus Inc., Arlington, Washington) captured the conjunctival cysts before (Figure 2.25-1A) and after incision (Figure 2.25-1B).

Clara returned 4 days later with cysts in the same location. She was educated that recurrence may be a possibility, in which case surgical intervention would be necessary. She understood and opted to have the lesions lanced one more time. This was done with a larger incision. Clara was instructed to use the antibiotic eye drops for a few more days. One week later, she reported that the cysts had not recurred. She continued to use artificial tears as needed.

Discussion

A conjunctival cyst is a benign tumor of the conjunctival epithelial cells that forms a fluid-filled sac. Hence it is a form of epithelial inclusion cyst.[1] Conjunctival cysts can develop spontaneously,

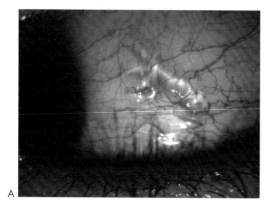

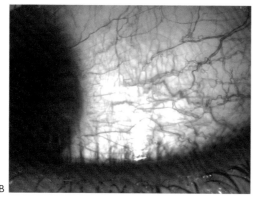

Figure 2.25-1   A, Conjunctival cysts OS.
B, Conjunctival cysts OS after being lanced with 27-gauge needle.

Abbreviation: OS, left eye.

as in this case, or following inflammation and trauma. In addition, ocular surgery can inadvertently deposit conjunctival epithelial cells into the lamina propria, which can subsequently proliferate into cysts.[2] Spontaneously developed cysts move freely under the conjunctiva, and can be removed via a small incision.[3] The diagnosis of conjunctival cyst is through clinical examination. Common symptoms are foreign body sensation and tearing with an apparent cyst that is visible to the patient. Differential diagnoses could include phlyctenular keratoconjunctivitis, pinguecula, and limbal dermoid, but retention cysts are quite distinct and are easily diagnosed because of the clear fluid-filled sac.

Histologically, nonkeratinizing conjunctival epithelium form the cysts. The clear fluid within the cavity often contains desquamated cellular debris, including inflammatory cells.[4] Although benign, the cyst can be uncomfortable and cosmetically displeasing. Lubricating eye drops can serve as supportive management, but prominent cysts must be drained or surgically removed. Lancing with a needle to drain the fluid will be successful in some cases, but recurrence is high because mere draining does not remove the conjunctival epithelial sac membrane. In Clara's case, the cyst had to be incised twice. Complete surgical resection, thermal cautery with radiofrequency, and argon laser photoablation are alternate methods of treatment. Small-incision removal of freely movable cysts without sutures has been performed successfully with staining dye.[5] Lancing the cyst is an appropriate first line of management. Subsequently, a topical antibiotic should be prescribed prophylactically. Occasionally, the needle may puncture a vein leading to a subconjunctival hemorrhage, which can be managed by applying pressure with a cotton-tipped applicator. A more recent method of extracting spontaneous conjunctival cysts using a 26-gauge needle attached to a 1-mL disposable syringe has also been reported. This method removes the conjunctival epithelial sac similar to surgical resection and minimizes recurrence.[6]

CLINICAL PEARLS

- Conjunctival cyst may occur in any part of the conjunctival anatomy but are more revealing and symptomatic in the bulbar conjunctiva. There is no predilection to race, gender, and age.

- Conjunctival cysts are usually asymptomatic and can typically be observed only. Stab incision with a needle may work in some cases, but recurrence is high. Surgical excision of the cyst may be necessary for large and symptomatic cysts.

- It is essential to rule out potential malignant conjunctival lesion such as lymphoma, or conjunctival melanoma.

REFERENCES

1. Shields CL, Shields JA. Tumors of the conjunctiva and cornea. *Surv Ophthalmol*. 2004;49:3-24.
2. Brownell RD. Bulbar subconjunctival epithelial cyst. *Am J Ophthalmol*. 1960;49:151-153.
3. Savar A, Nakra T. Freely mobile subconjunctival cyst. *Ophthalmology*. 2010;117:637.
4. Krachmer J, Mannis M, Holland E. Subepithelial neoplasms of the conjunctiva. In: Daniel Nelson J, Douglas Cameron J, eds. *Cornea, Fundamentals, Diagnosis* and *Management*. Vol 1. 3rd ed. Philadelphia, PA: Elsevier Mosby; 2010:488-489.
5. Eom Y, Ahn SE, Kang SY, et al. Sutureless small-incisionconjunctival cystectomy. *Can J Ophthalmol*. 2014;49:e17-e19.
6. Ikeda N, Ikeda T, Ishikawa H. In toto extraction of spontaneous conjunctival cysts without incision under slit-lamp microscopic view. *Can J Ophthalmol*. 2016;51(6):423-425.

2.26 Subconjunctival Hemorrhage

Lucy E. Kehinde, Rebekah Montes, and Susana C. Moreno

John, a 22-year-old African American male college student, presented for an emergency office visit due to acute redness in his right eye. This occurred shortly after he suffered blunt trauma to the eye while playing basketball earlier in the day. He recalled a sharp pain and noticed blood on the towel he used to wipe his face after he was poked in the eye with a finger. He now reported symptoms of dull pain with a severity of 5 on a scale from 0 to 10. John denied any changes in vision, light sensitivity, discharge or foreign body sensation. He was in good general health, did not take any medications and had no allergies to medication.

Clinical Findings

Unaided distance VA	OD: 20/20; OS: 20/25^{-2} (pinhole 20/20)
Confrontation visual fields	Full to finger counting OD and OS
Ocular motility	Full range of motion and smooth OU
Pupil evaluation	PERRL; no RAPD
Intraocular pressure (iCare)	OD: 8 mm Hg; OS: 11 mm Hg at 11:35 AM
Blood pressure	118/70 mm Hg RAS at 11:40 AM
Slit-lamp examination	OD: lids/lashes: 4 mm horizontal laceration and mild diffuse erythema of upper lid; cornea: clear, no abrasions; conjunctiva: nasal subconjunctival hemorrhage, no lacerations; iris: flat and intact; anterior chamber: 1+ cells, 1+ flare, no hyphema; lens: clear; angle: 4 × 4 OS: unremarkable
Fundus examination	OD: inferior lattice degeneration with atrophic holes, mild nasal and inferior commotio retinae; optic nerve: CD 0.5 × 0.5, distinct margins, well-perfused; macula: flat with even pigmentation; vasculature: normal course and caliber, no hemorrhages; vitreous: clear, no pigment cells OS: unremarkable

Abbreviations: CD, cup to disc; OD, right eye; OS, left eye; OU, both eyes; PERRL, pupils equal, round, reactive to light; RAPD, relative afferent pupillary defect; RAS, right arm sitting; VA, visual acuity.

Comments

John was diagnosed with a subconjunctival hemorrhage and traumatic iridocyclitis in the right eye. He was reassured that although the hemorrhage appeared severe, it would resolve completely without treatment in approximately 2 weeks. The importance of protective eyewear for sporting activities was emphasized to prevent future injury to the eyes and surrounding tissue. The uveitis was treated with 1 drop of atropine in the right eye, which was administered in office. John was also prescribed topical prednisolone acetate 1% for the right eye with an initial dosage of 4 times

268

a day for 1 week. This was followed by a gradual taper to 1 drop daily over the following 3 weeks. His intraocular pressures were measured weekly and remained stable throughout the course of treatment. The subconjunctival hemorrhage had resolved completely at a 2-week follow-up examination, and the uveitis had resolved by the third week after the injury.

Discussion

A subconjunctival hemorrhage often occurs following blunt trauma to the globe. However, other potential causes include mechanical rubbing of the eye, intraocular surgery or injections, and contact lens wear.[1] Patients using blood thinning medications or supplements that increase the risk of bleeding are more likely to develop a subconjunctival hemorrhage. In some cases, the hemorrhage can occur in association with an infection or tumor of the conjunctiva.[1,2] The accumulation of blood from ruptured capillaries between the clear conjunctival tissue and episclera can also result from the Valsalva maneuver, vomiting, coughing or sneezing, vascular disease or blood-clotting disorders (Figure 2.26-1).

Blood pressure should be checked as part of the evaluation of a patient presenting with a subconjunctival hemorrhage, as it can be associated with systemic vascular diseases such as hypertension, arteriosclerosis, or diabetes. A careful review of systems should also be performed, especially when there is no history of recent trauma. Systemic infections, for example, measles, influenza, malaria, and smallpox should be considered in febrile patients with subconjunctival hemorrhages.[2] In cases involving a suspected ocular infection, such as the coxsackie virus or types of enterovirus or adenovirus,[3] the lymph nodes in the head and neck should be palpated. Other systemic disorders that may be causative include liver diseases (eg, hepatitis or cirrhosis), particularly if the subconjunctival hemorrhages are recurrent. If these are suspected, then blood tests to assess liver function are essential. Laboratory work including a complete blood count (CBC), prothrombin time (PT), partial thromboplastin time (PTT), and measures of protein S and protein C should also be ordered if the patient has any signs or symptoms of blood abnormalities such as leukemia, anemia, platelet dysfunction, or clotting disorders.[4]

A subconjunctival hemorrhage following blunt trauma may present with other ocular complications such as traumatic cataract, disruption of corneal tissue, conjunctival laceration, hyphema, traumatic iridocyclitis or angle recession. In the posterior segment, commotio retinae, traumatic optic neuropathy or a retinal tear may be seen. Accordingly, a dilated fundus examination should be performed. In John's case, it was determined that the blood he noticed on the towel came from the small laceration on his right upper eyelid.

Most subconjunctival hemorrhages are not associated with any systemic disorder and are self-limiting. They typically resolve within 1 to 2 weeks, depending on the size. Cool compresses or artificial tears may be used to relieve any associated discomfort. A careful history and follow-up testing are required to rule out any underlying systemic disease that may require further treatment.

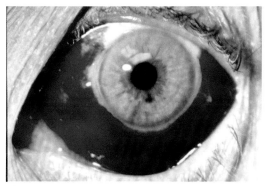

Figure 2.26-1   Large acute subconjunctival hemorrhage.

CLINICAL PEARLS

- Subconjunctival hemorrhages are self-limiting with complete resolution in 1 to 2 weeks.

- Complete a review of systems and check blood pressure of patients with subconjunctival hemorrhage as they commonly occur in patients with hypertension, arteriosclerosis, or other vascular disorders.

- Patients with recurrent subconjunctival hemorrhages should be referred for systemic evaluation and/or appropriate blood tests to assess for underlying diseases.

REFERENCES

1. Tarlan B, Kiratli H. Subconjunctival hemorrhage: risk factors and potential indicators. *Clin Ophthalmol.* June 2013;7:1160-1170.

2. Mimura T, Usui T, Yamagami S, et al. Recent causes of subconjunctival hemorrhage. *Ophthalmologica.* 2010;224(3):133-137.

3. Asbell PA, DeLuise VP, Bartolomei A. Viral conjunctivitis. In: Tabbara KF, Hyndiuk RA, eds. *Infections of the Eye.* Boston, MA: Listen Brown; 1996:462-463.

4. Onofrey BD, Skorin, L Jr, Holdeman NR. *Ocular Therapeutics Handbook: A Clinical Manual.* 3rd ed. Philadelphia, PA: Wolters Kluwer/Lippincott Williams & Wilkins; 2011.

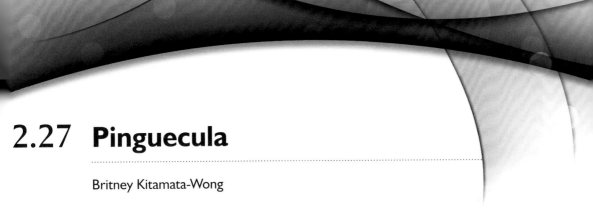

2.27 Pinguecula

Britney Kitamata-Wong

Lacey, a 36-year-old female, presented with a chief concern of soreness in each eye after removing her contact lenses. She was recently refitted into scleral contact lenses due to excessive movement of her previous corneal gas-permeable (GP) contact lenses, and had received her first pair of scleral contact lenses 3 days ago. She reported good vision and comfort during the day with the new lenses, achieving a maximum wear time of 13 hours. However, after removing the lenses, her eyes were red and sore on the nasal aspect of the conjunctiva in each eye. The symptoms resolved the following morning but would recur with subsequent lens wear. Lacey denied any issues with lens movement, fogging, eye pain, or light sensitivity. Her ocular history was positive for keratoconus, which was diagnosed 10 years ago. Her contact lens care system included a GP multipurpose solution for cleaning and disinfection and non-preserved saline solution for filling the lenses before application.

Clinical Findings

VA (through contact lenses)	OD: 20/15^{-3}; OS: 20/15^{-1}
Presenting CL Rx	OD: 18.2 mm diameter scleral lens with standard peripheral curves; base curve 47.00 D (7.18 mm); −5.25 sph; OS: 18.2 mm diameter scleral lens with standard peripheral curves; base curve 46.00 D (7.18 mm); −4.00 sph
Over-refraction	OD: Pl −0.50 × 105 (20/15); OS: Pl −0.50 × 075 (20/15)
Lens fit	OD: 175 micrometer central clearance/full limbal clearance/scleral alignment except mild blanching nasally; OS: 175 micrometer central clearance/full limbal clearance/scleral alignment except mild blanching nasally
Slit-lamp examination	OD: conjunctiva: 1.5 mm creamy round elevated lesion nasal bulbar conjunctiva, Grade 1+ nasal injection (Figure 2.27-1); cornea: (+) Fleischer ring, (−) striae, (−) scarring, (−) staining, (+) inferior thinning; OS: conjunctiva: 1.5 mm creamy round elevated lesion nasal bulbar conjunctiva, Grade 1+ nasal injection; cornea: (+) Fleischer ring, (−) striae, (−) scarring, (−) staining, (+) inferior thinning

Abbreviations: CL, contact lens; OD, right eye; OS, left eye; Pl, plano; Rx, prescription; sph, sphere; VA, visual acuity.

Comments

The diagnosis of pinguecula was discussed with Lacey along with alternative contact lens options. Since she had poor visual acuity (VA) with soft contact lenses and excessive movement with corneal GP lenses, Lacey preferred to continue with modified scleral contact lenses. To reduce pressure on

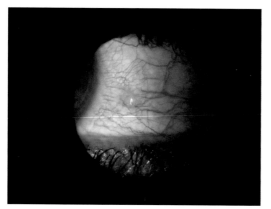

Figure 2.27-1   Elevated conjunctival lesion OD.
Abbreviation: OD, right eye.

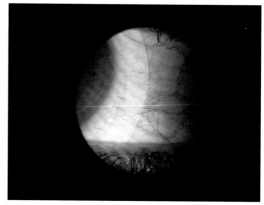

Figure 2.27-2   Reduction in conjunctival blanching with flatter scleral landing curves.

the nasal conjunctiva, new lenses were ordered with flatter peripheral (scleral landing) curves and were dispensed after arrival.

Lacey presented for a follow-up visit 2 weeks after the lenses were dispensed, and reported improvement in both redness and soreness following lens removal. The lenses were aligned over the nasal conjunctiva with minimal blanching (compression) (Figure 2.27-2).

Lacey was educated regarding her condition. Non-preserved artificial tears were recommended to minimize desiccation while wearing the lenses. A 2-week follow-up phone call indicated a significant improvement in redness and irritation at the end of the day. She was advised to return in 6 months for a contact lens progress evaluation, or sooner if symptoms arose.

Discussion

Pingueculae are the most common conjunctival lesions encountered in clinical practice.

They have a prevalence of approximately 48% in individuals older than 40 years,[1] although this can vary widely depending on the population, with a higher prevalence in rural communities.[2-4] Risk factors include sun exposure of more than 2 hours per day, increased age, and male gender. Alcohol consumption has been associated with increased risk of pinguecula,[1] although this is not found across all studies.[2-4]

Pingueculae are thought to arise from a combination of prolonged actinic (ultraviolet) exposure and environmental irritation from dust, heat, and desiccation.[5] Histopathology shows hyaline degeneration of the conjunctival substantia propria and fibrovascular proliferation,[6] leading to the thickened, elevated appearance. Pingueculae manifest as yellow or white lesions on the bulbar conjunctiva, most frequently on the nasal aspect. Mild hyperemia is often present.

Differential diagnoses include pterygium, conjunctival nevus, and ocular surface squamous neoplasia (OSSN).[5,7] Pterygia originate on the conjunctiva and cross the limbal border onto the cornea. Histopathology suggests that pingueculae can progress to pterygia[6] although this is somewhat controversial. Conjunctival nevi are discrete lesions that contain varying degrees of pigment and often have a cystic appearance.[7] Ocular surface squamous neoplasia is a broad category of conditions including conjunctival intraepithelial neoplasm (CIN), papilloma, and squamous cell carcinoma.[7] The size, shape, location, depth, and the presence or absence of feeder vessels should be documented in these conditions, which should be monitored with photographic documentation. When in doubt, a biopsy and referral to an anterior segment specialist should be considered.[5]

Pingueculae are usually slow growing with low risk of morbidity. Although most of the patients remain asymptomatic, some

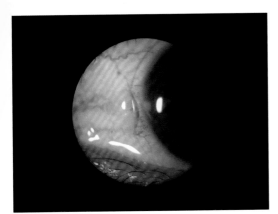

Figure 2.27-3   Notching the edge of a scleral gas-permeable contact lens to evade conjunctival pinguecula.

may develop redness, dryness, reduced tear breakup time, and inflammation. Treatment includes artificial tears, ultraviolet protection, and protection from environmental irritants. A short course of mild topical steroids can be used to reduce mild inflammation (pingueculitis). In more severe cases or for cosmetic restoration, surgical removal may be indicated.[5]

Pingueculae can cause significant challenges during contact lens fitting. Large lesions near the limbus can lead to decentration of soft contact lenses. Friction against these elevated regions from contact lens wear may exacerbate dryness and irritation. Non-preserved artificial tears are recommended to reduce dryness both during and after contact lens wear. Since the weight of a scleral contact lens is supported by the conjunctiva, fitting with flatter peripheral curves or custom edge modifications may be required to achieve proper alignment (Figure 2.27-3). Other contact lens options include refitting into a low modulus soft contact lens to minimize friction or a smaller diameter GP lens to avoid contact.

REFERENCES

1. Viso E, Gude F, Rodríguez-Ares MT. Prevalence of pinguecula and pterygium in a general population in Spain. *Eye.* 2011;25(3):350-357.
2. Fotouhi A, Hashemi H, Khabazkhoob M, Mohammad K. Prevalence and risk factors of pterygium and pinguecula: the Tehran Eye Study. *Eye.* May 2009;23(5):1125-1129.
3. Norn MS. Prevalence of pinguecula in Greenland and in Copenhagen, and its relation to pterygium and spheroid degeneration. *Acta Ophthalmol.* February 1979;57(1):96-105.
4. Le Q, Xiang J, Cui X, Zhou X, Xu J. Prevalence and associated factors of pinguecula in a rural population in Shanghai, Eastern China. *Ophthalmic Epidemiol.* April 2015;22(2):130-138.
5. Rapuano CJ. Conjunctival degenerations and mass lesions. In: Rapuano CJ, ed. *Color Atlas and Synopsis of Clinical Ophthalmology, Wills Eye Institute, Cornea.* 2nd ed. Philadelphia, PA: McGraw-Hill Companies Inc.; 2012.
6. Raizada IN, Bhatnagar NK. Pinguecula and pterygium (a histopathological study). *Indian J Ophthalmol.* 1976;24:16-18.
7. Othman IS. Ocular surface tumors. *Oman J Ophthalmol.* 2009;2(1):3-14.

2.28 **Pterygium**

Aaron Bronner

Danielle, a 43-year-old Hispanic female, presented with red irritated eyes, with the left eye affected more than the right. This was a long-standing issue, which Danielle thought began about a decade ago. She was also aware of a bump in her left eye that had partially grown over the iris, with a similar issue developing more recently on the right eye. Danielle reported irritation when she was in the wind or outdoors all day. In addition, she had noted a reduction in the vision of her left eye over the past 2 years. She had seen another eye doctor 2 years ago to see if these bumps could be removed, but was told that removal was not advisable. She was prescribed over-the-counter artificial tears in an attempt to slow advancement of the growth. Danielle continued using these drops but did not feel they were working. Her medical history was unremarkable.

Clinical Findings

Unaided distance VA	OD: 20/40; OS: 20/80 (pinhole 20/30)
Auto-refraction	OD: +0.50 −1.50 × 162 (20/20); OS: +3.00 −4.50 × 175 (20/40; pinhole 20/30)
Pupil evaluation	PERRL; no RAPD
Confrontation visual fields	Full to finger counting OD and OS
Intraocular pressure (iCare)	OD: 12 mm Hg; OS: 12 mm Hg at 10:15 AM
Slit-lamp examination	OD: 1+ nasal injection, 2.0 mm nasal pterygium (Figure 2.28-1); OS: 2+ nasal injection with a broad based 4.8 mm pterygium nasally, encroaching on visual axis (Figure 2.28-2)
Topography	OD: irregular astigmatism, moderate flattening in plane of pterygium (Figure 2.28-3); OS: irregular astigmatism, significant flattening in plane of pterygium (Figure 2.28-4)

Abbreviations: OD, right eye; OS, left eye; PERRL, pupils equal, round, reactive to light; RAPD, relative afferent pupillary defect; VA, visual acuity.

Comments

Danielle was diagnosed with an advanced progressive pterygium OS (Figure 2.28-4) and a moderate pterygium OD. Due to the severity of the growth in her left eye, together with the current impact on vision from the induced astigmatism and the potential for irreparable vision loss should further advancement occur, it was deemed necessary to remove this lesion surgically. Danielle was also given the option of removing the pterygium in her right eye, given that it was a source of chronic irritation and vision reduction (induced astigmatism). Danielle elected to pursue surgical treatment on the left eye only at this time, and to monitor the right eye for any further change. She would continue to use ocular lubricants to reduce irritation in her right eye to reduce irritation.

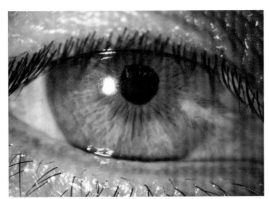

Figure 2.28-1   Moderate-sized nasal pterygium OD.
Abbreviation: OD, right eye.

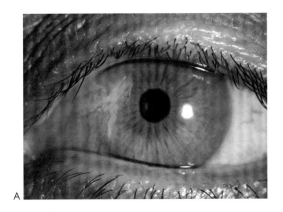

A

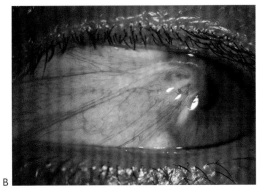

B

Figure 2.28-2   Large nasal pterygium OS.
Abbreviation: OS, left eye.

Discussion

The clinical diagnosis of a pterygium is generally an easy one to make. A pterygium is a wing-shaped or triangular fibrovascular growth originating in the interpalpebral conjunctiva and extending beyond the corneal limbus.

They are most commonly located on the nasal aspect of the limbus, but the temporal limbus may sometimes be affected, and occasionally double pterygia, found on both sides, may develop. The list of possible differential diagnoses is small and includes a trauma-induced pseudo-pterygium and ocular surface squamous neoplasia. In the case of trauma-induced pseudo-pterygium, a thin probe can be passed under the mass at the limbus, whereas a true pterygium is firmly attached and a probe cannot be passed under the lesion. Ocular surface squamous neoplasia are a group of conditions including squamous cell carcinoma and conjunctival intraepithelial neoplasia. These may also affect the interpalpebral limbal zone.

Many hours of exposure to sunlight without adequate ultraviolet protection is the primary risk factor for pterygium development.[1,2] The prevalence in at-risk black populations has been reported to be more than twice that found in Caucasians.[3] The nasal predilection probably results from incident temporal sunlight being totally internally reflected within the cornea, emerging onto the nasal limbus. Due to the concentration of the internally reflected light, its intensity may be 20 times greater than the incident temporal light, thereby increasing the oxidative effects in the nasal region.[1] This initiates a cascade of oxidative stress, cytokine and matrix metalloproteinase activity and fibroblast upregulation that may lead to pterygium genesis in genetically susceptible individuals.[1,2] Upregulation of inflammatory mediators leads to a chronically inflamed and irritated pterygium bed. As it crosses the limbus, the leading edge of the pterygium destroys Bowman's layer,[4] while it advances onto and conjunctivalizes the involved cornea. Visual changes can occur before the growth extends into the central axis, as flattening of the tissue results in mildly irregular, with-the-rule astigmatism. The destruction of Bowman's layer is critical when considering the appropriate time for surgical removal. Pathologies anterior to Bowman's layer can usually be removed without a scar. However, since pterygium genesis involves the dissolution of Bowman membrane, removal of these growths will leave a scar. The remaining scar will continue to impact vision through both opacification (if overlying

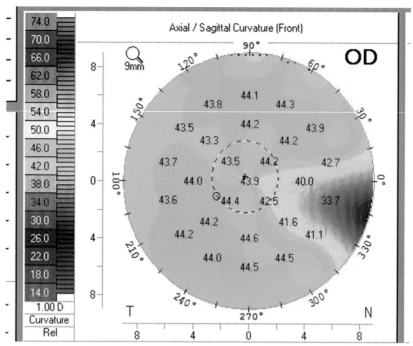

Figure 2.28-3   Corneal topography OD. Moderate flattening in the plane of the pterygium leading to with-the-rule astigmatism.

Abbreviation: OD, right eye.

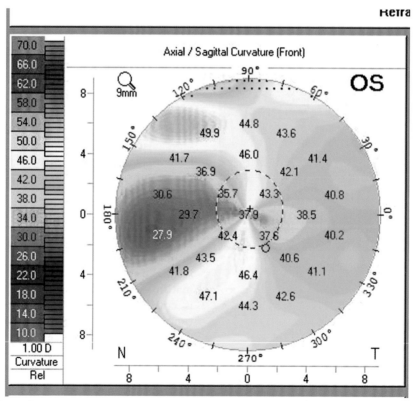

Figure 2.28-4   Corneal topography. Significant, somewhat irregular, flattening in the plane of the pterygium.

Abbreviations: OS, left eye.

the central axis) or with induced irregularity (if mid-peripheral). Accordingly, intervention should be encouraged prior to axial or even para-axial involvement. Significant reduction of pterygium-induced astigmatism usually occurs following their removal.

Conservative therapy of a stable, minimally symptomatic pterygium involves supportive treatment with lubrication and pulse dose of topical anti-inflammatory agents to control irritation and inflammation. If the irritation is poorly controlled with conservative therapy, vision is reduced and/or growth of the lesion occurs, then surgical removal should be considered. Treatment is the full removal of the lesion to the level of the sclera, followed by coverage with a conjunctival autograft harvested from the same eye (typically taken from the superior conjunctiva). The use of an autograft, as opposed to leaving a bare sclera, significantly lowers the risk of recurrence.[5] The autograft may be attached using tissue glue or sutured, although glue is easier to apply, and may be associated with a lower rate of recurrence.[6] Intraoperative application of mitomycin C, either with an autograft or alone, may also help reduce the risk of recurrence.[5] In the case of a recurrent pterygium, where a graft has already been used, the procedure is more difficult since harvesting a second graft may be impossible due to conjunctival fibrosis. In these cases, where a large or double pterygium is encountered, or where the amount of graft tissue required exceeds what is available, an amniotic membrane sheet may be applied. However, this technique is typically less successful than using an autograft.[5]

CLINICAL PEARLS

- In addition to irritation, a pterygium will cause increased astigmatism over time. This is often irregular and cannot be corrected satisfactorily with spectacles.

- Recurrent and double pterygium are more difficult to treat surgically, as the need for conjunctival graft tissue may exceed what is available.

REFERENCES

1. Coroneo MT, Girolama ND, Wakefield D. The pathogenesis of pterygia. *Curr Opin Ophthalmol.* 1999;10:282-288.
2. Chui H, Girolama NK, Wakefield D, Coronea MT. The pathogenesis of pterygium: current concepts and their therapeutic implications. *Ocul Surf.* 2009;6:24-43.
3. Luthra R, Nemesure BB, Wu S, et al. Frequency and risk factors for pterygium in the Barbados eye study. *Arch Ophthalmol.* 2001;119:1827-1832.
4. Chang R, Ching S. Corneal and conjunctival degenerations. In: Krachmer JH, Mannis MJ, Holland EJ, eds. *Cornea.* 2nd ed. St. Louis, MO: Mosby; 2004: 987-1004.
5. Kaufman SC, Jacobs DS, Lee Be, et al. Options and adjuncts in surgery for pterygium. A report by the American Academy of Ophthalmology. *Ophthalmology.* 2013;120:201-208.
6. Romano V, Cruciani M, Conti L, Fontana L. Fibrin glue versus sutures for conjunctival autografting in primary pterygium surgery. *Cochrane Database Syst Rev.* 2016;12:CD011308. doi:10.10002/14651858.CD011308.pub2.

2.29 Herpes Simplex Keratitis

Julia Canestraro

Anthony, a 36-year-old black male, presented with a unilateral, non-painful, red right eye. He reported that the red eye started approximately 2 to 3 weeks ago, with symptoms of photophobia, blurred vision, and a mild headache. He was seen by his primary care physician 1 week ago, who prescribed ciprofloxacin and azelastine drops to use twice a day OD. Anthony used the drops for 1 week, and since there was no resolution in the symptoms, he decided to stop taking the medication. His last eye examination was 3 years ago, where he was treated for herpes simplex keratitis in his right eye. The medical history was unremarkable.

Clinical Findings

Unaided distance VA	OD: 20/70 (pinhole 20/40); OS: 20/50 (pinhole 20/20⁻)
Pupil evaluation	PERRL; no RAPD
Ocular motility	Full and comitant: OD and OS
Confrontation visual fields	Full to penlight: OD and OS
Slit-lamp examination	OD: lids/lashes: mild edema superior lid; capped meibomian glands; conjunctiva: grade 1+ follicles superior and inferior palpebral conjunctiva, grade 2 injection, mild chemosis; cornea: approximately 4.5 mm vertical dendrite extending from 12 to 4 o'clock and crossing visual axis with surrounding stromal haze, (+) fluorescein staining of terminal bulbs; iris: flat and intact; anterior chamber: trace cells, no flare; angles: 4 × 4; corneal sensitivity: decreased. OS: lids/lashes: capped meibomian glands; conjunctiva: clear; cornea: clear; iris: flat and intact; anterior chamber: deep and quiet; angles: 4 × 4; corneal sensitivity: normal
Intraocular pressure (GAT)	OD: 15 mm Hg; OS: 15 mm Hg at 11:50 AM
Fundus examination	Unremarkable OD and OS

Abbreviations: GAT, Goldmann applanation tonometry; OD, right eye; OS, left eye; PERRL, pupils equal, round, reactive to light; RAPD, relative afferent pupillary defect; VA, visual acuity.

Comments

Anthony was diagnosed with recurrent herpes simplex conjunctivitis, epithelial and stromal keratitis, and iritis OD (see Figure 2.29-1). He was treated with trifluridine 1% 9 times a day OD, cyclopentolate twice a day OD, and oral acyclovir 400 mg 5 times a day. Steroid drops were deferred until the epithelial defect healed.

Anthony returned 2 days later with an improvement in symptoms and reported good compliance with the medications. Clinically, the presentation was similar to the first visit, except

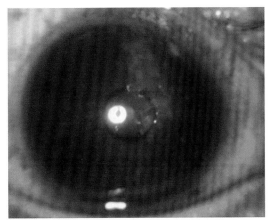

Figure 2.29-1   4.5-mm vertical dendrite of the corneal epithelium with surrounding stromal haze. The conjunctiva presented with significant injection.

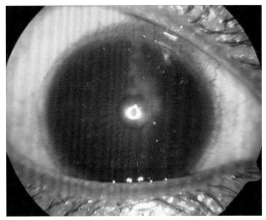

Figure 2.29-2   Resolved dendrite of the corneal epithelium with stromal haze. The conjunctival injection was resolving.

the dendrite appeared to be smaller in size. He was advised to continue all medications and to return in 1 week.

He returned 10 days later reporting good compliance with all medications. Visual acuity through pinhole was OD: 20/25⁻¹; OS: 20/25⁻¹. Slit-lamp examination showed a completely resolved epithelial defect with remaining stromal haze and a resolved iritis (see Figure 2.29-2). At this point, Anthony had completed his course of oral acyclovir. He was advised to taper the trifluridine 1% to 4 times a day, begin prednisolone acetate 1% 4 times a day OD and to discontinue the cyclopentolate.

Anthony was seen 4 more times over the next 6 weeks, during which time the steroid was slowly tapered along with the topical antiviral medication. On his last visit, his visual acuity (VA) was stable at OD: 20/25⁺²; OS: 20/20⁻³. A subepithelial scar remained in his right visual axis. He was prescribed prophylactic oral acyclovir 400 mg twice a day. Anthony was then lost to follow-up.

Discussion

An ocular history of herpes simplex keratitis with a clinical presentation of a unilateral, nonpainful, persistent redness in the same eye would lead to a likely diagnosis of recurrent herpes simplex keratitis. Approximately 50% to 80% of infections relating to the herpes simplex virus (HSV) are acquired before 30 years of age.[1] If a patient has 1 episode of either epithelial or stromal disease, then the chance of recurrence after 1, 2, and 10 years is 10%, 23%, and 50%, respectively.[1] The HSV is often passed via direct contact to skin or mucous membranes. There are 2 strains of the herpes virus, namely HSV-1 and HSV-2. It is HSV-1 that causes ocular involvement and resides in the trigeminal ganglion after the initial infection. Recurrences may be triggered by fever, hormonal changes, ultraviolet light, psychological stress, ocular trauma, and surgical manipulation of the trigeminal nerve.[2]

Both primary and secondary HSV infections can present as a blepharitis, conjunctivitis, epithelial keratitis, stromal keratitis, iritis, retinitis or any combination of the above.[2] Anthony presented with conjunctivitis, epithelial keratitis, stromal keratitis, and iritis. A typical HSV conjunctivitis exhibits hyperemia and follicles in the palpebral conjunctiva, which can often persist for 4 to 6 weeks after the initial infection.[3] An epithelial keratitis contains active viral cells, and will typically present with dendrites on the corneal surface. These dendrites present in a tree-like pattern with terminal end bulbs, where the edges are lined by heaped epithelial cells that stain with rose bengal and lissamine green and encase a central epithelial ulceration that stains with fluorescein. Stromal keratitis is an inflammation of the middle layers of the cornea, which presents as stromal haze and thickening. An associated iritis can best be seen with a conical beam in the slit lamp to view the cells in the anterior chamber. Since the herpes virus causes uveitis, elevated intraocular pressure (IOP) may be associated, although it was not found in this case.

The primary condition one should differentiate from herpes simplex is herpes zoster virus. Similar to herpes simplex, herpes zoster may also present with a follicular conjunctivitis, epithelial and stromal keratitis, iritis, and retinitis. A key differentiating factor is that herpes zoster keratitis will present with pseudodendrites, which can be differentiated from true dendrites in that they do not have end bulbs and do not stain with fluorescein. Typically, herpes zoster patients present with unilateral skin vesicles that often follow the trigeminal nerve dermatome.

The treatment for herpes simplex conjunctivitis is a topical antiviral agent such as trifluridine 1% 5 times a day or vidarabine ointment 3% 5 times a day, until resolution is complete (usually 7 to 14 days). The treatment for an epithelial keratitis is a topical antiviral[4] such as trifluridine 1% 9 times a day, ganciclovir gel 5 times a day or vidarabine ointment 3% five times a day. The topical antiviral should be continued for 7 to 14 days, tapered to 4 times a day for 4 days and then discontinued. Oral acyclovir 400 mg 5 times a day for 7 to 10 days may be used when drops cannot be instilled. There is no evidence that oral acyclovir, when accompanied by topical antiviral drugs, will prevent the development of stromal keratitis in patients with epithelial keratitis.[4] One may also consider gentle debridement of the epithelial lesion with a cotton-tipped applicator.[1] The treatment provided in this case was effective, but in retrospect, we would not have started oral acyclovir in addition to the topical antiviral. *Note that topical steroids should not be used with herpetic epithelial disease.*

Treatment of a stromal keratitis with or without a concurrent iritis should include a topical steroid such as prednisolone acetate 1% 4 times a day with a slow taper, antiviral prophylaxis such as trifluridine 1% 4 times a day or oral acyclovir 400 mg twice a day (which should be used concurrently during the steroid taper[2]), a cycloplegic agent twice or 3 times a day and aqueous suppressants in the presence of elevated IOP. Note that an antiviral alone is not adequate for the treatment of stromal keratitis. During the course of treatment, if additional signs, such as a deepening of the existing ulcer, a worsening anterior chamber reaction, or formation of a new infiltrate are observed, then the lesion should be cultured for bacterial or fungal involvement.

The visual prognosis for herpetic conjunctivitis, epithelial keratitis, and stromal keratitis is good provided proper and timely management is instituted. Approximately, 65% of patients with stromal keratitis had resultant VA of 20/40 or better after appropriate treatment.[2] In patients with recurrent herpetic stromal disease, a prophylactic dose of oral acyclovir 400 mg twice a day for at least 1 year has been shown to reduce the rate of recurrence.[5]

CLINICAL PEARLS

- Staining is important. Be aware of how sodium fluorescein, rose bengal, and lissamine green stain differently.

- Topical steroids should not be used with herpetic epithelial disease.

- In patients with recurrent herpetic stromal disease, a prophylactic dose of oral acyclovir 400 mg twice a day for at least 1 year has shown to reduce the rate of recurrence.

- There is no evidence that oral acyclovir prophylaxis 400 mg twice a day will prevent the development of stromal keratitis or uveitis in patients with herpetic epithelial keratitis.

REFERENCES

1. Barker NH. Ocular herpes simplex. *Br Med J Clin Evid.* 2008; https://www.ncbi.nlm.nih.gov/pmc/articles/PMC2907955/. February 8, 2017.
2. Liesegang TJ. Herpes simplex virus epidemiology and ocular importance. *Cornea.* 2001;20(1):1-13.
3. Darougar S, Wishart MS, Viswalingam ND. Epidemiological and clinical features of primary herpes simplex virus ocular infection. *Br J Ophthalmol.* 1985;69:2-6.
4. National Eye Institute. Clinical Studies Database: Herpetic Eye Disease Study (HEDS) II. https://clinicaltrials.gov/ct2/show/NCT00000139. February 8, 2017.
5. National Eye Institute. Clinical Studies Database: Herpetic Eye Disease Study (HEDS) I. www.nei.nih.gov/neitrials/viewStudyWeb.aspx?id=37. February 8, 2017.

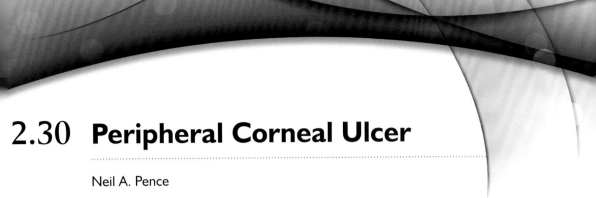

2.30 Peripheral Corneal Ulcer

Neil A. Pence

George, a 64-year-old male, presented with a red, mildly painful left eye. The eye was tender on awakening, and George acknowledged some crusting on the left lower lid and lashes. There was moderate photophobia when first opening the eye, but little at the time of the examination. He reported no other symptoms or concurrent acute illnesses.

A review of the patient's eye care record showed 2 previous urgent eye visits in the previous 5 months. On both occasions, George was found to have bacterial conjunctivitis. He had a history of keratoconus and was a long-time gas-permeable (GP) contact lens wearer. George's medical history was positive for sleep apnea. He used a continuous positive airway pressure (CPAP) device at night for this condition. He was diagnosed with Parkinson's disease 6 years ago.

Clinical Findings

Corrected distance VA (through spectacles)	OD: 20/40⁻ (pinhole 20/30); OS: 20/40 (pinhole 20/30)
Slit-lamp examination	OD: unremarkable; OS: conjunctiva: 2+ limbal redness mainly inferior nasally; mild bulbar conjunctival injection inferior and laterally; lids: slight crusting around 1-2 lashes on lower lid; mild thickening of lid margin, slight telangiectasia of posterior lid margin and inability to express meibum from nearly all meibomian glands (indicative of long-standing MGD); cornea: white 1.5 × 2.5 mm lesion noted at 7 o'clock roughly 1 mm inside the limbus; fluorescein staining showed very center stained immediately, and over time, the stain leached out over a wider area as it penetrated and diffused deeper into stroma; mild stipple staining was also noted over lower one-third of the cornea (indicative of epithelial drying or exposure keratitis). See Figure 2.30-1
	Anterior chamber: quiet, with no cells or flare OD and OS
Intraocular pressure (GAT)	OD: 17 mm Hg; OS: 17 mm Hg at 1:30 PM

Abbreviations: GAT, Goldmann applanation tonometry; MGD, meibomian gland dsyfunction; OD, right eye; OS, left eye; VA, visual acuity.

Comments

George was diagnosed with a peripheral corneal ulcer OS of suspected inflammatory and infiltrative etiology with a bacterial component.

The treatment plan was as follows:

1. An antibiotic–steroid combination, loteprednol etabonate 0.5% and tobramycin 0.3% ophthalmic suspension (Zylet) was prescribed for use 4 times a day OS.

2. Good lid hygiene was recommended to keep the lashes clean and remove any mattering.

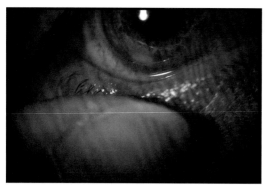

Figure 2.30-1   Note the peripheral corneal ulceration just inside the limbus at roughly 7 o'clock (stained with sodium fluorescein), and the limbal injection mainly inferiorly.

3. Two drops of 5% homatropine were instilled in the office.

4. A sample of non-medicated gel lubricating drops was provided to use at bedtime OU.

5. George was instructed not to wear a contact lens in his left eye.

6. He was instructed to return for a follow-up examination in 1 day.

At the 1-day follow-up visit, George reported no pain or discomfort and confirmed compliance with the treatment regimen. Findings were as follows:

Corrected distance VA (through spectacles)	OD: 20/40; OS: 20/40
Slit-lamp examination	OD: unremarkable; OS: conjunctiva: reduced inferior limbal redness, graded at 1+; lids and lashes: clear; Pupil: dilated and non-responsive; cornea: white lesion same size and appearance; tiny dot of central stain with fluorescein, but no leaching out with time
Intraocular pressure (GAT)	OD: 16 mm Hg; OS: 16 mm Hg at 9:15 AM

Abbreviations: GAT, Goldmann applanation tonometry; OD, right eye; OS, left eye; VA, visual acuity.

George was instructed to continue with the present treatment. Again, 1 drop of 5% homatropine was administered OS in the office. He was asked to return in 3 to 4 days, or sooner if his symptoms worsened.

At the 5-day follow-up visit, George reported his eye felt fine and that he wanted to return to GP contact lens wear. Slit-lamp examination revealed no limbal or bulbar redness, no corneal staining, and the white corneal lesion was beginning to fade. The plan was to continue the antibiotic/steroid drop 4 times a day for 2 more days, then twice a day for a further 7 days. He was told to wear his glasses for 2 more days, after which time he could resume GP wear. George was also told to continue using the lubricating gel at bedtime OU, and to continue good lid hygiene.

Discussion

Peripheral corneal ulcers tend to have a similar presentation. They are typically near the limbus, small and round with uniform borders. There is generally a central, full-thickness epithelial break. Redness tends to be localized to the limbus near the area of the ulcer. Symptoms can vary from painful to a mild foreign body sensation, and the amount of tearing can also vary.[1]

By comparison, central ulcers, that are more likely to be microbial keratitis, differ not only in location and depth, but they can be of any size, less round with more irregular margins, and are more likely to be accompanied by anterior chamber involvement. Redness is often more generalized, frequently additionally involving the bulbar conjunctiva.[2] Microbial keratitis ulcers are usually accompanied by greater pain and photophobia, lid edema, and a mucopurulent discharge.[3]

Peripheral corneal ulcers are most often infiltrative in origin. The numerous blood vessels at the limbus provide a rich source of white blood cells to send into the cornea in response to a challenge. With soft contact lenses, this is often created by toxins from *Staphylococcus aureus* found on the eyelids being trapped under the lens. Overnight wear of contact lenses will keep the toxins in 1 location. This triggers an inflammatory reaction, resulting in a corneal infiltrate that either migrates up or loosens the epithelial cells over it, causing a break in the epithelium. When this occurs as a result of contact lens wear, it is referred to as a contact lens peripheral ulcer (CLPU).[4]

Contact lens peripheral ulcers are most commonly seen where the lid margins cross the limbus (typically around 2, 5, 7, and 10 o'clock). Exposure to normal lid *Staphylococcus* as well as *Staphylococcus* by-products and toxins is greatest in these locations, and the limbus provides a rich supply of white blood cells. Accordingly, these areas are the optimal locations to trigger an inflammatory and infiltrative process within the cornea.

Contact lens peripheral ulcers have sometimes been referred to as "sterile" corneal ulcers, owing to their inflammatory, rather than infectious origin. Although clinical decision-making should consider the most likely underlying cause, in the case of corneal ulcers, one must also protect against the worst scenario, such as a pseudomonas infection. Therefore, while steroids will be needed to reduce inflammation, antibiotics are required to treat the possibility of microbial keratitis. If the lesion is at all suspicious for microbial keratitis, topical third- or fourth-generation fluoroquinolones are used, at least at the outset. Once it is clear that the condition is either not getting worse, or improving somewhat, steroids can be added.[5] If the ulcer is larger, more central, and more suspicious, then culturing should be considered. However, CLPUs are rarely cultured.

In George's case, the history of recent infections of likely bacterial origin given their successful treatment with tobramycin, and the fairly typical peripheral ulcer presentation led to a tobramycin–steroid combination drug being prescribed from the outset. The 1-day follow-up visit suggested that any infectious agent was being controlled, so this treatment plan was maintained. The antibiotic was not needed after the first week, but continuing the steroid may help to lessen the residual small and faint scar that remained after the resolution of the ulcer.

Any corneal insult can be assumed to cause some anterior segment reaction. Even in cases where no such reaction is visible, as was the case here, there may be a subclinical trace iritis. Instillation of cycloplegia during the first few days lessens the possibility of a lingering, low-grade, secondary iritis.

Of additional interest here was the use of a CPAP machine at night. These sometimes include a mask or small "pillows" that are inserted into the nostrils. Some masks can pull the lower eyelid down, thereby increasing the likelihood of incomplete lid closure and nighttime corneal exposure leading to ocular dryness. If positioned improperly, air can leak from the mask and blow across the eye, which will further exacerbate dry eye. Furthermore, there is a high association of floppy eyelid syndrome in obstructive sleep apnea patients, which will also increase corneal exposure during sleep due to lid laxity.[6] Indeed, the air pressure may be sufficient to force air back through the nasolacrimal ducts, out the puncta and into the eye. If the lower lid is pulled down while the pressure is being applied, it may be possible to observe bubbles emerging from the puncta. The continuous air flow, as well as the normal nasal flora being blown into the eye, place users of these machines at higher risk of not just dry eye but also ocular infections (see Chapter 2.16). All patients using a CPAP machine will benefit from instillation of a prophylactic, lubricating gel in both eyes at bedtime, and should be cautioned to the risk of dryness and infection.[6]

Finally, a brief comment about visual acuity (VA) in urgent case presentations. One should always attempt to obtain VA measurements, even when the patient is in pain and even reluctant to open their eye. Further, it is common to encounter contact lens wearers who report their spectacles are either old or not their current prescription. Therefore, the VA may be reduced through these glasses, and especially when the patient has keratoconus, such as was found here. However, clinicians should not simply accept that reduced VA is due to the glasses being "old" or corneal irregularity. At a minimum, the VA should be measured through a pinhole. If the current problem is affecting vision, then it is more serious and urgent in nature. George had corrected VA of 20/20⁻ when it was appropriate for him to restart wearing his GP contact lenses, that is, the same as prior to the incident. If VA is at least adequate to meet the patient's daily visual demands, then a refractive examination or prescription change should be delayed until after the pathology has cleared, and preferably 1 to 2 days after all medications have been stopped.

CLINICAL PEARLS

- Any significant corneal epithelial break is a cause for concern. Although most CLPUs are not infectious, they should always be considered as such and antibiotic treatment should be initiated.

- Inflammation is a common factor in CLPUs, so topical steroids will be useful once the lesion has been treated with antibiotics.

- Any corneal insult can be assumed to cause some anterior chamber reaction, so the use of a cycloplegic agent in the initial stages reduces the risk of a lingering, low-grade iritis.

- The use of CPAP machines to treat sleep apnea is associated with dry eye upon awakening, as well as an increased risk of ocular infection. The use of ocular lubricants at night is helpful for users of these devices.

REFERENCES

1. Silbert J. Is it an ulcer or an infiltrate? *Rev Optom*, July 3, 2007;144(6):91-101.
2. Holden BA, Sankaridurg PR, Jalbert I. Adverse events and infections: which ones and how many? In: Sweeney DF, ed. *Silicone Hydrogels: The Rebirth of Continuous Wear Contact Lenses*. Boston, MA: Butterworth-Heinemann; 2000:175-183.
3. Weissman BA, Giese M, Mondino BJ. Ulcerative bacterial keratitis. In: Silbert J, ed. *Anterior Segment Complications of Contact Lens Wear*. 2nd ed. Boston, MA: Butterworth-Heinemann; 2000:225-249.
4. Holden BA, Reddy MK, Sankaridurg PR, et al. Contact lens-induced peripheral ulcers with extended wear of disposable hydrogel lenses: histopathologic observations on the nature and type of corneal infiltrate. *Cornea*. September 1999;18(5):538-543.
5. Melton R, Thomas R. Corneal ulcers versus infiltrates. *Clin Refr Optom*. 2005;16:348-349.
6. Harrison W, Pence N, Kovacich S. Anterior segment complications secondary to continuous positive airway pressure machine treatment in patients with obstructive sleep apnea. *Optometry*. 2007;78:352-355.

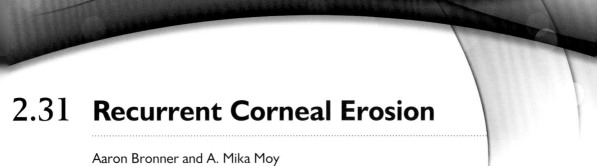

2.31　Recurrent Corneal Erosion

Aaron Bronner and A. Mika Moy

Devin, a 30-year old Caucasian male, complained of a sudden onset, painful, red left eye. He first noticed the pain when he awoke this morning. He graded the pain level as 6 out of 10 when he first awoke, but it had improved over the past 2 hours and was currently rated as 3 out of 10. He had instilled 0.05% tetrahydrozoline hydrochloride eye drops (Visine) in the left eye that morning. However, they stung badly and did not improve his symptoms. Devin reported a watery discharge from the eye, but no mucus. There was no history of contact lens wear. Devin thought that his left eye did occasionally feel dry and gritty on awakening. However, it had never been this severe before. He recalled a previous injury to his left eye approximately 1 year ago while playing basketball.

　Devin was otherwise in good health with no chronic illnesses or medications. He had no known drug allergies. There was no significant family, ocular, or medical history.

Clinical Findings

Unaided distance VA	OD: 20/20; OS: 20/20
Pupil evaluation	PERRL; no RAPD
Slit-lamp examination	OD: trace inspissated meibomian glands. Anterior chamber deep and quiet;
	OS: trace inspissated meibomian glands with a capped gland superiorly. Grade 1+ hyperemia 360° with enlarged tear lake (Figure 2.31-1). In white light, some corneal clouding from 2:00 to 4:00 (Figure 2.31-2) with positive and negative sodium fluorescein staining in that area (Figure 2.31-3). Anterior chamber deep and quiet
Intraocular pressure (GAT)	OD: 13 mm Hg; OS: 13 mm Hg at 1:00 PM
Fundus examination	Unremarkable: OD and OS

Abbreviations: GAT, Goldmann applanation tonometry; OD, right eye; OS, left eye; PERRL, pupils equal, round, reactive to light; RAPD, relative afferent pupillary defect; VA, visual acuity.

Comments

Devin was diagnosed with recurrent corneal erosion, which was likely secondary to a previous corneal abrasion received while playing basketball. His cornea was anesthetized with topical 0.5% tetracaine ophthalmic solution. The area was debrided, and a bandage contact lens fitted. Devin was prescribed 0.5% moxifloxacin ophthalmic solution to use 3 times a day to protect against infection. If the bandage contact lens did not manage the pain adequately, he was instructed to take 400 mg ibuprofen every 4 to 6 hours as needed. He was told to leave the bandage contact lens in place, and not to reposition the lens should it fall out. He was also instructed to not rub his

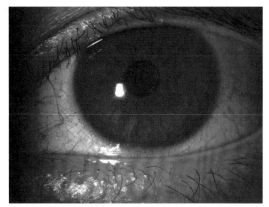

Figure 2.31-1   Low magnification, diffuse view of left eye. Note the hyperemia and large tear lake.

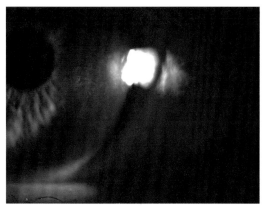

Figure 2.31-2   High magnification view of left cornea in white light. Note that the cornea is not perfectly clear.

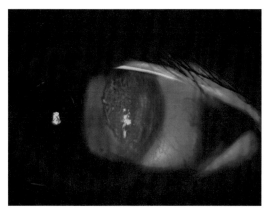

Figure 2.31-3   High magnification view of left eye. Note the positive and negative staining of the corneal epithelium.

eyes, to monitor any changes in his vision, and to return in 1 week.

Devin returned in 1 week and reported compliance with the instructions. The bandage contact lens was still in place and did not show any deposits. When viewed through the contact lens, the cornea appeared intact. The eye was flooded with non-preserved artificial tears and the bandage contact lens was removed with care. Instillation of sodium fluorescein showed trace positive and negative staining. Devin was instructed to discontinue the moxifloxacin and to use 0.5% sodium chloride ophthalmic ointment at bedtime for 1 month. The possibility of recurrence was discussed, and Devin was reassured that there were many other treatments that could be employed should the condition become more frequent.

Discussion

The differential diagnoses for a patient waking with a painful eye include nocturnal lagophthalmos, floppy lid syndrome, both sterile and microbial contact lens-related ulcerations, and recurrent corneal erosions. Although the corneal pain threshold of each patient is unique, the severity and acuteness of the pain from recurrent corneal erosion generally separates it from the other conditions described earlier, as it is both more severe and instantaneous when first opening the eyes. In cases where no obvious erosion is present, negative fluorescein staining patterns can help demarcate zones of healed microform erosions, which may heal in less than an hour and therefore be absent by the time the patient arrives for an examination. When faced with a symptomatic patient who does not exhibit any zones of positive staining, but does show areas of negative staining, then the tectonics of the epithelium in that area should be assessed with a sterile cotton-tipped applicator or Weck-Cel sponge (Beaver Visitec, Waltham, Massachusetts). If the epithelium rolls with light pressure, a poor or absent anchoring complex is revealed and this area will be involved in the patient's symptoms. An area that does not roll on palpation is uninvolved, even if negative staining exists. In cases where all evidence of erosion is absent, the ocular surface, including evaluation of lid tension and positioning, should be assessed fully to rule out other causes of morning discomfort.

Given Devin's symptoms, recurrent corneal erosion was suspected immediately and verified with the slit-lamp examination. As with approximately 45% to 67% of patients suffering from recurrent corneal erosion, he had a history of corneal trauma.[1] Approximately 20% to 30% of individuals develop the condition from epithelial basement membrane dystrophy.[2] The remaining cases do not have an identifiable risk factor.

As with all acute pathologies, once the diagnosis has been made, consideration should be given to both the early and later healing stages of the disease. In the case of recurrent corneal erosion, the acute healing process requires supporting reepithelialization of the abrasion and reducing pain, while preventing negative sequelae such as opportunistic microbial keratitis. Later considerations include the prevention of subsequent episodes.

In most cases, the early healing process involves the use of bandage soft contact lenses to reduce pain by protecting against the mechanical force of the upper lid as it moves over the ocular surface during each blink and allows more rapid reepithelialization. Increasingly, an amniotic membrane is being recommended for the treatment of recurrent corneal erosion on the basis of anecdotal reports that suggest its use may accelerate healing and prevent recurrence. Although there is no evidence on the ability of this modality to prevent subsequent episodes, an amniotic membrane seems a reasonable, albeit costly, substitute for a bandage lens in any corneal abrasion. For the prevention of opportunistic infection, an antibiotic should be provided while the epithelial defect persists. Given that infection would likely develop from the normal flora, the most appropriate therapy would have good coverage for these organisms; particularly, staphylococcal and streptococcal species. Depending on the original size, the erosion will generally heal in between 1 and 5 days, assuming no other stressors to the ocular surface.

Although treatment of the acute phase of recurrent corneal erosion is ongoing, thought should be given to the long-term prognosis and prevention of recurrence. The primary factor involved in the development of recurrent corneal erosion is the aberrant development of anchoring junctions between the corneal epithelial layers and Bowman's layer. These anchoring junctions take approximately 6 to 8 weeks to form so medical treatment to aid their development may be considered.[2] At its most conservative, long-term therapy involves the use of nocturnal bland or hypertonic ointments and should be the minimum applied strategy. Other medical approaches could involve the use of an amniotic membrane, chronic use of bandage soft contact lenses for up to 2 months (with the lens being changed at regular intervals), doxycycline with or without bandage lenses to reduce the influence of matrixmetalloproteinases or application of a topical steroid for 6 to 8 weeks (without a bandage contact lens). In case of repeated episodes, the patient should undergo one of the surgical or para-surgical procedures offered for recurrent corneal erosion. Anterior stromal puncture is a reasonable approach, assuming the abnormal anchoring complex lies away from the visual axis, as this procedure produces mild stromal scarring. However, epithelial debridement with diamond burr polishing or phototherapeutic keratectomy each appear to be more effective than stromal puncture, although both are also costlier.[3-5] Unfortunately, studies that have examined the long-term efficacy of treatments for recurrent corneal erosion have been poorly designed, and it is difficult to predict the optimum treatment for an individual patient.[6] It may be wise to follow a stepwise pattern favoring simpler and less expensive interventions initially and progressing to more complex therapies should recurrences persist. For example, start with a bandage soft contact lens together with instillation of doxycycline, and advance to debridement with diamond burr polishing if necessary. Only if both of these procedures are ineffective should phototherapeutic keratectomy be considered.

CLINICAL PEARLS

- Ask patients with suspected recurrent corneal erosion about previous episodes, as well as a history of corneal trauma.

- The treatment of recurrent corneal erosion involves 2 stages; the acute phase to minimize patient discomfort and prevent infection, followed by longer-term management to prevent subsequent episodes.

REFERENCES

1. Reidy JJ, Paulus MP, Gona S. Recurrent erosions of the cornea: epidemiology and treatment. *Cornea*. November 2000;19(6):767-771.
2. Hykin PG, Foss AE, Pavesio C, Dart JK. The natural history and management of recurrent corneal erosion: a prospective randomised trial. *Eye (Lond)*. 1994;8(Pt 1):35-40.
3. Das S, Seitz B. Recurrent corneal erosion syndrome. *Surv Ophthalmol*. January–February 2008;53(1):3-15.
4. Vo RC, Chen JL, Sanchez PJ, Yu F, Aldave AJ. Long-term outcomes of epithelial debridement and diamond burr polishing for corneal epithelial irregularity and recurrent corneal erosion. *Cornea*. 2015;34:1259-1265.
5. Stasi K, Chuck RS. Update on phototherapeutic keratectomy. *Curr Opin Ophthalmol*. July 2009;20(4):272-275.
6. Watson SL, Lee MH, Barker NH. Interventions for recurrent corneal erosions. *Cochrane Database*. 2012;12:CD001861. doi:10.1002/14651858.CD001861.

2.32 Ocular Effects of Amiodarone

Kelly Glass

Susan, a 69-year-old female, presented with complaints of blurred vision at distance and at near. She also reported ocular burning, irritation, and dryness. She noticed mucus and mattering coming from her eyes in the morning most days each week. She stated that these symptoms had become significantly worse during the past few months. Susan had not noticed any halos or glare in either eye. She was not currently wearing any glasses, as they were lost several months prior to the examination.

At her last eye examination 1 year ago, Susan was diagnosed with dry eye syndrome, as well as moderate non-proliferative diabetic retinopathy and clinically significant macular edema in both eyes. The patient had been referred to a retinal specialist but discontinued visits with the specialist shortly after the referral. Medical history included rheumatoid arthritis, type 2 diabetes mellitus (diagnosed 5 years ago), arrhythmia, and hypertension. Her most recent blood glucose was 244 mg/dL, and her last A_{1c} was 6.0%. Current medications included furosemide, carvedilol, lisinopril, insulin, amiodarone (200 mg once daily for the past year), and ocular lubricant used as needed, generally once or twice per day.

Clinical Findings

Unaided distance VA	OD: 20/60 (no improvement with pinhole); OS: 20/60 (no improvement with pinhole)
Present Rx	None
Confrontation visual fields	Full to finger count OD and OS
Pupil evaluation	PERRL; no RAPD
Subjective refraction	OD: −0.25 −0.50 × 156 (20/60); OS: −1.00 DS (20/60)
Near ADD	+2.00 OU (near VA: 20/40 OU)
Slit-lamp examination (Figure 2.32-1)	OD: 2+ meibomitis; mild superficial punctate keratitis on the inferior 1/3 of the cornea; mild whorl keratopathy seen as a horizontal line inferior to pupil; pseudophakia; otherwise unremarkable; OS: 2+ meibomitis; mild superficial punctate keratitis on the inferior 1/3 of the cornea; mild whorl keratopathy seen as a horizontal line inferior to pupil; pseudophakia; otherwise unremarkable
Intraocular pressure (GAT)	OD: 10 mm Hg; OS: 10 mm Hg at 9:00 AM

Fundus examination
(Figure 2.32-2)

OD: 0.3/0.3 CD ratio; healthy rim tissue with distinct disc margins; scattered microaneurysms and dot blot hemorrhages in all 4 quadrants; scattered hard exudates temporal and inferotemporal to fovea; macular edema within 1/3 disc diameter of the fovea; periphery intact;

OS: 0.3/0.3 CD ratio; healthy rim tissue with distinct disc margins; scattered microaneurysms and dot blot hemorrhages in all 4 quadrants; scattered hard exudates in macular region; macular edema within 1/3 disc diameter of the fovea; epiretinal membrane; periphery intact

Fluorescein angiography
(Figure 2.32-3)

Significant macular edema OS greater than OD

Abbreviations: CD, cup to disc; GAT, Goldmann applanation tonometry; OD, right eye; OS, left eye; OU, both eyes; PERRL, pupils equal, round, reactive to light; RAPD, relative afferent pupillary defect; Rx, prescription; VA, visual acuity.

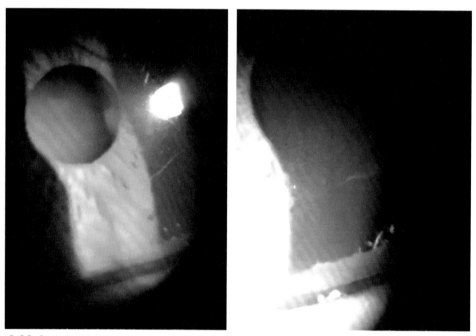

Figure 2.32-1   Whorl keratopathy.

Discussion

Susan had developed several systemic and ocular conditions, including diabetic retinopathy with clinically significant macular edema (causing Susan's decreased best corrected acuity), dry eye syndrome, and amiodarone keratopathy. To navigate your way through this multifactorial examination, it is important to be familiar with how systemic conditions affect the eyes, as well as potential ocular side effects of medications.

Susan was referred back to the retinal specialist for treatment of the diabetic retinopathy and macular edema. We emphasized the risk of vision loss if she did not comply with the recommendations. She was encouraged to control her blood glucose level more tightly and maintain follow-up visits with all health care specialists as indicated.

Susan was instructed to continue using artificial tears 4 times daily and warm compresses twice daily for 10 minutes to help alleviate dry eye symptoms. It is important to consider the

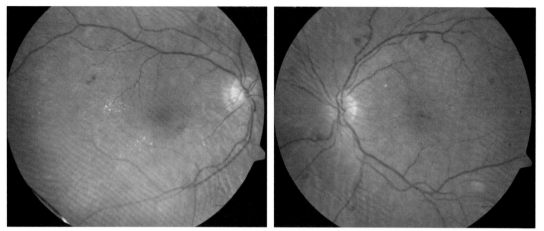

Figure 2.32-2 Fundus photos showing moderate diabetic retinopathy with macular edema in both eyes, as well as an epiretinal membrane in the left eye.

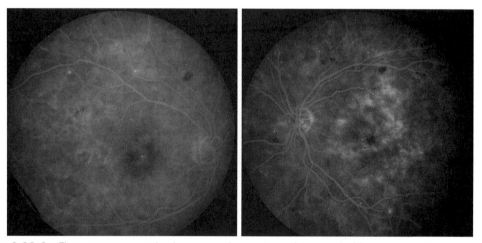

Figure 2.32-3 Fluorescein angiography showing significant edema of the macula OS greater than OD.
Abbreviations: OD, right eye; OS, left eye.

patient's medications as a potential cause of dry eye, as well as, hormonal, environmental, or dietary changes. Diuretics (eg, furosemide), beta-blockers (eg, carvedilol), lisinopril, and amiodarone have all been associated with dry eye.[1] Rheumatoid arthritis is also a potential source of dry eye. It was decided to treat the dry eye symptoms topically before making any changes to her medication regimen.

Amiodarone is an antiarrhythmic agent. This drug is linked to vortex keratopathy, a common side effect resulting in golden or grayish deposits that form inferiorly within the basal layer of the corneal epithelium in a whorl-like pattern extending toward the limbus. Vortex keratopathy seldomly creates a reduction in visual acuity or other ocular symptoms; however, in rare cases, the deposits can become dense enough to cause halos, glare, or vision impairment.[2] Susan's decrease in vision was felt to be a result of diabetic macular edema rather than amiodarone-induced whorl keratopathy. It is generally not necessary to discontinue amiodarone based solely on the presence of vortex keratopathy. If the drug is discontinued, corneal deposits typically regress within 3 to 20 months.[2]

Multiple studies suggest that vortex keratopathy secondary to amiodarone use occurs in nearly all patients.[3,4] It can occur as early as 1 to 2 weeks after initiation of amiodarone use but generally is seen after 1 to 4 months of amiodarone treatment. Vortex keratopathy can be divided into 3 stages. Stage 1 shows microdeposits in a horizontal line on the inferior cornea. Stage 2 is characterized by the horizontal line starting to develop arborizing lines. Stage 3 occurs when the whorl-like pattern is present extending into the visual axis. Susan's keratopathy was classified as stage 1 despite taking the medication for approximately 1 year. The mild nature may have been a result of lubricating drops flushing the amiodarone deposits from the corneal surface.[5]

When corneal verticillata is observed, Fabry disease, a glycosphingolipid metabolism disorder, should be included on the list of differentials. Inherited in an X-linked fashion, Fabry disease is typically diagnosed during childhood when a wide range of systemic symptoms are present, including pain in the extremities, kidney involvement, angiokeratomas, and neuropathy.[6] Because Susan had neither personal or family medical history of Fabry disease, nor did she have the characteristic symptoms of the disorder, it is safe to rule out this condition as a possible root cause of vortex keratopathy.

Besides amiodarone, several other medications are known to be responsible for producing whorl keratopathy. These include topical antibiotics tobramycin, gentamicin, and ciprofloxacin; antimalarial drugs chloroquine and hydroxychloroquine; and tamoxifen, indomethacin, and chlorpromazine.[2]

An additional differential diagnosis is Hudson-Stahli line, a linear formation of iron deposition typically located between the middle and lower thirds of the cornea, where the upper and lower eyelids come together. In addition, corneal irregularities, particularly after refractive surgery, can cause tears to pool resulting in iron depositing in the corneal epithelium. These patients, similar to those with whorl keratopathy, are generally asymptomatic. Susan had no history of refractive surgery or significant corneal irregularities except superficial punctate keratitis. In addition, her lesions were grayish

deposits compared to the brown appearance of Hudson–Stahli line.

Amiodarone has been linked to other ocular signs including lenticular opacities and optic neuropathy.[2] Optic neuropathy develops in 1% to 2% of amiodarone users within the initial year of treatment. However, in a serial study, Ingram and colleagues[7] observed no maculopathy in 105 patients taking amiodarone with a follow-up period ranging from 3 months to more than 7 years.

Amiodarone optic neuropathy is often characterized by gradual onset, slowly progressive vision loss with bilateral, persistent optic nerve edema.[8] If amiodarone-induced optic neuropathy is suspected, a dilated fundus examination, visual field, and nerve fiber layer optical coherence tomography (OCT) should be administered. Referral to the patient's primary care provider (PCP) or cardiologist is recommended to contemplate substitute drug therapy. Due to amiodarone's long half-life, disc swelling may endure for weeks to months after the medication is stopped. Vision loss associated with the optic neuropathy may be reversible with cessation of amiodarone therapy.[9] The manufacturers of amiodarone suggest routine eye evaluations to screen for optic neuropathy development but offer no specific follow-up time interval.[9] In Susan's case, there was no optic nerve edema, although she will continue to be monitored.

CLINICAL PEARLS

- Reduced visual acuity must always be explained. Perform an extra test or bring the patient back to determine the cause.

- It is important to be familiar with the ocular signs and symptoms associated with systemic conditions and medications.

REFERENCES

1. Askeroglu U, Alleyne B, Guyuron, B. Pharmaceutical and herbal products that may contribute to dry eyes. *Plast Reconstr Surg.* 2013;131(1):159-167.
2. Raizman MB, Hamrah P, Holland EJ, et al. Drug-induced corneal epithelial changes. *Surv Ophthalmol.* 2017;62(3):286-301.
3. Ingram DV. Ocular effects in long-term amiodarone therapy. *Am Heart J.* 1983;106(4):902-905.

4. Turk U, Turk BG, Yılmaz SG, Tuncer E, Alioğlu E, Dereli T. Amiodarone-induced multiorgan toxicity with ocular findings on confocal microscopy. *Middle East Afr J Ophthalmol*. 2015;22(2):258.

5. Ciancaglini M, Carpineto P, Zuppardi E, Nubile M, Doronzo E, Mastropasqua L. In vivo confocal microscopy of patients with amiodarone-induced keratopathy. *Cornea*. 2001;20(4):368-373.

6. Germain DP. Fabry disease. *Orphanet J Rare Dis*. 2010;5(1):30.

7. Ingram DV, Jaggarao NS, Chamberlain DA. Ocular changes resulting from therapy with amiodarone. *Br J Ophthalmol*. 1982;66(10):676-679.

8. Gokulgandhi MR, Vadlapudi AD, Mitra AK. Ocular toxicity from systemically administered xenobiotics. *Exp Opin Drug Metab Toxicol*. 2012;8(10):1277-1291.

9. Moorthy RS, Valluri S. Ocular toxicity associated with systemic drug therapy. *Curr Opin Ophthalmol*. 1999;10(6):438-446.

2.33 Cataract

Adam B. Blacker

Jerri, a 67-year-old female, complained of a film over her right eye, which seemed to be present all the time. This perception persisted even after blinking and seemed to be worse in the morning upon awakening. When Jerri put her glasses on she felt an immediate need to take them off and clean them, even though this did not improve her vision at all. Jerri first noticed the film approximately 6 months ago and stated that it was very annoying. She denied that straight lines ever appeared wavy or curved. Previous records indicated that Jerri had visual acuity (VA) of 20/20 in each eye 2.5 years ago. She had no history of ocular surgery. Her medical history was positive for systemic hypertension and elevated cholesterol.

Clinical Findings

Present Rx	OD: +1.50 −0.50 × 122 (20/200; pinhole 20/40⁻); OS: +1.00 −0.75 × 086 (20/25^{-2}; pinhole: 20/20); ADD: +2.00 OU (OD: 20/125; OS: 20/32; OU: 20/32)
Cover test (with present Rx)	Distance: orthophoria; near: orthophoria
Near point of convergence	11 cm/14 cm
Confrontation visual fields	Full to finger counting OD and OS
Pupil evaluation	PERRL; no RAPD
Retinoscopy	OD: −2.00 −1.50 × 072; OS: +1.50 −1.00 × 090
Subjective refraction	OD: −1.25 −1.75 × 093 (20/40); OS: +1.50 −1.00 × 090 (20/20)
Near ADD	+2.00 OU (20/20)
Brightness acuity testing	OD: 20/125; OS: 20/25
Intraocular pressure (GAT)	OD: 10 mm Hg; OS: 12 mm Hg at 12:04 PM
Slit-lamp examination	OD and OS: mild meibomian gland dysfunction with capping upper and lower lids; trace punctate fluorescein staining inferior cornea OD and OS; OD: lens: Grade 3 nuclear sclerosis, Grade 3+ posterior subcapsular cataract, Grade 1+ cortical cataract; OS: lens: trace nuclear sclerosis
Fundus examination	Unremarkable OD and OS

Abbreviations: GAT, Goldmann applanation tonometry; OD, right eye; OS, left eye; OU, both eyes; PERRL, pupils equal, round, reactive to light; RAPD, relative afferent pupillary defect; Rx, prescription.

Discussion

These clinical findings indicate that the decreased VA in Jerri's right eye is almost certainly due to the presence of the nuclear sclerotic and posterior subcapsular cataracts. Although this diagnosis is straightforward, the case management of this patient requires some thought.

It is estimated that approximately 17% of individuals elder than 40 years of age have a cataract in at least 1 eye.[1] The 3 most common types of cataracts are nuclear, cortical, and posterior subcapsular. These may present individually or in combination. Although all are associated with increasing age, development of cataracts has also been linked with trauma, diabetes, UV exposure, and steroid use.

Nuclear cataracts are typically the result of oxidation, resulting in darkening and hardening of the lens nucleus.[2] Optical absorption, rather than light scatter, leads to the reduction in VA with this type of cataract. Cortical cataracts occur when water infiltrates the lens cortex. This process takes place through osmosis after the cortical cell membranes are damaged. Hydrophilic ion levels increase, thereby attracting water into the lens.[3] This change creates light scattering similar to that found in posterior subcapsular cataracts. This latter type of opacity is thought to be formed by incompletely differentiated lens epithelial cells that migrate to the posterior pole.[4]

There is a prominent unilaterality in Jerri's case. It is common to see bilateral cataracts with asymmetric progression and symptoms, but this level of asymmetry presents a potential complication. Jerri has worn glasses for many years and considers them to be part of her "persona." She had several pairs of unique and fun frames. They are used, not only as a necessary vision device, but also as aesthetic accessories. Cataract surgery presents a problem for Jerri. Given the reduced VA, particularly under glare conditions as demonstrated by the brightness acuity test results, surgery should certainly be recommended. This would almost certainly be on the right eye only, even though the left lens exhibited trace nuclear sclerosis (which also affected her vision under glare testing). It is important that Jerri be educated on the likely outcome of cataract surgery. For example, if an emmetropic outcome is targeted, then this would reduce the need for her to wear glasses for distance viewing.

However, Jerri may also be left with anisometropia after treatment. Given the absence of a visually significant cataract in the fellow eye, the surgeon may consider seeking a low hyperopic endpoint similar to the refractive error in the left eye. This will minimize any vertical prism difference and aniseikonia in her postsurgical glasses. Jerri should be counseled to think about her corrective goals after surgery, and these should be communicated to the surgeon so as to minimize postsurgical complications.

Even if glasses were not prescribed at this visit, it is important to obtain precise measurements of VA and refractive error. Less-experienced clinicians may view these tests as unimportant, because the patient is being referred for surgery. However, precise findings are valuable in order to assess future improvements, as well as to aid in pre- and postsurgical management.

An additional aspect that may prove difficult in this case is the density of both the posterior subcapsular and nuclear sclerotic cataract. Opacified lenses make performing a dilated fundus examination more difficult. Because cataract extraction can increase the risk of a retinal tear or detachment,[5] the structural integrity of the retina must be evaluated before surgery. In cases of very dense cataracts, B-scan ultrasonography may be needed to rule out any gross retinal detachments.

CLINICAL PEARLS

- Cataract is a likely cause of a "film over the eye" that does not improve with blinking or after cleaning one's glasses.

- Tests such as a brightness acuity tester, potential acuity meter, and an optical coherence tomography (OCT) can all provide valuable information about the effect of the cataract on a patient's vision.

- Remember to compare the appearance of the cataract with VA to understand this relationship. Different types of cataracts have varying impacts on vision.

- Identify potential postsurgical complications, and discuss them with the surgeon and patient prior to treatment.

REFERENCES

1. Congdon N, Vingerling JR, Klein BE, et al. Prevalence of cataract and pseudophakia/aphakia among adults in the United States. *Arch Ophthalmol.* 2004;122(4): 487-494.
2. Jedziniak JA, Nicoli DF, Baram H, Benedek GB. Quantitative verification of the existence of high molecular weight protein aggregates in the intact normal human lens by light-scattering spectroscopy. *Invest Ophthalmol Vis Sci.* 1978;17(1):51-57.
3. Mathias RT, Rae JL, Baldo GJ. Physiological properties of the normal lens. *Physiol Rev.* 1997; 77(1):21-50.
4. Al-ghoul KJ, Novak LA, Kuszak JR. The structure of posterior subcapsular cataracts in the Royal College of Surgeons (RCS) rats. *Exp Eye Res.* 1998;67(2):163-177.
5. Care of the Adult Patient With Cataract, A.O.A.C.P. Guidelines, St. Louis, MO: American Optometric Association. 31-44. www.aoa.org. 1995. Accessed February 20, 2017.

2.34 Toric Multifocal Intraocular Lenses

Gurpreet K. Bhogal-Bhamra, Sai Kolli, and James S. Wolffsohn

Janet, a 58-year-old female physician, complained that her current vision was deteriorating. She wore mainly monovision soft contact lenses and reverted to progressive addition lenses (PALs) full-time on weekends. Although Janet had been wearing contact lenses for about 40 years, she reported that her vision was now becoming blurry at all distances. This made it hard to concentrate at times. Additionally, colors appeared less distinct. Although the vision with her spectacles was slightly better than with the contact lenses, she preferred not to wear glasses. Janet's general health was good and she was not taking any medications. She swam and played other sports regularly.

Clinical Findings

Unaided distance VA	OD: 20/120; OS: 20/200; OU: 20/100
Pupil evaluation	PERRL; no RAPD
Subjective refraction	OD: −2.75 −2.00 × 015 (20/20); OS: −2.50 −2.00 × 005 (20/25); ADD: +2.25 OU (20/30)
Intraocular pressure (NCT)	OD: 13 mm Hg; OS: 14 mm Hg at 10:40 AM
Slit-lamp examination	OD and OS: mild nuclear opacities (NO1, NC1 using Lens Opacities Classification System III), otherwise unremarkable
Dilated fundus examination	Unremarkable OD and OS
Ocular biometry (Zeiss IOLMaster 500, software version 7.3, Oberkochen, Germany)	OD: axial length: 24.61 mm; keratometry: 7.40 mm × 7.70 mm @ 013; anterior chamber depth: 3.35 mm; IOL power: +16.00; OS: axial length: 24.63 mm; keratometry: 7.41 mm × 7.76 mm @ 002; anterior chamber depth: 3.36 mm; IOL power: +16.25
Central corneal thickness (Pentacam)	OD: 505 nm; OS: 503 nm

Abbreviations: IOL, intraocular lens; NCT, noncontact tonometry; OD, right eye; OS, left eye; OU, both eyes; PERRL, pupils equal, round, reactive to light; RAPD, relative afferent pupillary defect; VA, visual acuity.

Comments

Janet had moderate myopia with astigmatism and early lens opacities. Given her desire for spectacle independence, she was interested in refractive lens exchange. Multifocal toric intraocular lens (IOL) implants were suggested and various types were discussed. The possibility of additional excimer laser surgery to fine-tune the postoperative refractive error was also discussed due to the current degree of astigmatism. Janet indicated that she wished to proceed with the surgery. The left eye was treated first followed by the right eye 3 weeks later.

Additional presurgical measurements were taken using Orbscan corneal analysis, corneal topography using placido rings, Pentacam Scheimpflug imaging (Oculus, Wetzlar, Germany; Figures 2.34-1A, B and 2.34-2) and central corneal thickness measured by Pentacam.

Zeiss ZCalc software (version 1.5) was used to calculate the required toric IOL, as well as the orientation of the incision. These output data are shown in Figure 2.34-3.

The trifocal toric IOLs implanted were as follows:

OD: Zeiss AT LISA tri toric 939 at axis 100°; OS: Zeiss AT LISA tri toric 939 at axis 88°.

Following surgery, Janet was prescribed ofloxacin (Exocin) 1 drop 4 times a day for 2 weeks, nepafenac (Nevanac) 1 drop 3 times a day for 4 weeks, and dexamethasone (Maxidex) 1 drop 6 times a day for 2 weeks with dexamethasone taper to 4 times a day for 2 weeks, then twice a day for 2 weeks. A follow-up visit was scheduled for 6 weeks after surgery.

At the follow-up examination 6 weeks after surgery, the following findings were obtained:

Unaided distance VA	OD: 20/20; OS: 20/20
Unaided near VA	OU: 20/30
Subjective refraction	OD:+0.25 −0.50 × 120 (20/20); OS: +0.50 −0.50 × 100 (20/20)
Slit-lamp examination	OD and OS: corneas clear, anterior chambers clear, IOLs clear and in situ with no rotation
Fundus examination	Unremarkable OD and OS

Abbreviations: IOLs, intraocular lenses; OD, right eye; OS, left eye; OU, both eyes; VA, visual acuity.

DISCUSSION

Moderate to high levels of astigmatism is present in approximately 15% to 20% of patients requiring cataract surgery. Often residual astigmatism is corrected with spectacles or contact lenses. However, residual astigmatism following cataract surgery has been shown to significantly impact daily life.[1] For higher levels of astigmatism, spectacle independence can be achieved by implantation of a toric, rather than a spherical, IOL. The axis markings are usually found as engravings on the periphery of toric IOLs to aid alignment. Accurate alignment is vital as rotation away from the correct axis can negate the intended correction. A deviation of 30° or more may even induce astigmatism.[2] Traditionally, needle or ink markings made by the surgeon on the limbus prior to surgery with the individual sitting upright to overcome the cyclorotation that occurs on lying down during surgery have been used for alignment purposes, but this crude method can lead to errors. Digital imaging techniques have now been implemented into biometry measurement systems for better alignment and visual outcomes.

Since their introduction in 1994,[3] the stability of toric IOLs has been of concern due to cases of rotation postimplantation requiring surgical repositioning.[4] When necessary, IOL repositioning should be performed early; preferably within 1 month after surgery. Various factors may influence the degree of rotation. Larger IOLs should be implanted with caution as rotation may occur through stretching of the capsular bag.[5] However, a larger capsular bag size warrants a larger IOL and has shown better stability.[6] A longer axial length has also been identified as a feature increasing the incidence of toric IOL rotation perhaps due to a lower corneal rigidity.[7] The haptic design may also play a role in stability, with plate-haptics showing a greater tendency to rotate than loop-haptics. Closed-loop, mini-loop, and Z-haptics have been introduced to provide greater stability in the capsular bag with promising results.[8-10] Newer IOL designs, such as the one used for Janet, offer multifocal options for astigmatic patients.

The use of advanced optics makes the visual outcome more susceptible to a combination of disturbances. Residual astigmatism may still sometimes remain following toric IOL implantation due to preoperative biometry errors,

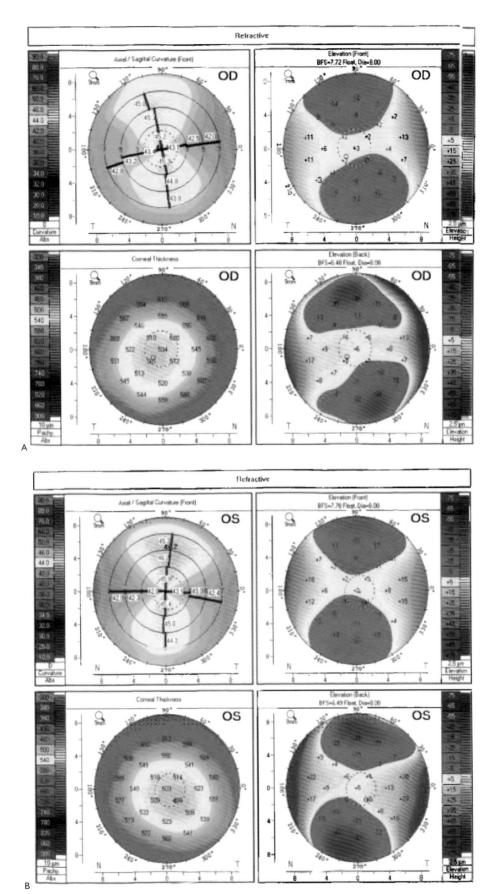

Figure 2.34-1 Pentacam corneal scans for the (A) right eye and (B) left eye.

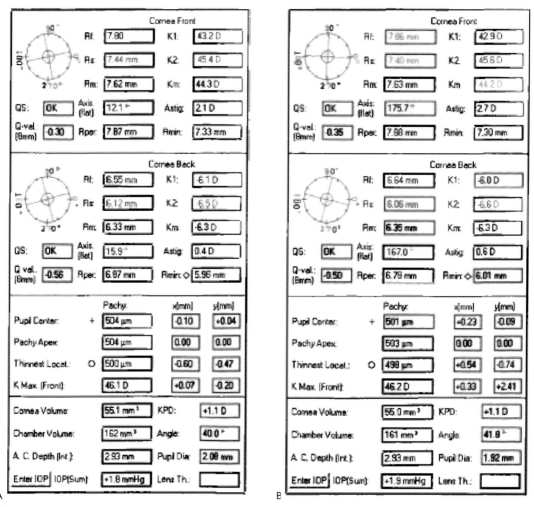

Figure 2.34-2 Pentacam corneal data for the (A) right eye and (B) left eye.

misaligned reference markings on the cornea or limbus, incorrect placement of the IOL or failing to account for surgically induced astigmatism.[11] It is, therefore, crucial to ensure all such factors are considered before surgery. Accurate biometry is paramount, particularly keratometry. It is a common practice to use several topographers to assess corneal astigmatism to give the surgeon confidence of the correct IOL power and axis to implant as topographers can differ markedly in their results. Figure 2.34-4 depicts a good biometry trace and a poor trace that would indicate the need for repeated measures and

perhaps using a different biometer before surgery. To increase accuracy when implanting toric IOLs, one should account for the total corneal astigmatism present (front and back surface) rather than basing calculations on keratometric values. This adjustment can reduce the level of residual astigmatism remaining after surgery.[11,12]

A trifocal toric IOL was prescribed for Janet to enhance her intermediate and near vision as her work required her to view digital displays extensively. She was very satisfied with the results and subsequent astigmatic laser surgery was not necessary.

Biometry preoperative (preop)

	Right (OD)	Left (OS)
Surgery date		
Examination date	14-Dec-2015	14-Dec-2015
AL-Measurement method	IOLMaster/Immersion US	IOLMaster/Immersion US
Axial length	24.61 mm	24.63 mm
Keratometry / n'	1.3375	1.3375
R_1/K_1	43.50 dpt / 12°	43.00 dpt /178°
R_2/K_2	45.50 dpt / 102°	45.30 dpt /88°
Anterior chamber depth	(from epithelium) 3.35 mm	(from epithelium) 3.36 mm
Target refraction (SE)	0.00 dpt	0.00 dpt
Incision orientation	180°	0°
SIA effect on incision axis	-0.50 dpt	-0.50 dpt
Recommendation	(Standard)	(Standard)
IOL type	AT LISA tri toric 939M | MP	AT LISA tri toric 939M | MP

Right (OD)

	Residual refraction				IOL refractive power		
	Sph. Equ. [D]	Sph [D]	Cyl [D]	A [°]	Sph. Equ. [D]	Sph [D]	Cyl [D]
	0.14	0.26	-0.24	10	15.50	14.00	3.00
	-0.22	-0.10	-0.24	10	16.00	14.50	3.00
	-0.58	-0.46	-0.24	10	16.50	15.00	3.00

Post-operative anterior chamber depth 4.63 mm
IOL axis 100°

Left (OS)

	Residual refraction				IOL refractive power		
	Sph. Equ. [D]	Sph [D]	Cyl [D]	A [°]	Sph. Equ. [D]	Sph [D]	Cyl [D]
	0.26	0.36	-0.21	178	15.75	14.00	3.50
	-0.10	0.00	-0.20	178	16.25	14.50	3.50
	-0.46	-0.37	-0.19	178	16.75	15.00	3.50

Post-operative anterior chamber depth 4.63 mm
IOL axis 88°

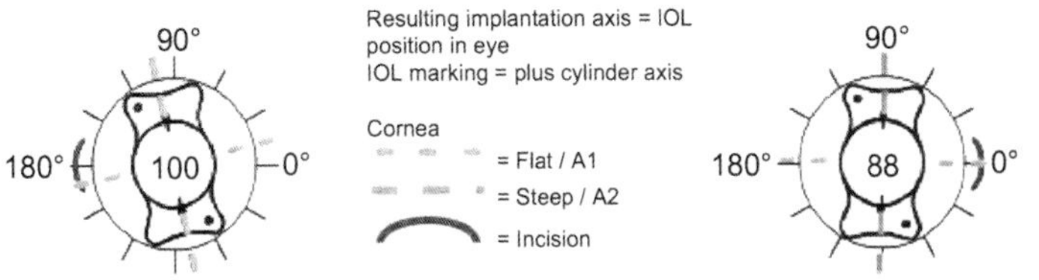

Resulting implantation axis = IOL position in eye
IOL marking = plus cylinder axis

Cornea
= Flat / A1
= Steep / A2
= Incision

Figure 2.34-3 Toric multifocal calculation calculated using Zeiss ZCalc software (version 1.5; Carl Zeiss, Oberkochen, Germany).

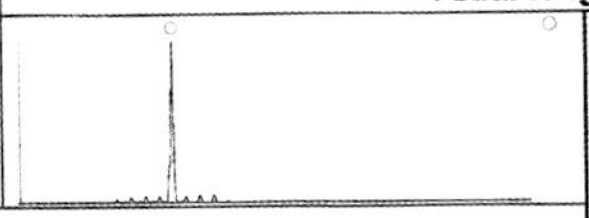

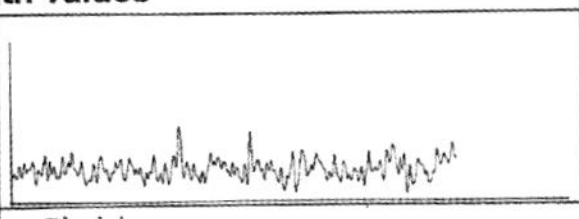

Axial length values

OD right — **OS** left

OD Phakic				OS Phakic			
Comp. AL: 23.08 mm		(SNR = 77.5)		Comp. AL: Evaluation!			(SNR = 4.5)
AL	SNR	AL	SNR	AL	SNR	AL	SNR
23.09 mm	13.7			34.61 mm	3.8	---	
23.03 mm	5.3			---		23.04 mm!	1.6
23.08 mm	11.6			---		18.39 mm!	1.6
23.07 mm	4.8			30.64 mm!	1.8	---	
23.10 mm	4.8			---		---	
23.07 mm	12.0			---		37.59 mm!	1.9
23.04 mm	4.1			---		---	
23.00 mm	6.1			---		20.72 mm!	1.6
23.09 mm	17.0			---		---	
23.09 mm	6.3			---		32.27 mm!	1.7

Keratometer values

MV: 43.55/44.18 D		SD: 0.00 mm		MV: 43.95/44.58 D		SD: 0.00 mm	
K1: 43.55 D x 165°		7.75 mm		K1: 43.95 D x 161°		7.68 mm	O X
K2: 44.18 D x 75°		7.64 mm		K2: 44.58 D x 71°		7.57 mm	O O
ΔK: +0.63 D x 75°				ΔK: +0.63 D x 71°			O O
K1: 43.55 D x 165°		7.75 mm		K1: 43.95 D x 159°		7.68 mm	O X
K2: 44.18 D x 75°		7.64 mm		K2: 44.58 D x 69°		7.57 mm	O O
ΔK: +0.63 D x 75°				ΔK: +0.63 D x 69°			O O
K1: 43.49 D x 165°		7.76 mm		---			O X
K2: 44.18 D x 75°		7.64 mm					O O
ΔK: +0.69 D x 75°							O O

Anterior chamber depth values

ACD: 2.64 mm					ACD: 2.78 mm				
2.69 mm	2.64 mm	2.64 mm	2.60 mm	2.53 mm	2.77 mm	2.76 mm	2.79 mm	2.79 mm	2.81 mm

White-to-white values

(* = value has been edited. ! = borderline value)

Figure 2.34-4 Biometry measures showing a good, accurate trace OD. A poor trace is seen OS, as a lens opacity restricted the axial length measurement and dry eye and lid closure impacted the keratometry findings.

Abbreviations: OD, right eye; OS, left eye.

CLINICAL PEARLS

- Accurate alignment of toric IOL designs is vital for a successful visual outcome. Clinicians should take advantage of digital technology offered to aid alignment. Moreover, biometry measures must be undertaken by skilled technicians with repeated and accurate corneal topography. It is best to use a range of instruments to determine ocular topography most accurately.

- Consideration should be given to the design features of the toric IOL, taking into account the loop design and the size of the implanted lens to ensure its stability.

- In cases of toric IOL rotation, repositioning should be performed within 4 weeks of implantation before significant fibrosis takes place.

- Patients should be counseled that residual astigmatism may still occur after toric IOL implantation, and additional laser treatment may be required to yield the desired results.

REFERENCES

1. Wolffsohn JS, Bhogal GK, Shah S. Effect of uncorrected astigmatism on vision. Surgical correction of astigmatism during cataract surgery. *J Cataract Refract Surg.* 2011;37(3):454-460.
2. Novis C. Astigmatism and toric lenses. *Curr Opin Ophthalmol.* 2000;11:47-50.
3. Shimzu K, Misawa A, Suzuki Y. Toric intraocular lenses: correcting astigmatism while controlling axis shift. *J Cataract Refract Surg.* 1994;20:523-526.
4. Wolffsohn JS, Buckhurst PJ. Objective analysis of toric intraocular lens rotation and centration. *J Cataract Refract Surg.* 2010;36:778-782.
5. Bylsma S. The STAAR Toric IOL: current technique and results with a plate-haptic lens that effectively neutralizes corneal astigmatism at the time of cataract surgery. *Cataract Refract Surg Today.* 2006;74-76.
6. Chang DF. Early rotational stability of the longer Staar toric intraocular lens. Fifty consecutive cases. *J Cataract Refract Surg.* 2003;29:935-940.
7. Shah GD, Praveen MR, Vasavada AR. Rotational stability of a toric intraocular lens: influence of axial length and alignment in the capsular bag. *J Cataract Refract Surg.* 2012;38:54-59.
8. Buckhurst PJ, Wolffsohn JS, Davies LN, et al. Surgical correction of astigmatism during cataract surgery. *Clin Exp Optom.* 2010;93(6):409-418.
9. De Silva DJ, Ramkissoon YD, Bloom PA. Evaluation of a toric intraocular lens with a Z-haptic. *J Cataract Refract Surg.* 2006;32:1492-1498.
10. Kent DG, Peng Q, Isaacs RT, et al. Mini-haptics to improve capsular fixation of plate-haptic silicone intraocular lenses. *J Cataract Refract Surg.* 1998;24:666-671.
11. Roach L. Clinical update toric IOLs: four options for addressing residual astigmatism. *EyeNet.* 2012;29-31.
12. Savini G, Næser K. An analysis of the factors influencing the residual refractive astigmatism after cataract surgery with toric intraocular lenses. *IOVS.* 2015;56(2):827-835.

2.35 Multifocal Intraocular Lenses

Gurpreet K. Bhogal-Bhamra, Sai Kolli, and James S. Wolffsohn

Josh, a 57-year-old male, presented with complaints of poor vision that had declined gradually over the last year. His symptoms seemed more debilitating in the evenings, and he reported significant glare from street lamps or headlights when driving at night. He was a professional cyclist, participating in races all year round. Race courses are often illuminated with bright overhead projection lights, which become troublesome with the onset of dusk and night time. During races, he needed to look at a global positioning satellite (GPS) data and timing system, as well as needing to be able to see clearly in the distance. The GPS device is located at a viewing distance of approximately 50 cm. His progressive addition lenses (PALs) are unsuitable for these demands, and instead, he wears multifocal contact lenses. However, his vision with contact lenses was still not adequate for cycling despite getting a new prescription. He was in good health, did not suffer any allergies, and was not taking any medications.

Clinical Findings

Unaided distance VA	OD: 20/50; OS: 20/50
Unaided near VA	OD: 20/150; OS: 20/200
Pupil evaluation	PERRL; no RAPD
Subjective refraction	OD: +1.50 −0.75 × 145 (20/30); OS: +1.25 −1.25 × 120 (20/30); ADD: +2.50 OU
Intraocular pressure (Pulsair NCT)	OD: 14 mm Hg; OS: 12 mm Hg at 10:40 AM
Slit-lamp examination	OD: cornea and anterior chamber: clear; posterior subcapsular lens opacity grade P2[a] OS: cornea and anterior chamber: clear; posterior subcapsular lens opacity grade P2[a]
Fundus examination	Unremarkable OD and OS
Biometry measures (Zeiss IOLMaster)	OD: axial length (mm): 24.30 mm; keratometry: 44.41 × 42.08 @ 006; anterior chamber depth: 3.69 mm; IOL power: +19.50; OS: axial length (mm): 24.20 mm; keratometry: 44.29 × 43.55 @ 004; anterior chamber depth: 3.55 mm; IOL power: +19.00
Contrast sensitivity test (Pelli-Robson)	OD: 1.20 log contrast sensitivity; OS: 1.35 log contrast sensitivity; OU: 1.35 log contrast sensitivity

Abbreviations: IOL, intraocular lens; NCT, noncontact tonometry; OD, right eye; OS, left eye; OU, both eyes; PERRL, pupils equal, round, reactive to light; RAPD, relative afferent pupillary defect; VA, visual acuity.

[a] Using the Lens Opacification Classification System, Version III (LOCSIII).

Comments

Josh was diagnosed with bilateral posterior subcapsular cataracts (PSCs). Despite visual acuity (VA) that met the legal requirements for driving, he reported that glare and poor near vision was significantly impacting his lifestyle. Options such as "accommodating" intraocular lenses (IOLs), monovision, and distance-focused IOLs with supplementary glasses for near vision were discussed. After weighing up the options, due to the impact on his activities of daily living, Josh chose bilateral, multifocal IOLs, as this would potentially satisfy the need for near vision during cycle races and allow independence from spectacles.

The postsurgical clinical findings were as follows:

Unaided distance VA	OD: 20/25; OS: 20/25
Unaided intermediate VA (50-60 cm)	OD: 20/50; OS: 20/50
Unaided near VA (40 cm)	OD: 20/50; OS: 20/50
Subjective refraction	OD: +0.75 sph (20/20); OS: +0.75 sph (20/20); ADD: +1.00 OU (OD: 20/30; OS: 20/30; OU: 20/30)

Abbreviations: OD, right eye; OS, left eye; OU, both eyes; sph, sphere; VA, visual acuity.

Discussion

Cataracts have long been associated with glare, often in the presence of good VA, due to intraocular light scatter. An early study reported 80% of subjects with PSCs find difficulty driving at night with much poorer glare disability than found in patients with cortical or nuclear opacities.[1] The Blue Mountains Eye Study reported that PSC caused the most reduction in contrast[2] and required earlier extraction compared with other types of cataract. The location of lens opacities may also differentially affect contrast sensitivity and light scatter.[2]

Where VA and symptoms do not appear to be concordant, glare testing may provide additional information on the quality of vision. Indeed, reduced glare or contrast sensitivity can provide a clinical justification for referral and surgical intervention.[3,4] In Josh's case, the Pelli-Robson contrast chart showed a lower contrast sensitivity threshold than expected for the patient's age, indicating poor visual quality in line with his symptoms. The Pelli-Robson chart offers a quick and standardized method for assessing contrast sensitivity.[3] A score of 2.0 is normal contrast sensitivity, while a score below 1.50 shows reduction and may suggest further investigation. Moreover, when combined with measurements of VA and visual fields, reductions, in contrast, can indicate a higher risk of road accidents.[5] For drivers presenting with cataracts, these tests, as well as those that assess glare may be beneficial in assessing their driving capability.

To meet the desire for spectacle independence, multifocal IOLs were suggested. Sometimes, monofocal IOLs can provide good near VA due to residual myopia, myopic astigmatism, and small pupils giving an increased depth of focus. These features can give a pseudo-accommodative range of 0.75 to 5.10 diopters.[6] A monovision correction is also an option to extend the range of focus, but in this case it was deemed unsuitable as Josh had previously found difficulty with this approach using contact lenses.

Multifocal IOLs split incoming light to provide different foci through diffractive or refractive optics. Refractive multifocal IOLs surfaces generally consist of concentric circles of varying power that provide superimposed images from distance and near foci. Refractive IOLs with asymmetrical segments of additional power are also now available. Diffractive multifocal IOLs utilize the Huygen-Fresnel principle by creating a diffraction grating with surface eschelets forming constructive and deconstructive interference. From the 2 images created on the retina, the brain selects the clearer one and suppresses the other. Light is lost during this process due to high order foci being beyond the useful power range, which leads to a reduction in contrast sensitivity. However, with the introduction of apodized or trifocal diffractive designs that combine diffractive and refractive surfaces, good VA and spectacle independence has been reported.[7-9] Bilateral multifocal IOL implantation is strongly recommended for better visual outcomes.[10,11]

The most common concern following multifocal implantation is the presence of glare and haloes, particularly under mesopic conditions. Fortunately, incorporating aspheric surfaces into the IOL design may improve such symptoms.[12] Accordingly, it is paramount to manage a patient's visual expectations. In this case, it was highlighted that glare and haloes may still occur following the cataract extraction due to the nature of the implants. It was emphasized that this would be very apparent at first, but previous experience suggests that symptoms will subside over time through adaptation.[13] Although, Josh was initially apprehensive, he understood the compromise to be made to achieve spectacle independence for cycling. Following surgery, minor complaints of haloes during night driving were made, but he did not find this as debilitating as before. A primary concern was to ensure that intermediate vision was restored using multifocal IOLs. Some reports have shown variability in intermediate vision among refractive multifocal IOLs.[14-18] To combat this, trifocal designs have been introduced, in which an additional intermediate power is incorporated to provide 3 foci. When assessing the suitability of multifocal IOL implantation, the degree of astigmatic error must also be considered. Residual astigmatism will cause a decrease in contrast sensitivity.[19] Therefore, it is vital to correct even small amounts of astigmatism during surgery for an optimal outcome. Surgery including relieving incisions or the option of toric multifocal IOLs may be considered in cases of higher astigmatism (see Chapter 2.34).

For successful refractive lens exchange with multifocal IOL implantation, thorough strong history and patient counseling are key. It is important to manage expectations of good vision at multiple distances with conversations stressing the potential compromises. It is also worthwhile to emphasize that the full benefit of multifocal implantation is generally evident only after bilateral treatment, to avoid any disappointment after surgery on the first eye. Confidence in the clinician is reinforced as possible complications are brought up while the patient is making the decision regarding surgery.

CLINICAL PEARLS

- When assessing cataracts for potential surgery, it is important to consider lifestyle impact in addition to VA. Referral for surgery should not be based solely on VA measurements.

- In cases of cataracts, particularly posterior subcapsular lens opacities, although the vision may appear acceptable in the clinical setting, patients may still complain of glare or poor quality of vision.

- The use of contrast sensitivity charts is advised to help warrant the decision for surgery.

- For successful refractive lens exchange with multifocal intraocular lens implantation, thorough strong history and counseling are important.

REFERENCES

1. Lasa MSM, Podgor MJ, Datiles MB III, et al. Glare sensitivity in early cataracts. *Br J Ophthalmol.* 1993;77:489-491.
2. Chua BE, Mitchell P, Cumming RG. Effects of cataract type and location on visual function: The Blue Mountains Eye Study. *Eye.* 2004;18:765-772.
3. Mäntyjärvi M, Laitinen T. Normal values for the Pelli-Robson contrast sensitivity test. *J Cataract Refract Surg.* 2001;27:261-266.
4. Shandiz JH, Derakhshan A, Daneshyarl A, et al. Effect of cataract type and severity on visual acuity and contrast sensitivity. *J Ophthalmic Vis Res.* 2011;6(1):26-31.
5. Decina LE, Staplin L. Retrospective evaluation of alternative vision screening criteria for older and younger drivers. *Accid Anal Prev.* 1993;25:267-275.
6. Menapace R, Findl O, Kriechbaum K, et al. Accommodating intraocular lenses: a critical review of present and future concepts. *Graefes Arch Clin Exp Ophthalmol.* 2007;245:473-489.
7. Berdeaux G, Viala M, de Climens R, et al. Patient-reported benefit of ReSTOR multi-focal intraocular lenses after cataract surgery: results of principal component analysis on clinical trial data. *Health Qual Life Outcomes.* 2008;6(10):1-9.

8. Javitt JC, Steinert RF. Cataract extraction with multifocal intraocular lens implantation – a multinational clinical trial evaluating clinical, functional, and quality-of-life outcomes. *Ophthalmology*. 2000;107: 2040-2048.

9. Chiam PJT, Chan JH, Haider SI, et al. Functional vision with bilateral ReZoom and ReSTOR intraocular lenses 6 months after cataract surgery. *J Cataract Refract Surg*. 2007;33:2057-2061.

10. Pineda-Fernandez A, Jaramillo J, Celis V, et al. Refractive outcomes after bilateral multifocal intraocular lens implantation. *J Cataract Refract Surg*. 2004;30:685-688.

11. Steinert RF. Visual outcomes with multifocal intraocular lenses. *Curr Opin Ophthalmol*. 2000;11:12-21.

12. Choi J, Schwiegerling J. Optical performance measurement and night driving simulation of ReSTOR, ReZoom, and Tecnis multifocal intraocular lenses in a model eye. *J Refract Surg*. 2008;24:218-222.

13. Vaquero-Ruano M, Encinas JL, Millan I, Hijos M, Cajigal C. AMO array multifocal versus monofocal intraocular lenses: long-term follow-up. *J Cataract Refract Surg*. 1998;24:118-123.

14. Bucci AF. Asymmetric implantation of multifocal IOLs may improve visual comfort in patients with cataracts and presbyopia. *Eurotimes*. 2006;11:9-16.

15. Alfonso JF, Fernandez-Vega L, Baamonde B, et al. Correlation of pupil size with visual acuity and contrast sensitivity after implantation of an apodized diffractive intraocular lens. *J Cataract Refract Surg*. 2007;33: 430-438.

16. Petermeier K, Szurman P. Subjective and objective outcome following implantation of the apodized diffractive AcrySof ReSTOR. *Ophthalmology*. 2007;104(5):399-404, 406-408.

17. Voskresenskaya A, Pozdeyeva N, Pashtaev N, et al. Initial results of trifocal diffractive IOL implantation. *Graefes Arch Clin Exp Ophthalmol*. 2010;248:1299-1306.

18. Carballo-Alvarez J, Vazquez-Molini JM, Sanz-Fernandez JC, et al. Visual outcomes after bilateral trifocal diffractive intraocular lens implantation. *BMC Ophthalmol*. 2015;15(26):1-8.

19. Ravalico G, Parentin F, Baccara F. Effect of astigmatism on multifocal intraocular lenses. *J Cataract Refract Surg*. 1999;25:804-807.

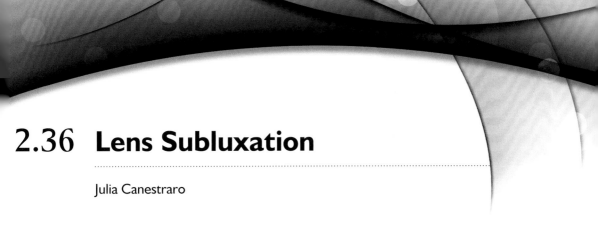

2.36 Lens Subluxation

Julia Canestraro

Robert, a 54-year-old Asian male, was referred by the emergency department with concerns of blurred vision OS. He reported a history of blunt trauma to the left side of his head with subsequent vision loss 6 months ago. He reported good vision in each eye before his injury. After the injury, he was seen at another eye clinic where he had a laser procedure performed OS. He was also told he needed cataract surgery, but did not return for follow-up. He denied any current pain, flashes or floaters. Robert's medical history was unremarkable except for a history of alcohol abuse. There was no family history of ocular disease.

Clinical Findings

Unaided distance VA	OD: 20/25; OS: 20/400
Pupil evaluation	OD: round and reactive; no RAPD; OS: minimal reaction to light, with sphincter tears 360°; no RAPD
Ocular motility	Full and comitant OD and OS
Confrontation visual field	OD: full to penlight; OS: constriction 360°
Subjective refraction	OD: Pl −0.50 × 090 (20/20); OS: −4.25 −4.00 × 090 (20/70: no improvement with pinhole)
Slit-lamp examination	OD: lids/lashes: capped meibomian glands, debris on lashes; conjunctiva: clear; cornea: clear; iris: flat and intact; anterior chamber: deep and quiet; angles: 3 × 3. OS: lids/lashes: capped meibomian glands, debris on lashes; conjunctiva: clear; cornea: clear; iris: sphincter tears at 2, 3, 5, 10 to 1 o'clock, patent laser iridotomy at 3 o'clock; anterior chamber: deep and quiet; angles: 2 × 2
Intraocular pressure (GAT)	OD: 16 mm Hg; OS: 22 mm Hg at 11:00 AM After dilation: OD: 19 mm Hg; OS: 32 mm Hg at 1:00 PM
Gonioscopy	OD: open to ciliary body 360°, flat approach, no iris processes; OS: no structures seen with compression 360°, bowed iris
Fundus examination	OD: 0.65 V/0.60 H; lens: trace nuclear sclerosis; vitreous: syneresis; periphery: flat and intact 360°; no phacodonesis (see Discussion section); OS: 0.70 V/0.65 H; lens: 1+ nuclear sclerosis, 1 posterior subcapsular cataract, lens subluxated temporally with no zonules visible nasally (see Figure 2.36-1); vitreous: syneresis; periphery: flat and intact 360°; positive phacodonesis (see Discussion section)

Abbreviations: GAT, Goldmann applanation tonometry; H, horizontal; OD, right eye; OS, left eye; Pl, plano; RAPD, relative afferent pupillary defect; V, vertical; VA, visual acuity.

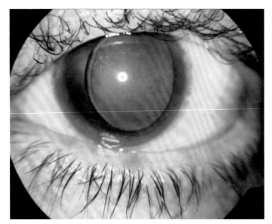

Figure 2.36-1   Retroillumination of the lens viewed after dilation. The lens is subluxated temporally, with no zonules visible.

Comments

Robert was diagnosed with mild traumatic lens subluxation and suspected glaucoma OS. He had a low risk for pupillary block, given that he had a patent iridotomy OS. However, intraocular pressures (IOPs) were elevated and so he was prescribed timolol 0.5% twice a day, OS. Given his poor visual acuity (VA), he was referred for surgical consultation, for intervention of the subluxated lens, and advised to return for an IOP check and glaucoma testing.

He was seen 2 weeks later and reported good compliance with the timolol. Distance VA and entrance testing were unchanged from the previous visit. Other findings were as follows:

Intraocular pressure (GAT)	OD: 17 mm Hg; OS: 19 mm Hg at 10:15 AM
24-2 SITA-standard visual field (Figure 2.36-2)	OD: (size III target): unreliable, superior nasal edge defects, significant cluster inferior temporal, inconsistent with optic nerve appearance; OS: (size V target): unreliable, superior temporal cluster, inconsistent with optic nerve appearance
Optic nerve OCT (Figure 2.36-3)	OD: good quality, borderline temporal thinning; OS: poor quality, superior temporal thinning, consistent with optic nerve appearance

Abbreviations: GAT, Goldmann applanation tonometry; OCT, optical coherence tomography; OD, right eye; OS, left eye.

Intraocular pressure was improved in the left eye with the medication. Although the optic nerve Optical coherence tomography (OCT) correlated with the optic nerve appearance in the left eye, the visual field was unreliable. Robert was advised to continue with the current medication and to return in 6 weeks for repeat imaging. He had a pending appointment with a cataract specialist. Unfortunately, Robert was subsequently lost to follow-up.

Discussion

Most frequently, traumatic lens subluxation results from zonular disruption via coup–contrecoup injury. Trauma accounts for more than half of all lens displacement/subluxation cases.[1] Blunt force can also cause disruption of the iris root, ciliary body, and lens capsule. First, one must determine whether the lens has been subluxated or dislocated. A subluxated lens has partial disruption of the zonules, whereas a dislocated lens exhibits complete disruption of the zonules, so that the lens is fully displaced either to the anterior or posterior chambers. The degree of lens subluxation may be categorized into 3 groups, namely: mild (lens edge uncovers 0% to 25% of the dilated pupil), moderate (lens edge uncovers 25% to 50% if the dilated pupil), and severe (lens edge uncovers >50% of the dilated pupil).[2] Focal trauma or congenital defects tend to cause localized damage to the zonules, whereas systemic conditions may cause diffuse zonular defects.[2] Based on the clinical presentation of this case, it is clear that Robert presented with a mild traumatic lens subluxation.

Subtle lens subluxation is most easily seen in retroillumination through a dilated pupil.

OD Single Field Analysis — Central 24-2 Threshold Test

Fixation Monitor:	Gaze/Blind Spot	
Fixation Target:	Central	
Fixation Losses:	12/17 XX	
False POS Errors:	22% XX	
False NEG Errors:	31%	
Test Duration:	09:44	
Fovea:	Off	

Stimulus:	III, White
Background:	31.5 asb
Strategy:	SITA-Standard
Pupil Diameter:	3.8 mm *
Visual Acuity:	
Rx:	+2.50 DS

Date:	Oct 18, 2016
Time:	9:36 AM
Age:	54

Threshold values (30°):

```
           14  24   24  <0
       21  25  26   27  27  25
   10  26  28  27   27  29  25  24
13 28  27  28  31   28  33  31   6
 3 19  30  27  30   28  29   8  27
   28  30  30  29   28  28  20  16
       28  29  29   28  28  22
           23  31   28  23
```

Total Deviation

```
          -13  -4   -3 -29
      -7  -4  -4   -2  -2  -3
  -19 -4  -3  -5   -4  -1  -5  -5
-14  -1 -5  -4  -2  -5   1      -24
-24 -11 -1 -5  -3  -4  -3      -3
   -2 -1  -2  -3   -4  -4 -11 -14
      -2  -2  -2   -3  -3  -8
          -6   1   -2  -7
```

Pattern Deviation

```
          -12  -2   -1 -27
      -6  -3  -2   -1   0  -1
  -18 -2  -1  -3   -3   0  -4  -3
-13  0 -3  -3   0  -3   2      -22
-23 -9  1  4  -2  -3  -2      -1
    0  0 -1  -2   -3  -2  -9 -13
       0  0 -1   -1  -1  -7
          -4   3   0  -6
```

GHT:	Outside Normal Limits
VFI:	92%
MD:	-4.67 dB P < 0.5%
PSD:	5.34 dB P < 0.5%

*** Excessive High False Positives ***

::	P < 5%
	P < 2%
	P < 1%
■	P < 0.5%

Figure 2.36-2 A. 24-2 visual field OD. A standard size III target was used. B. 24-2 visual field OS. A size V target was used.

Abbreviations: OD, right eye; OS, left eye.

It is also useful to check for the presence of phacodonesis. Although the patient is in the slit lamp, view the lens with retroillumination and gently bang on the base of the slit lamp with your hand. This will cause the lens to vibrate if it is not bound tightly to the zonules. Other symptoms may include monocular diplopia and decreased VA from induced lenticular astigmatism and myopia when viewing through the lens periphery.[2] Elevated IOP may occur if vitreous

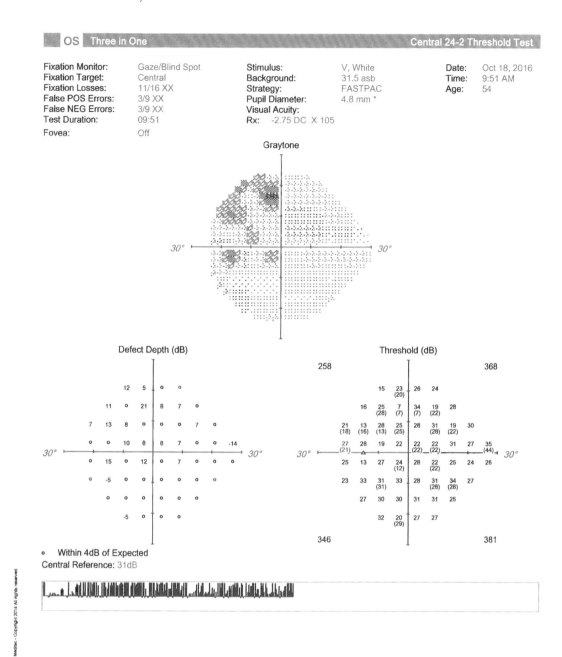

Figure 2.36-2 (Continued)

blocks the angle, or if previous trauma caused an angle recession.[2] It is important to check for pupillary block that can cause acute secondary glaucoma from iris lens apposition.[3] As Robert had an iridotomy in his affected eye, this eliminated the likelihood of pupillary block. However, because he presented with elevated

IOPs in the presence of a patent iridotomy, we prescribed an IOP lowering medication. Given a history of trauma, it was also important to check for retinal breaks.

Other etiologies of lens subluxation should be considered during the case history. For example, questions about family and medical

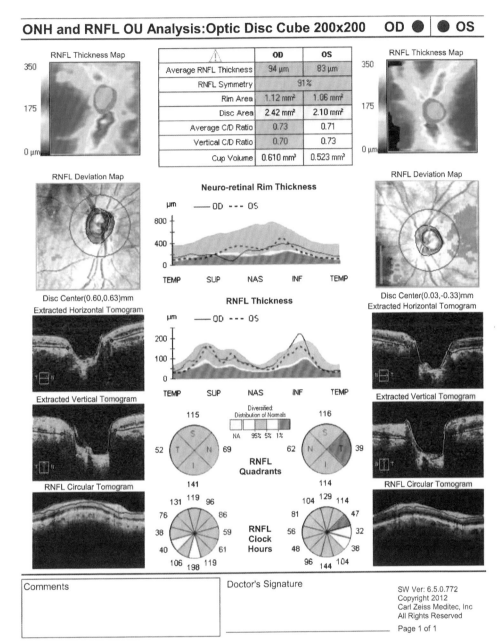

Figure 2.36-3   Optic nerve optical coherence tomography of each eye.

history (including cardiac and other connective tissue disorders) may help to identify the following conditions: Marfan's syndrome, homocystinuria, Ehlers-Danlos syndrome, Weill-Marchesani syndrome, sulfite oxidase deficiency, and congenital aniridia syndrome.[2] If any of these are suspected, the patient should be referred to their physician, as they are often accompanied by serious medical complications. Pseudoexfoliation syndrome is the most common cause of adult onset lens subluxation, after trauma.[2]

Treatment depends on the severity of the subluxation/dislocation and the resulting VA. If a patient is asymptomatic and has mild lens subluxation with normal IOP, then no intervention is indicated. Should they experience monocular diplopia, a prosthetic contact lens can be fitted to block the "second pupil," alternatively one can prescribe fogging or occluding spectacles, or pilocarpine to eliminate the diplopia. If a patient has moderate to severe lens subluxation and vision is degraded, surgical intervention is warranted. Although our patient only had mild subluxation, given that he also had decreased VA and poor visual quality, a surgical consultation was pursued. Placement of an intraocular lens (IOL) will depend on the extent of damage to the zonules and lens capsule. The surgeon may choose between a posterior chamber, sulcus or anterior chamber IOL.[2] For acute presentations, where the lens is completely dislocated into the anterior chamber, the patient should be dilated, placed in the supine position and their head positioned so as to manipulate the lens into the posterior chamber. Once the lens is repositioned, instill 1% pilocarpine in office. Once the dilation is reversed, the lens will not be able to fall back into the anterior chamber again. The patient will need to continue the pilocarpine 4 times a day and be referred for an iridotomy and surgical consultation as soon as possible. A lens in the anterior chamber poses a serious risk to the corneal endothelial cells and therefore corneal integrity.[4] If the lens is dislocated into the posterior chamber, with normal IOP and no inflammation, and there is an intact capsule, then no intervention is needed. Otherwise, the lens must be removed surgically.

CLINICAL PEARLS

- Case history is important. Ask regarding recent trauma and systemic or familial conditions. This information will narrow down the differential diagnoses and aid in the treatment plan.

- Perform gonioscopy and check for pupillary block and elevated IOP. These signs require immediate referral for an iridotomy.

- The management is driven by patient symptoms, unless the lens poses a direct threat to the cornea or retina (such as a dislocated lens in the anterior chamber or vitreous with a ruptured capsule).

REFERENCES

1. Kubal WS. Imaging of orbital trauma. *Radiographics.* 2008;28(6):1729-1739.
2. Hoffman RS, Snyder ME, Devgan U, et al. Management of the subluxated crystalline lens. *J. Cataract Refract Surg.* 2013;39:1904-1915.
3. Dagi LR, Walton DS. Anterior axial lens subluxation, progressive myopia, and angle-closure glaucoma: recognition and treatment of atypical presentation of ectopia lentis. *J AAPOS.* August 2006;10(4):345-350.
4. Kawashima M, Kawakita T, Shimazaki J. Complete spontaneous crystalline lens dislocation into the anterior chamber with severe corneal endothelial cell loss. *Cornea.* May 2007;26(4):487-489.

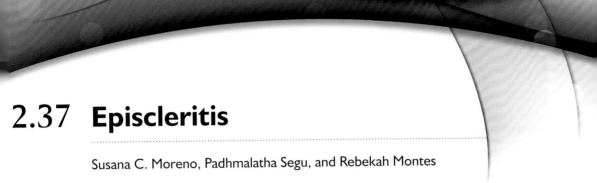

2.37 Episcleritis

Susana C. Moreno, Padhmalatha Segu, and Rebekah Montes

Ali, a 12-year-old Middle Eastern male, presented with an acute, red, right eye, which was first noticed 3 days ago. He reported no pain, photosensitivity, decrease in vision, itching, foreign body sensation, or discharge. There was no recent history of exposure to a red eye. Ali reported no recent fever, illness, injury, or prior contact lens wear. He instilled an unknown, over-the-counter eye drop that provided no relief. Ali denied taking any other medications. His parents believed the red eye was due to "playing too much video games at home." His past medical and ocular histories were unremarkable. No medication or environmental allergies were noted.

Clinical Findings

Unaided distance VA	OD: 20/20; OS: 20/20
IOP (NCT)	OD: 15 mm Hg; OS: 18 mm Hg at 10:00 AM
Confrontation fields	Full to finger counting OD and OS
Ocular motility	Full OU
Pupil evaluation	PERRL; no RAPD
Slit-lamp examination	OD: bulbar conjunctiva: 3+ sectoral inferior nasal injection, (−) nodules, (−) chemosis; OS: bulbar conjunctiva: trace diffuse injection; OD and OS: lacrimal system: tear film normal; eyelashes: trace anterior blepharitis; palpebral conjunctiva: trace inferior papillae; cornea, iris, lens, anterior chamber, angle and vitreous: unremarkable
Fundus examination	Unremarkable OU

Abbreviations: IOP, intraocular pressure; NCT, noncontact tonometry; OD, right eye; OS, left eye; OU, both eyes; PERRL, pupils equal, round, reactive to light; RAPD, relative afferent pupillary defect; VA, visual acuity.

Comments

Ali was diagnosed with simple episcleritis (Figure 2.37-1) and prescribed 1 drop of loteprednol etabonate (Lotemax) OD 4 times a day for 1 week. He was advised to return for care in 4 days or sooner if symptoms worsened. The family was educated on the nature of his condition and recommended an appointment with his physician to rule out systemic disease. The parents were instructed to limit his use of electronic devices as using them for long periods of time may cause ocular dryness. As with any case of acute red eye, both Ali and his parents were educated on the importance of practicing good lid hygiene, frequent hand washing, and replacing bed linens to prevent ocular complications or the spread of infection. Lid scrubs were prescribed every morning in both eyes and Ali was advised to avoid eye rubbing. At his 4-day follow-up visit, the redness had improved and no new symptoms or increase in intraocular pressure (IOP) were observed. The topical corticosteroid was tapered to twice a day OD for 1 additional week and discontinued thereafter.

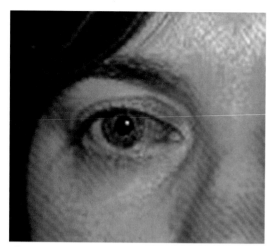

Figure 2.37-1   Example of episcleritis.

Discussion

Episcleritis is an acute, self-limiting, generally benign inflammation of the episclera and occurs more frequently in young- to middle-aged women (Figure 2.37-1). Presentation is unilateral in 70% of cases. However, bilateral involvement is more common in children and often mistaken for conjunctivitis with a stronger association of systemic disease. The etiology is unknown in most cases, but is believed to be immune mediated, and occasionally associated with systemic disease. Symptoms may include minimal eye pain, foreign body sensation, and possibly reduced visual acuity (VA). Clinical signs include a bright red or salmon pink hemorrhage (visible in natural light) on the bulbar conjunctiva. The superficial episcleral vessels are injected and the redness can be sectoral (70% of the time), diffuse, or rarely, nodular. The vessels are easily mobile when palpated with a cotton-tipped applicator, and blanch following the instillation of topical 10% phenylephrine. Small peripheral corneal opacities are present in approximately 10% of cases.[1]

The distinction between episcleritis and scleritis is important to determine the appropriate treatment, and when monitoring for ocular complications during follow-up care. In general, patients with scleritis tend to be older, in their 50s, and will often present with decreased VA, anterior uveitis, peripheral ulcerative keratitis, and ocular hypertension. Episcleritis will rarely present with similar signs and/or progress to scleritis. Connective tissue or vascular diseases are more frequent in patients with scleritis. In contrast, more frequent secondary complications in patients with episcleritis include rosacea, atopy, or foreign body sensation.[2] Episcleritis generally responds well to topical anti-inflammatory agents such as corticosteroids, whereas scleritis typically requires systemic medications, such as oral nonsteroidal anti-inflammatory drugs (NSAIDs), oral corticosteroids, or in some cases immunosuppressive medications.[3]

Episodes of episcleritis are commonly mild, transient, and subside without treatment, usually within 2 to 21 days. Most patients can be treated with cold compresses and iced artificial tears. However, in a significant number of cases, episcleritis can be associated with a systemic disorder. Treatment should then include management of the underlying condition. Therefore, a careful review of systems should be performed on all patients at the initial assessment.[4] Although benign, in children it is important to rule out systemic diseases such as lupus erythematosus, inflammatory bowel disease, rheumatic fever, juvenile idiopathic arthritis, spondyloarthropathy, and polyarteritis nodosa.[5] Underlying etiologies in adults may also include Wegener's granulomatous, infectious diseases such as herpes zoster, herpes simplex, Lyme disease, syphilis, hepatitis B, and bacterial or fungal conditions. Trauma and thyroid disease have also been associated with episcleritis.[6]

A thorough ophthalmic examination is required at each visit to detect concurrent eye disease, such as ocular rosacea, keratoconjunctivitis sicca, and atopic keratoconjunctivitis. Each of these conditions require specific treatment (eg, oral doxycycline for rosacea, topical mast cell stabilizers for atopy) to prevent the recurrence of episcleritis. Any allergens or irritants should be eliminated, particularly in the atopic patients.[4] Simple episcleritis is more common than nodular episcleritis in children and adults. Because it is a self-limiting cause of "red eye," episcleritis can easily be mistaken for conjunctivitis, which is common in childhood.[5]

As discussed previously, supportive therapy, such as cold compresses and iced artificial tears, help relieve symptoms through vasoconstriction and lubrication. Topical NSAIDs are no more effective than placebo.[3] Complications of long-term topical steroid therapy, such as glaucoma, cataract formation, and susceptibility to infections should be considered in patients with recurrent benign idiopathic episcleritis. The use of systemic NSAIDs may be beneficial in these cases. Over-the-counter oral NSAIDs (eg, naproxen sodium 200 mg twice daily) are usually effective and well tolerated by patients. Treatment for a period of usually 6 months is required to prevent recurrences.[4]

In summary, episcleritis in most cases is benign and self-limiting; however, it should be monitored closely for ocular complications secondary to concurrent eye disease or for underlying systemic conditions when a positive review of systems is noted.

CLINICAL PEARLS

- The key to differentiating between episcleritis and scleritis is pain. They may have similar appearances, but a patient with scleritis will often present with significant pain.

- Instillation of topical phenylephrine will blanch the vessels in episcleritis but not in scleritis.

REFERENCES

1. Sen H, Nida MD. Chapter 3. Episcleritis, scleritis and keratitis. In: Larson T, ed. *Color Atlas & Synopsis of Clinical Ophthalmology Wills Eye Institute*. Philadelphia, PA: Lippincott Williams & Wilkins; 2012:13-15.
2. Sainz De La Maza M, Molina N, Gonzalez-Gonzalez LA, Doctor PP, Tauber J, Foster CS. Clinical characteristics of a large cohort of patients with scleritis and episcleritis. *Ophthalmology*. 2012;119(1):43-50.
3. Jabs DA, Mudun A, Dunn JP, Marsh MJ. Episcleritis and scleritis: clinical features and treatment results. *Am J Ophthalmol*. 2000;130(4):469-476.
4. Akpek EK, Uy HS, Christen W, Gurdal C, Foster S. Severity of episcleritis and systemic disease association. *Ophthalmology*. 1999;106(4):729-731.
5. Read RW, Weiss AH, Sherry DD. Episcleritis in childhood. *Ophthalmology*. 1999;106(12):2377-2379.
6. Michaud L. Chapter 10. Immune disease, episcleritis. In: Onofrey BE, Skorin L, Holdeman NR, eds. *Ocular Therapeutics Handbook: A Clinical Manual*. Philadelphia, PA: Wolters Kluwer/Lippincott Williams & Wilkins Heath; 2011:276-279.

2.38 Herpetic Anterior Uveitis

Rosalynn H. Nguyen-Strongin

Alex, a 47-year-old male, presented with decreased vision for the last 6 weeks with transient eye pain, headaches, and redness in the right eye only. The patient had been seen by urgent care and his primary care provider, and had been given an "antibiotic drop" for "conjunctivitis." However, the drop had not been helping. There was no significant personal or family medical history. The patient's eye history included a retinal detachment in the right eye with status post cryopexy many years ago.

Clinical Findings

Distance VA (with current glasses)	OD: 20/400 (no improvement with pinhole); OS: 20/20
Confrontation visual fields	Full to finger counting OD and OS
Pupil evaluation	OD: pupil 4 mm in dim illumination and 3 mm in bright illumination, slight irregular shape, and sluggish reactivity; no RAPD; OS: pupil 3 mm in dim illumination and 2 mm in bright illumination, round, and brisk reactivity; no RAPD
Ocular motility	Full OD and OS
Intraocular pressure (Tonopen)	OD: 41 mm Hg; OS: 14 mm Hg at 3:25 PM
Slit-lamp examination	OD: cornea exhibited 1+ keratic precipates, 4+ cells in the anterior chamber and deep (open angles), 1+ nuclear sclerotic with 3+ posterior subcapsular cataract; OS: clear cornea, deep and quiet anterior chamber, 1+ nuclear sclerotic cataract
Fundus examination	OD: CD 0.25/0.25, clear and distinct rim tissue, flat and avascular macula, normal vessels, supratemporal and inferior cryopexy and laser scars, vitreous clear with status post pars plana vitrectomy. Hazy view of fundus due to cataract; OS: CD 0.25/0.25, clear and distinct rim tissue, flat and avascular macula, normal vessels, intact and normal peripheral retina

Abbreviations: CD, cup to disc; OD, right eye; OS, left eye; RAPD, relative afferent pupillary defect; VA, visual acuity.

Comments

Alex was diagnosed with granulomatous anterior uveitis in the right eye. Prednisolone acetate (Pred Forte) 1% ophthalmic suspension was prescribed, to be instilled every 2 hours in the right eye. The elevated intraocular pressure (IOP) in the right eye also suggested ocular hypertension or uveitic glaucoma. To address the elevated IOP, dorzolamide-timolol ophthalmic solution was prescribed to be instilled twice a day in the right eye. The following laboratory tests were ordered: HLA subtype B27 antigen, erythrocyte sedimentation rate (ESR), C-reactive protein, herpes simplex virus 1 & 2 immunoglobulin type G (IgG), herpes simplex virus 1 & 2 immunoglobulin type M (IgM), angiotensin-converting enzyme (ACE), rapid plasma reagin (RPR), and antinuclear antibody (ANA) titer.

At the 1-week follow-up examination, Alex reported he was doing much better. He no longer had pain or redness in his right eye. The vision in this eye was still blurry, but slightly improved. Alex reported that he had completed all of the laboratory work that had been ordered, but the results were not yet available.

At the 1-week follow-up visit, the findings were as follows:

Distance VA (with current glasses)	OD: 20/200 (no improvement with pinhole); OS: 20/20
Pupil evaluation	OD: pupil 4 mm in dim illumination and 3 mm in bright illumination, slight irregular shape, and sluggish reactivity; no RAPD; OS: pupil 3 mm in dim illumination and 2 mm in bright illumination, round, and brisk reactivity; no RAPD
Intraocular pressure (iCare)	OD: 13 mm Hg; OS: 16 mm Hg at 4:09 PM
Slit-lamp examination	OD: cornea exhibited 1+ keratic precipates, 2+ cells in anterior chamber and deep open angles, 1+ nuclear sclerotic with 3+ posterior subcapsular cataract; OS: clear cornea, deep and quiet anterior chamber, 1+ nuclear sclerotic cataract

Abbreviations: OD, right eye; OS, left eye; RAPD, relative afferent pupillary defect; VA, visual acuity.

Comments

With the anterior chamber inflammation and IOP improving but not completely resolved in the right eye, the same treatment regimen was maintained. However, because there was still a great deal of inflammation and white blood cells in the anterior chamber and visual acuity (VA) was still poor, oral steroids were also initiated. The current treatment plan now comprised: prednisolone acetate (Pred Forte) drops every 2 hours OD, dorzolamide-timolol twice a day OD and oral methylprednisolone (Medrol) 4 mg tablet once per day.

At the 2-week follow-up examination, Alex was no longer symptomatic apart from blurry vision in his right eye. The patient's laboratory results were also reviewed at this visit (Table 2.38-1).

The clinical findings at the 2-week follow-up visit were as follows:

Distance VA (with current glasses)	OD: 20/150 (no improvement with pinhole); OS: 20/20
Pupil evaluation	OD: pupil 4 mm in dim illumination and 3 mm in bright illumination, slight irregular shape, and sluggish reactivity; no RAPD; OS: pupil 3 mm in dim illumination and 2 mm in bright illumination, round, and brisk reactivity; no RAPD
Intraocular pressure (Tonopen)	OD: 16 mm Hg; OS: 17 mm Hg at 4:12 PM
Slit-lamp examination	OD: cornea exhibited 1+ keratic precipates, deep and quiet anterior chamber, 1+ nuclear sclerotic with 3+ posterior subcapsular cataract; OS: clear cornea, deep and quiet anterior chamber, 1+ nuclear sclerotic cataract

Abbreviations: OD, right eye; OS, left eye; RAPD, relative afferent pupillary defect; VA, visual acuity.

Table 2.38-1   Uveitis Laboratory Panel Results

Test	Value	Result Interpretation
Angiotensin converting enzyme	20 U/L	Negative
Rapid plasma reagin (Syphilis)	Non-reactive	Negative
Antinuclear antibody	Negative	Negative
Erythrocyte sedimentation rate	2 mm/h	Negative
C-reactive protein	<0.10 mg/dL	Negative
Human leukocyte antigen-B27	Negative	Negative
Herpes simplex virus 1 immunoglobulin G	>5.00	Positive
Herpes simplex virus 1 immunoglobulin M	Negative	Negative
Herpes simplex virus 2 immunoglobulin G	<0.90	Negative
Herpes simplex virus 2 immunoglobulin M	Negative	Negative
Chest x-rays	Normal	Negative

Because the anterior chamber was deep and quiet, Alex was told to discontinue the methylprenisolone 4 mg tablets and the prednisolone acetate was tapered to 3 times a day OD. He was instructed to continue the dorzolamide-timolol twice a day OD. The laboratory results were negative for all suspected conditions apart from herpes simplex virus 1 (HSV1) immunoglobulin type G. Because HSV1 immunoglobulin type G was positive and HSV immunoglobulin type M was negative, it was determined that no active infection was present. Also, Alex did not exhibit any apparent signs or symptoms of herpes simplex infection. Therefore, acyclovir oral tablets were not prescribed. The final diagnosis was presumed herpetic granulomatous anterior uveitis with mild uveitic glaucoma of the right eye.

Alex was instructed to return for monthly monitoring. Based on consultation with an ophthalmologist, cataract extraction with intraocular implant surgery was suggested as this could improve his vision in the right eye. However, the visual prognosis was still uncertain given the history of retinal detachment repair. Unfortunately, because Alex was a new patient to the clinic, we did not know his best-corrected VA after the retinal repair. Most corneal specialists and cataract surgeons agree that for patients with an ocular history like Alex, it is standard management to have a quiet anterior chamber for at least 3 months before cataract surgery could be performed.[1] This is due to risk of reactivation of the virus as well as an increase in anterior chamber inflammatory response that commonly results from cataract surgery.

Discussion

Uveitis is a general term to describe inflammation of the uveal tract, which includes the iris, ciliary body, and choroid. This inflammation can also be described in terms of its location, that is, anterior or posterior. Anterior uveitis will affect the iris and/or ciliary body, whereas posterior uveitis will impact the choroid and retina. In addition, uveitis may be non-granulomatous or granulomatous. Ocular histopathology can help differentiate between the 2 subtypes. For example, granulomatous uveitis commonly presents with large mutton-fat keratic precipitates deposited on the corneal endothelium and larger inflammatory cell types (epitheloid cells and macrophages) in the anterior chamber. Also, granulomatous uveitis is usually more indicative of systemic inflammation than the non-granulomatous condition. Therefore, it is imperative to determine the etiology underlying the inflammation. Common chronic systemic conditions that can cause uveitis include arthritis, HLA-B27 diseases, and sarcoidosis. In addition to systemic inflammation, uveitis may also be associated with infection and trauma.

Anterior herpetic uveitis accounts for 5% to 10% of all uveitic cases where inflammation is caused by either the herpes simplex or varicella zoster viruses.[2] It is an elusive type of inflammation with a variety of presentations. At times, a herpetic uveitis may be accompanied by corneal findings, such as dendrites from an active keratitis. At other times, such as in this case, there may be no corneal signs. Although keratitis may not be present, iris irregularities and iris atrophy can still be common clinical features.[3]

Regarding herpetic uveitis, ocular involvement is almost always unilateral and more often presents as the granulomatous type of the condition. In Alex's case, keratic precipitates were found on the inferior cornea of the right eye only. In addition, ocular hypertension and/or glaucoma are present in 90% of the cases.[4] This may be attributed to the association found between herpetic infections and trabeculitis due to an increased intraocular pressure from inflammatory materials blocking the trabecular meshwork.[5] The finding is consistent with Alex, given that the highest IOP before treatment was 41 mm Hg. Although the clinical findings described earlier are adequate to make the diagnosis of herpetic uveitis, antigen testing is recommended. When managing intraocular pressures in these patients, it is important to avoid prostaglandins to treat elevated IOP as they may aggravate or induce uveitis.[6]

In summary, the treatment of herpetic uveitis is similar to other uveitis etiologies with the use of steroids (topical, oral, or both) to control inflammation. It is important to comanage with the primary care physician when oral steroid treatment is initiated, because these medications can adversely affect the blood pressure and glucose levels. Also, due to the high prevalence of increased IOPs, clinicians should meticulously monitor and treat (as necessary) for glaucoma. Herpetic infections are chronic in nature, and recurrence and reactivation of the virus is always a concern. Patients with frequent recurrences, as well as immunocompromised patients, may benefit from long-term maintenance therapy of oral acyclovir (400 to 800 mg/d).[7]

CLINICAL PEARLS

- If you encounter a chronic red eye with pain that is not responding to antibiotics or allergy/dry eye medications, then assess for uveitis.

- Always assume uveitis has a systemic etiology until proven otherwise by ordering appropriate laboratory tests and imaging.

- Educate patients that uveitis may be recurrent and require lifelong monitoring and management.

REFERENCES

1. Sykakis E, Karim R, Parmar DN. Management of patients with herpes simplex virus eye disease having cataract surgery in the United Kingdom. *J Cataract Refract Surg.* 2013;8:1254-1259.
2. Siverio Junior CD, Imai Y, Cunningham ET. Diagnosis and management of herpetic anterior uveitis. *Int Ophthalmol Clin.* 2002;42:43-48.
3. Van der Lelij A, Ooijman FM, Kijlstra A, Rothova A. Anterior uveitis with sectoral iris atrophy in the absence of keratitis: a distinct clinical entity among herpetic eye diseases. *Ophthalmology.* 2000;107:1164-1170.
4. Sungur GK, Hazirolan D, Yalvac IS, Ozer PA, Aslan BS, Duman S. Incidence and prognosis of ocular hypertension secondary to viral uveitis. *Int Ophthalmol.* 2010;30:191-194.
5. Hogan MJ, Kimura SJ, Thygeson P. Pathology of herpes simplex keratouveitis. *Trans Am Ophthalmol Soc.* 1963;61:75-99.
6. Fechtner RD, Khouri AS, Zimmerman TJ, et al. Anterior uveitis associated with latanoprost. *Am J Ophthalmol.* 1998;126:37-41.
7. The Herpetic Eye Disease Study Group. A controlled trial of oral acyclovir for the prevention of stromal keratitis or iritis in patients with herpes simplex virus epithelial keratitis. *Arch Ophthalmol.* 1997;115:703-712.

2.39 Toxoplasmosis

Jerome Sherman

Maria, a 35-year-old Hispanic female, complained of light sensitivity in her left eye that has been increasing over the past several weeks. She reported that her vision had previously been very good in each eye, but now noticed a slight haze in her left eye when compared with the right one. Maria had a history of recurrent eye infections in her left eye that had been treated with an unknown medication in Mexico about 10 years ago.

Clinical Findings

Best-corrected distance VA	OD: 20/20$^+$; OS: 20/20
Pupil evaluation	PERRL; no RAPD
Ocular motility	Full OU
Slit-lamp examination	OD: unremarkable; OS: 1+ cells and flare, all else unremarkable

Fundus examination
  (Figures 2.39-1 and
  2.39-2)
	OD: unremarkable;
	OS: very hazy vitreous, especially anterior and superior to the disc. 4 lesions observed superior to the optic disc. The 2 most peripheral lesions oval in shape, 3 × 1 disc diameters in size with well-pigmented borders. A third round lesion, nearly 2 disc diameters in size but less pigmented than the more peripheral lesions. A fourth, smaller, nonpigmented lesion seen closer to the disc, grey in color, and appeared elevated with blurred borders.

Abbreviations: OD, right eye; OS, left eye; OU, both eyes; PERRL, pupils equal, round, reactive to light; RAPD, relative afferent pupillary defect; VA, visual acuity.

Comments

The three pigmented lesions were typical of old, inactive retinochoroiditis scars due to toxoplasmosis. In contrast, the smaller circular gray lesion with blurred borders closest to the disc was characteristic of an active toxoplasmosis lesion. Reactivated areas are often near or contiguous with old lesions, as was found in this case.

Active toxoplasmosis is almost always associated with an overlying vitritis, resulting in a blurred view of the retina. The cells and flare observed in the anterior chamber represent a "spillover" inflammation from the active retinal lesion. Presumed ocular histoplasmosis syndrome is a much less common etiology for this type of retinal lesion and rarely results in a vitritis.

Because the appearance of the lesions was so characteristic of toxoplasmosis, systemic testing with collection of ocular specimens via a vitreal "tap" was not considered necessary to reach a diagnosis. Fundus imaging was performed. It is valuable to know the patient's HIV status because toxoplasmosis is an opportunistic infection associated with immunodeficiency. Maria was HIV negative.

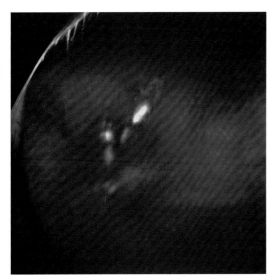

Figure 2.39-1 At the initial presentation, 4 lesions superior to the optic disc were observed in this ultra-wide field image. The blur is due to the overlying vitritis. The lesion closest to the disc is new and active because it is unpigmented and has very blurred borders.

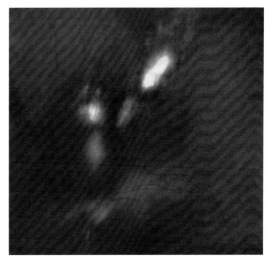

Figure 2.39-3 After successful treatment, the fundus image is clearer and reveals more detail because the overlying vitritis has resolved.

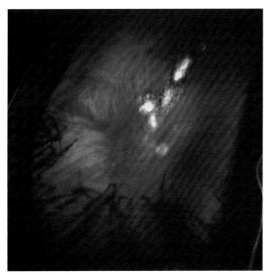

Figure 2.39-2 A magnified view of Figure 2.39-1. The 3 pigmented lesions are old and inactive.

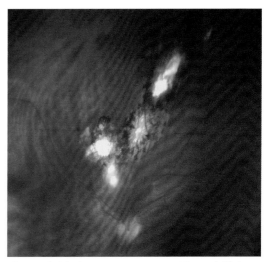

Figure 2.39-4 A magnified view of Figure 2.39-3. Now, the lesion closest to the disc has well-defined borders. It will become pigmented over the next year or so, making it similar in appearance to the 3 older lesions.

Maria was treated with pyrimethamine (Daraprim), double sulfa (ie, 2 sulfa drugs in 1 pill), and an oral steroid (prednisone). In addition, cyclopentolate eye drops were prescribed to treat the iritis. Maria was re-evaluated 2 weeks later and only minor improvement was observed. However, after 2 months, the vitritis had lessened considerably (Figures 2.39-3 and 2.39-4), and the previously active gray, poorly defined lesion now appeared white with minimal pigment superiorly. In addition, the borders of the lesion were much more clearly defined. The dosages of medications were tapered and subsequently discontinued. Maria has not had another reactivation of this condition.

This fourth lesion, that is, the smallest lesion located closest to the optic disc, appeared to represent the third reactivation of this condition. Any future activation located inferior to this lesion will threaten the optic disc directly, with the possibility of significant vision loss. In patients with average levels of pigmentation, these lesions typically become pigmented in about 1 year, with pigmentation starting at the periphery and eventually filling the entire lesion. Therefore, the degree of pigmentation provides a gross indication of the age of the lesion. Careful follow-up is recommended in these cases. Providing an Amsler grid for the patient to use at home can be valuable, especially in cases where the macula is threatened.

Discussion

Ocular toxoplasmosis is the most common cause of infectious posterior uveitis in many countries around the world, as well as most regions of the United States.[1] As shown here, in most cases the diagnosis can be made by the clinical findings alone. In the past, it was thought that active ocular toxoplasmosis represented a reactivation of an infection acquired transplacentally from the mother. However, more recently, it has been shown that acquired infections occur more often than previously suspected.[2]

When used, confirmatory laboratory testing relies on the analysis of serum or intraocular samples (such as vitreous) for antibody detection. However, polymerase chain reaction testing is becoming more widely available for the direct identification of parasite DNA within the eye, and the sensitivity of this test is improving with new methods of detection. Polymerase chain reaction testing is a technique that amplifies either a single or multiple copies of a DNA segment by several orders of magnitude. This can generate millions of copies of a particular DNA sequence.

Although the classic, triple-drug therapy of pyrimethamine (Daraprim), sulfadiazine, and a corticosteroid is an effective choice of treatment, alternative regimens, including single-agent treatment with trimethoprim–sulfamethoxazole (Bactrim), intravitreal injection of clindamycin with dexamethasone, or a combination of azithromycin with pyrimethamine, have all been shown to be effective against ocular toxoplasmosis. However,

this classic treatment is not without risk. Administration of pyrimethamine requires weekly monitoring of blood cell and platelet counts, as well as the coadministration of folinic acid to protect against leukopenia and thrombocytopenia. Similarly, sulfadiazine may cause a severe allergic reaction, which can be life-threatening in some patients. Moreover, the cost of these drugs is high, and they are not readily available in some areas.[1] In addition, the use of these drugs is unsafe in pregnant women, and there is no liquid formula for pediatric patients. Compliance can be difficult, as patients need to take up to 10 pills per day.[3,4] Given these issues, safer and simpler therapies for ocular toxoplasmosis have received increasing attention. The use of the trimethoprim–sulfamethoxazole combination is now preferred by many practitioners due to improved patient compliance, faster resolution of chorioretinitis, and better final visual acuity (VA). Trimethoprim–sulfamethoxazole is well tolerated for long-term prophylaxis in high-risk patients such as those with AIDS and low CD4 counts. Intravitreal injections of clindamycin and dexamethasone provide high concentrations of therapeutic agents into the vitreous cavity and retina while avoiding most systemic side effects. The oral regimen of pyrimethamine and azithromycin has also been reported to have excellent efficacy against ocular toxoplasmosis, with significantly lower side effects than the pyrimethamine and sulfadiazine combination. New developments in diagnosis and treatment have significantly improved our ability to prevent or significantly limit vision loss from ocular toxoplasmosis.

CLINICAL PEARLS

- Active toxoplasmosis lesions that threaten the optic disc or macula should be treated.

- Lesions in other areas of the retina, such as the mid-periphery can be watched without treatment until the overlying vitritis subsides, and the borders of the lesion become well defined.

REFERENCES

1. Cornell PJ, Winston JV, Rimmer TG. UCLA Community-Based Uveitis Study Group. Causes of uveitis in the general practice of ophthalmology. *Am J Ophthalmol*. 1996;121:35-46.
2. Gilbert RE, Stanford MR. Is ocular toxoplasmosis caused by prenatal or postnatal infection? *Br J Ophthalmol*. 2000;84(2):224-226.
3. Dodds E. Ocular toxoplasmosis: clinical presentation, diagnosis and therapy. In: *Focal points: Clinical Modules for ophthalmologists*. Vol XVII. San Francisco, CA: American Academy of Ophthalmology; 1999.
4. Soheilian M, Ramezani A, Azimzadeh A, et al. Randomized trial of intravitreal clindamycin and dexamethasone versus pyrimethamine, sulfadiazine, and prednisolone in treatment of ocular toxoplasmosis. *Ophthalmology*. January 2011;118(1):134-141.

2.40 Sarcoidosis

Sarah MacIver

Maya, a 40-year-old Indian female, presented with a red, elevated bump on the temporal conjunctiva of her left eye. She reported that the bump started 3 weeks ago as a much smaller, painless lesion. The swelling had worsened progressively over the past 10 days and had become extremely painful over the past 3 days. Maya described the pain as a deep and boring ache and rated it at 6 on a pain scale from 0 to 10. The pain was worse if she touched the area over the elevation. In addition, she reported mild photophobia. Maya was able to control the pain somewhat with 400 mg ibuprofen. There were no associated symptoms such as discharge or change in her vision.

Her ocular history that was positive for 2 prior episodes of acute non-granulomatous anterior uveitis. The first episode was 6 years ago and occurred in the right eye. The second, most recent, episode was in the left eye, and it had resolved 8 months ago. A full blood work panel specific for uveitis was performed after the second episode of uveitis.

Maya's last physical examination was 8 months ago (at the time of the last uveitis episode) and was unremarkable other than she was anemic. She was not taking any medications.

Clinical Findings

Unaided distance VA	OD: 20/20; OS: 20/20
Confrontation visual fields	Full to finger counting OD and OS
Pupil evaluation	PERRL; no RAPD
Ocular motility	Full, OU
Retinoscopy	OD: +1.00 sph; OS: +1.25 sph
Subjective refraction	OD: Pl −0.25 × 030 (20/20); OS: Pl −0.25 × 030 (20/20)
Near ADD	+1.00 OU (20/20)
NRA/PRA	+0.50/−0.50
Intraocular pressure (GAT)	OD: 18 mm Hg; OS: 16 mm Hg at 5:30 PM
Slit-lamp examination	OD: conjunctiva: clear; angle: 1 × 1; cornea: ghost keratic precipitates; anterior chamber: deep and quiet; iris: flat and intact, no nodules;
	OS: conjunctiva: sectoral injection and engorgement of conjunctival vessels over lesion on temporal conjunctiva, edematous episclera (Figure 2.40-1). Nodule 1.5 mm—tender to palpation, immobile; angle: 1 × 1; cornea: ghost keratic precipitates; anterior chamber: deep and quiet; iris: flat and intact, no nodules
Fundus examination	Unremarkable OD and OS

Abbreviations: GAT, Goldmann applanation tonometry; NRA, negative relative accommodation; OD, right eye; OS, left eye; OU, both eyes; PERRL, pupils equal, round, reactive to light; Pl, plano; PRA, positive relative accommodation; RAPD, relative afferent pupillary defect; sph, sphere; VA, visual acuity.

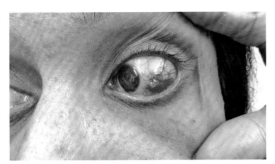

Figure 2.40-1   Presentation of temporal lesion.

Comments

One drop of 2.5% phenylephrine was instilled into the left eye, which improved the injection by 50%. Nevertheless, injected scleral vessels were still apparent (Figure 2.40-2).

A diagnosis of non-necrotizing nodular anterior scleritis was made. Treatment comprised difluprednate ophthalmic emulsion (Durezol) 0.05% 4 times a day in the left eye, indomethacin 50 mg/d oral and ranitidine (Zantac) 150 mg twice a day oral. Poor resolution of the lesion was noted 1 week after initiation of treatment

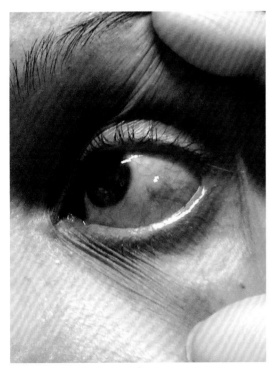

Figure 2.40-2   Lesion following insertion of phenylephrine. Note that there is residual fluorescein in the eye.

so oral prednisone 50 mg/d was added. One week after starting the oral prednisone, the lesion had improved. The oral prednisone was tapered by 10 mg/d and discontinued.

Additional systemic testing was arranged to rule out other causes of nodular scleritis. Blood work and Tuberculin test were found to be unremarkable. The chest x-ray revealed bilateral nodularity/lymphadenopathy in the hilium. The nodule is calcified azygous lymph node suggestive of an old granuloma. A diagnosis of presumed sarcoidosis was made. Maya was referred to internal medicine for further management of the systemic condition.

Discussion

Maya presented with a non-necrotizing nodular anterior scleritis and a history of recurrent non-granulomatous anterior uveitis. Underlying systemic disease is found in up to 50% of patients with scleritis.[1] The most common etiologies for anterior scleritis include systemic vasculitis, connective tissue disease, and infection. Laboratory testing had been ordered 8 months ago to rule out these underlying causes (Table 2.40-1). Given the history of recurrent non-granulomatous anterior uveitis, laboratory and diagnostic testing to investigate other systemic causes of inflammation were ordered (Table 2.40-2).

While it is well recognized that sarcoidosis should be considered whenever granulomatous inflammation is found, the ubiquitous nature of this disease suggests that it should be considered whenever a systemic inflammatory etiology is suspected.[2] Indeed, some studies suggest that a non-granulomatous uveitis may be a more common presentation of anterior uveitis in sarcoidosis.[3]

Sarcoidosis is a multisystem, granulomatous systemic disease that can affect almost any organ in the body. But, most commonly it targets the lungs, lymph nodes, skin, heart, liver, muscles, and the eyes.[4] Pathogenesis is due to the initiation of an inflammatory response characterized histologically by the presence of noncaseating granulomas. Initially, macrophages release cytokines such as tumor necrosis factor (TNF)-alpha and interleukin that cause infiltration of T-helper lymphocytes.[5]

Table 2.40-1   Sampling of Primary Laboratory Results Following Second Episode of Non-granulomatous Anterior Uveitis With Results Outside of the Laboratory Reference Range Highlighted.

Blood Chemistry Parameter	Result	Reference Ranges
Hemoglobin	121 g/L	115-160 g/L
Hematocrit	0.378 L/L	0.37-0.47 L/L
Red blood cell (RBC) count	4.95×10^{12}/L	3.80-5.50×10^{12}/L
Mean corpuscular volume (MCV)	76 fL	80-98 fL
Mean corpuscular hemoglobin (MCH)	24.4 pg	27.0-32.0 pg
White blood cell (WBC) count	11.0×10^9/L	4-11.0×10^9/L
Absolute neutrophil count	8.2×10^9/L	1.6-7.5×10^9/L
RBC morphology	Normal	
Platelet count	360×10^9/L	140-400
Erythrocyte sedimentation rate (ESR)	22 mm/h	0-12 mm/h
Rheumatoid factor	<20 kU/L	<20
Antinuclear antibody (ANA) panel	Negative	
High sensitivity C-reactive protein (hs-CRP)	2.3 mg/L	>8.0 mg/L
Glucose serum fasting	4.7	3.6-6.0 mmol/L
Ferritin	17 μg/L	31-300 μg/L
Vitamin B12	188 pmol/L	>221 pmol/L
HLA B27	Negative	

Table 2.40-2   Secondary Serology Testing Ordered to Rule Out Additional Underlying Causes of Sarcoidosis

Blood Chemistry Parameter	Possible Underlying Cause
Hepatitis B/C	Hepatitis (infectious)
Bartonella henselae	Lyme disease (infectious)
Venereal disease research laboratory (VDRL)	Syphillis (infectious)
Uric acid	Infectious disease
Complement C3/C4	Systemic lupus erythematosus
Perinuclear antineutrophil cytoplasmic antibodies (p-ANCA)	vasculitis
Cytoplasm antineutrophil cytoplasmic antibodies (c-ANCA)	Wegener granulomatosis
TB skin test	Tuberculosis
Chest x-ray	Tuberculosis

Maya's results were unavailable.

The lymphocytes stimulate further release of cytokines and recruit other inflammatory cells to the site of inflammation forming granulomas. However, the underlying cause of the inflammatory response is still unknown. Some have postulated that it may arise from an antigen to an infection or an environmental trigger. Alternatively, it may be due to an inherited or acquired abnormality of the immune system.[6]

A definitive diagnosis of sarcoidosis can only be made when the biopsy confirms the presence of a noncaseating, granulomatous, noninfectious, non-necrotic, inflammatory process. Other diseases that cause granulomatous lesions, including tuberculosis, must to be ruled out. Common biopsy sites in sarcoidosis include the skin, peripheral lymph nodes, and lungs.[7]

Clinically, a presumed diagnosis is often made in lieu of a definitive diagnosis because of the invasive nature of the biopsy. The presumed diagnosis is made on the basis of characteristic clinical findings, confirmatory laboratory and other diagnostic test results.[4,8] A chest x-ray/computed tomography (CT) scan and serum angiotensin-converting enzyme (ACE) are the most commonly ordered tests. Imaging of the chest with CT scan or x-ray is recommended to evaluate for bilateral hilar adenopathy with or without parenchymal infiltrates. Bilateral hilar adenopathy is a hallmark sign of sarcoidosis and is found in 90% of patients with sarcoidosis.[6] Serum ACE is secreted by granulomas. It is elevated in approximately 60% of patients and shows a positive correlation with the degree of active pulmonary disease.[7] However, other conditions such as diabetes, chronic renal disease, asbestosis, leprosy, and tuberculosis can also elevate ACE levels.

Many patients with sarcoidosis are asymptomatic at the time of diagnosis, and the condition is only recognized after abnormal chest x-ray or laboratory results. Most patients with symptomatic sarcoidosis will have respiratory symptoms, while others may have more generalized signs and symptoms such as fever, anemia, fatigue, and/or weight loss.[6]

Ocular involvement in sarcoidosis is common; found in 20% to 50% of patients.[9,10] African American and Caucasian individuals develop more anterior and posterior segment disease, respectively.[3] Ocular manifestations often occur early in the disease and may be one of the first presenting signs.[10] Any ocular structure can become involved (Table 2.40-3[8,10]).

Anterior uveitis is one of the most common ocular manifestations of saroidosis. The classic appearance is a chronic, bilateral, granulomatous anterior uveitis with large, mutton-fat keratic precipitates. However, unilateral, acute and nongranulomatous anterior uveitis may also occur. Acute, anterior uveitis of limited duration with small keratic precipitates is observed in 15% to 45% of patients with ocular sarcoidosis.[10]

Asymptomatic patients with hilar adenopathy do not generally require systemic therapy. Individuals with symptomatic pulmonary or eye disease will usually be treated with corticosteroids.[8,10] Ocular therapy is tailored to the severity of the ocular disease. Acute,

Table 2.40-3   Ocular Manifestations in Sarcoidosis

Ocular Manifestations	
Anterior segment	• Acute nongranulomatous or chronic granulomatous anterior uveitis* • Iris nodules* • Nodular infiltration of the trabecular meshwork* • Conjunctival granulomas • Nodular scleritis • Episcleritis • Band keratopathy • Nonspecific conjunctivitis • Keratitis
Posterior segment	• Chorioretinal granulomas* • Vitritis with snowball opacities* • Retinal periphlebitis* • Candlewax drippings and yellow "waxy spots"* • Retinal arteritis • Venous occlusion and neovascularization • Optic neuritis • Retro-bulbar or chaismal lesions leading to optic atrophy
Orbital disease	• Dacroadenopathy* • Lacrimal gland granulomas* • Orbital granulomas • Extra-ocular muscle lesions

The most common manifestations are marked with an asterisk.[2,8]

anterior inflammation is usually managed successfully with topical corticosteroids. If stronger, more localized treatment is indicated, then the inflammation usually responds well to periocular injections. Systemic corticosteroids may be indicated in severe chronic anterior or posterior uveitis. The inflammation from sarcoidosis generally responds favorably to high doses of steroid, which may be tapered slowly. Cyclosporin and other immunosuppressive agents have also been shown to be successful for the long-term treatment of chronic inflammation, but more research is required before they become the standard of care.[11]

The dosage of systemic corticosteroids is usually decided in consultation with the managing physician. It may be adjusted based on the clinical signs and symptoms, as well as pulmonary function tests, chest x-ray findings, and serum ACE levels. In sarcoid patients exhibiting ocular manifestations, the goal is to control the inflammation and prevent permanent visual impairment that may arise from cystoid macular edema, glaucoma, and cataract. The prognosis is dependent on the severity of the inflammation, although many patients show remission several years following diagnosis.[2,11]

CLINICAL PEARL

- Sarcoidosis is an inflammatory condition that may cause granulomatous uveitis. However, it may cause ocular inflammation via alternative pathways. This diagnosis should be considered whenever uveitis with a systemic inflammatory etiology is suspected.

REFERENCES

1. Sainz de la Maza M, Molina N, Gonzalez-Gonzalez LA, et al. Clinical characteristics of a large cohort of patients with scleritis and episcleritis. *Ophthalmology*. 2012;119:43-50.
2. Cowan C. Chapter 7.15 Sarcoidosis. In: Yanoff M, Duker J, eds. *Ophthalmology*. 3rd ed. London, UK: Elsevier Saunders; 2014:753-757.
3. Evans M, Sharma O, LaBree L, Smith RE, Rao NA. Differences in clinical findings between Caucasians and African Americans with biopsy-proven sarcoidosis. *Ophthalmology*. 2007;114:325-333.
4. Chan CC, Wetzig RP, Palestine AG, et al. Immunohistopathology of ocular sarcoidosis: report of a case and discussion or immunopathogenesis. *Arch Ophthalmol*. 1987;105:1398-1402.
5. Iannuzzi MC, Rybicki BA, Teirstein AS. Sarcoidosis. *N Engl J Med*. 357:2153-2165, 2007.
6. Whitcup S. Chapter 22: Sarcoidosis. In: Nussenblatt R, Whitcup S, eds. *Uveitis: Fundamentals and Clinical Practice*. Los Angeles, CA: Mosby Elsevier; 2010: 278-287.
7. Stavrou P. *Ocular Sarcoidosis. Uveitis*. Waltham, MA: The Ocular Immunology and Uveitis Foundation. http://www.uveitis.org/wp-content/uploads/2017/05/ocular_sarcoidosis.pdf. Accessed April 1, 2017.
8. Khanna A, Sidhu U, Bajwa G, Malhotra V. Pattern of ocular manifestations in patients with sarcoidosis in developing countries. *Acta Ophthalmol Scand*. 2007;85:609-612.
9. Pefkianaki M, Androudi S, Praidou A, et al. Ocular disease awareness and pattern of ocular manifestation in patients with biopsy-proven lung sarcoidosis. *J Ophthalmic Inflamm Infect*. 2011;1:141-145.
10. Baughman R, Nunes H. Therapy for sarcoidosis: evidence-based recommendations. *Expert Rev Clin Immunol*. 2012;8:95-103.

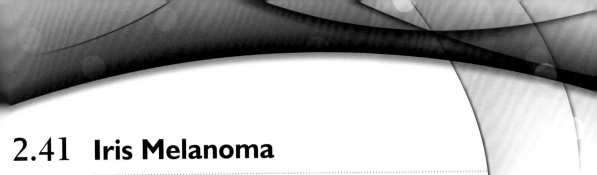

2.41   Iris Melanoma

Lorne Yudcovitch

Steve, a 53-year-old Caucasian male, was referred for evaluation of a "spot" on his right eye that had been present for the past 5 months. History included removal of a corneal foreign body several years ago (the patient was unsure as to which eye), asthma, and a family history of cancer. Steve was currently taking trazodone, lithium, and albuterol sulfate inhaler (Ventolin), a nicotine patch and triamcinolone cream. He reported no allergies to medication, consumption of 1 to 2 alcoholic beverages per day and smoked a pack of cigarettes daily.

Clinical Findings

General observation	Normal facial symmetry, with no atypical skin pigmentation or lesions
Unaided distance VA	OD: 20/15; OS: 20/15
Present Rx (reading glasses)	OD: +1.50 sph; OS +1.50 sph
Ocular motility	Full, smooth and equal in all fields of gaze OU; no pain or diplopia reported
Confrontation visual fields	Full to finger counting OD and OS
Pupil evaluation	PERL; no RAPD, OD: slight elongation of pupil from 1 o'clock to 7 o'clock
Subjective refraction	OD: +0.50 sph (20/15) OS: +0.25 −0.25 × 085 (20/15) ADD: +1.00 OU (20/20)
Intraocular pressure (NCT)	OD: 14 mm Hg; OS: 15 mm Hg at 8:55 AM
Slit-lamp examination	OD raised light brown 3.5 mm × 3.5 mm mass on the iris at the 7 o'clock region, approximately 0.5 mm from the pupil border (Figure 2.41-1). Mild vascularization noted along the edge of the mass. Pupil elongation from 1 o'clock to 7 o'clock, with no ectropion uveae noted; OS: unremarkable
Fundus examination	Unremarkable OD and OS
Gonioscopy	OD: elevation of the mass located near the pupillary ruff. Mild vasculature noted in the angle at the 7 o'clock position. Otherwise a flat iris approach and visible ciliary body seen in all quadrants OS: unremarkable
Anterior segment OCT	OD: spectral-domain anterior segment OCT performed on several sections of the iris mass showed notable (over 1 mm) thickening anteriorly and posteriorly, with minimal hyporeflectivity or cavitation (Figure 2.41-2). The lesion appeared to be localized to the iris, without extension into the ciliary body or angle

B-scan ultrasound

OD: low and high gain imaging showed no other apparent abnormalities in the globe (Figure 2.41-3)

Prior photographs

On request, the patient produced a self-portrait photograph taken at 18 years of age (Figure 2.41-4). Although the photo quality was poor, under high magnification the iris pigmentation can be seen at 7 o'clock, consistent with the location in the current examination

Abbreviations: NCT, non-contact tonometry; OCT, optical coherence tomography; OD, right eye; OS, left eye; OU, both eyes; PERRL, pupils equal, round, reactive to light; RAPD, relative afferent pupillary defect; Rx, prescription; sph, sphere; VA, visual acuity.

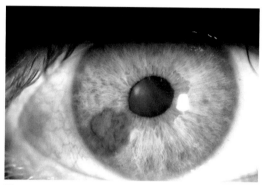

Figure 2.41-1   Iris mass on the patient's right eye. Note the slight pupil corectopia toward the mass.

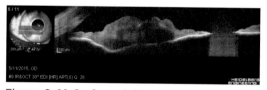

Figure 2.41-2   Spectral-domain anterior segment optical coherence tomography cross section of the iris mass.

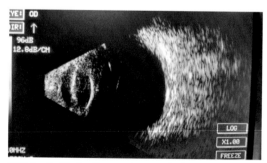

Figure 2.41-3   B-scan ultrasound of patient's right eye, showing no apparent abnormalities.

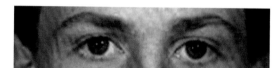

Figure 2.41-4   Age 18 self-portrait (magnified). Despite the reduced quality of the magnified image, the pigmentation of right iris is visible at the 7-o'clock position.

Comments

Based on the clinical findings of a growing mass, the potential of an iris melanoma was discussed with the patient. He was promptly referred to an ocular oncologist for biopsy and potential treatment. Fluorescein angiography by the ocular oncologist revealed hyperfluorescent sentinel (feeder) vessels within the lesion, and fine-needle aspiration with cytological evaluation indicated spindle cells consistent with a malignant iris melanoma.

Steve opted for brachytherapy treatment over sectoral tissue excision or enucleation. A radioactive Iodine-125 plaque was sutured over the eye for 4 days followed by postsurgical monitoring, with reduction of the iris mass to 0.7 mm thickness with no posterior extension. Genetic biopsy showed a gene expression profile (GEP) class 1B (ie, low risk of metastasis—see Discussion section); however, a pulmonary nodule was identified on computerized tomography lung imaging. This is being monitored along with periodic liver imaging, as the liver is the most common site for metastasis from an ocular melanoma.

Discussion

Ocular melanomas comprise only 3.7% of all melanoma cases in the United States, with an incidence of 6 per million people. They represent the second most common melanoma, skin melanomas as the most common. Caucasian patients have a much higher prevalence than other ethnicities. Of the ocular melanomas, uveal melanomas have an incidence of 4.9 per million, and iris melanomas comprise only a 3% to 10% of uveal melanomas. The average age at which an iris melanoma is diagnosed is between 40 and 50 years.[1] There is no predilection for gender or a particular eye. The main differentials of iris melanoma are iris nevus or iris cyst. The prevalence of these conditions (irrespective of age) is nevus (42%), iris pigment epithelium cyst (19%), and melanoma (17%).[2]

Iris melanomas can be well circumscribed or diffuse. The former manifestation often appears on the inferior section of the iris. They are commonly yellow, tan or brown. The surface may be flat or raised, and they can thicken either anteriorly or posteriorly. A diffuse iris melanoma may appear as a unilateral, flat, dark iris (acquired heterochromia) and may lead to secondary glaucoma. This type of glaucoma can be difficult to treat, and on rare occasions can cause eye pain due to high intraocular pressure (IOP). Diffuse iris melanomas have a higher metastatic risk than localized, well-demarcated iris melanomas. A nasal location, extension into the ciliary body, and pigment dispersion are all associated with an increased metastatic risk.[3]

The following are criteria in the clinical diagnosis of an iris melanoma[4]:

1. Greater than 3 mm in diameter and 1 mm in thickness
2. Replaces the iris stroma
3. At least 3 of the following features:

   a. photographic documentation of growth,
   b. secondary glaucoma,
   c. secondary cataract,
   d. prominent vascularity, and
   e. ectropion iridis.

This case exhibited the first 2 criteria, as well as 2 elements of the third (growth and vascularity). Although ectropion iridis was not present, corectopia was noted. The risk of conversion from an iris nevus to a melanoma is increased with any of the following factors: (a) patient is younger than 40 years; (b) history of hyphema; (c) tumor has an inferior location; (d) a diffuse appearance; (e) ectropion uveae; or (f) tumor has a feathery margin.[5]

The following tests that can help differentiate iris and ciliary body melanomas from cysts or nevi include:

1. Biomicroscopy, including photo documentation and review of old photographs
2. Globe transillumination (melanomas may appear dark, while cysts are clear)
3. Dilated fundus examination including scleral indentation
4. Ultrasonic biomicroscopy and/or anterior segment OCT
5. B-scan ultrasonography (can assess for ciliary body/more posterior melanomas)
6. Fluorescein angiography of iris (not commonly performed in ophthalmic practice)
7. Aqueous paracentesis (to check for metastasis)
8. Fine-needle aspiration biopsy (for cytology/pathology study)

Genetic testing is now an extremely important component in the management of any ocular melanoma. Available genetic testing can provide prognostic information on the risk of metastasis from ocular melanoma using a GEP. Results are divided into following 3 classes, namely:

1. Class 1A: Very low risk (2% chance of metastasis over 5 years)
2. Class 1B: Low risk (21% chance of metastasis over 5 years)
3. Class 2: High risk (72% chance of metastasis over 5 years)

Ideally, genetic testing should precede treatment, as prognostic indicators of metastasis and mortality may dictate more conservative or aggressive therapies (eg, brachytherapy vs enucleation). However, the Collaborative Ocular Melanoma Study (COMS) observed similar 5-year mortality rates (18% to 19%) for medium-sized choroidal melanomas with either treatment regimen.[6]

CLINICAL PEARLS

- An iris melanoma may be differentiated from a nevus if it has a diameter greater than 3 mm or thickness greater than 1 mm, replaces the iris stroma, and exhibits one of the following features: photographic documentation of growth, secondary glaucoma, secondary cataract, prominent vascularity, or ectropion iridis.

- Anterior segment OCT is helpful in determining the thickness and extension the lesion.

- Genetic testing of melanomas can be used to predict the risk of mortality.

REFERENCES

1. Waheed NK, Jayne RP, Crawford CM, et al. Iris Melanoma. In: Taravella M, ed. *Drugs and Diseases*. Medscape. http://emedicine.medscape.com/article/1208624-overview. 2016. Accessed October 3, 2017.
2. Shields CL, Kancherla S, Patel J, et al. Clinical survey of 3680 iris tumors based on patient age at presentation. *Ophthalmology*. February 2012;119(2):407-414.
3. Demirci H, Shields CL, Shields JA, Eagle RC Jr, Honavar SG. Diffuse iris melanoma: a report of 25 cases. *Ophthalmology*. August 2002;109(8):1553-1560.
4. Shields JA, Sanborn GE, Augsburger JJ. The differential diagnosis of malignant melanoma of the iris. A clinical study of 200 patients. *Ophthalmology*. June 1983;90(6):716-720.
5. Shields CL, Kaliki S, Hutchinson A, et al. Iris nevus growth into melanoma: analysis of 1611 consecutive eyes: the ABCDEF guide. *Ophthalmology*. April 2013;120(4):766-772.
6. Onken MD, Worley LA, Char DH, et al. Collaborative Ocular Oncology Group report number 1: prospective validation of a multi-gene prognostic assay in uveal melanoma. *Ophthalmology*, epub. The Collaborative Ocular Melanoma Study: an overview. 2012;119: 1-8.

2.42 Ciliary Body Melanoma

Joanne Caruso

John, a 53-year-old white male, presented for an eye examination because he had failed his Department of Motor Vehicles vision screening. His last eye examination had been 3 years ago. He had a history of long-standing decreased vision in his left eye secondary to a grenade flash when he was 25 years old. Three years ago, the visual acuity (VA) in his right eye was recorded as 20/20. John did not have any complaints of flashes, floaters, or double vision. He did not take any medications nor had any medical issues. He did not have any known allergies to medications. However, he felt that his vision had decreased in his right eye and wanted to get new glasses to renew his driver's license.

Clinical Findings

Current Rx	OD: −1.50 −2.00 × 170 (20/70) OS: −2.75 −1.50 × 180 (20/60)
Unaided near VA	OD: 20/25; OS 20/50
Confrontation visual fields	Full to finger counting OD and OS
Pupil evaluation	PERRL; no RAPD
Retinoscopy	OD −1.00 −2.50 × 015 OS −2.75 −1.50 × 180
Subjective refraction	OD −1.00 −2.50 × 030 (20/25⁻) OS −2.75 −1.50 × 180 (20/50⁻)
Slit-lamp examination	OD: iris pushed forward between 5 and 7 o'clock with an area of injected iris vessels at the inferior angle. Iris transillumination showed cyst formation. Otherwise unremarkable; OS: unremarkable
Intraocular pressure (GAT)	OD: 15 mm Hg; OS: 15 mm Hg at 1:25 PM
Fundus examination	OD: dark cyst (possible ciliary body melanoma) inferior retina. Otherwise unremarkable; OS: unremarkable

Abbreviations: GAT, Goldmann applanation tonometry; OD, right eye; OS, left eye; PERRL, pupils equal, round, reactive to light; RAPD, relative afferent pupillary defect; Rx, prescription; VA, visual acuity.

Comments

John was tentatively diagnosed with a ciliary body melanoma in the right eye (Figure 2.42-1). An appointment was made for him to see a retinal specialist the following day for further testing.

At the ophthalmologic follow-up visit, the diagnosis of ciliary body melanoma was confirmed. The lesion measured 13 mm horizontal × 12 mm vertical on the scleral surface. Ultrasound revealed a maximum height of 7 mm (Figure 2.42-2). Proton beam radiation was recommended. Surgical

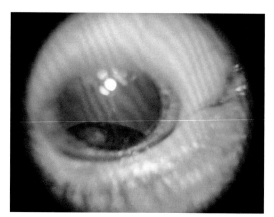

Figure 2.42-1   Dilated view with dark cyst (ciliary body melanoma) visible inferiorly.

localization of the lesion was performed. Tantalum rings were sutured around the borders after they were defined by transillumination to aim the proton beam directly at the tumor. Despite treatment with proton beam irradiation, John passed away 3 years after the initial diagnosis from systemic metastases.

Discussion

John presented for an eye examination because he failed the Department of Motor Vehicles vision screening required to renew his driving license. At the initial examination, despite a 40° change in the cylinder axis of the right eye, the VA could not be corrected to 20/20. This should never be ignored. Typically, the axis of astigmatism does not change so dramatically. Slit-lamp evaluation showed the iris being pushed forward, while iris transillumination and dilated fundus examination revealed a dark-colored mass. This was confirmed subsequently as a ciliary body melanoma.

Ciliary body melanomas are rare ocular tumors. About 3% to 5% of all melanomas develop in the uveal tract of which 85% to 90% are choroidal, 5% to 8% involve the ciliary body, and 3% to 5% are iris lesions.[1] Uveal melanomas, arising from uveal pigment cells (melanocytes), are the most common intraocular malignancy in adults.[2] Most uveal melanomas are seen in patients between 50 and 80 years (mean age at detection is 58 years). They are most prevalent in Caucasian/Non-Hispanic whites (6 per million) and have a 30%

higher frequency in males than females.[1] About 50% of patients will develop metastases.[1] The most common metastatic sites are the liver (60.5%), lungs (24.4%), skin/soft tissue (10.9%), and bone (8.4%).[1] The overall rate of survival from initial diagnosis is 69% at 5 years, 55% at 15 years, and 51% at 25 years; however, following the development of metastatic disease, median overall survival is approximately 13.4 months, with only 8% surviving 2 years.[1]

Because of their hidden location behind the iris, ciliary body melanomas are often large when first detected. When present, they are usually discovered during a routine eye evaluation. The prognosis tends to be poor and metastatic rate tends to be high because of late discovery. Prognosis will vary with tumor size, location, and genetic profile.[2,3] Timely detection and treatment are extremely important for preserving a patient's vision and preventing systemic metastases.

Ciliary body melanomas are usually globular in shape, have a smooth inner surface and, as noted earlier, are usually large when detected. The initial clinical signs may include sentinel vessels (dilated episcleral blood vessels in the same quadrant as the tumor), pressure on the crystalline lens leading to anterior lens displacement and secondary astigmatism, lens subluxation, and/or lens opacity. A dark epibulbar mass may be seen due to extension of the tumor through the scleral emissary vessels. The tumor pushing the iris root into the anterior chamber may cause anterior displacement of the iris. Anterior segment inflammation may be caused by tumor necrosis. If the tumor is very large, it can cause iris neovascularization, secondary glaucoma, dense cataract, ring melanoma (360° ring of tumor around the ciliary body), and/or a retinal detachment due to posterior extension of the tumor.[4]

A ciliary body melanoma may be diagnosed by slit-lamp biomicroscopy, indirect ophthalmoscopy, B-Scan ultrasonography, computed tomography (CT) scan, and magnetic resonance imaging (MRI).[3,5] Baseline systemic evaluation (a complete physical evaluation including blood work up [complete blood count (CBC), serum liver panel]); chest x-ray; and CT, MRI or ultrasound of abdominal organs (especially the liver) are performed to rule out systemic metastases.[5]

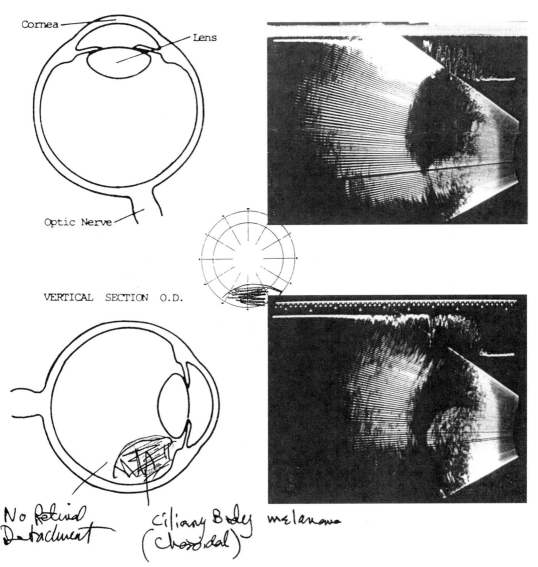

HORIZONTAL SECTION O.D.

Cornea

Lens

Optic Nerve

VERTICAL SECTION O.D.

No Retinal Detachment

Ciliary Body (Choroidal) melanoma

Figure 2.42-2   Ultrasound of ciliary body melanoma inferiorly. No retinal detachment seen.

Treatment options include observation (if small or dormant tumors are present or in patients who cannot undergo treatment due to poor health), enucleation, radiation therapy (plaque radiotherapy, proton beam irradiation, gamma knife, and stereotactic radiosurgery), microsurgical resection, laser therapy, cryotherapy, multimodal therapy or exenteration.[5]

Although ciliary body melanomas are rare, it is very important for the eye care professional to assess the anterior and posterior segment carefully, especially in a patient whose refractive correction has changed significantly and VA is worse than 20/20. As illustrated here, the underlying cause may be life-threatening.

CLINICAL PEARL

- Evaluate the ocular health of the patient carefully if there is an unexplained change in the axis of astigmatism, and best-corrected VA is worse than 20/20.

ACKNOWLEDGMENT

I would like to acknowledge the assistance of Peter Lou, MD, Boston, Massachusetts with this case.

REFERENCES

1. Krantz BA, Dave N, Komatsubara KM, Marr BP, Carvajal RD. Uveal melanoma: epidemiology, etiology, and treatment of primary disease. *Clin Ophthalmol (Auckland, NZ)*. 2017;11:279-289.
2. Carvajal RD, Schwartz GK, Tezel T, Marr B, Francis JH, Nathan PD. Metastatic disease from uveal melanoma: treatment options and future prospects. *Br J Ophthalmol*. 2017;101(1):38-44.
3. Rodríguez A, Dueñas-Gonzalez A, Delgado-Pelayo S. Clinical presentation and management of uveal melanoma. *Mol Clin Oncol*. 2016;5(6):675-677.
4. Caruso J, Pietrantonio J, Capone R. *Ciliary Body Melanoma*, Grand Rounds Poster Session. Orlando, FL: American Academy of Optometry; December 14, 1991.
5. Duker JS, Yanoff S. *Ophthalmology*. 4th ed. London, UK: Elsevier/Saunders. 2013;8(2):801-809.

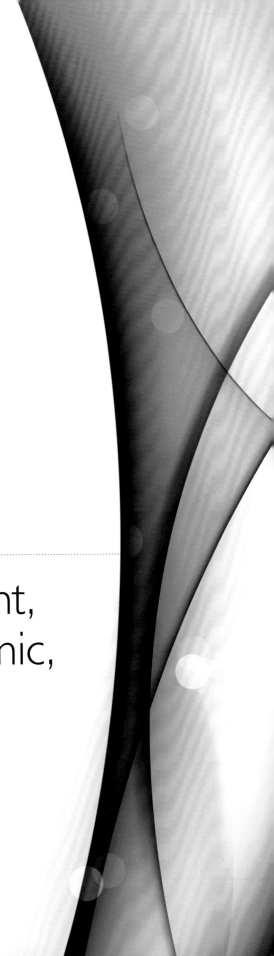

SECTION 3

Posterior Segment, Neuro-Ophthalmic, and Systemic Conditions

Lead section editor: DENISE GOODWIN

3.1 Dry Age-Related Macular Degeneration

Angela V. Shahbazian

Lynne, an 82-year-old Caucasian female, presented with a complaint of not being able to see as well as she used to. She was having difficulty reading books and needed more light to accomplish this. She also noted that when going from light to dark conditions, it took a long time for her eyes to adjust. These symptoms had a slow onset over the previous 5 years. She was retired and still very active but was concerned about being safe while driving at night or through dark tunnels.

She had been seen regularly by an ophthalmologist who performed her cataract surgery 5 years ago. This was her first time at our clinic, and she hoping to get a second opinion regarding the cause of the vision loss. Medical history was positive for hypertension and hypothyroidism, which were well controlled with amlodipine and levothyroxine. She did not smoke cigarettes but drank alcohol 2 to 3 times per month.

Clinical Findings

Habitual distance VA	OD: 20/25; OS: 20/20
Present Rx	OD: −1.00 −0.75 × 142 OS: −1.75 −0.50 × 025 ADD: +2.50 OU (OD: 20/25; OS: 20/20)
Cover test	Distance: 2Δ XP; near: 4Δ XP
Confrontation visual fields	Full to finger counting OD and OS
Pupil evaluation	PERRL; no RAPD
Retinoscopy	OD: −0.75 −0.75 × 142 OS: −1.75 −0.50 × 025
Subjective refraction	OD: −0.75 −0.75 × 142 (20/20) OS: −1.75 −0.50 × 025 (20/20)
Near ADD	+2.50 OU (20/20)
Slit-lamp examination	OD: mild blepharitis; posterior chamber IOL, status post YAG capsulotomy; otherwise unremarkable OS: mild blepharitis; posterior chamber IOL, status post YAG capsulotomy; otherwise unremarkable
Intraocular pressure (GAT)	OD: 13 mm Hg; OS: 12 mm Hg at 2:52 PM
Fundus examination (Figure 3.1-1)	OD: 0.2/0.2 CD ratio; healthy rim tissue with distinct disc margins; extensive intermediate drusen and a few large drusen in the macula with pigmentary changes superior to fovea; normal vasculature; periphery intact OS: 0.2/0.2 CD ratio; healthy rim tissue with distinct disc margins; extensive intermediate drusen and a few large drusen in the macula with pigmentary changes superior to fovea; normal vasculature; periphery intact

Amsler grid	OD: no metamorphopsia; OS: no metamorphopsia
Photostress recovery	OD: 6 min 30 s OS: 6 min 45 s
Fundus autofluorescence (Figure 3.1-2)	OD: scattered areas of hyperautofluorescence in reticular pattern, particularly superior to fovea OS: scattered areas of hyperautofluorescence in reticular pattern, particularly superior to fovea
Macular OCT (Figure 3.1-3)	OD: Normal foveal contour; no subretinal fluid; irregularity of interdigi- tation zone; disruption of ellipsoid zone in areas of pigmentary changes OS: Normal foveal contour; no subretinal fluid; irregularity of interdigi- tation zone; disruption of ellipsoid zone in areas of pigmentary changes
Contrast sensitivity in standard luminance (Mars chart)	OD: 1.68 log Weber contrast sensitivity (normal) OS: 1.44 log Weber contrast sensitivity (moderate loss)
Contrast sensitivity in low luminance (measured with NoIR dark gray fit-over glasses with 4% transmission and Mars chart)	OD: 0.88 log Weber contrast sensitivity (severe loss) OS: 0.88 log Weber contrast sensitivity (severe loss)

Abbreviations: CD, cup to disc; GAT, Goldmann applanation tonometry; IOL, intraocular lens; OCT, optical coherence tomography; OD, right eye; OS, left eye; OU, both eyes; PERRL, pupils equal, round, reactive to light; RAPD, relative afferent pupillary defect; Rx, prescription; sph, sphere; VA, visual acuity; XP, exophoria; YAG, yttrium-aluminum-garnet.

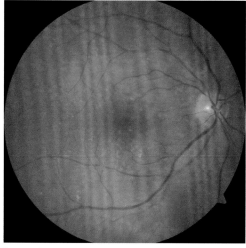 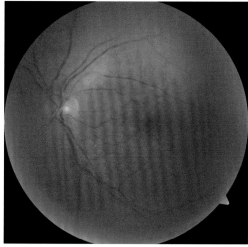

Figure 3.1-1   Fundus photos showing intermediate and large drusen, as well as pigmentary changes in the macular area of both eyes.

Discussion

Lynne's fundus examination and optical coherence tomography (OCT) were consistent with age-related macular degeneration (AMD). She was advised to monitor her vision with an Amsler grid at home on a daily basis and to return to the clinic immediately if she noticed metamorphopsia. She was also advised to take the Age-Related Eye Disease Study 2 (AREDS 2) vitamin formula daily to reduce the chances of developing advanced disease. Finally, the

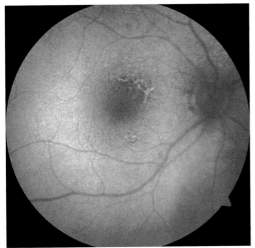
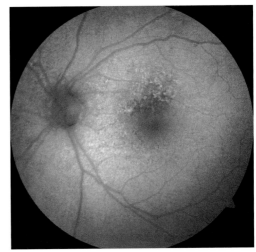

Figure 3.1-2   Fundus autofluorescence showing hyperautofluorescence in the macular area of both eyes.

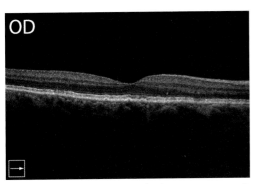
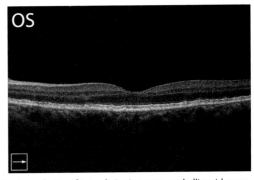

Figure 3.1-3   Macular optical coherence tomography showing irregularity of interdigitation zone and ellipsoid zone consistent with drusen. Note small, bright areas in outer nuclear layer nasal to the fovea in the right eye, consistent with pigment migration.

importance of adequate lighting and proper light placement when reading was discussed. Lynne was advised that her contrast sensitivity was not safe for driving at night or in low-light conditions.

Age-related macular degeneration is the leading cause of legal blindness for the elderly in industrialized nations. The etiology is not fully understood, but it is clear that the disease develops in part due to dysfunction of the retinal pigment epithelium (RPE) in disposing of cellular waste from the photoreceptors, as well as inflammation at the level of the RPE, Bruch's membrane, and choriocapillaris. Risk factors for the disease include older age, family history, and presence or history of smoking cigarettes. It is more common in lightly pigmented individuals.

The hallmark sign for this condition is drusen: deposits between the RPE and Bruch

membrane. On fundus examination, drusen typically appear within the macula as small yellow spots, which can have distinct borders (hard drusen) or indistinct borders (soft drusen). Another common sign of AMD is pigment mottling within the macula, which can vary from slight pigment irregularity to large pigment clumps.

The severity of the disease is characterized by the number and size of drusen, as well as the presence of pigment mottling. As a general rule, patients with more, larger, or soft drusen, or those with pigment mottling have more advanced disease. Early AMD is characterized as having small- or a few intermediate-sized drusen. Intermediate AMD is defined as extensive intermediate-sized drusen, 1 large drusen, or geographic atrophy not involving the fovea. As the disease worsens, patients can develop areas of RPE atrophy (geographic atrophy) within the macula, creating scotomas in the patient's central visual field that correspond to these areas of atrophy. While most patients develop some of the clinical signs mentioned earlier without developing advanced disease, approximately 10% to 15% of patients with AMD have advanced disease, defined as central geographic atrophy or choroidal neovascularization (CNV).[1]

Patients with early or intermediate macular degeneration are likely to have good visual acuity (VA; 20/40 or better), while patients with advanced macular degeneration generally have significantly worse acuity, even to the point of being legally blind. Because there is such a significant difference in VA between patients with and without advanced disease, research has sought to determine which clinical signs indicate a higher risk of developing advanced disease and what treatment is available to prevent its development.

The AREDS Research Group examined the effectiveness of a selection of high-dose vitamins and zinc in preventing advanced disease. The authors concluded that supplements of high-dose zinc, copper, vitamin C, vitamin E, and beta carotene reduced the chances of developing advanced disease by approximately 25% for patients with intermediate AMD or patients who already have advanced disease in the contralateral eye.[2] A follow-up study (AREDS2) found that lutein and zeaxanthin could replace beta carotene in the formulation with no change in effectiveness.[3] This modified AREDS2 formula is considered safer since beta carotene supplements increase the risk of lung cancer in smokers.

Disease severity is monitored through VA testing and fundus examination with photography. Patients with intermediate AMD should be directed to take the AREDS2 formula if there are no contraindications and to monitor their vision with the Amsler grid daily. Patients should be advised to return to clinic immediately if sudden onset blur or metamorphopsia is noted, as this could be a sign of CNV. If CNV is suspected, patients should receive an immediate referral to a retinal specialist for treatment, as visual outcomes are generally improved with earlier treatment.[4] Unfortunately, there is currently no treatment for dry AMD or geographic atrophy. Patients with central geographic atrophy are likely to have severely reduced VA and should be referred to a low-vision specialist.

Because patients may experience visual difficulties despite normal visual acuity, supplementary testing can provide valuable information regarding visual function. For example, patients with normal visual acuity can have a notably abnormal response on the photostress recovery test or contrast sensitivity testing. The recovery time on the photostress recovery test is prolonged for patients with AMD,[5] and this test can help quantify patient complaints of difficulty adapting from light to dark conditions. Contrast sensitivity worsens as AMD progresses,[6] and this change can be detected earlier in the disease when tested under low luminance conditions.[7]

Macular degeneration should be differentiated from other diseases that exhibit yellow lesions or mottling at the macula, particularly the pattern dystrophies, which are inherited and appear symmetric between the 2 eyes. Pigment mottling alone can also appear in a variety of diseases, including cone dystrophy and retinal toxicity from chloroquine or hydroxychloroquine. A thorough case history and careful fundus examination are required to make the correct diagnosis.

New technology can detect retinal changes not easily observed with color fundus photographs. Fundus autofluorescence can highlight areas of abnormal retinal function (seen as hyperautofluorescence), as well as areas of geographic atrophy not easily detected in color photographs (seen as hypoautofluorescence). Macular OCT and fluorescein angiography are valuable for visualizing subretinal abnormalities that may indicate CNV. Genetic testing is available to determine a patient's risk for developing advanced disease, and studies are being conducted to find new treatment that targets the pathology caused by these genes.

CLINICAL PEARL

- Patients with macular degeneration can have measurably worse vision even if their VA is 20/20.

REFERENCES

1. Klein R. Prevalence of age-related macular degeneration in the US population. *Arch Ophthalmol.* 2011;129(1):75-80.
2. Age-Related Eye Disease Study Research Group. A randomized, placebo-controlled, clinical trial of high-dose supplementation with vitamins C and E, beta carotene, and zinc for age-related macular degeneration and vision loss: AREDS report no. 8. *Arch Ophthalmol.* 2001;119(10):1417-1436.
3. Chew EY, Clemons TE, Sangiovanni JP, et al. Secondary analyses of the effects of lutein/zeaxanthin on age-related macular degeneration progression: AREDS2 report No. 3. *JAMA Ophthalmol.* 2014;132(2):142-149.
4. Boyer DS, Antoszyk AN, Awh CC, Bhisitkul RB, Shapiro H, Acharya NR. Subgroup analysis of the MARINA study of ranibizumab in neovascular age-related macular degeneration. *Ophthalmology.* 2007;114(2):246-252.
5. Neelam K, Nolan J, Chakravarthy U, Beatty S. Psychophysical function in age-related maculopathy. *Surv Ophthalmol.* 2009;54(2):167-210.
6. Kleiner RC, Enger C, Fine SL. Contrast sensitivity in age-related macular degeneration. *Arch Ophthalmol.* 1988;106(1):55-57.
7. Maynard ML, Zele AJ, Feigl B. Mesopic Pelli-Robson contrast sensitivity and MP-1 microperimetry in healthy ageing and age-related macular degeneration. *Acta Ophthalmol.* 2016;94(8):e772-e778.

3.2 Wet Age-Related Macular Degeneration

Kelly Glass

Gerald, a 77-year-old male, presented for a general eye examination. He noticed blurred vision in his left eye for several years primarily when viewing objects in the distance. He was a retired mechanic and watched television several hours each day. Ocular history was remarkable for wet age-related macular degeneration (AMD) in the left eye and cataract surgery in both eyes less than 1 year ago. Gerald also had a choroidal nevus in the left eye that had been stable for several years. He took hydrochlorothiazide for hypertension and ipratropium bromine/albuterol (Combivent Respimat) for chronic obstructive pulmonary disease. Gerald smoked cigarettes (1 pack per day) and was a social drinker.

Gerald discontinued his Avastin injection appointments with a retinal specialist 4 to 5 months ago. He was told by the doctor that his condition was improving, but subjectively he did not notice any changes in his vision. He was growing frustrated with the AMD treatments.

Clinical Findings

Habitual distance VA	OD: 20/20; OS: 20/80 (no improvement with pinhole)
Present Rx	OD: +0.50 −0.50 × 095 OS: +0.50 −0.50 × 167 ADD: +2.50 OU (20/20 OU)
Cover test	Orthophoria at distance; 6Δ exophoria at near
Ocular motility	Full range of motion OD and OS
Confrontation visual fields	Full to finger counting OD and OS
Pupil evaluation	PERRL; no RAPD
Retinoscopy	OD: Pl −0.50 × 098; OS: +0.50 −0.50 × 167
Subjective refraction	OD: +0.50 −0.50 × 095 (20/20) OS: +0.50 −0.50 × 167 (20/80)
Near ADD	+2.50 OU (20/20 OU)
Amsler grid	OD: no metamorphopsia or scotomas OS: central metamorphopsia and scotoma
Slit-lamp examination	OD: mild posterior blepharitis; nasal pinguecula; posterior chamber IOL centered and clear; otherwise unremarkable OS: mild posterior blepharitis; nasal pinguecula; posterior chamber IOL centered and clear; otherwise unremarkable
Intraocular pressure (GAT)	OD: 12 mm Hg; OS: 12 mm Hg at 10:13 AM

Fundus examination (Figure 3.2-1)   OD: 0.3/0.3 CD ratio; healthy rim tissue with distinct disc margins; 1+ macular drusen; mildly tortuous blood vessels with venous beading, no artery/vein nicking; peripheral retina intact

OS: 0.3/0.3 CD ratio; healthy rim tissue with distinct disc margins; subretinal hemorrhage inferior to the fovea; mildly tortuous blood vessels with venous beading, no artery/vein nicking; choroidal nevus approximately 2 disc diameters in size with overlying drusen (stable from 2 years prior); peripheral retinal otherwise intact

Macular OCT   OD: mild drusen present

OS: significant thickening of the macula; disruption of Bruch membrane with associated RPE detachment and subretinal edema (Figure 3.2-2)

Abbreviations: CD, cup to disc; GAT, Goldmann applanation tonometry; IOL, intraocular lens; OCT, optical coherence tomography; OD, right eye; OS, left eye; OU, both eyes; PERRL, pupils equal, round, reactive to light; Pl, plano; RAPD, relative afferent pupillary defect; RPE, retinal pigment epithelium; Rx, prescription; VA, visual acuity; XP, exophoria.

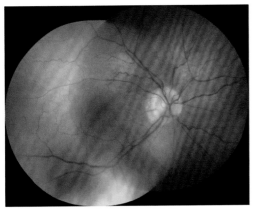
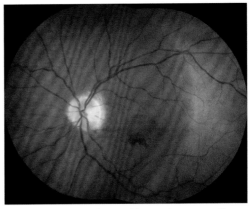

Figure 3.2-1   Fundus photography showing 1+ macular drusen OD. There is a subretinal hemorrhage, as well as a choroidal nevus OS.

Abbreviations: OD, right eye; OS, left eye.

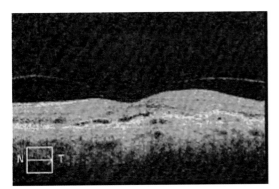

Figure 3.2-2   Macula optical coherence tomography (OCT) of the left eye showing macular thickening and subretinal fluid within the macula.

Discussion

Gerald had several ocular conditions, the most urgent being wet AMD in the left eye. He was told that the vision loss and other findings were consistent with wet AMD and that ocular injections would decrease the risk of further decline in his vision. Gerald agreed to be seen again by the retinal specialist for additional treatment. He was offered a referral to a counselor to cope with the visual diagnosis, but the patient declined. He was scheduled for a 2-month follow-up examination to ensure continuity of care. Gerald was given an Amsler grid for daily monitoring of each eye and was educated on its proper use, as well as the importance of monitoring the Amsler grid at home.

In addition to the wet AMD, Gerald was diagnosed with a pinguecula in each eye and was educated about the importance of wearing sunglasses to protect from wind and ultraviolet light. He was given a sample of rewetting drops to use 4 times daily. The choroidal nevus was stable from photographs taken 2 years ago, so no intervention was necessary. Finally, Gerald had dry AMD in the right eye. To reduce the risk of conversion to wet AMD, it was recommended that he take an Age-Related Eye Disease Study (AREDS) 2 supplement and was encouraged to stop smoking.

Age-related macular degeneration is the primary cause of legal blindness in North Americans who are 65 years of age or older. AMD is divided into 2 types: dry AMD (also known as nonexudative or non-neovascular AMD) and wet AMD (also called exudative or neovascular AMD). Approximately 10% to 15% percent of cases involve progression from dry AMD to the more advanced and visually damaging wet form.[1]

The hallmark of wet AMD is the formation of choroidal neovascularization, new irregular blood vessels growing into the subretinal pigment epithelium or subretinal space. Oxygen-deprived retinal cells produce a protein called vascular endothelial growth factor (VEGF), which in turn prompts the growth of new retinal blood vessels. Due to their aberrant nature, these neovascular vessels easily break and leak, producing intraretinal, subretinal, or subretinal pigment epithelium edema. This process can create scarring, leading to severe central vision loss.

Wet macular degeneration can be subdivided into 2 categories: occult and classic. The occult type is characterized by indistinct subretinal neovascularization generating less discrete leakage compared with the classic type. Occult AMD is typically accompanied by mild vision loss. The second, more visually devastating form of AMD, is the classic type. This involves distinct outlines of neovascular subretinal growth and observable scarring.

The fundus may appear normal despite the presence of choroidal neovascularization,

particularly if the only sign present is subretinal fluid. Alternatively, fundus biomicroscopy may reveal perceptible retinal elevation from underlying fluid or blood. Well-defined, classic choroidal neovascularization appears on optical coherence tomography (OCT) as hyperreflective regions, either under the RPE or in the subretinal space, that form a dome-shape or flat formation. Occult choroidal neovascularization will cause a flat separation between the retinal pigment epithelium (RPE) and choroid. Either type may be accompanied by retinal edema or an RPE detachment as fluid or blood leaks out of the newly formed blood vessels. Optical coherence tomography is a useful tool to provide information about the activity of neovascular membranes, optimize treatment regimens, and decrease the number of injections in neovascular AMD patients.[2] Additionally, OCT is instrumental in objectively tracking subretinal fluid changes and differentiating AMD from other conditions that create fluid accumulation in the macula, including central serous retinopathy.

Pharmaceutical drugs that inhibit VEGF, such as aflibercept (Eylea), ranibizumab (Lucentis), and bevacizumab (Avastin), have transformed neovascular AMD treatment. Stability of the condition, visual acuity (VA) improvements, and reduced macular fluid can be achieved in the majority of patients receiving this therapy.[2-5] The Comparison of Age-Related Macular Degeneration Treatments Trials (CATT) study group[6] compared the efficacy of ranibizumab and bevacizumab in advanced neovascular AMD. They concluded that ranibizumab efficacy is equivalent to bevacizumab in both monthly and as-needed dosing. The study also confirmed that substantial improvement in visual acuity can be accomplished with as-needed injections compared to monthly injections.

Patients receiving routine intraocular injections may become frustrated with the AMD treatment process. Some patients report discomfort days after the treatment sessions. Nonsteroidal anti-inflammatory drug (NSAID) may be prescribed to reduce the length of posttreatment discomfort.[7] Knowledge of what the patient experiences when undergoing wet AMD treatment is critical, as this may assist future strategies aimed at maximizing compliance. It is important to discuss and reevaluate treatment expectations with wet AMD patients to prevent anxiety and improve quality of life.[8]

CLINICAL PEARLS

- Reeducating the patient is often necessary to maximize compliance in individuals with a chronic ocular condition.

- The fundus may appear normal despite the presence of choroidal neovascularization. Visual changes, including metamorphopsia, should cause the clinician to have a high suspicion for neovascularization.

REFERENCES

1. O'Connell SR, Bressler NM. Age-related macular degeneration. In: Regillo CD, Flynn HW, Brown GC, eds. *Vitreoretinal Disease*. 1st ed. New York, NY: Thieme; 1999:213-240.

2. Lalwani GA, Rosenfeld PJ, Fung AE, et al. A variable-dosing regimen with intravitreal ranibizumab for neovascular age-related macular degeneration: year 2 of the PrONTO study. *Am J Ophthalmol*. 2009;148(1):43-58.

3. Brown DM, Kaiser PK, Michels M, et al. Ranibizumab versus verteporfin for neovascular age-related macular degeneration. *N Engl J Med*. 2006;355(4):1432-1444.

4. Heier JS, Brown DM, Chong V, et al. Intravitreal aflibercept (VEGF trap-eye) in wet age-related macular degeneration. *Ophthalmology*. 2012;119(12):2537-2548.

5. Martin DF, Maguire MG, Fine SL, et al. Ranibizumab and bevacizumab for treatment of neovascular age-related macular degeneration: two-year results. *Ophthalmology*. 2012;119(7):1388-1398.

6. CATT Research Group, Martin DF, Maguire MG, et al. Ranibizumab and bevacizumab for neovascular age-related macular degeneration. *N Engl J Med*. 2011;364(20):1897-1908.

7. Rifkin L, Shlomit S. Shortening ocular pain duration following intravitreal injections. *Eur J Ophthalmol*. 2012;22(6):1008-1012.

8. Boyle J, Vukicevic M, Koklanis K, et al. Experiences of patients undergoing repeated intravitreal anti-vascular endothelial growth factor injections for neovascular age-related macular degeneration. *Psychol Health Med*. January 9, 2017;23:1-14.

3.3 Diabetic Retinopathy

Munish Sharma

Alejandro, a 47-year-old Hispanic male, presented with floaters and flashes in the right eye. He stated that these symptoms had been progressing slowly over a period of 4 to 6 months and had recently been associated with glare, making it difficult to drive at night. He had never had an eye examination and reported using +2.50 D over-the-counter readers for near work. He was diagnosed with diabetes 14 years ago. He was supposed to be using both glipizide and metformin to control the diabetes, but he discontinued both the medications against medical advice couple months prior to the exam for financial reasons. He was not monitoring his blood glucose at home, and his last blood glucose was unknown. He reported an HbA1c of around 9% 1 week earlier, the lowest it had been in years. He was diagnosed with hypertension 5 years ago and was started on lisinopril, which he had not been able to afford for the past few months. He was a construction worker but had been unable to find work for the past 6 months.

Clinical Findings

Unaided distance VA	OD: hand motion; OS: 20/80
Near habitual VA (+2.50 OTC)	OD: hand motion; OS: 20/50
Cover test	Distance: 1Δ EP, 3Δ left HP;
	Near (with +2.50 OTC): 4Δ XP, 3Δ left HP
Confrontation visual fields	Could not be performed OD; full to finger counting OS
Pupil evaluation	Equal and round with minimal reaction to light (4 mm in dark, 3 mm in light) OU; 2+ RAPD OD
Keratometry	OD: 43.25 @ 96/43.75 @ 006; OS: 43.00 sph; mires clear and regular OD and OS
Retinoscopy	OD: −0.75 −0.75 × 105; OS: −1.00 −0.50 × 063
Subjective refraction	OD: not performed; OS: −1.00 −0.50 × 080 (20/50)
Near ADD	+1.50 OU (near VA: 20/50 OU)
Intraocular pressure (GAT)	OD: 11 mm Hg; OS: 11 mm Hg at 3:30 PM
Slit-lamp examination	OD: temporal pinguecula; otherwise unremarkable with no iris neovascularization
	OS: temporal pinguecula; otherwise unremarkable with no iris neovascularization
Fundus examination (Figure 3.3-1)	OD: 0.3/0.3 CD ratio; dense neovascularization of the optic nerve with overlying fibrovascular bands; significant macula edema with exudative material surrounding fovea; neovascularization elsewhere involving the superior temporal arcades over 1 disc diameter in size; scattered hemorrhages throughout posterior pole; preretinal and vitreous hemorrhages; peripheral tractional retinal detachment superiorly

OCT of the macula
    (Figure 3.3-2)

OS: 0.3/0.3 CD ratio; dense neovascularization of the optic nerve with overlying fibrovascular bands; mild macula edema with exudative material temporally within 1/3 disc diameter of fovea; neovascularization elsewhere superior and inferior to disc; scattered hemorrhages throughout posterior pole; intraretinal microvascular abnormalities (IRMA) nasal to disc; floaters; peripheral retina intact

OD: significant traction and intraretinal edema in the macular area

OS: mild macular edema with retinal exudates present

Abbreviations: CD, cup to disc; EP, esophoria; GAT, Goldmann applanation tonometry; HP, hyperphoria; OCT, optical coherence tomography; OD, right eye; OS, left eye; OTC, over the counter; OU, both eyes; RAPD, relative afferent pupillary defect; sph, sphere; VA, visual acuity; XP, exophoria.

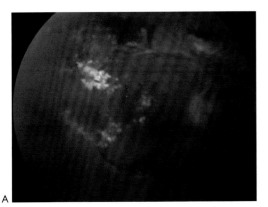
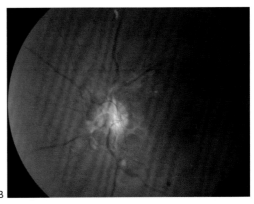

A   B

Figure 3.3-1   Retinal photos showing exudation, hemorrhages, neovascularization, and tractional detachment of the right eye (A) and neovascularization of the disc of the left eye (B).

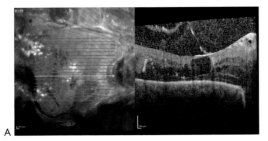
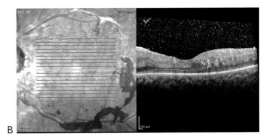

A   B

Figure 3.3-2   Macular optical coherence tomography showing significant edema and macular traction of the right eye (A) and mild edema with exudates within one-third disc diameter of the fovea in left eye (B).

Comments

Alejandro was referred to a retinal specialist who confirmed neovascularization of the disc and neovascularization elsewhere, as well as diffuse capillary non-perfusion involving most of the retina in each eye with fluorescein angiography (Figure 3.3-3). The patient received an intravitreal anti-vascular endothelial growth factor (VEGF) injection (Avastin) in the left eye on the same day and was scheduled to undergo a pars plana vitrectomy with retinal detachment repair of the right eye.

During the pars plana vitrectomy, triamcinolone was used for vitreous visualization to assist with vitrectomy. The fibrovascular traction tissue was dissected and removed with limited peripheral retinectomy to flatten the retina followed by Perfluoron liquid silicon oil exchange with silicon oil tamponade as vitreous

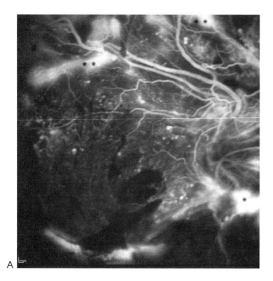

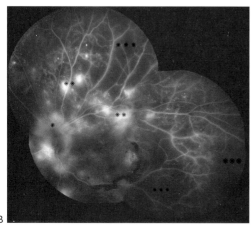

Figure 3.3-3 Fluorescein angiography demonstrating microaneurysms, neovascularization of the disc*, and neovascularization elsewhere**, as well as diffuse capillary nonperfusion***.

substitute. Also, intraoperative endolaser panretinal photocoagulation was completed.

Alejandro was examined the next day and 1 week after the retinal detachment surgery. Vision remained unchanged. At the 1- and 2-month follow-up visits, Alejandro had residual macular edema in the right eye and additional intravitreal Avastin injections were administered. Alejandro had a significant decrease in macular edema at the 3-month follow-up visit. At that time panretinal photocoagulation was performed in the right eye to address the residual proliferative diabetic retinopathy (PDR). Best-corrected visual acuity (VA) after 4 months was 20/200 OD and 20/30 OS.

Discussion

According to the Centers for Disease Control, 23.1 million people, or 7.2% of the US population, has been diagnosed with diabetes.[1] Diabetes can be classified into 4 general categories (Table 3.3-1) utilizing the criteria for diagnosis listed in Table 3.3-2.[2]

Diabetic retinopathy, found in nearly 35% of those with diabetes, is the leading cause of blindness among working adults.[3] Additionally, 7.0% of people with diabetes have PDR, 6.8% have diabetic macular edema (DME), and 10.2% have vision-threatening diabetic retinopathy.[3] Diabetic retinopathy is associated with duration of diabetes, hyperglycemia, hypertension, hyperlipidemia, and genetic factors.[4] Despite optimal control of blood

Table 3.3-1	Classifications of Diabetes
Type 1 diabetes	Due to pancreatic beta-cell destruction, usually leading to absolute insulin deficiency
Type 2 diabetes	Due to a progressive insulin secretory defect and insulin resistance
Gestational diabetes	Diabetes diagnosed in the second or third trimester of pregnancy that is not overt diabetes
Diabetes due to other causes	Monogenic diabetes syndromes such as neonatal diabetes and maturity-onset diabetes of the young, diseases of the exocrine pancreas such as cystic fibrosis, and drug- or chemical-induced diabetes such as in the treatment of HIV/AIDS or after organ transplantation

Table 3.3-2	Criteria for Diabetes and Prediabetes Diagnosis

A patient can be diagnosed with diabetes if any one of the following criteria is met:

- HbA1c ≥6.5%

- Fasting plasma glucose ≥126 mg/dL (7.0 mmol/L). Fasting is defined as no caloric intake for at least 8 h

- Two-hour plasma glucose ≥200 mg/dL (11.1 mmol/L) during an oral glucose tolerance test

- Random plasma glucose ≥200 mg/dL (11.1 mmol/L) in a patient with classic symptoms of hyperglycemia or hyperglycemic crisis

A patient is categorized to be at increased risk of diabetes (prediabetes) if any one of the following criteria is met:

- HbA1c 5.7%-6.4%

- Fasting plasma glucose 100-125 mg/dL (5.6-6.9 mmol/L)

- Two-hour plasma glucose with the oral glucose tolerance test 140-199 mg/dL (7.8-11.0 mmol/L)

glucose, the majority of diabetic patients will develop retinopathy over time. Several biochemical markers, including inflammation, growth factors, and hormones, have been found responsible for development of diabetic retinopathy.[5]

The link between hyperglycemia-induced retinopathy is related to the following 4 pathways[6-8]: polyol pathway, advanced glycation end products pathway, protein kinase C, and pathway hexosamine pathway. These 4 pathways ultimately result in hypoxia that causes upregulation of growth factors and cytokines such as VEGF, angiopoietins, tumor necrosis factor, interleukins, and matrix metalloproteinases, which contribute to vascular dysfunction and breakdown of the blood retinal barrier by breakdown of endothelial cell junctional complexes, pericyte loss, and thickening of the basement membrane.[4]

Diabetic retinopathy occurs due to abnormalities in the retinal circulation. This is initially classified as non-proliferative diabetic retinopathy (NPDR), evident as microaneurysms (focal vascular weakness), intraretinal hemorrhages (vascular leakage), hard exudates (lipid and protein deposition), cotton wool spots (area of retinal nerve fiber layer [RNFL] infarction), intraretinal microvascular abnormalities (vascular remodeling),

and venous beading (irregular vein caliper). Neovascularization may develop representing progression to PDR. The neovascularization commonly involves the retina, optic nerve, or iris and may lead to vision-threatening complications, such as vitreous hemorrhage, tractional retinal detachment, or neovascular glaucoma. Classification of diabetic retinopathy is based on the following severity[9,10]:

- Mild NPDR: Only microaneurysms with no other signs

- Moderate NPDR: More than microaneurysms but less than severe NPDR

- Severe NPDR: Any of the following changes with no signs of PDR:

  - Four quadrants of severe intraretinal hemorrhages and microaneurysms (US definition) or more than 20 intraretinal hemorrhages in each of 4 quadrants (international definition)

  - Two or more quadrants of venous beading

  - One or more quadrants of intraretinal microvascular abnormalities (IRMA)

- Proliferative diabetic retinopathy: One of the following:

  - Neovascularization of the disc (NVD) or neovascularization elsewhere (NVE)

  - Vitreous or preretinal hemorrhages

- High-risk PDR: Characterized by 1 or more of the following:

  - Neovascularization of the disc greater than one-fourth to one-third disc area in size (Early Treatment of Diabetic Retinopathy Study [ETDRS] standard photograph 10A)

  - Neovascularization of the disc less than one-fourth disc area in size with fresh vitreous or preretinal hemorrhage present

Patients in any of the aforementioned severity stages can develop macular edema (defined as retinal thickening within 2 disc diameters (DDs) of the center of the macula). This can progress to clinically significant macular edema (CSME) if 1 of the following is present[10,11]:

- Thickening of the retina ≤500 micrometer (1/3 DD) from the center of the macula

- Hard exudates ≤500 micrometer (1/3 DD) from the center of the macula with thickening of the adjacent retina

- A zone or zones of retinal thickening ≥1 DD in size, any portion of which is ≤1 DD from the center of the macula

Early detection of retinal abnormalities is essential in preventing diabetic retinopathy and macular edema–related loss of vision. Screening recommendations for patients with diabetes are as follows[2,10,11]:

- Type 1 diabetes: First evaluation within 5 years after onset of diabetes and annual follow-up until they develop retinopathy.

- Type 2 diabetes: First evaluation at the time of diabetes diagnosis and annual follow-up until they develop retinopathy.

- Women with preexisting diabetes planning pregnancy or who have become pregnant: First evaluation before pregnancy or early in first trimester of pregnancy with follow-up every 3 to 12 months if they have no retinopathy to mild/moderate NPDR and follow-up every 1 to 3 months if they develop severe NPDR or worse.

Frequency of follow-up once the patient develops diabetic retinopathy is not only dependent on the grade of the retinopathy, but also on the type of treatment and patient's response to treatment (Table 3.3-3).[11]

Management of blood glucose is critical in reducing microvascular complications, including diabetic retinopathy. Tight and continuous blood glucose control (HbA1c less than 7% is a common target) has been shown to reduce diabetic retinopathy. Additionally, management of blood pressure and cholesterol levels is also helpful in reducing ocular complications.

In spite of recent advances in management of diabetic retinopathy, there are several management challenges.[12] Diabetic retinopathy

Table 3.3-3	Recommended Time Line for Follow-up Visits in Those With Diabetic Retinopathy		
	No Macular Edema, mo	Macular Edema (No CSME), mo	CSME[a], mo
Mild NPDR	12	4-6	2-4
Moderate NPDR	6-8	4-6	2-4
Severe NPDR	3-4	2-3	2-3
Very severe NPDR	2-3	2-3	2-3
Non-high risk PDR	2-3	2-3	2-3
High risk PDR	2-3	1-2	1-2

Abbreviations: CSME, clinically significant macular edema; NPDR, non-proliferative diabetic retinopathy; PDR, proliferative diabetic retinopathy.

[a] Follow-up is typically monthly for the first year of treatment if intravitreal anti-VEGF injections are given.

management can be divided into 2 categories based on the key pathology addressed: DME management and PDR management.

Diabetic Macular Edema Management

Focal or grid laser has been the standard of care for the treatment of DME since the ETDRS demonstrated reduction of moderate vision loss by 50% or more following this treatment.[12] Intravitreal triamcinolone was introduced as an alternative, but monotherapy with intravitreal triamcinolone showed no long-term benefit in visual acuity (VA) improvement.[12,13] Recently, intravitreal anti-VEGF has become the first line of management for DME.[12,14] Diabetic macular edema involving the center of macula is managed aggressively, even before VA is affected or the edema becomes clinically significant.[12,13] Treatment is generally based on the initial VA.[14,15] Either bevacizumab or ranibizumab (0.3 mg in the United States and 0.5 mg in Europe) is used for patients with VA of 20/40 or better because of its lower cost. In eyes with VA of 20/50 or worse, aflibercept is used because of its greater efficacy. Risks relating to intravitreal injection, such as endophthalmitis or retinal detachment, though rare, are serious.[14]

Although anti-VEGF monotherapy results in better visual outcome and greater decrease in macular thickness,[16] laser treatment still has value as adjunctive therapy.[12] It produces a synergistic effect that lasts longer (resulting in the need for fewer injections) and increases in effectiveness over time while injections have more stable long-term results. Macular thickness may be further reduced when laser treatment is combined with anti-VEFG injections.[12] Furthermore, combination therapy may reduce the chance of secondary engorgement of the laser burns, as the prompt effect of the antiangiogenic drying the macula reduces the intensity of the laser required.[12] Macular laser is applied as focal laser spots (spot size 50 to 100 micrometer) or as a grid laser. Focal laser is performed around microaneurysms, IRMA, and short capillary segments that show focal fluorescein leakage. Grid laser is usually applied diffusely to an area of 500 to 3000 μm superiorly, nasally, and inferiorly from the center of macula and 500 to 3500 μm temporal to the fovea, avoiding the areas 500 μm from the center of the macula and within 500 μm of the disc margin. Newer technologies such as imaged-guided photocoagulation systems and short-pulse lasers may improve laser outcomes.[12]

Proliferative Diabetic Retinopathy Management

Pan-retinal photocoagulation (PRP) has been the standard of care for PDR since the Diabetic Retinopathy Study showed that timely PRP of high-risk PDR decreases the risk of severe vision loss by more than 50%.[10,11,14] Laser photocoagulation obliterates the ischemic mid-peripheral retina and downregulates the VEGF synthesis promoting regression of neovascularization. Unfortunately, the same obliterative process leads to permanent loss of peripheral vision and reduced night vision as complications from PRP.

Intravitreal anti-VEGF injections lead to involution of neovascularization but the effect of a single injection is transient with recurrence of neovascularization in approximately 12 weeks.[17] Baseline PRP has been compared with intravitreal anti-VEGF (ranibizumab) given at baseline and repeated every 4 weeks on an as-needed basis.[17] Patients receiving ranibizumab had better best-corrected VA, less peripheral visual field sensitivity loss, fewer vitrectomies, and a lower incidence of DME over the 2-year duration of the study. Also, these patients needed fewer injections in year 2, suggesting some disease modification with ranibizumab therapy. Patient compliance with anti-VEGF therapy is an important factor in obtaining this outcome, and other anti-VEGF options, including bevacizumab and aflibercept are potential off-label alternatives to ranibizumab.

Most patients with neovascularization of the iris respond to PRP and anti-VEGF treatment, but some patients need vitrectomy for management of non-resolving PDR and neovascularization of the iris. Additional indications for vitrectomy include the follwing[10,18]:

- Macula-threatening tractional retinal detachment (particularly of recent onset)
- Combined traction–rhegmatogenous retinal detachment

- Vitreous or preretinal hemorrhage precluding PRP
- Non-resolving macular edema

Vitrectomy in these patients is usually a very involved process as was in the case of Alejandro. Vitrectomy must be combined with lensectomy and silicon oil tamponade for anatomical success.[18]

CLINICAL PEARLS

- Symptoms of flashes of light do not always indicate retinal detachment.
- Untreated diabetic retinopathy can lead to irreversible loss of vision.

REFERENCES

1. National Diabetes Statistics Report. Estimates of diabetes and its burden in the United States. Centers for Disease Control and Prevention Web site. https://www.cdc.gov/diabetes/pdfs/data/statistics/national-diabetes-statistics-report.pdf. 2017. Accessed October 16, 2017.
2. American Diabetes Association. Standards of medical care in diabetes-2017 abridged for primary care providers. *Clin Diabetes*. 2017;35(1):5-26.
3. Yau JW, Rogers SL, Kawasaki R, et al. Global prevalence and major risk factors of diabetic retinopathy. *Diabetes Care*. 2012;35(3):556-564.
4. Das A, McGuire PG, Rangasamy S. Diabetic macular edema: pathophysiology and novel therapeutic targets. *Ophthalmology*. 2015;122(7):1375-1394.
5. Ahsan H. Diabetic retinopathy—biomolecules and multiple pathophysiology. *Diabetes Metab Syndr*. 2015;9(1):51-54.
6. Lorenzi M. The polyol pathway as a mechanism for diabetic retinopathy: attractive, elusive, and resilient. *Exp Diabetes Res*. 2007;2007:61038.
7. Mathebula SD. Polyol pathway: a possible mechanism of diabetes complications in the eye. *Afr Vis Eye Health*. 2015;74(1), Art. #13, 5 pages. http://dx.doi.org/10.4102/aveh.v74i1.13.
8. Safi SZ, Qvist R, Kumar S, Batumalaie K, Ismail IS. Molecular mechanisms of diabetic retinopathy, general preventive strategies, and novel therapeutic targets. *BioMed Res Int*. 2014;2014:801269.
9. Wilkinson CP, Ferris FL, Klein RE, et al. Proposed international clinical diabetic retinopathy and diabetic macular edema disease severity scales. *Ophthalmology*. 2003;110(9):1677-1682.
10. American Academy of Ophthalmology Retina/Vitreous Panel. *Preferred Practice Pattern® Guidelines. Diabetic Retinopathy*. San Francisco, CA: American Academy of Ophthalmology; 2016. Available at: www.aao.org/ppp. Accessed September 27, 2017.
11. American Optometric Association Evidence-Based Optometry Guideline Development Group. *Eye Care of the Patient With Diabetes Mellitus*. Approved by the AOA Board of Trustees, February 7, 2014.
12. Distefano LN, Garcia-Arumi J, Martinez-Castillo V, Boixadera A. Combination of anti-VEGF and laser photocoagulation for diabetic macular edema: a review. *J Ophthalmol*. 2017;2017:2407037.
13. Diabetic Retinopathy Clinical Research Network. A randomized trial comparing intravitreal triamcinolone acetonide and focal/grid photocoagulation for diabetic macular edema. *Ophthalmology*. 1449;115(9):1447-1449.
14. Stewart MW. Treatment of diabetic retinopathy: recent advances and unresolved challenges. *World J Diabetes*. 2016;7(16):333-341.
15. Diabetic Retinopathy Clinical Research Network, Wells JA, Glassman AR, et al. Aflibercept, bevacizumab, or ranibizumab for diabetic macular edema. *N Engl J Med*. 2015;372(13):1193-1203.
16. Rajendram R, FraserBell S, Kaines A, et al. A 2-year prospective randomized controlled trial of intravitreal bevacizumab or laser therapy (BOLT) in the management of diabetic macular edema: 24-month data: report 3. *Arch Ophthalmol*. 2012;130(8):972-979.
17. Jorge R, Costa RA, Calucci D, Cintra LP, Scott IU. Intravitreal bevacizumab (avastin) for persistent new vessels in diabetic retinopathy (IBEPE study). *Retina*. 2006;26(9):1006-1013.
18. Diabetic Retinopathy Clinical Research Network Writing Committee, Haller JA, Qin H, et al. Vitrectomy outcomes in eyes with diabetic macular edema and vitreomacular traction. *Ophthalmology*. 2010;117(6):1093.e3.

3.4 Cystoid Macular Edema

Munish Sharma

Donald, a 68-year-old Caucasian male, was referred for evaluation by his cataract surgeon for inadequate vision improvement in the right eye after cataract surgery. He had cataract surgery in the right eye 6 weeks ago and surgical notes indicated the surgery was complicated by floppy iris syndrome leading to posterior capsular rupture. Past ocular history was otherwise unremarkable, and he was using over-the-counter readers for near work. He had been diagnosed with diabetes 10 years ago, which was well controlled with metformin. His last blood glucose was 110 mg/dL, and he had an HbA1C of 7% during the preoperative evaluation. Additionally, he had hypertension that was controlled with lisinopril and benign prostate hyperplasia that was treated with tamsulosin (Flomax).

Clinical Findings

Unaided distance VA	OD: 20/80 (no improvement with pinhole); OS: 20/25
Subjective refraction	OD: Pl −0.50 × 060 (20/70) OS: Pl −0.50 × 120 (20/20) ADD: +2.50 (20/60 OD; 20/20 OS)
Cover test	Distance: orthophoria; near: 3Δ XP
Confrontation visual fields	Full to finger counting OD and OS
Pupil evaluation	PERRL; no RAPD
Intraocular pressure (GAT)	OD: 11 mm Hg; OS: 11 mm Hg at 3.30 PM
Slit-lamp examination	OD: 3 mm well healed cataract surgery incision on the temporal cornea; IOL in sulcus with open posterior capsule; otherwise unremarkable OS: Grade 1 nuclear sclerosis; otherwise unremarkable
Fundus examination (Figure 3.4-1)	OD: 0.3/0.3 CD ratio; healthy rim tissue with distinct disc margins; macular edema involving lower half of the fovea; normal vasculature; periphery intact OS: 0.3/0.3 CD ratio; healthy rim tissue with distinct disc margins; fovea flat and dry; normal vasculature; periphery intact
Macular OCT (Figure 3.4-2)	OD: significant macular edema OS: no macular edema present
Fluorescein angiography (Figure 3.4-3)	OD: petaloid pattern leakage in the macular area OS: unremarkable

Abbreviations. CD, cup to disc; GAT, Goldmann applanation tonometry; IOL, intraocular lens; OCT, optical coherence tomography; OD, right eye; OS, left eye; PERRL, pupils equal, round, reactive to light; RAPD, relative afferent pupillary defect; VA, visual acuity; XP, exophoria.

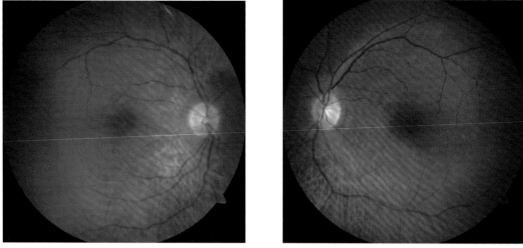

Figure 3.4-1 Edema involving inferior macula of the right eye.

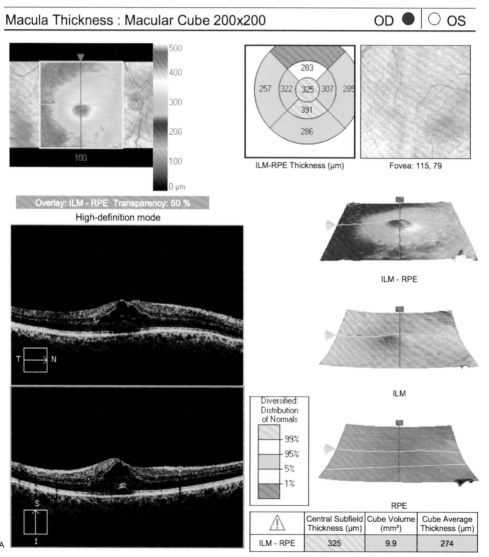

Figure 3.4-2 Optical coherence tomography showing macular edema in the right eye (A). The left eye (B) has normal macular thickness.

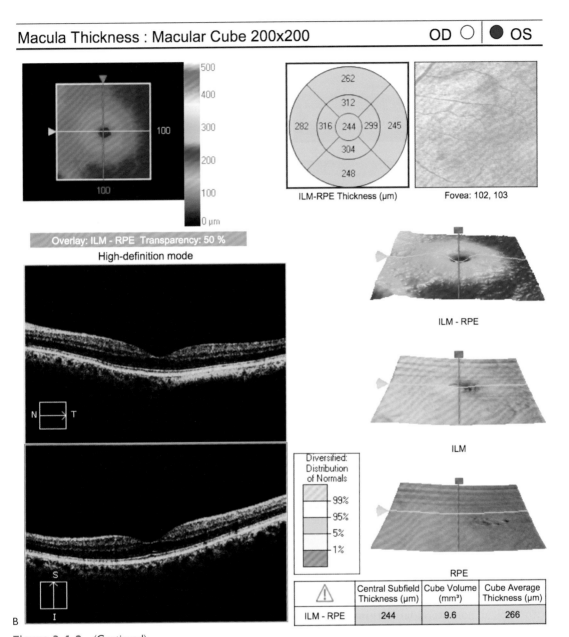

Macula Thickness : Macular Cube 200x200   OD ○ | ● OS

ILM-RPE Thickness (µm)   Fovea: 102, 103

Overlay: ILM - RPE Transparency: 50 %
High-definition mode

ILM - RPE

ILM

Diversified:
Distribution
of Normals

99%
95%
5%
1%

RPE

⚠	Central Subfield Thickness (µm)	Cube Volume (mm³)	Cube Average Thickness (µm)
ILM - RPE	244	9.6	266

B

Figure 3.4-2   (Continued)

Comments

Optical coherence tomography and fluorescein angiography confirmed the clinical diagnosis of cystoid macular edema (CME). The patient was started on topical bromfenac 0.09% (Bromday) once daily OD and difluprednate 0.05% (Durezol) 4 times a day OD. He was asked to return in 2 weeks to assure resolution of the macular edema.

Follow-up Visits (2 and 6 Weeks Following the Initial Examination)

At the 2-week follow-up visit, Donald reported good compliance and no adverse reactions to the medications. He had significant improvement of the macular edema on OCT, and his best-corrected visual acuity (VA) improved to 20/25. Intraocular pressure was 13 mm Hg OD and 11 mm Hg

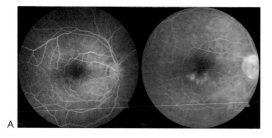

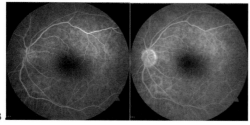

Figure 3.4-3 Fluorescein angiography demonstrating leakage of fluid in the right macula (A) consistent with cystoid macular edema. No edema is present in the left eye (B).

OS. He was advised to continue both topical medications for 2 additional weeks followed by a taper of the Durezol to twice daily for 2 additional weeks. He was asked to return in 4 weeks.

At the 6-week follow-up visit, there was a complete resolution of the macular edema confirmed with macular OCT (Figure 3.4-4). Best-corrected VA was 20/20−. All topical medications were discontinued at that time.

Discussion

Donald developed postoperative pseudophakic CME in the right eye, which resolved over time with topical non steroidal anti-inflammatory drugs (NSAIDs) and corticosteroids. There were several risk factors in this case including Flomax-associated floppy iris syndrome with the consequential complication of posterior capsular rupture during cataract surgery. This, in the presence of diabetes, compounded his risk of developing CME.

Cystoid macular edema following cataract surgery is also known as Irvine-Gass syndrome. Cystoid macular edema is one of the most common complications of otherwise uncomplicated cataract surgery,[1] and it is the leading cause of unexpected postoperative vision loss.[2]

The incidence of CME following cataract surgery varies depending on the method of detection (clinical, angiographic, or OCT),[3,4] but it has decreased with the advent of modern cataract surgery techniques to as low as 1.2%.[5] In contrast, clinically significant macular edema (CSME) occurs postoperatively in up to 56% of diabetic patients with mild-to-moderate non-proliferative diabetic retinopathy but no diabetic macular edema preoperatively.[1]

In addition to cataract surgery, CME is associated with several other ocular conditions. Various mechanisms have been implicated in the development of CME. These include vascular instability either due to ischemia (associated with retinal vein occlusion and diabetes) or dystrophy (with retinitis pigmentosa and retinal telangiectasia), retinal degeneration (associated with age-related macular degeneration), mechanical forces (implicated with vitreomacular traction), operating microscope phototoxicity (following ocular surgery), and topical prostaglandin analogue therapy (with glaucoma).[2,6] The most accepted mechanism for CME following cataract surgery is inflammation (post-uveitis) triggered either with leukotrienes via the lipoxygenase pathway or with prostaglandins via the cyclooxygenase pathway. This inflammation leads to disruption of the blood-retinal barrier and leakage of perifoveal capillaries.[2,7] The resultant fluid generally accumulates as intraretinal cysts in the inner nuclear and outer plexiform layers of the macula producing a petaloid pattern following the distribution of Henle's fiber layer. Edema of the outer nuclear layer and subretinal area has been reported. The CME generally starts 6 to 8 weeks following cataract surgery but can occur as early at week 2.

Although CME may resolve spontaneously, it carries a risk of permanent impairment of central acuity or loss of contrast sensitivity.[7] Corticosteroids and topical NSAIDs, either as monotherapy or combined therapy, are the first-line treatment approach.[2,7] When this approach is ineffective, intravitreal application of corticosteroids or anti-vascular endothelial growth factor agents may be an option.[7] Additionally, prophylaxis with topical steroids and NSAIDs is known to decrease the odds of

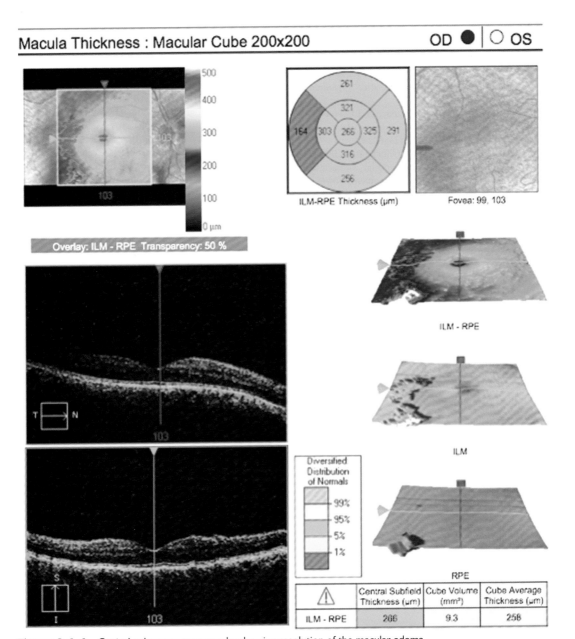

Figure 3.4-4 Optical coherence tomography showing resolution of the macular edema.

developing CME postoperatively, especially in high-risk patients including those with diabetic retinopathy, recent uveitis, complicated cataract surgery, and those with a history of retinal vein occlusion.[1,6,7]

For Donald's left eye, Flomax was discontinued 2 weeks prior to surgery, and the patient was prophylactically started on topical NSAIDs and steroids. The patient had a better intraoperative dilation and a faster visual recovery with no CME in the left eye.

CLINICAL PEARLS

- Complicated cataract surgery, as well as diabetes, can put the patient at a higher risk of developing macular edema following the surgery.

- Prophylaxis with topical steroids and NSAIDs is known to decrease the odds of developing CME postoperatively, especially in high-risk patients.

REFERENCES

1. Wielders LHP, Lambermont VA, Schouten JSAG, et al. Prevention of cystoid macular edema after cataract surgery in nondiabetic and diabetic patients: a systematic review and meta-analysis. *Am J Ophthalmol.* 2015;160(5):968-981.
2. Grzybowski A, Sikorski BL, Ascaso FJ, Huerva V. Pseudophakic cystoid macular edema: update 2016. *Clin Interv Aging.* 2016;11:1221-1229.
3. Wetzig PC, Thatcher DB, Christiansen JM. The intracapsular versus the extracapsular cataract technique in relationship to retinal problems. *Trans Am Ophthalmol Soc.* 1979;77:339-347.
4. Levitz L, Reich J, Roberts TV, Lawless M. Incidence of cystoid macular edema: femtosecond laser-assisted cataract surgery versus manual cataract surgery. *J Cataract Refract Surg.* 2015;41(3):683-686.
5. Chu CJ, Johnston RL, Buscombe C et al. Risk factors and incidence of macular edema after cataract surgery: a database study of 81984 eyes. *Ophthalmology.* February 2016;123(2):316-323.
6. Lim BX, Lim CH, Lim DK, Evans JR, Bunce C, Wormald R. Prophylactic non-steroidal anti-inflammatory drugs for the prevention of macular oedema after cataract surgery. *Cochrane Database Syst Rev.* November 1, 2016;11:CD006683.
7. Sheppard JD. Topical bromfenac for prevention and treatment of cystoid macular edema following cataract surgery: a review. *Clin Ophthalmol (Auckland, NZ).* 2016;10:2099-2111.

3.5 Central Serous Retinopathy

Amiee Ho

Lexi, a 44-year-old African American female, presented with a complaint of a constant black dot in the center of her vision for the past 2 days. In addition, she mentioned blur at near, as well as headaches located temporally on both sides of the head over the past 2 days. She denied seeing flashes of light, floaters, or a curtain over her vision.

She reported that she was generally in good health, but she was under a lot of stress. Her brother was incarcerated a few months ago, and she had taken custody of her brother's 2 small children. Since that time, she had noted her hair falling out, flaking skin, and painful, irregular menses. She was not experiencing lactation. She was being treated by her naturopathic doctor for thyroid and adrenal gland dysfunction. She reported taking herbal supplements, including bilberry, eyebright, turmeric, ginger, garlic, adrenal support, and maca extract. She was not using any systemic or topical corticosteroids. She denied a personal or family history of hypertension, diabetes, glaucoma, or blindness.

Clinical Findings

Unaided distance VA	OD: 20/25 (no improvement with pinhole); OS: 20/20
Pupil evaluation	PERRL; no RAPD
Extraocular muscles evaluation	Smooth, accurate, and full OU
Confrontation visual fields	Full to finger counting OD and OS
Slit-lamp examination	OD: unremarkable OS: unremarkable
Intraocular pressures (GAT)	OD: 13 mm Hg; OS: 14 mm Hg at 2:20 PM
Fundus examination (Figure 3.5-1)	OD: 0.4/0.4 CD ratio; healthy rim tissue with distinct disc margins; 1 disc diameter macular edema involving the fovea; normal vasculature; periphery intact OS: 0.4/0.4 CD ratio; healthy rim tissue with distinct disc margins; fovea flat and dry; normal vasculature; periphery intact
Amsler grid	OD: no wavy lines or missing areas; black spot noted temporal to fixation OS: no wavy lines or missing areas
Red desaturation	Right eye was lighter (80%) compared to the left eye
Color testing (Ishihara)	8/8 plates correctly identified OD and OS
Visual fields (Humphrey 30-2 SITA-Fast, Figure 3.5-2)	OD: no significant defects OS: no significant defects
Macular OCT (Figure 3.5-3)	OD: edema involving the outer retinal layers OS: normal foveal thickness and architecture

Abbreviations: CD, cup to disc; GAT, Goldmann applanation tonometry; OCT, optical coherence tomography; OD, right eye; OS, left eye; OU, both eyes; PERRL, pupils equal, round, reactive to light; RAPD, relative afferent pupillary defect; VA, visual acuity.

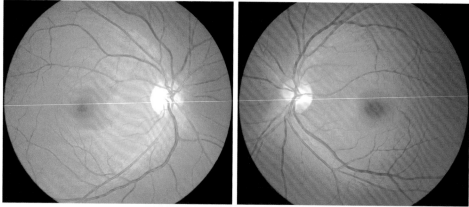

Figure 3.5-1   Fundus photos showing edema in the macular area of the right eye. The left eye was unremarkable.

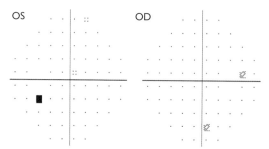

Figure 3.5-2   The visual field demonstrated no significant defects of either eye.

Follow-up Visits (4 Weeks, 3 Months, and 6 Months Following the Initial Examination)

Laboratory testing results	CBC, cortisol, luteinizing hormone, prolactin, growth hormone, TSH, T3, and T4 levels were within normal limits. Follicle stimulating hormone was high at 64.6 mIU/mL (norm 1.5-17.7)
Visual acuity (at 6 months)	OD: 20/20; OS: 20/20
Refraction (at 6 months)	OD: +0.75 −0.50 × 092 (20/20+); OS: +0.50 sph (20/15); ADD: +1.00 (20/20 OU)

Macular OCT (at 6 months, Figure 3.5-4)	OD: no edema; disruption of the RPE and photoreceptors in the foveal area OS: unremarkable

Abbreviations: CBC, complete blood count; OCT, optical coherence tomography; OD, right eye; OS, left eye; OU, both eyes; RPE, retinal pigment epithelium.

Discussion

Lexi's fundus appearance and optical coherence tomography (OCT) were consistent with central serous retinopathy (CSR). Generally, this is a self-limiting condition. However, due to the reported thyroid and adrenal cortex dysfunction, as well as other symptoms the patient was experiencing, including irregular menses, we were concerned about a pituitary lesion. For this reason, we performed a visual field and laboratory testing. Each of the systems causing Lexi's symptoms are regulated by the pituitary gland. For example, adrenocorticotropic hormone is released by the anterior pituitary gland. This then travels to the adrenal cortex causing corticosteroid release into the blood stream. Excess exogenous or endogenous corticosteroids can result in CSR, and increased endogenous corticosteroids due to pituitary adenoma has been reported.[1] Lexi's follicle stimulating hormone (FSH), which is also controlled by the pituitary gland, was high,

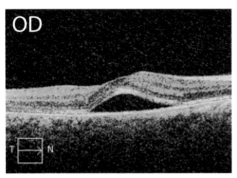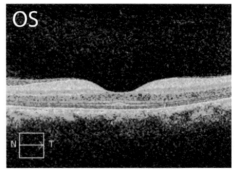

Figure 3.5-3   Macular optical coherence tomography demonstrating macular edema consistent with central serous retinopathy.

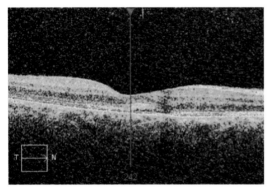

Figure 3.5-4   Macular optical coherence tomography of the right eye 6 months after the onset of her symptoms showing mild retinal pigment epithelium and photoreceptor disruption.

but there were no other indicators of pituitary dysfunction. Thyroid-stimulating hormone, which when released from the pituitary gland will cause T3 and T4 release from the thyroid gland, was normal. Her prolactin level was also normal, consistent with her report of lack of lactation. We recommended that she see a gynecologist for further evaluation of the FSH level and irregular menses, but she wanted to continue care with her naturopathic doctor. In addition, we prescribed single-vision reading glasses, which helped with her headaches. The headaches were most likely due to impending presbyopia, as well as the strain from not being able to use both eyes together during the acute stages of CSR.

In CSR, fluid accumulates in the macular region underneath the neurosensory retina forming a subsensory retinal detachment. In addition, fluid can accumulate underneath

the retinal pigmented epithelium to form pigmented epithelial detachments, observed in 53% to 100% of CSR cases.[2]

Men are more likely to be affected by CSR than women. Between 72% and 88% of CSR cases occur in men.[2] Traditionally, the age range is estimated to be 25 to 50 years[3]; however, more recent studies suggest a higher mean age range of 39 to 51 years.[2] Women with CSR tend to be slightly older. Central serous retinopathy occurs more frequently during pregnancy, particularly during the third trimester, and generally resolves spontaneously after delivery.[4] Although the prevalence in ethnic groups is controversial, some studies have found that CSR is more prevalent and severe among the Asian population, with atypical bilateral and multifocal presentations.[2] The incidence is also high in the Caucasian and Hispanic groups. African Americans seem to have the lowest incidence; however, when CSR is observed in African Americans, the condition tends to be more visually devastating and severe.[2]

There is an increased likelihood of CSR occurring in patients with increased corticosteroid concentrations, whether it be from exogenous or endogenous origins.[3] Exogenous sources can include oral, intravenous, nasal, or topical steroids. Endogenous sources may arise from increased psychological or physiologic stress (as seen with a type A personalities), a medical condition such as Cushing syndrome, or transient hormone changes in pregnancy. As mentioned earlier, increased endogenous corticosteroids due to pituitary adenoma has been reported. There is a higher incidence of

CSR in patients with rheumatic or inflammatory conditions such as systemic lupus erythematosus.[3] This is likely due to a combination of systemic steroid treatment and inflammatory events that weaken the choroid and retinal pigment epithelium (RPE).[5] Other possible conditions associated with CSR include cardiovascular disease, hypertension, sympathetic–parasympathetic imbalance, gastroesophageal disorders, and obstructive sleep apnea.[2] Finally, CSR is commonly idiopathic in nature.

Diagnosis of CSR is made by completing a thorough case history and dilated fundus examination. A macular OCT scan should be performed to confirm the diagnosis, looking for intact retinal layers with subretinal fluid accumulation. Further diagnostic testing, including fundus autofluorescence, fluorescein angiography, and indocyanine green angiography, can be helpful to support the diagnosis. Fundus autofluorescence detects RPE lipofuscin and will show a diminished scan signal (hypoautofluorescence) in the areas corresponding to the subretinal detachment and/or pigmented epithelial detachment.[2] Fluorescein angiography images ocular vasculature and will highlight areas responsible for the edema.[2] Indocyanine green angiography images the choroidal vasculature and will show delayed initial filling of arteries and choriocapillaris (hypofluorescence), in addition to dilation of the large choroidal vessels in the affected areas.[2]

Various studies have discovered an increase in choroidal thickness in eyes that have been affected by CSR.[2] This choroidal thickening is postulated to be a result of focal or diffuse dilation of large choroidal vessels. More anterior to the large dilated choroidal vessels are small and medium choroidal vessels that are often found to be atrophied.[2] It is postulated that the vessel atrophy is due to compressive damage from enlarged outer choroidal vessels. The atrophy of the small and medium choroidal vessels reduce RPE adhesion causing hydro-ionic

dysregulation and, ultimately, atrophy of the RPE.[2] Eventually, these alterations of the choroidal anatomy cause focal RPE barrier breakdown allowing fluid to seep under the retina or RPE, leading to CSR.[2]

Central serous retinopathy generally has a good prognosis for a spontaneous recovery to at least 20/30 visual acuity or better.[3] Therefore, close observation is usually a sufficient management. Prognosis can be worse if there is recurrent CSR, multiple or large areas of detachment, or a prolonged course of recovery.[3] In these poorer prognostic cases, referring the patient for laser photocoagulation treatment, verteporfin photodynamic therapy, or intravitreal anti-vascular endothelial growth factor (VEGF) injections can be beneficial.[2,3]

CLINICAL PEARLS

- Central serous retinopathy is generally idiopathic, but endogenous or exogenous corticosteroid levels can cause the condition.

- Listen to the patient to uncover clues that might aid in your investigation of the patient's chief concern.

REFERENCES

1. Giovansili I, Belange G, Affortit A. Cushing disease revealed by bilateral atypical central serous chorioretinopathy: case report. *Endocr Pract.* 2013;19(5):e129-e133. doi:10.4158/ep12389.cr.
2. Daruich A, Matet A, Dirani A, et al. Central serous chorioretinopathy: recent findings and new physiopathology hypothesis. *Prog Retin Eye Res.* 2015;48:82-118. doi:10.1016/j.preteyeres.2015.05.003.
3. Ehlers JP, Shah CP. *The Wills Eye Manual: Office and Emergency Room Diagnosis and Treatment of Eye Disease.* New Delhi, India: Wolters Kluwer; 2010.
4. Chumbley LC, Frank RN. Central serous retinopathy and pregnancy. *Am J Ophthalmol.* 1974;77(2):158-160. doi:10.1016/0002-9394(74)90667-9.
5. Tarabishy AB, Ahn E, Mandell BF, Lowder CY. Central serous retinopathy. *Arthritis Care Res.* 2011;63(8):1075-1082. doi:10.1002/acr.20485.

3.6 Hydroxychloroquine Retinopathy

Anna K. Bedwell and Jared Staats

Patricia, a 63-year-old Caucasian female, presented for hydroxychloroquine (Plaquenil) screening following a recommendation from her rheumatologist. She had been taking hydroxychloroquine 200 mg twice a day for the past 8 years to treat rheumatoid arthritis. She reported her weight at 160 pounds (72.6 kg) which put her daily dose at 5.51 mg/kg.

Patricia had no visual complaints. At the time of the examination, she was homeless and had been in and out of halfway houses. Her last eye examination was about 3 years ago, but she did not remember the location so we were unable to get previous records. She reported no past eye problems or family history of any eye disease, including glaucoma or vision loss. In addition to the hydroxychloroquine, she was taking levothyroxine for hypothyroidism and sertraline for depression.

Clinical Findings

Unaided distance VA	OD: 20/20; OS: 20/20
Cover test	Orthophoria distance and near
Confrontation visual fields	Full to finger counting OD and OS
Pupil evaluation	PERRL; no RAPD
Retinoscopy	OD: +0.25 sph; OS: +0.50 sph
Subjective refraction:	OD: +0.25 sph (20/15); OS: +0.50 sph (20/20)
Near ADD	+2.50 OU (20/20)
Slit-lamp examination	OD: unremarkable OS: unremarkable
Intraocular pressure (GAT)	OD: 15 mm Hg; OS: 15 mm Hg at 11:02 AM
Fundus examination (Figure 3.6-1)	OD: 0.7v/0.6 CD ratio with inferior notch; pigment dropout inferotemporal to fovea; normal vasculature; periphery flat and intact; OS: 0.45/0.45 CD ratio; healthy rim tissue with distinct disc margins; pigment dropout inferotemporal to fovea; normal vasculature; periphery flat and intact
Fundus autofluorescence (Figure 3.6-2)	OD: mild hypoautofluorescence inferotemporal to fovea; OS: hypoautofluorescence inferotemporal to fovea
Nerve fiber layer OCT (Figure 3.6-3)	OD: extensive retinal nerve fiber layer thinning superiorly and inferiorly; OS: extensive retinal nerve fiber layer thinning superiorly and inferiorly

Macula OCT (Figure 3.6-4)	OD: extensive perifoveal retinal thinning; loss of the outer nuclear layer temporally, as well as disruption of the interdigitation and ellipsoid zones temporally; OS: extensive perifoveal retinal thinning; significant loss of the outer nuclear layer, interdigitation zone, and ellipsoid zone temporally
Visual field (10-2 SITA-standard, Figure 3.6-5)	OD: diffuse depression, greatest in the superior nasal quadrant; mean deviation: −8.58 dB; OS: dense depression in superior nasal quadrant, moderate depression in superior temporal quadrant; mean deviation: −12.98 dB

Abbreviations: CD, cup to disc; GAT, Goldmann applanation tonometry; OCT, optical coherence tomography; OD, right eye; OS, left eye; OU, both eyes; PERRL, pupils equal, round, reactive to light; RAPD, relative afferent pupillary defect; sph, sphere; v, vertical; VA, visual acuity.

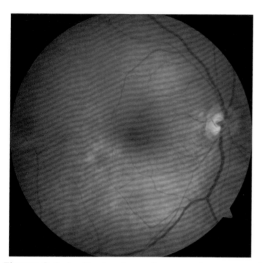
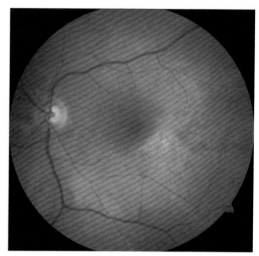

Figure 3.6-1   Fundus photos demonstrating paramacular pigmentary changes in both eyes.

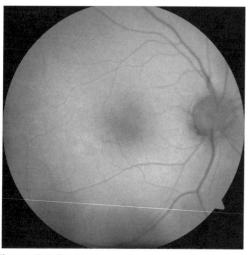
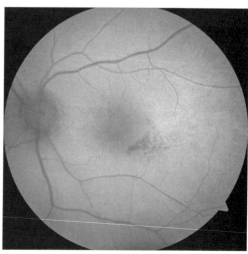

Figure 3.6-2   Fundus autofluorescence showing hypoautofluorescence inferior temporal to macula, greater in the left eye.

ONH and RNFL OU Analysis:Optic Disc Cube 200x200　　OD ● | ● OS

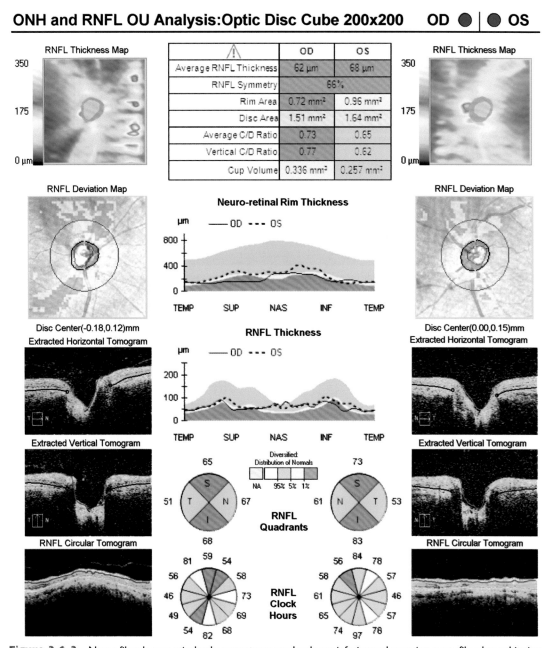

⚠	OD	OS
Average RNFL Thickness	62 µm	68 µm
RNFL Symmetry	66%	
Rim Area	0.72 mm²	0.96 mm²
Disc Area	1.51 mm²	1.64 mm²
Average C/D Ratio	0.73	0.65
Vertical C/D Ratio	0.77	0.62
Cup Volume	0.336 mm³	0.257 mm³

Figure 3.6-3 Nerve fiber layer optical coherence tomography shows inferior and superior nerve fiber layer thinning in both eyes.

Discussion

Following the American Academy of Ophthalmology recommended protocol, Patricia had a dilated fundus examination, spectral domain optical coherence tomography (OCT), fundus autofluorescence, and 10-2 automated visual field.[1] Her fundus examination and macular OCT were consistent with hydroxychloroquine retinopathy in both eyes. Because we were unable to get previous records, a preexisting retinal abnormality could not be ruled out. However, given that the examination findings were consistent with hydroxychloroquine retinopathy, it was felt that it would be in Patricia's best interest to discontinue the medication. These findings were

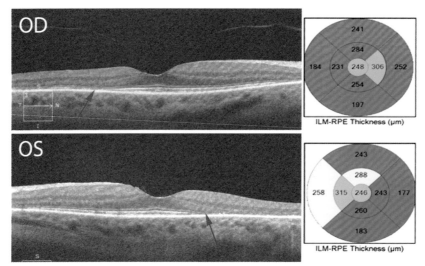

Figure 3.6-4 Disruption of the outer retinal layers is evident in both eyes with macular optical coherence tomography.

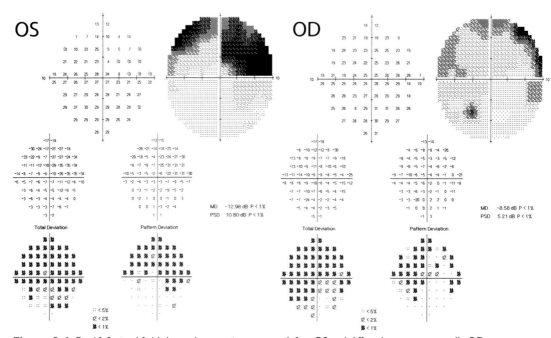

Figure 3.6-5 10-2 visual field showed a superior arcuate defect OS and diffuse loss greater nasally OD.

Abbreviations: OD, right eye; OS, left eye.

communicated to her rheumatologist, and she was taken off hydroxychloroquine and started on etanercept (Enbrel).

In addition to the hydroxychloroquine retinopathy, the optic nerve appearance and nerve fiber layer OCT were highly suspicious for normotensive glaucoma. It was difficult to differentiate the 2 conditions based on the 10-2 visual field alone. Inferior temporal fibers, those presumed to be involved in the hydroxychloroquine retinopathy, in this case, travel around the fovea to enter the inferior optic disc. The inferior disc is also a common site of damage from glaucoma. Given that the superior arcuate defect was worse in the left eye despite the more advanced cupping in the right eye, it is likely that the visual field loss was at least partially due to hydroxychloroquine retinopathy. At a later visit, a 30-2 visual field was performed, which showed that the visual field loss extended beyond 10° of fixation. Gonioscopy (which showed that the angle was open to ciliary body with minimal trabecular meshwork pigmentation and no evidence of angle recession) and pachymetry (559 micrometer OD and 566 micrometer OS) showed no further glaucoma risk factors. Ultimately, due to the optic nerve characteristics of the right eye, the patient was prescribed latanoprost (1 drop in each eye at night) for normal tension glaucoma.

Chloroquine is a 4-aminoquinilone drug used across the world for the treatment and prevention of malaria. Its analogue, hydroxychloroquine, is also used commonly to treat rheumatological and dermatological conditions. Retinal toxicity, which occurs by a mechanism that is still poorly understood, is an uncommon consequence of these medications. With a daily dose between 4.0 and 5.0 mg/kg, the risk of toxicity after 5, 10, and 20 years of treatment years is less than 1%, less than 2%, and nearly 20%, respectively.[2] The risk of retinal toxicity increases with a daily dose over 5.0 mg/kg (>2.3 mg/kg for chloroquine).[1,2] Other risk factors for maculopathy include duration of use over 5 years, renal disease, concomitant tamoxifen use, or preexisting macular disease.[1,2] This patient had 2 risk factors: 8 years of hydroxychloroquine use and daily dosage of 5.51 mg/kg.

Patients with hydroxychloroquine toxicity are often asymptomatic in the early stages. However, as the condition progresses they may report paracentral scotomas. Visual acuity is generally not affected until later in the disease process.

Current technology allows for an early diagnosis prior to the classical appearance of bull's eye pigment changes, that is, a ring of parafoveal depigmentation with foveal sparing. Fundus examination alone should not be used as a screening tool, because other methods, such as spectral domain (SD) OCT, visual field, multifocal electroretinography (ERG), and fundus autofluorescence, can detect retinal involvement earlier.[1]

The characteristic sign of toxicity on spectral domain OCT is retinal thinning, specifically dropout of the ellipsoid zone in the parafovea with preservation of the foveal photoreceptors.[3] This can advance to retinal pigment epithelium (RPE) disruption. There are generally no significant changes of the inner retinal anatomy. Photoreceptor damage is generally parafoveal, but Asian patients may have damage more peripherally, closer to the arcades.[4]

Visual field loss classically starts within 10° of fixation (most often between 2° and 6°) and develops into a ring scotoma. Approximately 10% of patients with early toxicity exhibit an obvious ring scotoma despite no apparent abnormality on SD OCT.[3] This emphasizes the need for repeated visual field testing to confirm visual field loss and the need for additional objective testing such as fundus autofluorescence or multifocal ERG.

Fundus autofluorescence will initially show hyperautofluorescence pericentrally. This may be present prior to changes on OCT. Once RPE is lost, hypoautofluorescence will occur.

Multifocal ERG evaluates electrophysiologic activity in the retina to provide a topographic measurement of retinal function. In hydroxychloroquine retinopathy, multifocal ERG shows pericentral loss demonstrated by an increased R1/R2 ratio (the average of the pericentral amplitudes, R2, is reduced compared to the amplitude of the central reading, R1).[5]

The most recent screening recommendations call for a baseline fundus examination to establish any confounding ocular condition. A visual field or OCT may also be helpful. If the patient has no other risk factors, annual screening can be deferred until the patient has been taking the medication for 5 years.[1] Screenings should include an automated visual field and spectral domain OCT.[1] A 10-2 visual field is most useful, but those of Asian descent should additionally have a 24-2 or 30-2 visual field performed.[1,4] Any visual field loss should be confirmed by an objective test. Other objective tests, including multifocal ERG and fundus autofluorescence, may also be useful.

Congenital or acquired macular disease should be considered as a differential for hydroxychloroquine retinopathy. Specifically, macular degeneration, chronic macular hole, central areolar choroidal dystrophy, benign concentric annular dystrophy, Stargardt disease, and cone-rod dystrophy can develop a bull's eye maculopathy.[6] In Patricia's case, congenital macular disease would likely have manifested earlier in life. Previous records would have helped to support this, but they could not be obtained. The absence of drusen helped to rule out macular degeneration, and the OCT was not consistent with a macular hole. Lack of family history of vision impairment, as well as having no visual symptoms and normal visual acuities, make central areolar choroidal dystrophy, benign concentric annular dystrophy, Stargardt disease, and cone-rod dystrophy less likely. This, in addition to her history of 8 years of hydroxychloroquine use, narrowed our suspicion to hydroxychloroquine retinopathy.

Vision loss from hydroxychloroquine is irreversible, and maculopathy can worsen even after the drug is discontinued. Fortunately, Patricia did not show progression over 1 year of follow-up. Patients with moderate or severe maculopathy are at greater risk for progression compared with those without visible RPE abnormalities.[7] This emphasizes the importance of early detection to minimize functional vision loss.

CLINICAL PEARL

- A patient can present with 2 separate causes of visual field loss. Each disease must be managed while keeping the other in mind.

REFERENCES

1. Marmor MF, Kellner U, Lai TY, Melles RB, Mieler WF. Recommendations on screening for chloroquine and hydroxychloroquine retinopathy (2016 revision). *Ophthalmology*. 2016;123(6):1386-1394.
2. Melles RB, Marmor MF. The risk of toxic retinopathy in patients on long-term hydroxychloroquine therapy. *JAMA Ophthalmol*. 2014;132(12):1453-1460.
3. Marmor MF, Melles RB. Disparity between visual fields and optical coherence tomography in hydroxychloroquine retinopathy. *Ophthalmology*. 2014; 121(6):1257-1262.
4. Melles RB, Marmor MF. Pericentral retinopathy and racial differences in hydroxychloroquine toxicity. *Ophthalmology*. 2015;122(1):110-116.
5. Lyons JS, Severns ML. Detection of early hydroxychloroquine retinal toxicity enhanced by ring ratio analysis of multifocal electroretinography. *Am J Ophthalmol*. 2007;143(5):801-809.
6. Ehlers JP, Shah CP. *The Wills Eye Manual: Office and Emergency Room Diagnosis and Treatment of Eye Disease*. 5th ed. Philadelphia, PA: Lippincott; 2008.
7. Marmor MF, Hu J. Effect of disease stage on progression of hydroxychloroquine retinopathy. *JAMA Ophthalmol*. 2014;132(9):1105-1112.

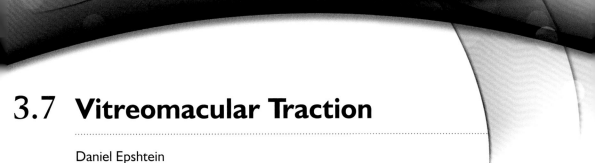

3.7 Vitreomacular Traction

Daniel Epshtein

Amy, a 74-year-old South Asian female, presented with dryness and intermittent blur in both eyes, which was incompletely relieved with artificial tears 2 times a day in both eyes. She had experienced these symptoms since having cataract surgery 2 years ago and had attempted to self-medicate with over-the-counter artificial tears. Amy also reported a small bubble in the central vision of both eyes. She had first noted this 4 months prior and denied any change since onset. Medical history was positive for type 2 diabetes and hypertension, which were controlled with metformin and lisinopril, respectively. She reported her last fasting blood glucose as 134 mg/dL and HbA1c as 7.4%.

Clinical Findings

Unaided distance VA	OD: 20/30 (no improvement with pinhole); OS: 20/30+ (pinhole 20/25^{-2})
Present Rx	+2.50 D over-the-counter reading glasses
Blood pressure	136/80 mm Hg
Confrontation visual fields	Full to finger counting OD and OS
Pupil evaluation	PERRL; no RAPD
Subjective refraction	OD: Pl −0.50 × 090 (20/30); OS: Pl −0.50 × 090 (20/25)[a]
Near ADD	+2.50 OU (20/30 at near)
Slit-lamp examination	OD: mild meibomian gland dysfunction with lid notching; trace superficial punctate keratitis inferiorly; corneal incision scars temporally and superiorly; centered IOL with trace posterior capsular haze OS: mild meibomian gland dysfunction with lid notching; trace superficial punctate keratitis inferiorly; corneal incision scars temporally and inferiorly; centered IOL with trace posterior capsular haze
Intraocular pressure (GAT)	OD: 18 mm Hg; OS: 19 mm Hg at 2:32 PM
Fundus examination	OD: 0.6/0.6 CD ratio; healthy rim tissue with distinct disc margins; fovea flat and dry with no foveal reflex; mild arteriolar attenuation; posterior vitreous detachment present; periphery intact OS: 0.6/0.6 CD ratio; healthy rim tissue with distinct disc margins; fovea flat and dry with no foveal reflex; mild arteriolar attenuation; posterior vitreous detachment present; periphery intact

Macular OCT (Figure 3.7-1)   OD: vitreous traction of the inner retina layers in the foveal area; outer nuclear layer, ellipsoid zone, interdigitation zone, and RPE/Bruch's complex have mild disruption

OS: vitreous traction of the inner retina layers in the foveal area; outer nuclear layer, ellipsoid zone, and interdigitation zone are intact

Abbreviations: CD, cup to disc; D, diopters; GAT, Goldmann applanation tonometry; IOL, intraocular lens; OCT, optical coherence tomography; OD, right eye; OS, left eye; OU, both eyes; PERRL, pupils equal, round, reactive to light; RAPD, relative afferent pupillary defect; RPE, retinal pigment epithelium; Rx, prescription; VA, visual acuity.

ª Fluctuations in vision during the refraction were noted.

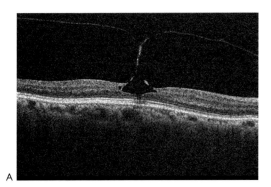

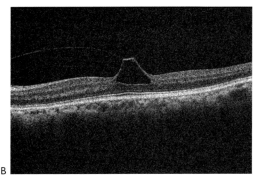

Figure 3.7-1 Vitreomacular traction is seen in the right (A) and left (B) eye. There is mild disruption of the outer retinal layers in the right eye.

Comments

Amy had several ocular issues that needed to be evaluated. Her complaint of dryness and fluctuating vision was felt to be due to meibomian gland dysfunction. We recommended warm compresses once daily in both eyes and gave her a prescription for cyclosporine ophthalmic emulsion 0.05% (Restasis) to be used twice daily in both eyes. She was told to discontinue the use of artificial tears. Although the dryness was causing inferior punctate keratitis, this was not felt to account for the decreased best-corrected visual acuities (VAs).

The patient's vasculopathic history was mildly uncontrolled but no significant ocular manifestations were noted. Strict blood pressure and glucose control were stressed to the patient and a consultation letter was written to the patient's primary care doctor.

Although trace posterior capsular haze was noted in both eyes, it was not thought to be the etiology of the reduced vision due to the symmetric and extremely mild haze. This was contrary to the asymmetrically reduced visual acuity.

Fundoscopy revealed loss of a foveal reflex, a nonspecific sign of maculopathy, and a possible etiology of the reduced vision. Due to the patient's complaint of metamorphopsia, reduced vision, and loss of a foveal reflex, a macular optical coherence tomography (OCT) was performed. The macular OCT revealed vitreomacular traction in both eyes with mild outer retinal disruption in the right eye. The patient was apprised of all findings and educated on the risks and benefits of intervention. The patient reported that she was not too bothered by the visual disturbance; therefore, no intervention was deemed necessary. The patient was asked to follow-up in 3 months, at which time her dry eye would also be assessed.

Follow-up Visit (3 Months Following the Initial Examination)

Amy reported compliance and relief of the dryness with Restasis but admitted to not completing the warm compresses. She reported improved subjective vision and that the central bubble in her vision had begun to fade.

Unaided distance VA	OD: 20/25; OS: 20/25
Pinhole distance VA	OD: 20/25; OS: 20/25
Slit-lamp examination	OD: no superficial punctate keratitis; otherwise stable from previous visit OS: no superficial punctate keratitis; otherwise stable from previous visit
Intraocular pressure (GAT)	OD: 19 mm Hg; OS: 20 mm Hg at 8:32 AM
Fundus examination	OD: stable from previous visit OS: stable from previous visit
Macular OCT (Figure 3.7-2)	OD: no vitreomacular traction; break in the internal limiting membrane and disruption of Henle's fiber layer; mild disruption of the outer nuclear layer, ellipsoid zone, and interdigitation zone OS: no vitreomacular traction; disruption of the internal limiting membrane with cystic spaces within Henle's fiber layer; outer nuclear layer, ellipsoid zone, and interdigitation zone are intact

Abbreviations: GAT, Goldmann applanation tonometry; OCT, optical coherence tomography; OD, right eye; OS, left eye; VA, visual acuity.

Discussion

Macular OCT revealed spontaneous release of the vitreomacular traction with resultant improvement in the retinal disruption. This correlated to improvement in the patient's metamorphopsia. Small pseudocysts remained, but no treatment was required. Additionally, with the dry eye treatment, Amy had

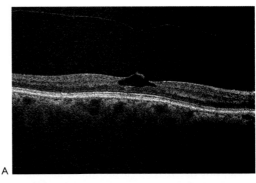
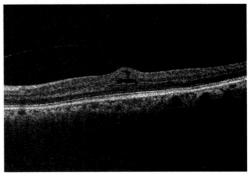

Figure 3.7-2 The vitreomacular traction has released, but pseudocysts involving the inner retinal layers remain. Right eye (A) and left eye (B).

subjective improvement in her ocular comfort and vision that correlated with her improved corneal appearance. Although it would be difficult to definitively differentiate the etiology of her decreased best-corrected vision, the asymmetric visual acuity seemed to correspond to the asymmetric retinal disruption, whereas the corneal findings were symmetric and not affecting the central cornea. The posterior capsular haze was stable at the follow-up visit and thus was considered a contributor, but not the main etiology, of the decreased vision.

Vitreomacular traction is a sequela of age-related vitreous degeneration that can be accelerated in eyes that have undergone surgery or trauma or those with significant myopic elongation.[1] The typical result of age-related vitreous degeneration is a posterior vitreous detachment. Occasionally, persistent adhesion between the vitreous and retina remains following a posterior vitreous detachment. This is called vitreomacular adhesion. This causes no retinal distortion and patients will be asymptomatic. Approximately one-third of those with vitreomacular adhesion will go on to develop vitreomacular traction.[2] Vitreomacular traction is a type of vitreomacular interface disease characterized by retinal disruption due to excessive adhesion between the vitreous and macula.[3]

Patients with vitreomacular traction may be asymptomatic, or they may report blurred vision, distorted vision, metamorphopsia, or central photopsias. Vitreomacular traction may be difficult to detect by fundus examination alone, but the vitreous attachment and disruption of the foveal anatomy are easily identified with OCT. Vitreomacular traction is classified as either focal (adhesion size of $\leq 1500\ \mu m$) or broad (adhesion size of $\geq 1500\ \mu m$), and as isolated or concurrent depending on the presence of comorbid retinal disease. Retinal changes seen on OCT include foveal detachment, pseudocyst formation, foveal contour irregularity, and epiretinal membrane.[3,4]

Vitreomacular traction can result in a full-thickness macular hole. This occurs when the tractional forces associated with the vitreomacular adhesion create a pseudocyst in the foveal region. If the pseudocyst expands into the outer retinal layers, degeneration of retinal tissue occurs. The roof of the pseudocyst then detaches creating the macular hole. A small macular hole may repair itself if the vitreomacular traction is released early. A lamellar macular hole can be caused by the same process, but there will be a defect involving the inner retina only while the photoreceptor layer will remain intact.

Vitreomacular traction can spontaneously release. The probability of spontaneous resolution of isolated vitreomacular traction as assessed by OCT ranges from 26% to 43%.[5,6] Therefore, before more invasive treatment is recommended, observation is often recommended for at least 3 months, especially in cases with mild subjective complaints. In cases where patients have severe symptoms associated with vitreomacular traction or if the traction is causing enlargement of a macular hole, treatment may be necessary. Treatment options include pars plana vitrectomy or pharmacologic vitreolysis with an intravitreal injection of ocriplasmin (Jetrea).

CLINICAL PEARLS

- Patients often present with multiple signs and symptoms. A careful examination of the entire visual pathway, including a refraction and cornea, lens, and retinal evaluation can help determine proper management.

- Patients with vitreomacular traction may report blurred vision, distorted vision, metamorphopsia, or central photopsias; however, they are commonly asymptomatic.

REFERENCES

1. Johnson MW. Posterior vitreous detachment: evolution and complications of its early stages. *Am J Ophthalmol.* 2010;149(3):371-382.
2. Theodossiadis GP, Chatziralli IP, Sergentanis TN, Datseris I, Theodossiadis PG. Evolution of vitreomacular adhesion to acute vitreofoveal separation with special emphasis on a traction-induced foveal pathology. A prospective study of spectral-domain optical coherence tomography. *Graefes Arch Clin Exp Ophthalmol.* 2014;253(9):1425-1435.
3. Duker JS, Kaiser PK, Binder S, et al. The International Vitreomacular Traction Study Group classification of vitreomacular adhesion, traction, and macular hole. *Ophthalmology.* 2014;120(12):2611-2619.
4. Steel DHW, Lotery AJ. Idiopathic vitreomacular traction and macular hole: a comprehensive review of pathophysiology, diagnosis, and treatment. *Eye.* 2013;27:S1-S21.
5. Dimopoulos S, Bartz-Schmidt KU, Gelisken F, Januschowski K, Ziemssen F. Rate and timing of spontaneous resolution in a vitreomacular traction group: should the role of watchful waiting be re-evaluated as an alternative to Ocriplasmin therapy? *Br J Ophthalmol.* 2014:1-4.
6. Theodossiadis GP, Grigoropoulos VG, Theodoropoulou S, Datseris I, Theodossiadis PG. Spontaneous resolution of vitreomacular traction demonstrated by spectral-domain optical coherence tomography. *Am J Ophthalmol.* 2014;157(4):842-851.

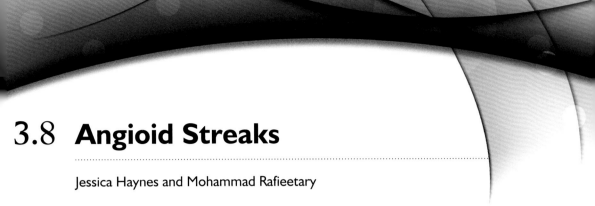

3.8 Angioid Streaks

Jessica Haynes and Mohammad Rafieetary

Adam, a 50-year-old Pakistani male, presented with a chief concern of visual distortion in the right eye that had been consistently present for 1 week. He reported that straight lines had a curve or dip in them. This was particularly bothersome at his job where he worked as a computer programmer. He had no complaints with vision of the left eye. He reported no significant personal or family ocular history. Medical history included depression, high cholesterol, acid reflux, and seasonal allergies, for which he was taking sertraline, divalproex, simvastatin, pantoprazole, and azelastine nasal spray. He reported no family history of medical illness. He denied drinking, smoking, or illicit drug use. He had no known drug allergies.

Clinical Findings

Best-corrected visual acuity	OD: 20/20; OS: 20/20
Confrontation visual fields	Full to finger counting OD and OS
Extraocular motilities	Full range of motion with no pain or diplopia OU
Pupil evaluation	PERRL; no RAPD
Intraocular pressure (Tonopen)	OD: 11 mm Hg; OS: 12 mm Hg at 9:30 AM
Slit-lamp evaluation	OD: trace cortical lens opacities; otherwise unremarkable OS: trace cortical lens opacities; otherwise unremarkable
Fundus examination (Figure 3.8-1)	OD: 0.3/0.3 CD ratio; healthy rim tissue with distinct disc margins; peripapillary pigment abnormalities with linear areas of hyperpigmentation extending from the optic nerve into the macular area; subretinal hemorrhage inferior nasal to fovea with gray elevated region superior to the hemorrhage; 2 disc diameter congenital hypertrophy of the RPE in the superior temporal midperipheral retina OS: 0.3/0.3 CD ratio; healthy rim tissue with distinct disc margins; peripapillary pigment abnormalities with linear areas of hyperpigmentation extending from the optic nerve into the macular area; fovea flat and dry; no peripheral retinal abnormalities
Peripapillary OCT (Figure 3.8-2)	OD: disruption of Bruch membrane with overlying hyperreflectance and thickening, suggestive of choroidal neovascular membrane and/or subretinal hemorrhage; hyporeflective regions consistent with serous fluid adjacent to and overlying this area OS: RPE disruption and breaks in Bruch membrane
Fundus autofluorescence (Figure 3.8-3)	OD and OS: linear regions of hypoautofluorescence suggesting RPE atrophy; patchy areas of hyperautofluorescence suggesting the RPE is undergoing metabolic stress

Fluorescein angiography
(Figure 3.8-4)

OD: early hyperfluorescence along areas of linear hyperpigmentation with minimal increase in fluorescence into later stages; early hyperfluorescence in the area superior to the subretinal hemorrhage with increased fluorescence throughout later stages

OS: early hyperfluorescence in the areas of linear hyperpigmentation with minimal increase in fluorescence into later stages

Abbreviations: CD, cup to disc; OCT, optical coherence tomography; OD, right eye; OS, left eye; OU, both eyes; PERRL, pupils equal, round, reactive to light; RAPD, relative afferent pupillary defect; RPE, retinal pigment epithelium.

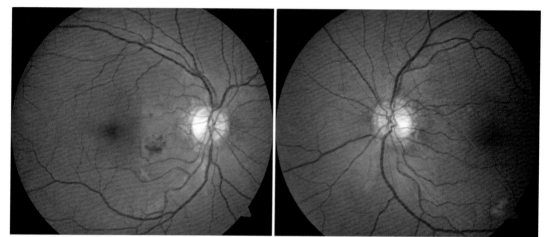

Figure 3.8-1 Fundus photography of patient with angioid streaks in both eyes and choroidal neovascularization nasal to fovea in the right eye.

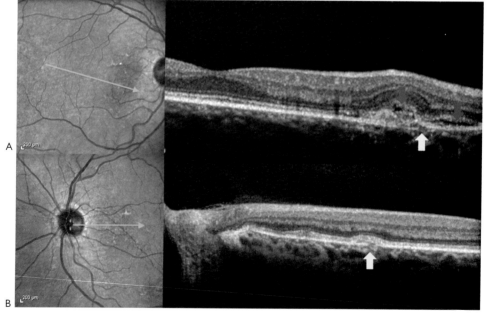

Figure 3.8-2 A, Optical coherence tomography (OCT) of the right eye showing a choroidal neovascular membrane with overlying and adjacent areas of subretinal fluid (red arrows) and a crack in Bruch membrane (yellow arrow). B, OCT of left eye showing a break in Bruch membrane (yellow arrow) corresponding to a larger angioid streak with overlying retinal pigment epithelium disruption.

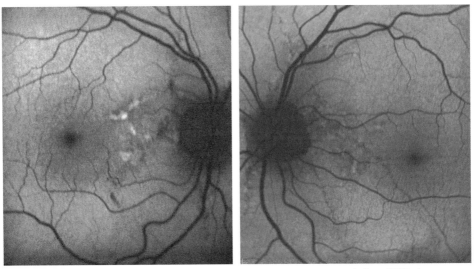

Figure 3.8-3   Fundus autofluorescence showing linear areas of retinal pigment epithelium (RPE) disruption as well as regions of RPE disruption outside of areas of visible angioid streaks in both eyes.

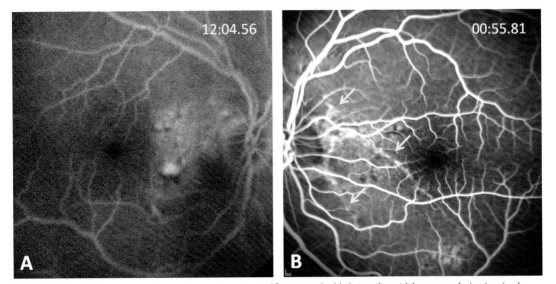

Figure 3.8-4   A, Late stage fluorescein angiography at 12 minutes highlighting choroidal neovascularization (red arrow) resultant from angioid streaks. B, Fluorescein angiography at 1 minute shows window-type defects in the regions of angioid streaks (yellow arrows).

Discussion

This patient has angioid streaks, which represent cracks or breaks in Bruch membrane. They are believed to develop because of abnormal elastin structure or increased calcification of Bruch membrane causing it to become brittle.[1]

Angioid streaks present as bilateral, deep, jagged lines of pigment abnormalities radiating away from the optic nerve. The coloration of angioid streaks varies depending on the pigmentation of the retina. In more darkly pigmented eyes they appear medium to dark brown. In more lightly pigmented eyes they are reddish or light brown. They can become darker with time, as there is increased disruption in the retinal pigment epithelium (RPE).[1] Patients often have abnormal, irregular pigmentation surrounding the optic nerve in a serrated pattern. These pigment alterations can be striking in appearance or subtle. A red-free filter can be utilized to improve visualization of angioid streaks.

On optical coherence tomography (OCT), angioid streaks show alteration of the Bruch membrane–RPE complex. Actual breaks in Bruch membrane can often be visualized. Optical coherence tomography imaging can also be helpful in identifying development of choroidal neovascular membranes.[2]

On fluorescein angiography, angioid streaks appear as a window defect with linear areas of hyperfluorescence. Since the RPE is disrupted, the fluorescent signal coming from the choroid appears brighter. Areas of choroidal neovascularization show increased fluorescence that continues to leak into late phases.[1]

Fundus autofluorescence, which is used to image the RPE by using the autofluorescent properties of lipofuscin, can also be helpful in identifying angioid streaks. Healthy RPE gives a uniformly fluorescent signal. Retinal pigment epithelium that is unhealthy can no longer properly metabolize lipofuscin, leading to lipofuscin buildup. This results in a hyperautofluorescent signal. If there is sufficient damage to cause atrophy of the RPE, there will be less lipofuscin present resulting in a hypoautofluorescent signal. Angioid streaks result in linear areas of alteration in this signal that can cause both hyper- and hypo-autofluorescence. Fundus autofluorescence may also show diffuse RPE abnormalities not visible on fundus examination.[3]

In addition to the aforementioned technologies, one can monitor angioid streaks with careful dilated fundus examinations and Amsler grid testing. Serial fundus photography is also beneficial in documenting progression of angioid streaks. If there is evidence or suspicion of choroidal neovascularization, referral to a retinal specialist for additional testing or treatment is required.

Angioid streaks are frequently associated with systemic disease but can occur idiopathically. All patients with newly diagnosed angioid streaks should undergo an appropriate systemic workup.[1] The acronym "PEPSI" is helpful in remembering the most common systemic associations of angioid streaks: **P**seudoxanthoma elasticum, **E**hlers-Danlos syndrome, **P**aget disease of bone, **S**ickle cell disease and other hemoglobinopathies, and **I**diopathic. Pseudoxanthoma elasticum is the most commonly associated systemic disease. These patients often develop yellowish papules or plaques on the skin of the neck and areas of flexure such as the elbows. They may also have cardiovascular and gastrointestinal complications.[1] Ehlers-Danlos syndrome is a group of disorders affecting connective tissue. It can be present with a wide array of complications, such as joint hyperlaxity, skin hyperextensibility, and cardiovascular complications.[4] Paget disease is a chronic bone disease with abnormal bone remodeling. These patients have increased risk of bone fracture and arthritis, among other systemic complications.[5] Individuals with sickle hemoglobinopathies may experience symptoms, such as fatigue, pain in the arms and legs, and swelling in the feet and hands, or they may be entirely asymptomatic.[6] They may also present with sickle cell retinopathy.

Angioid streaks themselves rarely result in visual disturbances unless they run underneath the fovea. Retinal pigment epithelium alterations in patients with angioid streaks can progress with time, and there is no current therapy or treatment for this process.[1] Due to breaks in Bruch membrane, choroidal neovascularization develops in up to 86% of patients with angioid streaks. These patients commonly report metamorphopsia. Left untreated, centrally located choroidal neovascularization often results in a poor visual outcome. Many therapies have been considered for choroidal neovascularization, but the treatment of choice at this time is intravitreal anti-vascular endothelial growth factor (VEGF) agents. These therapies have been shown to improve or stabilize visual acuity in many patients with resultant choroidal neovascularization associated with angioid streaks, but long-term therapy for recurrences is often required.[7]

The length of time from the development of choroidal neovascularization to the initiation of treatment is an important factor in visual prognosis.[7] Patients with angioid streaks should be carefully monitored for development of choroidal neovascularization and educated to monitor their vision monocularly with Amsler grid. Patients must understand to report immediately if visual changes are detected.

Because Bruch membrane is more fragile, patients with angioid streaks have a higher risk of choroidal rupture with even mild blunt trauma. Patients should be instructed to wear protective eyewear when playing sports or other activities where trauma is possible.

In this case, the patient was found to have no associated systemic abnormalities. He was treated with anti-VEGF agents with good response, but 4 years later he continued to have choroidal neovascularization recurrences that required maintenance treatment in the right eye. He later developed choroidal neovascularization in the left eye that required periodic anti-VEGF treatment as well.

CLINICAL PEARLS

- Patients with angioid streaks should be educated about the importance of monitoring central vision due to the potential for development of choroidal neovascularization.

- Patients with angioid streaks should be cautioned regarding increased risk of choroidal rupture from blunt trauma.

- The most common systemic condition associated with angioid streaks is pseudoxanthoma elasticum.

REFERENCES

1. Georgalas I, Tservakis I, Papaconstaninou D, Kardara M, Koutsandrea C, Ladas I. Pseudoxanthoma elasticum, ocular manifestations, complications and treatment. *Clin Exp Optom.* 2011;94(2):169-180.
2. Charbel Issa P, Finger RP, Holz FG, Scholl HP. Multimodal imaging including spectral domain OCT and confocal near infrared reflectance for characterization of outer retinal pathology in pseudoxanthoma elasticum. *Invest Ophthalmol Vis Sci.* 2009;50(12):5913-5918.
3. Finger RP, Charbel Issa P, Ladewig M, Götting G, Holz FG, Scholl HP. Fundus autofluorescence in pseudoxanthoma elasticum. *Retina.* 2009;29(10):1496-1505.
4. Malfait F, Wenstrup R, De Paepe A. Clinical and genetic aspects of Ehlers-Danlos syndrome, classic type. *Genet Med.* 2010;12(10):597-605.
5. Lalam RK, Cassar-Pullicino VN, Winn N. Paget disease of bone. *Semin Musculoskelet Radiol.* 2016;20(3):287-299.
6. Lovett PB, Sule HP, Lopez BL. Sickle cell disease in the emergency department. *Emerg Med Clin North Am.* 2014;32(3):629-647.
7. Finger RP, Charbel Issa P, Schmitz-Valckenberg S, Holz FG, Scholl HN. Long-term effectiveness of intravitreal bevacizumab for choroidal neovascularization secondary to angioid streaks in pseudoxanthoma elasticum. *Retina.* 2011;31(7):1268-1278.

3.9 Retinitis Pigmentosa

Jeung Hyoun Kim

Nina, a 38-year-old African American female, presented with distance blur for the past 6 months. She also complained of difficulty seeing at night (nyctalopia). On questioning, she admitted she had become clumsier, frequently bumping into objects around the house, particularly at night. She had not had an eye examination since she was a child. Past ocular and medical histories were unremarkable, and she was taking no medications. She did not have any remarkable family medical or ocular history.

Clinical Findings

Unaided distance VA	OD: 20/25 (pinhole 20/20); OS: 20/40 (pinhole 20/30)
Cover test	Orthophoria at distance and near
Confrontation visual fields	OD: full to finger count OS: superior and inferior temporal defect
Pupil evaluation	PERRL; trace RAPD OS
Subjective refraction	OD: −0.25 sph (20/20); OS: −0.25 −0.25 × 090 (20/30)
Slit-lamp examination	OD: unremarkable OS: unremarkable
Intraocular pressure (GAT)	OD: 16 mm Hg; OS: 15 mm Hg at 2:47 PM
Fundus examination (Figure 3.9-1)	OD 0.3/0.3 CD ratio; pink and healthy rim tissue with distinct disc margins; fovea flat and dry; normal vasculature; periphery intact
	OS 0.2/0.2 CD ratio; pale rim tissue with distinct disc margins and peripapillary atrophy; fovea flat and dry; arterial attenuation with perivascular pigmentary changes; extensive pigmentary changes denser superiorly than inferiorly extending to mid-periphery

Abbreviations: CD, cup to disc; GAT, Goldmann applanation tonometry; OD, right eye; OS, left eye; PERRL, pupils equal, round, reactive to light; RAPD, relative afferent pupillary defect; sph, sphere; VA, visual acuity.

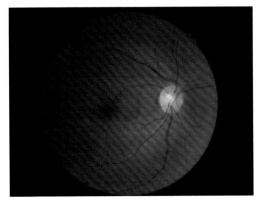 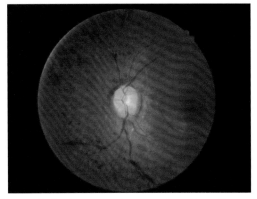

Figure 3.9-1   Typical signs of retinitis pigmentosa, including bone-spicule pigmentary changes, artery attenuation, and disc pallor, can be seen in the left eye. The right fundus does not show signs of RP.

Follow-up Visit and Supplementary Testing (1 Week Following the Initial Examination)

Visual fields (24-2 SITA-fast, Figure 3.9-2)	OD: scattered defects greater superiorly OS: significantly depressed overall visual field
Flash electroretinogram (ERG)	Scotopic ERG demonstrated reduced amplitude of both a- and b-waves with normal implicit time in both eyes. The reduction was greater in the left eye compared to the right eye (Figure 3.9-3A). Photopic flash ERG demonstrated reduced amplitude of the a-wave and borderline abnormal amplitude and implicit time for the b-wave for both eyes. The reduction was greater in the left eye compared to the right eye (Figure 3.9-3B). Flicker ERG demonstrated normal amplitude for the right eye and subnormal amplitude for the left eye (Figure 3.9-3C).

Abbreviations: OD, right eye; OS, left eye.

Discussion

Nina presented with classic signs and symptoms of retinitis pigmentosa (RP) unilaterally. Her funduscopic findings included the classic triad of RP: waxy pallor of the optic nerve, arterial attenuation, and bone-spicule like pigmentary changes. Classically RP manifests in both eyes, although it can be asymmetric.[1] In this case, the clinical presentation appeared unilateral; however, the flash electroretinogram (ERG) showed bilateral, yet asymmetric, involvement.

Retinitis pigmentosa is one of the most common inherited retinal conditions. It is considered a rod–cone dystrophy where the rod photopigments are initially affected and the cone photopigments are affected eventually as the disease progresses. Its prevalence is estimated to be 1:3000 to 1:5000. The inheritance pattern can be autosomal dominant, autosomal recessive, or X-linked, although it can occur sporadically without any genetic predisposition. More than 100 genes have been identified, most frequently affecting the phototransduction pathway.

Patients with RP typically present with concerns of decreased night vision or difficulty with dark adaptation. This can be attributed to the death of rod photoreceptors, which in turn causes release of pigment by the retinal pigment epithelium (RPE) creating a bone spicule formation in the mid and far periphery of the retina. The death of these photoreceptors creates a ring-shaped scotoma in the peripheral visual field. In most forms of generalized RP, patients lose 50% of their remaining visual

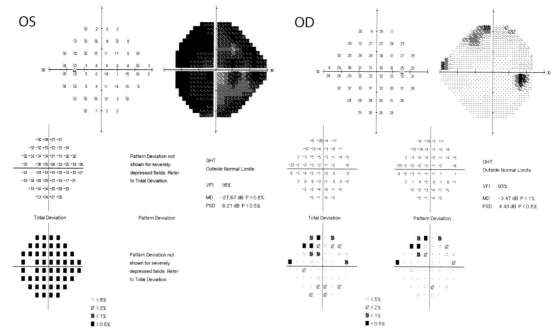

Figure 3.9-2   Superior arcuate visual field loss and mild loss inferiorly in the right eye. Severe overall depression of the left visual field.

field every 5 years. Patients may be asymptomatic until they develop tunnel vision with the loss of peripheral visual field.[2] The prognosis of RP is highly variable. Patients with X-linked RP tend to exhibit a worse prognosis, developing legal blindness due to the residual visual field being less than 20° in the better-seeing eye by the fourth decade.[3]

For a suspected rod–cone dystrophy such as RP, it is important to take baseline electrophysiology and visual fields. Flash ERG will confirm the diagnosis and also serve as a monitoring tool to measure rod and cone function.

Flash ERG is a diagnostic tool to measure the electrical activity in the retina in response to specific light stimuli. This light stimulus elicits a biphasic waveform that consists of 2 components: the a- and b-waves. The a-wave refers to the first prominent negative component and is generated by the photoreceptor cells. The b-wave refers to the subsequent positive component and is generated by inner retinal cells such as bipolar cells and Muller cells. For each component, 2 characteristics are clinically important: amplitude and implicit time. The amplitude refers to the size of each peak measured from a reference point. Implicit

time refers to the duration to reach the peak of each component measured from the onset of the stimulus.[4]

Flash ERG can be used to objectively measure retinal photoreceptor function. Depending on the test conditions, it can isolate specific photoreceptor function and associated inner retinal function. It can be performed under scotopic conditions after dark adaptation to evaluate rods and associated inner retinal function or under photopic conditions after light adaptation to evaluate cones and associated inner retinal function. In addition, a flicker at 30 Hz, rather than a single flash, can be presented to elicit the macular cone response.[4]

In conjunction with flash ERG, visual field testing is a powerful tool to monitor functional vision. Visual field loss begins with a ring scotoma pattern in the early stage and progresses to become quite severe. A small area of inferior temporal visual field is often spared even in the moderately advanced stage.[5] Instruments that test the entire visual field, such as the Goldmann perimeter, are useful since RP patients will often show mid-peripheral field loss not tested on traditional automated visual field testing.

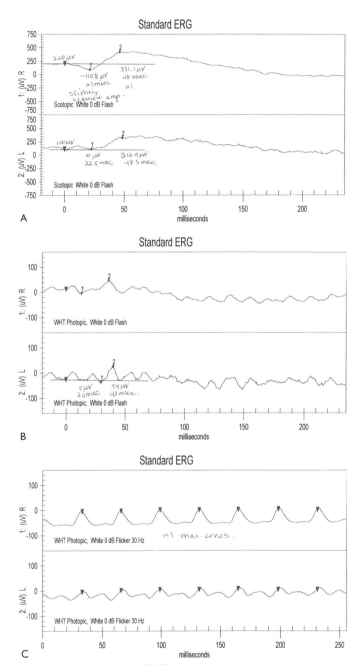

Figure 3.9-3 Scotopic flash electroretinogram (ERG) (A) shows slightly reduced amplitude in right eye and significantly reduced amplitude in the left eye. Photopic flash ERG (B) also demonstrates reduced amplitude in each eye. The 30 Hz flicker ERG (C) shows a normal amplitude for the right eye and subnormal amplitude for the left eye. The right eye is shown in the upper graph and the left eye is shown in the lower graph for each type of ERG.

In addition to electrophysiology and visual field, a dilated fundus examination should be performed every 1 to 2 years, at minimum, to monitor for ocular complications such as cystoid macular edema or posterior subcapsular cataract.

Typically, RP is considered a bilateral condition. On rare occasions, it can manifest unilaterally, in which case one would need to rule out other treatable ocular conditions that can mimic RP. Any previous insult to the retina such as trauma, infection, retinal detachment, intraocular foreign body, inflammation, or vascular occlusions can masquerade as a unilateral RP. Often, suspected cases of unilateral RP will manifest in the fellow eye eventually.[6] In the case of true unilateral RP, the condition should be monitored for at least 5 years to rule out asymmetric RP cases.[6,7]

Due to its hereditary nature, pedigree analysis and genetic counseling are helpful to discuss the risk of having progeny with RP and predict the prognosis. A low vision consultation and mobility training should be considered when necessary. Vitamin A treatment has been shown to be beneficial for certain types of RP, such as typical RP and Usher's syndrome. Other antioxidant treatments have not been consistently successful with RP patients. With the advancement of molecular and genetic technology, gene therapy is likely to become a promising treatment option for the future.[6]

CLINICAL PEARLS

- Although manifestations of RP can be atypical, such as asymmetric or sectoral involvement, it is important to remember the bilateral and progressive nature of this condition.

- When possible, order flash ERG along with a full field visual field to confirm the diagnosis and to monitor the progression of the condition.

REFERENCES

1. Bowling B. *Kanski's Clinical Ophthalmology: A Systematic Approach.* 8th ed. Philadelphia, PA: Saunders; 2015.
2. Massof RW, Finkelstein D. A two-stage hypothesis for the natural course of retinitis pigmentosa. *Adv Biosci.* 1987;62:29-58.
3. Berson EL, Sandberg MA, Rosner B, Birch DG, Hanson AH. Natural course of retinitis pigmentosa over a three-year interval. *Am J Ophthalmol.* 1985;99:240-251.
4. Daphne L. McCulloch DL, Marmor MF, et al. ISCEV Standard for full-field clinical electroretinography (2015 update). *Documenta Ophthalmologica.* 2015;130(1):1-12.
5. Fishman GA, Bozbeyoglu S, Massof RW, Kimberling W. Natural course of visual field loss in patients with type 2 Usher syndrome. *Retina.* 2007;27(5):601-608.
6. Alexander LJ. *Primary Care of the Posterior Segment.* 3rd ed. New York, NY: McGraw Hill; 2002.
7. Weller JM, Michelson G, Juenemann AG. Unilateral retinitis pigmentosa: 30 years follow-up. *BMJ Case Rep.* 2014; bcr2013202236.

3.10 Retinal Vein Occlusion

Jessica Haynes, Roya Attar, and Mohammad Rafieetary

Gloria, a 76-year-old white female, presented with a chief concern of poor vision in the right eye for 1 week. She reported dimness, blurriness, and a dark circle in the center of her vision. She could no longer read small print or see detail with her right eye. The symptoms were constantly present and did not fluctuate.

Gloria had a past ocular history of macular degeneration in each eye and also reported a family history of macular degeneration in her mother. She reported no other personal or family ocular history. Medical history included hypertension, high cholesterol, acid reflux, and hypothyroidism. She had been diagnosed with hypertension 25 years ago, and she reported that her blood pressure was currently well controlled. She was taking the following medications: aspirin 81 mg per day, clonidine 0.1 mg 4 times per day, hydrochlorothiazide 12.5 mg per day, fenofibrate 160 mg per day, pravastatin 40 mg per day, pantoprazole 40 mg per day, levothyroxine 25 mg one half capsule per day, and iCaps Age-Related Eye Disease Study 2 (AREDS2) formulation vitamins daily.

Gloria was a former smoker but had discontinued smoking 10 years ago. She denied alcohol or drug use. She had no known drug allergies. Her mood and affect were normal.

Clinical Findings

Habitual distance VA	OD: 20/200^{+2} (no improvement with pinhole); OS: 20/40 (no improvement with pinhole)
Habitual Rx	OD: −0.25 −2.75 × 075; OS: −0.75 −1.25 × 115; ADD: +2.25 OU
Blood pressure	149/87 mm Hg RAS
Confrontation visual fields	Full to finger counting OD and OS
Extraocular motilities	Full range of motion with no pain or diplopia OU
Pupil evaluation	PERRL; no RAPD
Intraocular pressure (Tonopen)	OD: 14 mm Hg; OS: 13 mm Hg at 9:55 AM
Slit-lamp examination	OD: 2+ nuclear sclerosis and 2+ peripheral cortical lens opacities; otherwise unremarkable
	OS: 2+ nuclear sclerosis and 2+ peripheral cortical lens opacities; otherwise unremarkable
Fundus examination (Figure 3.10-1)	OD: 0.3/0.3 CD ratio; mildly hyperemic optic nerve with flame shaped hemorrhages extending from the nerve; multiple flame and blot shaped hemorrhages within the macula and extending into all peripheral quadrants; macular edema was present, as well as mildly visible soft drusen partially obscured by the hemorrhages and macular edema; moderately dilated and tortuous veins in all quadrants

	OS: 0.3/0.3 CD ratio; healthy rim tissue with distinct disc margins; vascular loop versus shunt vessels located along the nasal disc margin; macula demonstrated mixture of small- to large-sized drusen with no hemorrhage present; mild increase in arterial light reflex; periphery intact
Fluorescein angiography (Figure 3.10-2)	OD: arm to retina time 18 s. Prolonged arteriovenous transit time. Early blockage from retinal hemorrhages. Early hyperfluorescence of the optic disc with continued leakage in later phases. Early leakage in petaloid appearance around fovea with continued leakage in later phases. Mild hyperfluorescence around veins in late phases. No capillary non-perfusion evident with wide-angle visualization.
	OS: perifoveal microaneurysms present exhibiting mild leakage in late phase
Macular OCT (Figure 3.10-3):	OD: macular edema with central foveal thickness of 996 microns. Mildly visible RPE disruption and drusen present.
	OS: no macular edema. Drusen present.

Abbreviations: CD, cup to disc; OCT, optical coherence tomography; OD, right eye; OS, left eye; OU, both eyes; PERRL, pupils equal, round, reactive to light; RAPD, relative afferent pupillary defect; RAS, right arm sitting; Rx, prescription; VA, visual acuity.

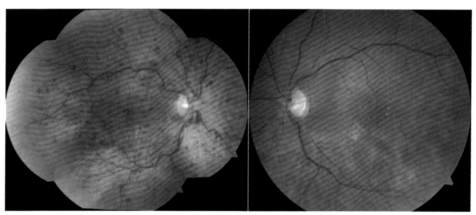

Figure 3.10-1 Central retinal vein occlusion in the right eye demonstrated by flame-shaped and blot hemorrhages throughout the retina. Small to large drusen are seen in the macula of the left eye.

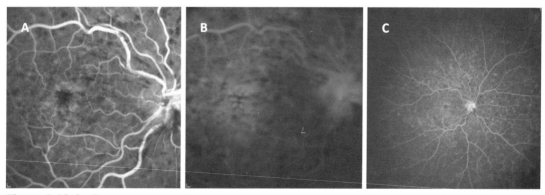

Figure 3.10-2 Fluorescein angiography shows hypofluorescence in the areas of retinal hemorrhages, mild hyperfluorescence of the optic disc, and leakage in petaloid appearance around fovea in the early stage (A). In the late stage (B) there is continued leakage around the optic disc and macula. No capillary non-perfusion evident with wide-angle visualization (C).

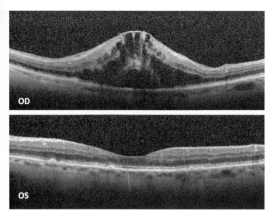

Figure 3.10-3 Macular optical coherence tomography demonstrating significant macular edema of the right eye (top). Drusen, seen as moderately reflective deposits below the retinal pigment epithelium, are present in the left eye (bottom).

Discussion

Gloria was diagnosed with central retinal vein occlusion (CRVO). Central retinal vein occlusion is a relatively common retinal vascular disease characterized by reduced outflow through the central retinal vein. Clinically, it presents with unilateral loss of vision ranging from mild to severe. A dilated fundus examination will reveal diffuse retinal hemorrhages in all 4 quadrants of the retina, as well as dilated, tortuous retinal veins. Other findings include cotton-wool spots, disc edema and hemorrhages, macular edema, and collateral or shunt vessels. Central retinal vein occlusion can cause retinal ischemia, resulting in neovascularization of the optic disc, retina, iris, or angle.[1-4]

Although the classification is not standardized, and each individual case may not conform to the classification, CRVO has traditionally been described as either ischemic or nonischemic. Ischemic CRVO typically presents with poor visual acuity (VA), often worse than 20/200, and a marked relative afferent pupillary defect (RAPD). Clinically, it has more extensive retinal hemorrhages, a greater number of cotton-wool spots, worse disc edema, and greater non-perfusion on fluorescein angiography when compared with nonischemic cases. Visual prognosis in ischemic CRVO is guarded, and visual recovery is limited by the large degree of retinal ischemia.

There is a higher risk of neovascular complication as ischemia leads to increased levels of vascular endothelial growth factors (VEGF), promoting new vessel formation.

Nonischemic CRVO typically does not cause an RAPD and acuities are generally 20/200 or better, correlating with the density and distribution of retinal hemorrhages and macular edema. Visual acuity often improves as the macular edema regresses; however, chronic macular edema can cause sustained visual damage.

Since CRVO is a chronic condition and not just an isolated event, retinal ischemia can worsen with time. Ultimately vision is limited by the extent of ischemia, as well as complications of neovascularization such as vitreous hemorrhage, tractional retinal detachment, and neovascular glaucoma.

The most common risk factor for CRVO is systemic hypertension. Other risk factors include diabetes mellitus, hyperlipidemia, atherosclerosis, smoking, inflammatory disorders, hypercoagulation diseases, glaucoma, and use of oral contraceptives.[4,5] Central retinal vein occlusion does not have a racial predilection but is slightly more frequent in males than females. Although CRVO has been reported in all age groups, more than 90% of CRVO cases occur in patients older than 50 years.[5]

Several factors are involved in appropriate assessment of CRVO. In addition to a thorough history and ocular examination, including dilated ophthalmoscopy, a number of ancillary tests should be considered. These include OCT and fluorescein angiography. Optical coherence tomography testing aids in the detection of macular edema and is extremely useful in monitoring the effectiveness of treatment for macular edema. Fluorescein angiography can evaluate the degree of retinal ischemia, giving insight into the risk of neovascularization.

While emphasis on the posterior segment is important, careful examination of anterior segment structures is also required in CRVO patients. Gonioscopy is warranted to rule out neovascularization of the angle.[6] It is suggested to perform gonioscopy 3 months from the initial presentation due to the high incidence of anterior segment neovascularization at that time. Close evaluation of the iris and documentation of the absence of iris neovascularization is good practice, as iris neovascularization can present subtly.

Ophthalmic treatment of CRVO is aimed at reducing the risk of neovascularization and decreasing macular edema. In the past decade, there has been a paradigm shift for treatment of macular edema. Intravitreal injections of VEGF inhibitors have greatly improved the visual outcome. These include bevacizumab (Avastin), ranibizumab (Lucentis), and aflibercept (Eylea).[4,7] Intravitreal injections of steroids such as triamcinolone and dexamethasone are also utilized in the management of macular edema, although the preferred treatment is generally anti-VEGF agents. This is largely due to the drastically favorable side effect profile of anti-VEGF agents over steroids.[7] Panretinal photocoagulation (PRP) and anti-VEGF agents are both utilized, often in combination, for treatment of the neovascular component of the condition. In addition, surgical intervention may be necessary for neovascular sequelae.

Management of underlying conditions is critical to improve the ocular outcome and reduce comorbidities. Hypertension and other vasculopathic disorders, as well as glaucoma, should be managed appropriately. If the etiology is unclear, a systemic workup is necessary, including laboratory tests for a hypercoagulative state. Although anticoagulants such as aspirin may be needed for systemic management of the underlying conditions, these do not alter the course of the CRVO in a positive or negative way.

Due to Gloria's age and long-term history of hypertension, additional medical workup was not pursued in this case. The patient's primary care provider (PCP) was notified of her new condition, and it was recommended that she return to her PCP to ensure adequate control of her blood pressure. The patient's macular edema was treated with bevacizumab (Avastin) intravitreal injections. One month following the first intravitreal injection, Gloria showed improved acuity to 20/70 in the right eye and significant improvement in macular edema with a reduced foveal thickness of 205 micrometers. She reported subjective improvement in visual function with resolution of the dark circle in her vision. She did not develop retinal or anterior segment neovascularization, but the macular edema became recurrent and chronic. The patient received a total of 14 anti-VEGF injections over the subsequent 7 years with final visual acuity in the right eye of 20/200.

CLINICAL PEARLS

- Central retinal vein occlusion is a common cause of painless unilateral vision loss.

- Ocular complications of macular edema and neovascularization must be addressed in patients with CRVO.

REFERENCES

1. Hayreh SS, Podhajsky PA, Zimmerman MB. Natural history of visual outcome in central retinal vein occlusion. *Ophthalmology*. 2011;118(1):119-133.
2. Gerstenblith AT, Rabinowitz MP. *The Wills Eye Manual: Office and Emergency Room Diagnosis and Treatment of Eye Disease*, 6th ed. Philadelphia, PA: Lippincott Williams & Wilkins; January 2013.
3. Wong TY, Scott IU. Retinal-vein occlusion. *N Engl J Med*. 2010;363(22):2135-2144.
4. Kiire CA, Chong V. Managing retinal vein occlusion. *Br Med J*. 2012;344:e499.
5. Citirik M, Haznedaroglu IC. Clinical risk factors underlying the occurrence of retinal vein occlusion. *Int J Ophthalmic Res*. 2016;2(1):91-95.
6. The Central Vein Occlusion Study Group. Natural history and clinical management of central retinal vein occlusion. *Arch Ophthalmol*. 1997;115:486-491.
7. Danzmann L, Pielen A, Bajor A. Anti-VEGF therapy for retinal vein occlusion. *Int J Ophthalmic Res*. 2016; 2(1):110-116.

3.11 Retinal Artery Occlusion

Jeffrey D. Perotti

Michael, a 57-year-old Caucasian male, presented with a sudden onset of inferior visual loss in his left eye that started 3 days ago. There had been no changes in symptoms since onset, and he noticed the symptoms mainly when he sat to read or play the piano. He reported no changes in distance or near visual acuity (VA) and no flashes, floaters, headaches, or additional secondary complaints.

Michael reported a 10-year history of hypertension with no additional systemic conditions. He also reported no prior ocular conditions or significant family history. He reported taking hydrochlorothiazide for hypertension, claimed no medical allergies, and was a regular tobacco user.

Clinical Findings

Unaided distance VA	OD: 20/20; OS: 20/20−
Extraocular muscle motilities	Full and accurate OD and OS
Cover test	Orthophoric at distance and near
Pupil evaluation	PERRL; mild RAPD OS
FDT screening visual fields	OD: unremarkable OS: inferior defect
Blood pressure	128/76 mm Hg RAS
Slit-lamp examination	OD: unremarkable, with no Shafer sign noted in the anterior vitreous OS: unremarkable, with no Shafer sign noted in the anterior vitreous
Intraocular pressure (GAT)	OD: 13 mm Hg; OS: 13 mm Hg at 9:42 AM
Fundus examination (Figure 3.11-1)	OD: 0.2/0.2 CD ratio; healthy rim tissue with distinct disc margins; fovea flat and dry with positive foveal light reflex; normal vasculature; periphery intact OS: 0.2/0.2 CD ratio; healthy rim tissue with distinct disc margins; fovea flat and dry with positive foveal light reflex; retinal ischemia and edema superior to the macula and within the vascular arcades; no embolus noted; periphery intact
Visual fields (24-2 SITA fast, Figure 3.11-2)	OD: unremarkable OS: central scotoma inferiorly that respects the horizontal midline

Abbreviations: CD, cup to disc; FDT, Frequency Doubling Technology; GAT, Goldmann applanation tonometry; OD, right eye; OS, left eye; PERRL, pupils equal, round, reactive to light; RAPD, relative afferent pupillary defect; RAS, right arm sitting; VA, visual acuity.

Comments

Michael was diagnosed with a superior branch retinal artery occlusion (BRAO) in his left eye and educated about his clinical findings, including the likelihood that inferior vision loss in his left eye

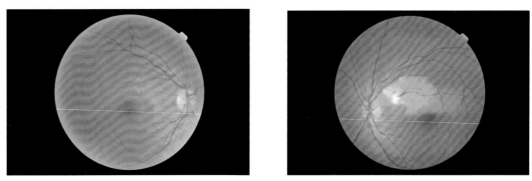

Figure 3.11-1   Fundus photos showing retinal ischemia in the left eye.

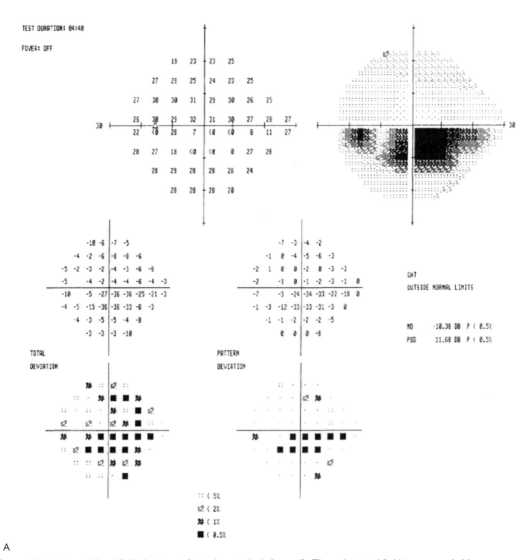

A

Figure 3.11-2   A, Visual field showing inferior loss in the left eye. B, The right visual field is unremarkable.

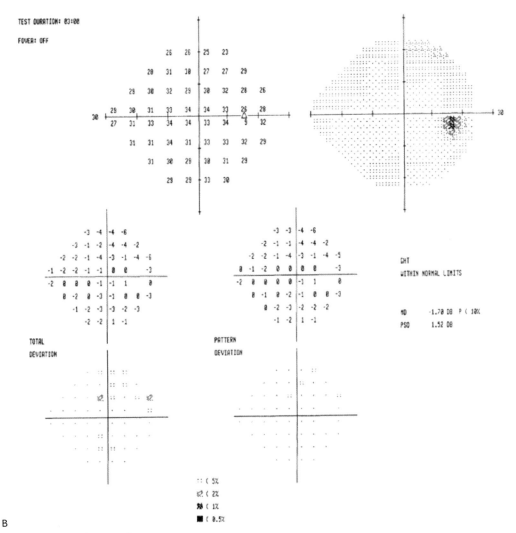

TEST DURATION: 03:00

FOVER: OFF

TOTAL
DEVIATION

PATTERN
DEVIATION

GHT
WITHIN NORMAL LIMITS

MD   -1.78 DB P (10%
PSD   1.52 DB

:: (5%
☒ (2%
▨ (1%
■ (0.5%

B

Figure 3.11-2 (Continued)

would be permanent. On further questioning, Michael reported he had not taken his blood pressure medicine for several months. During that time, he occasionally self-monitored his blood pressure and reported it to have been extremely high. One month prior to his current eye care examination, he made an appointment with his primary care provider (PCP) who reinstated his hypertension medication. The PCP later confirmed Michael's blood pressure to be 194/96 mm Hg and that medical therapy was successfully reinitiated.

After discussion with the PCP, Michael was referred to a cardiologist for additional testing. In the interim, Michael was encouraged to maintain good blood pressure control and to discontinue tobacco use. A cardiovascular workup, including tests to rule out diabetes and hyperlipidemia, a complete blood count (CBC) with differential, and a prothrombin time/activated partial thromboplastin time (PT/PTT) was requested. Other tests included an erythrocyte sedimentation rate (ESR), C-reactive protein (CRP), and platelet count to rule out giant cell arteritis, and a carotid Doppler and echocardiogram (ECG) to rule out sources of retinal emboli.[1] Michael's PCP reported that all of these tests came back negative.

Michael returned to our clinic 6 weeks after the initial visit for a follow-up examination. Although VA remained 20/20 in both eyes, he still reported inferior vision loss and trouble reading. The edema had dissipated leaving a significant nerve fiber layer defect, which corresponded to the stable visual field defect. We reviewed quality-of-life issues with him and scheduled an appointment with our vision rehabilitation service to determine if tools or techniques were available to improve his performance in reading.

Discussion

The presence of sudden inferior vision loss results in several differential diagnoses that must be ruled out. The first of these, retinal detachment, is made unlikely by the fact that the patient experienced no flashes or floaters and had no Shafer sign. Retinal detachment was ultimately ruled out on dilated examination. Next, giant cell arteritis causing arteritic ischemic optic neuropathy should also be considered in the differential. This diagnosis was ultimately excluded by a negative ESR and CRP. Based on symptoms, as well as the area of retinal ischemia, a diagnosis of BRAO was confirmed.

Retinal artery occlusion can be thought of as a stroke of the eye. It is most commonly caused by an embolism from either the carotid arteries or the heart. The occlusion may occur at the level of the central retinal artery (central retinal artery occlusion [CRAO]) or within one of the retinal arterial branches (branch retinal artery occlusion [BRAO]). Other causes of artery occlusion include giant cell arteritis and hypercoagulopathy.

Vision loss associated with retinal artery occlusion is sudden and painless. If seen within hours of the occlusion, the retina may appear normal. With time edema develops, appearing as grayish-white retinal tissue within the area normally supplied by the involved blood vessel. In the case of CRAO, there may be overall retinal whitening due to retinal edema with relative sparing of the macular tissue, which is supplied by choroidal vasculature, creating the classic cherry red spot appearance. In addition, up to 50% of the population have a cilioretinal artery.[2] This artery bypasses the retinal circulation and supplies the macular area. In cases of CRAO, patients with a cilioretinal artery may retain central areas of vision. Narrowing of the retinal blood vessels and cotton wool spots are also commonly seen in retinal artery occlusions.

An embolus is a common cause of arterial blockage in retinal artery occlusion. It is important to look for emboli in the retina downstream from the area of ischemia and to realize that emboli have the potential to migrate after the initial occlusive event. In our current case, no embolus was found. Emboli are typically cholesterol (Hollenhorst plaque), platelet-fibrin, or calcific in composition. If visible, the appearance of the embolus can aid in determining the etiology. Cholesterol plaques are yellow and refractile in nature and typically indicate carotid artery disease. Calcific material is more white and non-refractile. It is commonly found in larger arteries near the optic nerve and originates from either carotid atherosclerosis or calcified heart valves. Platelet-fibrin emboli are a pale white color and are associated with both carotid and cardiac disease.

In a recent study, 30% of patients with BRAO presented with greater than 50% ipsilateral internal carotid stenosis, 66% showed the presence of carotid plaques, and 42% presented with an embolic source identified via echocardiogram.[3] Therefore, in consultation with a cardiologist, supplemental testing should be performed to potentially identify a source of the retinal embolism. Carotid ultrasound can identify internal carotid atherosclerosis. An irregular pulse may be indicative of atrial fibrillation, which is an additional potential source of retinal emboli. Echocardiography can rule out this and other cardiac conditions.

Optical coherence tomography appearance of retinal areas affected by retinal artery occlusion depends on the chronicity of the condition. An acute artery occlusion demonstrates thickening of the inner retinal layers without intraretinal cystic spaces. With time, atrophy may manifest itself as thinning of the inner retinal layers. Optical coherence tomography angiography or fluorescein angiography can be used to demonstrate loss of capillary perfusion to the affected area.[4]

Studies have demonstrated a strong correlation between retinal artery occlusion and cardiovascular and cerebrovascular risk factors such as diabetes mellitus, hypertension, hyperlipidemia, transient ischemic attack, cerebrovascular accident, carotid artery disease, coronary artery disease, and tobacco smoking. In addition, those who have had a retinal artery occlusion are almost twice as likely to experience acute coronary syndrome.[5] Therefore, treatment and management of retinal artery occlusion is generally directed toward identifying and mitigating these underlying risk factors. An ESR and CRP is critical to rule out giant cell arteritis as a cause of retinal artery occlusion in patients elder than 60 years, and younger patients should undergo laboratory testing for coagulopathy or connective tissue disease that may cause vasculitis. If coagulopathy is found, anticoagulation therapy may be warranted. Carotid endarterectomy may be necessary if significant carotid stenosis is present. Fortunately, a vascular workup in this case did not identify significant systemic disease beyond hypertension.

Unfortunately, there is no current treatment for retinal artery occlusion that provides proven benefit to the patient.[6] Common treatment modalities are generally directed toward dislodging the retinal embolus and restoring perfusion to the affected retina, a process that should start within 4 hours of the onset of the occlusive event to reduce the risk permanent vision loss.[2,6] The need to initiate treatment immediately has hampered the ability to conduct large-scale studies on potential treatment modalities. A partial list of common treatment modalities includes ocular massage, induction of vasodilation by rebreathing exhaled carbon dioxide in a bag, lowering intraocular pressure, and antiplatelet thrombolysis with tissue plasminogen activator (tPA), a medication used to help resolve ischemic strokes. Spontaneous recovery of vision can occur, but vision loss is often permanent. Referral to vision rehabilitation services can assist patients with quality-of-life issues.

CLINICAL PEARL

- A retinal artery occlusion should be considered a stroke of the eye. As such, it generally indicates the presence of systemic cardiovascular and cerebrovascular issues, which should be ruled out emergently.

REFERENCES

1. Branch retinal artery occlusion. In: Bagheri N, Wajda BN, ed. *The Wills Eye Manual: Office and Emergency Room Diagnosis and Treatment of Eye Disease.* 7th ed. Philadelphia, PA: Wolters Kluwer; 2017.
2. Varma, DD, Cugati C, Lee AW, Chen CS. A review of central retinal artery occlusion: clinical presentation and management. *Eye.* 2013;27:688-697.
3. Hayreh SS, Podhajsky PA, Zimmerman MB. Retinal artery occlusion: associated systemic and ophthalmic abnormalities. *Ophthalmology.* 2009;116:1928-1936.
4. Coady PA, Cunningham ET, Vora RA, et al. Spectral domain optical coherence tomography findings in eyes with acute ischaemic retinal whitening. *Br J Ophthalmol.* 2015;99:586-592.
5. Chang Y-S, Chu C-C, Weng S-F, et al. The risk of acute coronary syndrome after retinal artery occlusion: a population-based cohort study. *Br J Ophthalmol.* 2015; 99:227-231.
6. Hayreh SS. Acute retinal arterial occlusive disorders. *Prog Retin Eye Res.* September 2011;30(5):359-394.

3.12 **Peripheral Retinal Lesions**

Kyla S. Duchin and Priscilla A. Lenihan

Mark, a 52-year-old Caucasian male, presented for a routine eye examination. He was satisfied with his corrected vision but was interested in obtaining a new pair of eyeglasses. He wore prescription eyeglasses for distance and used +1.00 over-the-counter readers for near work. On questioning, he denied flashes of light or floaters in his vision. He had not had an eye examination in 8 years and no past eye records were available for review. Mark had no known family history of ocular disease and denied a history of eye injuries or surgeries. Mark's medical history was significant for erectile dysfunction for which he took sildenafil.

Clinical Findings

Habitual distance VA	OD: 20/25; OS: 20/20
Habitual Rx	OD: −0.25 −0.50 × 095; OS: −0.25 −0.75 × 072
Confrontation visual fields	Full to finger counting OD and OS
Cover test	Orthophoria at distance; 4Δ XP at near
Extraocular muscles	Smooth, accurate, full, and extensive OD and OS
Pupil evaluation	PERRL; no RAPD
Subjective refraction	OD: −0.25 −0.75 × 100 (20/20); OS: −0.25 −1.00 × 080 (20/20)
	ADD: +1.75 OU
Intraocular pressure (non-contact tonometry)	OD: 18 mm Hg; OS: 17 mm Hg 2:21 PM
Slit-lamp examination	OD: unremarkable
	OS: unremarkable
Fundus examination	OD: 0.3/0.3 CD ratio; healthy rim tissue with distinct disc margins; fovea flat and dry; normal vasculature; horseshoe tear in the nasal retina with no subretinal fluid and minimal surrounding pigment; no Shafer sign or vitreous detachment
	OS: 0.3/0.3 CD ratio; healthy rim tissue with distinct disc margins; fovea flat and dry; normal vasculature; periphery intact

Abbreviations: CD, cup to disc; OD, right eye; OS, left eye; OU, both eyes; PERRL, pupils equal, round, reactive to light; RAPD, relative afferent pupillary defect; Rx, prescription; VA, visual acuity; XP, exophoria.

Discussion

Mark presented to our clinic for a routine comprehensive examination wishing only to obtain an updated pair of eyeglasses. It was only after having a dilated fundus examination that a horseshoe tear was found incidentally. He was diagnosed with an asymptomatic horseshoe retinal tear in the right eye. We educated him on the signs and symptoms of retinal detachment, including new onset floaters, flashes of light, or loss of vision. He was advised to return to our clinic immediately if any of these symptoms occurred. We recommended that Mark be seen by a retinal specialist within 1 month and referred him to a local provider. He was seen by the retina specialist 6 weeks after the initial examination. The retina specialist also noted the small nasal horseshoe tear in the right eye posterior to a prominent oral bay with minimal pigmentation present. Mark was advised that a long-standing asymptomatic tear may remain stable, but laser retinopexy was recommended. Mark declined treatment, preferring to monitor the retinal tear, and he was referred back to our office. All findings remained stable 6 months after his initial presentation. We continue to monitor this asymptomatic retinal tear annually with dilated fundus examinations.

A horseshoe tear, also known as a flap or U-shaped tear, is a full thickness, U-shaped break in the neurosensory retina that occurs due to vitreous traction (Figure 3.12-1). A flap of torn retinal tissue forms where the retina remains attached to the vitreous gel. Pigment associated with a retinal break indicates that the break is not acute. The pigment can serve as a barrier preventing liquid vitreous from entering the subretinal space and causing a retinal detachment. As with other defects in the retina, these tears can be symptomatic or asymptomatic. A symptomatic break is one that is associated with new onset flashes and/or floaters or one that occurs due to vitreoretinal traction in a patient with a new posterior vitreous detachment (PVD). The incidence of asymptomatic retinal tears is unclear; however, retinal tears are found in approximately 10% to 15% of patients with a symptomatic PVD.[1,2]

Treatment for retinal tears involves the prompt creation of a chorioretinal adhesion surrounding the retinal break using either photocoagulation or cryotherapy. Because only approximately 5% of eyes with asymptomatic horseshoe tears will progress to retinal detachment,[3-5] these tears are often observed carefully. Conversely, as many as half of symptomatic retinal breaks with persistent vitreoretinal traction will lead to a clinical retinal detachment.[6-8] When treatment is applied, the risk of retinal detachment is reduced to less than 5%.[7,8]

In addition to symptomatic and asymptomatic retinal tears, other peripheral retinal lesions can be precursors to retinal detachment including lattice degeneration, cystic retinal tufts, atrophic holes, and operculated breaks.

Lattice Degeneration

Lattice degeneration (Figure 3.12-2), present in 6% to 8% of the population,[9] is a peripheral area of retinal thinning associated with overlying vitreous liquefaction and firm vitreoretinal adhesions at the margins. Lattice degeneration is typically oval in shape running in bands parallel to the ora serrata. Round holes are frequently found within lattice degeneration. Although the presence of lattice degeneration increases the risk of retinal detachment, prophylactic treatment is not recommended.[9]

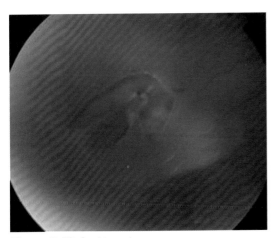

Figure 3.12-1 Horseshoe tear.

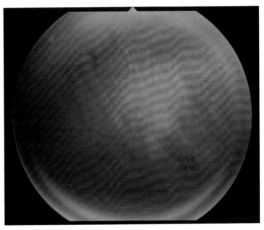

Figure 3.12-2 Lattice degeneration.

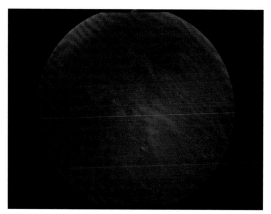

Figure 3.12-3   Retinal tuft.

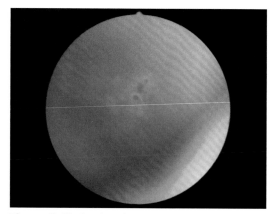

Figure 3.12-4   Atrophic retinal holes.

Retinal Tufts

Retinal tufts (Figure 3.12-3) are small, congenital lesions in the peripheral retina where the retina is firmly attached to the overlying vitreous cortex. These lesions are usually white, slightly elevated, and may have associated pigmentation. They are sometimes the cause of a retinal tear following a PVD.[10] Because the risk of retinal detachment due to cystic retinal tufts is very low, prophylactic treatment is not recommended; however, careful monitoring with annual dilated fundus examination is advised.[11]

Atrophic Holes

Full thickness retinal defects that are unrelated to vitreoretinal traction are called atrophic retinal breaks or holes (Figure 3.12-4). These can be associated with lattice degeneration or they can be in the area of an otherwise normal appearing retina. Again, the risk of retinal detachment is very low and prophylactic treatment is not recommended.[10]

Operculated Retinal Break

In the case of an operculated retinal break, retinal tissue at the site of vitreoretinal traction is pulled completely away from the retina (the operculum) leaving a defect in the retina. Even in the case of symptomatic operculated breaks, a retinal detachment is unlikely to occur unless the vitreous remains adherent to the surrounding retina.[6] When a symptomatic operculated retinal break forms during a PVD, the traction in the area of the retinal break is eliminated.

In addition to retinal lesions described earlier, myopia, intraocular surgery, trauma, a history of retinal detachment in the fellow eye, or a strong family history of retinal detachments are all risk factors for retinal detachment. Having more than 1 risk factor may additionally increase the risk of retinal detachment.[10]

Regarding our patient, Mark was asymptomatic and did not have any additional risk factors for retinal detachment; therefore, careful monitoring for retinal detachment was an acceptable approach. Mark was scheduled for a 6-month follow-up, thoroughly educated on the signs and symptoms of a retinal detachment, and advised to return to clinic immediately if symptoms were to occur.

CLINICAL PEARL

- A dilated fundus examination is critical in recognizing findings that may put the patient at increased risk of retinal detachment.

REFERENCES

1. Linder B. Acute posterior vitreous detachment and its retinal complications. *Acta Ophthalmol.* 1966(suppl 87):1-108.
2. Tasman WS. Posterior vitreous detachment and peripheral retinal breaks. *Trans Am Acad Ophthalmol Otolaryngol.* 1968;72:217-224.
3. Byer NE. What happens to untreated asymptomatic retinal breaks, and are they affected by posterior vitreous detachment? *Ophthalmology.* 1998;105:1045-1050.
4. Byer NE. Rethinking prophylactic therapy of retinal detachment. In: Stirpe M, ed. *Advances in Vitreoretinal Surgery.* New York, NY: Ophthalmic Communications Society; 1992:399-411.

5. Neumann E, Hyams S. Conservative management of retinal breaks. A follow-up study of subsequent retinal detachment. *Br J Ophthalmol.* 1972;56:482-486.

6. Davis MD. Natural history of retinal breaks without detachment. *Arch Ophthalmol.* 1974;92:183-194.

7. Shea M, Davis MD, Kamel I. Retinal breaks without detachment, treated and untreated. *Mod Probl Ophthalmol.* 1974;12:97-102.

8. Colyear BH Jr, Pischel D. Preventive treatment of retinal detachment by means of light coagulation. *Trans Pac Coast Otoophthalmol Soc Annu Meet.* 1960; 41:193-217.

9. Byer NE. Long-term natural history of lattice degeneration of the retina. *Ophthalmology.* 1989;96:1396-1401; discussion 1401-1402.

10. American Academy of Ophthalmology. *Preferred Practice Pattern. Posterior Vitreous Detachment, Retinal Breaks, and Lattice Degeneration.* San Francisco, CA: American Academy of Ophthalmology. https://www.aao.org/preferred-practice-pattern/posterior-vitreous-detachment-retinal-breaks-latti-6. October 2014. Accessed April 11, 2018.

11. Andrean SD, Eliott D. Prophylaxis for retinal detachment. *Review of Ophthalmology.* https://www.reviewofophthalmology.com/article/prophylaxis-for-retinal-detachment. Published July 15, 2005. Accessed April 11, 2018.

3.13 Rhegmatogenous Retinal Detachment

Amiee Ho

Carrie, a 49-year-old female, presented with concerns of persistent floaters in the right eye for the past 7 weeks, as well as an enlarging gray spot at the bottom of her vision in the right eye for the past 5 days. She had been evaluated and diagnosed with an acute posterior vitreous detachment (PVD) 7 weeks ago. At that time, the retina had no breaks, tears, or holes, and she was told to return immediately if she noticed any changes in her vision, including flashes of light, new floaters, or vision loss. She had no complaints with her left eye.

Ocular history was significant for LASIK 15 years ago in both eyes. She had approximately 4.00 D of myopia in each eye prior to the LASIK procedure. Medical history was significant for hypercholesterolemia, allergies, postnasal drip, and a chronic cough. She was taking simvastatin for hypercholesterolemia. Family medical and ocular histories were noncontributory.

Clinical Findings

Unaided distance VA	OD: 20/50 (no improvement with pinhole); OS: 20/20
Pupil evaluation	Equal, round, reactive to light OD and OS with a trace relative afferent pupillary defect OD
Extraocular muscle motilities	Smooth, accurate, full, and extensive OU
Confrontation fields	OD: moderate constriction of inferior nasal quadrant
	OS: full to finger counting
Slit-lamp examination	OD: unremarkable
	OS: unremarkable
Intraocular pressures (Tonopen)	OD: 10 mm Hg; OS: 12 mm Hg at 4:20 PM
Fundus examination (Figure 3.13-1)	OD: 0.1/0.1 CD ratio; healthy rim tissue with distinct disc margins; mild subretinal fluid in fovea; retinal detachment from 8:00 to 1:00 with horseshoe tear at 10:30
	OS: 0.1/0.1 CD ratio; healthy rim tissue with distinct disc margins; fovea flat and dry; normal vasculature; periphery intact

Abbreviations: CD, cup to disc; OD, right eye; OS, left eye; OU, both eyes; VA, visual acuity.

Comments

Carrie was urgently referred to a retinal specialist where she was treated with pneumatic retinopexy and then a pars plana vitrectomy and scleral buckle the following day. She subsequently developed an epiretinal membrane in the right eye, and 4 months following the retinal surgery needed surgical

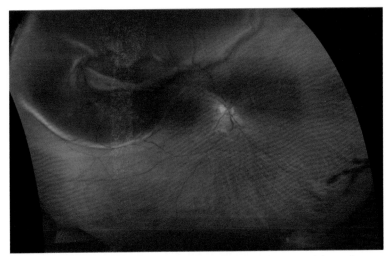

Figure 3.13-1   Fundus image of the right eye showing large retinal detachment with horseshoe tear.

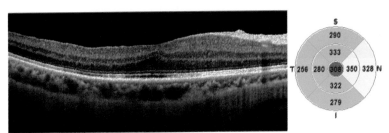

Figure 3.13-2   The macular optical coherence tomography performed 2 years following retinal detachment surgery and one and a half years following the epiretinal membrane peel shows loss of the foveal contour, as well as slight disruption of the interdigitation zone within the fovea.

removal of the epiretinal membrane because it was producing traction on the macula and reducing vision. Nearly 1 year after the retinal detachment she underwent uncomplicated cataract extraction in the right eye. Two years following the retinal detachment visual acuity was 20/30 in the involved eye. She continued to have disruption of the ellipsoid zone in the foveal area (Figure 3.13-2), as well as retinal scarring consistent with the scleral buckle (Figure 3.13-3).

Discussion

This patient presented with multiple risk factors for retinal detachment, most notably myopia and PVD. Even in low myopes ranging from 1 to 3 D, the risk of developing a rhegmatogenous retinal detachment is increased 4-fold,[1] and this risk continues to escalate as the level of myopia increases.[2]

Although a natural aging process, a PVD has the potential to cause a retinal detachment. Typical cases of acute PVD without any findings of retinal breaks or tears will have a low 2% to 5% risk of developing a retinal break or tear within weeks after the initial symptoms.[3] Aside from myopia and PVD, other risk factors for retinal detachment include cataract surgery, ocular trauma, previous personal or family history of a retinal detachment, peripheral retinal degenerations such as lattice or retinoschisis, and ocular diseases such as uveitis, diabetic retinopathy, and retinopathy of prematurity. Retinal detachment can occur at any age, but it is more common after the age of 40 years.[4] It is more common in men, and Caucasians are affected more than African Americans.[4]

A retinal detachment occurs at the potential space between the neurosensory retina and the retinal pigment epithelium (RPE). This

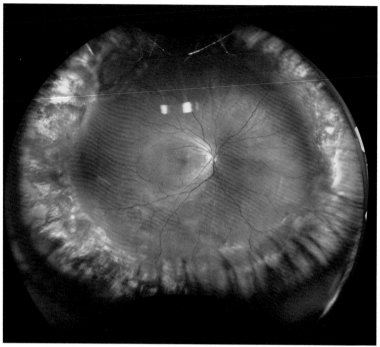

Figure 3.13-3   Fundus image of the right eye showing peripheral retinal scarring 360°, consistent with a scleral buckle.

space is present due to the way the eye forms embryologically. The embryologic cup, which forms the retina and RPE, invaginates forming 2 layers. The inner layer eventually forms the neural retina, and the outer layer will become the RPE. The 2 layers come together, but a potential space remains between the neural retina and RPE. Although the RPE and neural retina remain apposed by hydrostatic forces and interdigitations, there is no physical attachment between the 2 retinal layers. This potential space allows physical separation and fluid accumulation between the neural retina and the RPE during a retinal detachment.

The separation can happen in 3 ways. The most common is rhegmatogenous retinal detachment, which is a break or tear in the retina that allows fluid to seep between the retina and RPE, causing the separation of these 2 entities. The least common is tractional retinal detachment, which is a by-product of the contraction of scar tissue on the retinal surface pulling the retina away from the RPE. Finally, exudative retinal detachment is the accumulation of fluid from underneath of retina due to inflammatory conditions or trauma.

A thorough history is necessary to identify risk factors for retinal detachment. Common symptoms of retinal detachment include photopsia, floaters, a curtain over the vision, visual field loss, or decrease in central vision (if the macula is involved). Photopsia can also be caused by vitreoretinal traction secondary to a PVD. This needs to be differentiated from photopsia associated with migraine aura, postural hypotension, or transient ischemic attack. Floaters can be caused by vitreal clumping, hemorrhage, or glial tissue on the vitreous cortex.

To diagnose the retinal detachment, a clinician must be able to appreciate the separation of the retina from the RPE. On dilated fundus examination, this appears as a raised, corrugated area of the retina. It is important to look for a hole or tear in the retina where the fluid was able to enter between the RPE and neural retina. Be sure to look for the presence of dispersed pigment in the vitreous (ie, Shafer sign) or a vitreous hemorrhage. Scleral indentation can aid in recognizing peripheral retinal breaks. A large retinal detachment can cause a relative afferent pupillary defect. Hypotony is a common finding with retinal detachment so take note of asymmetric intraocular pressures of more than 4 to 5 mm Hg between the eyes. B-scan ultrasound may be necessary if a media opacity, such as a vitreous hemorrhage, prevents adequate viewing of the retina.

Once a retinal detachment is detected, a timely referral is key to getting the patient treated. There is more urgency in cases where the macula is still attached but is being imminently threatened by the advancing area of the retinal detachment. These cases need immediate referral with surgical treatment within 24 hours. Most other retinal detachment cases can be repaired within 2 to 4 days.

Current treatment options include laser photocoagulation, cryotherapy, scleral buckle, pars plana vitrectomy, and pneumatic retinopexy. Laser photocoagulation uses a laser to scar the retina around the outer edges of the detachment to seal it off. Cryotherapy works in a similar fashion but uses intense cold to freeze the retina to cause scarring. Treatment with a scleral buckle involves placing a band around the eye to mitigate the pull of the retina from the RPE, allowing the retina to settle back in place. The vitreous often causes retinal traction promoting further detachment, so performing a pars plana vitrectomy eliminates this force by removing the vitreous gel in the eye and replacing it with a gas or oil bubble. Pneumatic retinopexy introduces a gas bubble into the vitreous cavity to help physically push the retina back in place. Pneumatic retinopexy is often used in conjunction with cryotherapy or laser photocoagulation. The aim of these surgical treatments is to seal off the detached area of retina, minimize retinal traction, and stabilize the condition to prevent further detachment and vision loss.

If the macula is not involved and the patient has been treated in a timely fashion, prognosis is usually very good. However, these patients are at a 15% risk of developing a retinal detachment in the other eye, and this chance increases from 25% to 30% after cataract extraction.[5]

CLINICAL PEARL

- A macula-on retinal detachment is an emergent situation and should be referred to a retinal specialist immediately.

REFERENCES

1. Eye Disease Case-Control Study Group. Risk factors for idiopathic rhegmatogenous retinal detachment. *Am J Epidemiol*. 1993;137:749-757.
2. Bernheim D, Rouberol F, Palombi K, et al. Comparative prospective study of rhegmatogenous retinal detachments in phakic or pseudophakic patients with high myopia. *Retina*. 2013;33(10):2039-2048.
3. Dayan MR, Jayamanne DG, Andrews RM, Griffiths PG. Flashes and floaters as predictors of vitreoretinal pathology: is follow-up necessary for posterior vitreous detachment? *Eye*. 1996;10(4):456-458.
4. Facts about retinal detachment. National Institute of Health: National Eye Institute (NEI) Web site. https://nei.nih.gov/health/retinaldetach/retinaldetach. Last reviewed October 2009. Accessed February 9, 2017.
5. Pandya H. Retinal detachment. Practice essentials, background, pathology. Medscape Web site. http://emedicine.medscape.com/article/798501-overview. Updated November 22, 2016. Accessed February 9, 2017.

3.14 Horner Syndrome

Kirk L. Halvorson

Hilde, a 37-year-old white female, was referred by the emergency department with recent onset, left-sided headaches, unequal pupils, and ptosis. She had been seen in the emergency department 1 day prior where they performed a head computed tomography (CT) scan and complete blood count (CBC) with differential, each of which was unremarkable. Hilde was discharged and told to have further evaluation by an eye care provider due to unequal pupils and headaches. At the time of the eye examination, Hilde had unremarkable medical and ocular histories. She did not report trauma, was not taking any medications, and had no known allergies.

Clinical Findings

Unaided distance VA	OD: 20/20; OS: 20/25−
Pupil evaluation	OD: 3 mm in bright light, 5 mm in dim light; round and reactive to light
	OS: 2.5 mm in bright light, 3 mm in dim light; round and reactive to light with slight lag on dilation
	No RAPD
Ocular motility	Unrestricted in all gazes OD and OS
Confrontation visual fields	Full to finger counting OD and OS
Eyelid margin to corneal reflex distance (Figure 3.14-1)	OD: 4 mm; OS: 2 mm
Intraocular pressure (GAT)	OD: 12 mm Hg; OS: 10 mm Hg at 10:30 AM
Slit-lamp examination	OD: unremarkable
	OS: mild ptosis; diffuse grade 1 conjunctiva injection; otherwise unremarkable
Fundus examination	OD: 0.3/0.3 CD ratio; healthy rim tissue with distinct disc margins; fovea flat and dry; normal vasculature; periphery intact
	OS: 0.3/0.3 CD ratio; healthy rim tissue with distinct disc margins; fovea flat and dry; normal vasculature; periphery intact
Visual field (30-2 SITA-fast)	OD: no defects
	OS: no defects

Abbreviations: CD, cup to disc; GAT, Goldmann applanation tonometry; OD, right eye; OS, left eye; RAPD, relative afferent pupillary defect; VA, visual acuity.

Comments

Based on clinical findings, Horner syndrome was the most likely diagnosis. Normally this would have been differentiated from physiologic anisocoria with pharmacologic testing. However, due

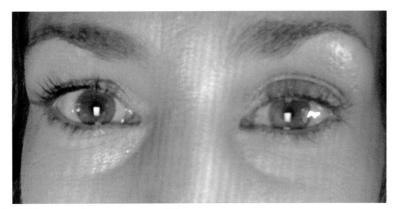

Figure 3.14-1 Mild ptosis with anisocoria in the left eye.

to a lack of resources, pharmaceutical confirmation could not be performed. Horner syndrome was diagnosed based on the ptosis, miosis, and dilation lag. With the recent onset headache, internal carotid artery dissection was suspected as the cause. After consulting with the radiologist, a CT and CT angiography of head and neck were ordered. Findings were consistent with a dissection of both the right and left internal carotid arteries (Figure 3.14-2).

Discussion

Hilde was referred by the emergency department for a pupil abnormality, which turned out to be a very serious condition. Because she presented with left-sided miosis, mild ptosis, and mild injection, Horner syndrome was high on the list of differential diagnoses. With limited pharmaceuticals available, the radiology department was consulted, and Hilde was sent back to the hospital for a repeat CT and CT angiography of the head and neck. Bilateral internal carotid dissection was diagnosed.

After consultation, Hilde was sent immediately to a neurologist for further management, which included antiplatelet therapy. She had an magnetic resonance imaging (MRI) and magnetic resonance angiography (MRA) 1 week later (Figure 3.14-3), which confirmed bilateral carotid artery dissection with an aneurysmal component of the right dissection. The MRI also revealed a signal abnormality that likely represented a subacute, mild

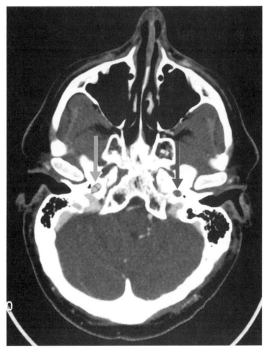

Figure 3.14-2 Axial-computed tomography angiography showing bilateral internal carotid artery dissection. The right internal carotid artery (blue arrow) shows an irregular blood vessel wall and intimal flap. The left internal carotid artery (red arrow) has an irregular wall and reduced lumen size.

ischemic injury in the vascular distribution of the left internal carotid artery. After approximately 3 months of therapy, her carotid artery dissections healed spontaneously. She was sent for further laboratory testing to look for any potential underlying systemic associations. This workup was unrevealing.

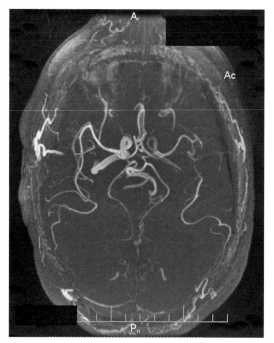

Figure 3.14-3 Magnetic resonance angiography showing decreased flow of the left internal carotid artery.

Although Horner syndrome, sometimes called oculosympathoperesis, manifests as an ocular entity, it really is a neurologic finding that could represent a larger issue. The sympathetic pathway is long, and lesions can affect it anywhere along its first-order, second-order, or third-order neurons. The typical Horner syndrome patient presents with ptosis, miosis, and anhidrosis, but symptoms may vary depending on where the lesion is located.

A lesion of the sympathetic pathway will result in pupil miosis on the affected side. Anisocoria is more evident in dim compared with bright illumination. Anisocoria associated with Horner syndrome is usually 1.0 to 1.5 mm, and the miotic pupil exhibits a dilation lag.[1] Here, the involved pupil takes longer to dilate following the removal of a light source. This is evidenced by the magnitude of anisocoria being greater 5 seconds after the removal of the light source compared with the magnitude 15 seconds after the light source is removed. Because sympathetic innervation to the eyelids involves Muller muscle rather than the levator, ptosis is mild. Patients can also exhibit an inverse ptosis where the inferior lid is raised slightly.

The first-order, central neuron starts at the hypothalamus and travels through the brainstem to synapse at the cervicothoracic spinal cord (C8 to T2). This first-order nerve can be affected by stroke, tumor, or demyelinating disorders. Lesions along this pathway may also cause vertigo, ataxia, dysphagia, weakness, sensory deficit, or diplopia.[1]

The second-order preganglionic nerve leaves the cervical spinal cord, passes along the apex of the lung, and travels superiorly to synapse in the superior cervical chain ganglia. Second-order deficits can occur as a result of trauma from forceps delivery, chest tube placement, or coronary artery bypass because the nerve courses through the brachial plexus and over the lung apex.[1] A CT of the chest may be indicated if a patient with Horner syndrome has ipsilateral arm pain, as it can also be associated with malignancy at the apex of the lung, called Pancoast syndrome.

The third-order, postganglionic nerve leaves the superior cervical ganglion and follows the internal carotid artery to the cavernous sinus. There, sympathetic fibers travel briefly with the abducens nerve before joining the ophthalmic division of the trigeminal nerve. From here sympathetic fibers travel with branches of the trigeminal nerve to the iris dilator muscle, as well as the conjunctival and choroidal blood vessels. Sympathetic fibers going to the iris dilator, Muller muscle, and sweat glands of the medial forehead travel within the internal carotid artery plexus. Fibers innervating sweat glands and blood vessels serving the remainder of the face branch off and follow the external carotid artery. For this reason, a postganglionic Horner syndrome generally does not cause facial anhidrosis other than at the ipsilateral medial forehead.

Carotid artery dissection is a major concern when dealing with a third-order (postganglionic) Horner syndrome. Dissection occurs when there is an intimal tear splitting the arterial wall layers, resulting in a hematoma within the artery wall. Approximately 45% of patients with carotid artery dissection present with pain involving the face, head, or neck. It is usually spontaneous or caused by trauma.[2] Some systemic conditions can be associated with carotid artery dissection such as Ehlers-Danlos syndrome, Marfan syndrome, autosomal dominant polycystic kidney disease, osteogenesis imperfecta type 1, fibromuscular dysplasia, and syphilis.[1,3] The major concern for patients with carotid artery dissection is the high risk of cerebral infarction, often within a few weeks after onset, even though the risk of death is low.[2] Although painful, Horner syndrome is the most common ophthalmic finding with internal carotid artery dissection, transient monocular vision loss, permanent vision loss (due to ischemic optic neuropathy, ocular ischemic syndrome, or retinal artery occlusion), or cranial nerve palsies may also occur.[1,2]

Other entities can lead to postganglionic Horner syndrome such as a space-occupying lesion, otitis media, or pathology within the cavernous sinus. One should be suspicious of lesions in the cavernous sinus or orbital apex if multiple cranial nerves are involved. Congenital Horner syndrome makes up 5% of cases of Horner syndrome and can present with heterochromia. It is thought that the sympathetic system controls pigment formation in early development.[1] Unilateral facial flush, also known as harlequin sign, is another possible finding in congenital cases.

Historically, diagnostic pharmaceutical testing included topical cocaine (2% to 10%) to diagnose a Horner syndrome followed by hydroxyamphetamine to differentiate between preganglionic and postganglionic involvement. Cocaine works by blocking the reuptake of norepinephrine. This will cause pupil dilation in normal eyes. Because Horner syndrome is caused by a dysfunction of the sympathetic pathway, cocaine will not dilate an affected eye no matter where the lesion is located along the pathway. More recently, because of its commercial availability, apraclonidine (0.5% or 1.0%) is used to confirm a diagnosis of Horner syndrome. Apraclonidine, an alpha agonist that primarily works on alpha-2 receptors, is generally used to control intraocular pressure (IOP); however, it does have weak alpha-1 receptor activity. The drop is not strong enough to cause dilation of the pupil in a normal eye, but due to the hypersensitivity caused by denervation, it will cause pupil dilation of 1.0 to 4.5 mm, as well as reversal of ptosis, in a Horner syndrome patient.[1,4] The hypersensitivity usually takes about 2 weeks to develop after initial damage, but a positive apraclonidine test has been reported as early as 36 hours following the onset of the condition.[4,5]

Hydroxyamphetamine can be used to differentiate if a lesion is affecting the preganglionic (first- or second-order) nerves or the postganglionic (third-order) nerve. It is important to wait at least a day after cocaine or apraclonidine testing, in order to get reliable results with hydroxyamphetamine. Hydroxyamphetamine will cause release of norepinephrine if norepinephrine is available at the nerve ending. For norepinephrine to arrive at the nerve ending, there must be a healthy connection between the cell body and the synapse. Because of this, hydroxyamphetamine will not cause pupil dilation if the postganglionic axon is damaged but will dilate the pupil when there is a preganglionic lesion, which prevents stimulation of the healthy postganglionic nerve. Phenylephrine 1% has also been shown to cause mydriasis in postganglionic Horner syndrome. Like apraclonidine, the dilation occurs secondary to denervation hypersensitivity.

For cases of painful, postganglionic Horner syndrome, such as with Hilde, CT and CT angiography or MRI and MRA is warranted. Patients diagnosed with carotid artery dissection are typically treated with heparin followed by warfarin, and spontaneous resolution is usually seen within 3 months. When a patient exhibits persistent ischemia, surgical intervention with ligation of the carotid artery or percutaneous balloon angioplasty may be warranted.[3]

CLINICAL PEARLS

- Have a strong suspicion for internal carotid artery dissection if a Horner syndrome is associated with pain.

- Apraclonidine will cause dilation of a Horner pupil, as well as reversal of the ptosis, due to hypersensitivity of the damaged nerve.

REFERENCES

1. Walton KA, Buono LM. Horner syndrome. *Curr Opin Ophthalmol*. 2003;14:357-363.
2. Biousse V, Touboul PJ, D'Andlejan-Chatillon J, et al. Ophthalmological manifestations of internal carotid artery dissection. *Am J Ophthalmol*. 1998;126;565-577.
3. Schievink W. Spontaneous dissection of the carotid and vertebral arteries. *N Engl J Med*. 2001;344:898-906.
4. Smit DP. Pharmacological testing in Horner's syndrome – a new paradigm. *S Afr Med J*. 2010;100:738-740.
5. Davagnanam I, Fraser CL, Miszkiel K, Daniel CS, Plant GT. Adult Horner's syndrome: a combined clinical, pharmacological, and imaging algorithm. *Eye*. 2013;27:291-298.

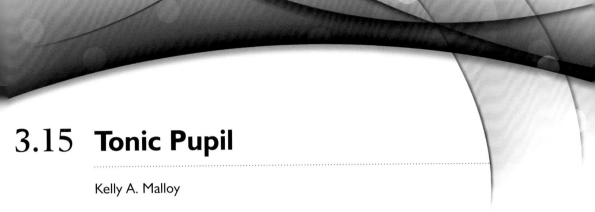

3.15 Tonic Pupil

Kelly A. Malloy

Vanessa, a 53-year-old woman, presented for a comprehensive eye examination. She reported that her last eye examination was 4 years ago where she was informed of an abnormality with her pupils. At that time, she was referred to a neurologist for further evaluation. The neurologist recommended neuroimaging, but the patient did not complete the recommended workup.

Vanessa felt her vision was good in each eye. She denied any diplopia, ptosis, transient vision loss, headache, or other neurologic symptoms. She had a history of trauma at a young age. When she was 9 years old, she was an unrestrained passenger in a car that was involved in an accident. She flew into the dashboard and lost consciousness for a few moments. She was hospitalized with an apparent broken nose, and she reported that both eyes were bruised and swollen shut.

Vanessa was in good health. She denied diabetes, hypertension, or any other health problems, including infectious or inflammatory disease. She was not taking any prescription medications.

Clinical Findings

Entering distance visual acuity	OD: 20/20; OS: 20/20
Color vision (Ishihara)	OD: 14/14; OS: 14/14
Confrontation visual fields	Full to finger counting and red targets OD and OS
Pupil evaluation (Figure 3.15-1)	OD: pupil diameter of 2.75 mm in bright and 2.75 mm in dim with no reaction to light; 2+ reaction to near target
	OS: irregular pupil shape; pupil diameter of 2.75 mm × 3.25 mm in bright and 2.75 mm × 3.25 mm in dim (measurements are vertical × horizontal) with no reaction to light; 2+ reaction to near target
	Due to lack of pupillary reaction to light binocularly, we were unable to assess for an RAPD
Extraocular motilities	Full in all positions of gaze; no nystagmus OU
Cover test	Orthophoria; comitant in all positions of gaze
Anterior segment examination	OD: sectoral paralysis and stromal spread present. No appreciation of stromal streaming due to lack of light reactivity. Anterior segment health otherwise unremarkable.
	OS: asymmetry of pupillary border (Figure 3.15-2). Sectoral paralysis and stromal spread present. No appreciation of stromal streaming due to lack of light reactivity. Anterior segment health otherwise unremarkable.
Fundus examination	OD: 0.35/0.35 CD ratio; healthy rim tissue with no pallor and distinct disc margins; fovea flat and dry; normal vasculature
	OS: 0.35/0.35 CD ratio; healthy rim tissue with no pallor and distinct disc margins; fovea flat and dry; normal vasculature

Neurologic examination   Normal cranial nerve, motor, sensory, and coordination testing; decreased deep tendon reflexes bilaterally

Diagnostic pupil testing (30 min after instillation of 0.125% pilocarpine OU, Figure 3.15-3)   Pupil sizes in bright illumination: OD: 2.25 mm; OS: 2.25 mm × 2.75 mm

Pupil sizes in dim illumination: OD: 2.25 mm; OS: 2.25 mm × 2.75 mm

Abbreviations: CD, cup to disc; OD, right eye; OS, left eye; OU, both eyes; RAPD, relative afferent pupillary defect.

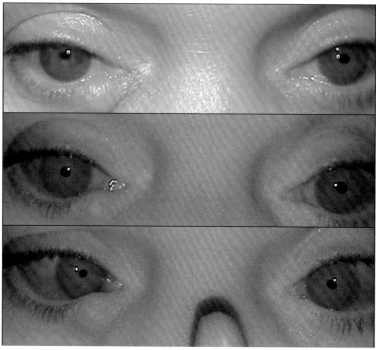

Figure 3.15-1   Pupils in bright (top) and dim (middle) illumination and with an accommodative target (bottom).

Discussion

Vanessa presented with bilaterally nonreactive pupils. This pupil abnormality was noted by a previous doctor 4 years ago, which prompted the recommendation of neuroimaging and neurologic consultation, neither of which were completed.

To determine if further workup, including neuroimaging, is warranted, it is first necessary to determine the nature of the clinical presentation. A very important aspect of this case is not only that the pupils do not react to a light stimulus but also that the pupils react better to an accommodative target. This is indicative of light–near dissociation.

Because there are a handful of conditions that can cause light–near dissociation (see Chapter 3.16), determining the exact etiology is essential.[1-2] A very helpful aspect of this case is that the pupils have an irregular shape, which should prompt the clinician to consider the possibility of tonic pupil. Under slit-lamp magnification, there were 2 hallmark features of tonic pupil: areas of sectoral paralysis and stromal spread. These can be identified by the linear, rather than circular, pupil border and by asymmetry of the tightness of the iris folds. Because the pupils were not reactive, there was no evidence of the third hallmark slit-lamp feature of tonic pupil: stromal streaming. This occurs due to

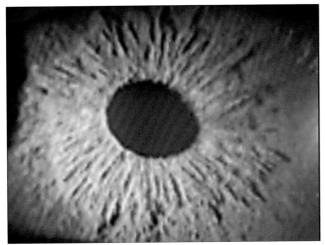

Figure 3.15-2   Left pupil demonstrating sector paralysis with flattened pupil margin from 1 to 3 o'clock, as well as stromal spread with less pronounced iris folds from 2 to 3 o'clock.

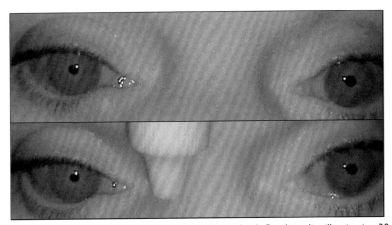

Figure 3.15-3   Pupils in dim illumination prior to drop instillation (top). Pupils in dim illumination 30 minutes after instillation of 0.125% pilocarpine (bottom).

segmental contraction of the areas of the iris sphincter that have relatively normal innervation. The contracting areas pull on the weaker areas of the iris. Stromal streaming can be seen by turning the slit-lamp light off and then on quickly while watching for irregular, segmental iris movement. The iris will seem to constrict in a concentric pattern rather than moving radially toward the center of the pupil.

The parasympathetic system is affected in tonic pupil. The preganglionic fibers travel with cranial nerve III as part of the efferent light reflex pathway. These preganglionic fibers synapse in the ciliary ganglion (within the orbit). The postganglionic parasympathetic fibers then travel with the short ciliary nerves (within the retrobulbar and suprachoroidal space) to the iris sphincter and ciliary body muscles. Tonic pupil occurs when there is damage to the ciliary ganglion or possibly the short ciliary nerves. Because the parasympathetic fibers innervate the ciliary body as well as the iris sphincter, patients may report blur at near due to an impaired ability to accommodate. Vanessa was presbyopic, so she did not notice this symptom; she was already wearing a full add in her glasses.

Normally about 97% of the postganglionic parasympathetic fibers innervate the ciliary body muscle, while the other 3% travel to the pupil.[3] Therefore, with damage, there is a greater proportion of pupillary fiber damage compared to the proportion of accommodative fiber damage. This is the basis for better pupillary reaction to an accommodative stimulus than to a light stimulus (light–near dissociation) in tonic pupil. As healing of the nerve occurs over time, some nerve fibers originally intended for the ciliary body muscle aberrantly grow to innervate the iris sphincter muscle. Although the pupils continue to react poorly to a light stimulus because of damage to the pupillary fibers, they react better to a near stimulus because some of the previous accommodative fibers are now also working to constrict the pupil when looking at a near target. Accommodative function typically improves as regeneration occurs.

Because innervation to the iris sphincter is impaired, an acute tonic pupil will be relatively large in diameter and may cause symptoms of photophobia or difficulty with dark adaptation. However, the tonic pupil often gets smaller as nerve fibers regenerate and these symptoms improve. Vanessa's tonic pupils were relatively small so she did not exhibit the typical concerns associated with an acute presentation.

Diagnostic testing using 0.125% pilocarpine was performed to confirm the tonic pupil diagnosis. This dilute percentage is made by combining 1 drop of 1% pilocarpine and 8 drops of saline. After 30 minutes, Vanessa's pupils were smaller than the pre-drop measurements, bilaterally. Lack of pupillary constriction would indicate a negative test for tonic pupil, and pupillary constriction, as seen in this case, indicates a positive test for tonic pupil.[4] Because this test involves a supersensitivity reaction, the cornea should not be touched, and no other drops should be instilled before doing this test.

Early in the process, when tonic pupils are large, the differential diagnosis will include pharmacologic dilation and cranial III palsy. In these cases, 0.125% pilocarpine would be used to rule out a tonic pupil. If there is no constriction, then 1% pilocarpine would be used to test for pharmacologic dilation. A pharmacologically dilated pupil would not constrict

with 1% pilocarpine because the receptors are already bound by the dilating agent. In contrast, other etiologies of a dilated, nonreactive pupil, such as a cranial nerve III palsy, would constrict with 1% pilocarpine.[4]

Other causes of irregular, nonresponsive pupils must be taken into consideration. Argyll Robertson pupil, typically due to neurosyphilis, may be a consideration as it can also present with light–near dissociation. This differential was considered in this case, but Argyll Robertson pupils are typically very miotic, measuring 2.5 mm or less. Although Vanessa's pupils were relatively small, they were still slightly larger than 2.5 mm. She also had slit-lamp features more consistent with tonic pupil. Nevertheless, syphilis can be a cause of tonic pupil and was therefore ruled out with laboratory testing.[1]

Once the diagnosis of tonic pupil has been made, the etiology must be determined. Note that the term Adie tonic pupil has not yet been used; the more appropriate term is simply tonic pupil.[2] Adie tonic pupil is reserved for an idiopathic tonic pupil, which is a diagnosis of exclusion. Other documented etiologies of tonic pupil are many and include orbital processes (tumor, trauma, surgery) and systemic diseases (diabetes, syphilis, sarcoid, autoimmune disease, Lyme disease, and a paraneoplastic process).[5-6] These processes should be ruled out before calling it an Adie tonic pupil. Adie tonic pupil is typically unilateral at onset but may become bilateral. The fact that this case is a bilateral presentation makes an orbital process unlikely. A systemic cause is also less likely as this had been noted for at least 4 years, and no other symptoms of associated disease had been noticed. Despite this, a systemic cause still needs to be considered.

A neurologic examination can be helpful in determining the cause of tonic pupil. Some causes of tonic pupil have been shown to affect not only the ciliary ganglia, but also the dorsal root ganglia, resulting in diminished deep tendon reflexes. This has been noted with Adie tonic pupil, and if present in association with tonic pupil, is termed Adie syndrome.[2] This has been postulated to be the result of either a virus or indolent neuronal degeneration.[7] However, this combination of findings is not pathognomonic for Adie syndrome because it has also been noted in other causes of tonic pupil, such as Sjögren syndrome, which is thought to cause an autoimmune ganglionitis.[5]

Due to her history and clinical presentation, it was thought that Vanessa likely had Adie syndrome. Because of the bilateral presentation, and apparent stability over time, an orbital mass was not likely; neuroimaging was, therefore, not indicated. However, laboratory testing was ordered to rule out systemic causes of tonic pupil. This included HbA1c, rapid plasma reagin (RPR), fluorescent treponemal antibody absorption (FTA-ABS), angiotensin-converting enzyme (ACE), antinuclear antibody (ANA), and Lyme titer. All laboratory results were reported to be within normal ranges.

Vanessa had dark irides, and her pupils were relatively small; therefore, she was not bothered by the cosmetic appearance of the tonic pupil. Because the condition was bilateral and she was already wearing bifocals, she was not symptomatic of accommodative issues. However, if patients with tonic pupils are symptomatic, they may benefit from unequal adds, early initiation of bifocals, or even cosmetic contact lenses to hide noticeable anisocoria.

Clinically, it is important to check pupillary reaction to a near accommodative target any time the pupils either do not respond to light or respond less briskly than expected for the patient's age. Light–near dissociation is a very important clinical finding that can be instrumental in determining a diagnosis. It is important to realize that the mechanism for light–near dissociation does differ among its various causes.

CLINICAL PEARLS

- If the pupils do not react well to a light stimulus, check for reaction to a near stimulus.

- Use the slit lamp to look for telltale features that distinguish tonic pupil from other causes of light–near dissociation.

REFERENCES

1. Thompson HS, Kardon RH. The Argyll Robertson pupil. *J Neuroophthalmol.* 2006;26(2):134-138.
2. Kelly-Sell M, Liu GT. "Tonic" but not "Adie" pupils. *J Neuroophthalmol.* 2011;31(4):393-395.
3. Warwick R. The ocular parasympathetic nerve supply and its mesencephalic sources. *J Anat.* 1954;88:71-93.
4. Antonio-Santos AA, Santo RN, Eggenberger ER. Pharmacological testing of anisocoria. *Expert Opin Pharmacother.* 2005;6(12):2007-2013.
5. Bhagwan S, Bhagwan B, Moodley A. Bilateral tonic pupils as the initial manifestation of Sjögren's syndrome. *Neuroophthalmology.* 2015;39(5):248-252.
6. Peyman A, Kabiri M, Peyman M. Tonic pupil, a paraneoplastic neuro-ophtalmological disease associated with occult breast cancer. *Breast J.* 2015;21(5):543-544.
7. Thompson HS, Burmeister LF, Meek ES. A search for serum antibodies in Adie's syndrome. *Albrecht Von Graefes Arch Klin Exp Ophthalmol.* 1977;205(1):29-32.

3.16 Light–Near Disassociation

Kelsey L. Moody

Virginia, a 45-year-old female, was referred for evaluation of anisocoria. Virginia denied any changes in her ocular appearance; however, she did note occasional vertical double vision that went away when covering an eye. The double vision started after a car hit her 6 years ago. Virginia sustained substantial injuries to the right side of her body, including a large laceration to the right side of her head, a punctured lung, a hip injury, and memory loss. While she was in the hospital she was told of an abnormality to her eyes and pupils. Over time, the double vision improved but never completely resolved.

Virginia felt that her vision was good in each eye. She experienced frontal headaches, which had improved since she received her new glasses a few months ago. The headaches had reduced to approximately once per month and resolved with over-the-counter nonsteroidal anti-inflammatory drugs (NSAIDs). She denied any vision loss, eye pain, lid droop, or any other neurologic symptoms.

Virginia reported good overall health. The only positive medical condition was anemia, for which she took iron supplements. She denied ever being told of diabetes, hypertension, or infectious or inflammatory disease.

Clinical Findings

Aided distance VA	OD: 20/20; OS: 20/20
Habitual Rx	OD: −0.50 sph; OS: −0.75 sph
Cover test	Distance: 2Δ exophoria in primary position with varying amounts of exo and hyper deviation in eccentric gazes (see Figure 3.16-1); near: 4Δ exophoria
Confrontation visual fields	Full to finger counting OD and OS
Pupil evaluation	OD: 3.25 mm in bright, 3.5 mm in dim; 1+ reaction to light, 2+ reaction to near target
	OS: 2.0 mm in bright, 3.0 mm in dim; 3+ reaction to light, 2+ reaction to near target
	No relative afferent pupillary defect
Color vision (Ishihara)	14/14 plates OD and OS
Ductions	Supraduction: OD: 60%; OS: 100%
	Infraduction: OD: 100%; OS: 100%
	Abduction: OD: 100%; OS: 100%
	Adduction: OD: 100%; OS: 100%
	Diplopia noted on up gaze and left gaze; eyelid elevation OD was present on down gaze and adduction
Worth 4-dot	Fusion at distance, intermediate, and near
Palpebral apertures	OD: 7 mm; OS: 8 mm

Exophthalmometry	OD: 21 mm; OS: 20 mm (base: 97 mm)
Intraocular pressure (GAT)	OD: 15 mm Hg; OS: 15 mm Hg at 9:47 AM
Slit-lamp examination	OD: unremarkable
	OS: unremarkable
Fundus examination	OD: unremarkable
	OS: unremarkable

Abbreviations: GAT, Goldmann applanation tonometry; OD, right eye; OS, left eye; Rx, prescription; sph, sphere; VA, visual acuity; XP, exophoria.

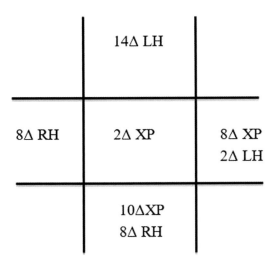

Figure 3.16-1   Cover test results in different positions of gaze.

Discussion

Virginia was initially referred for evaluation of anisocoria. Anisocoria can be a physiologic, mechanical, or neurologic problem affecting the pupillary size. Physiologic anisocoria, seen in 15% to 30% of the population, may be more evident in dim illumination, but the difference in pupil size between the 2 eyes should measure the same in bright and dim illumination. Mechanical abnormalities, such as posterior synechiae, tears of the iris, or surgical trauma, should be ruled out as they are easy to identify and are generally benign.[1,2]

Once it is determined that the anisocoria is not physiologic or mechanical, the next step is to determine if the anisocoria is greater in bright or dim illumination. This difference occurs due to an imbalance of the sympathetic and parasympathetic systems. Sympathetic fibers innervate the iris dilator and parasympathetic fibers (traveling as a part of the oculomotor nerve) innervate the iris sphincter. Damage to the sympathetic fibers causes anisocoria greater in dim illumination because the involved pupil does not dilate well. Damage to the parasympathetic fibers causes anisocoria greater in bright illumination because the affected pupil does not constrict as well as the normal pupil. Virginia had a difference in pupillary size of 1.25 mm in bright illumination and 0.50 mm in dim illumination indicating a parasympathetic problem.[1,2]

Following pupillary size measurements, the direct pupillary response to light should be evaluated. If there is a poor or absent response to light, it is important to check the pupillary reaction to a near accommodative target. It is normal if the pupillary reaction to light is greater than or equal to the pupillary reaction to a near stimulus. If the pupil reacts better to a near target, the patient has light–near dissociation. Light–near dissociation narrows down the differential diagnosis to 1 of 5 conditions: a blind eye, Argyll Robertson pupil, tonic pupil, dorsal midbrain syndrome, or aberrant regeneration of cranial nerve III.[2]

Virginia had normal visual acuity, so we can rule out a blind eye. Argyll Robertson pupil usually presents with bilateral, small, pinpoint pupils (less than 2.5 mm in size) even in dim illumination. Virginia's condition was unilateral and her pupils were moderately sized making this an unlikely diagnosis. Neurosyphilis is the most common cause of Argyll Robertson pupil.[3]

Tonic pupil is an important differential, but this generally causes sector paralysis of the iris sphincter, which is seen on slit-lamp examination as vermiform pupillary movements. If tonic pupil was still a concern, it can be ruled out by instilling a drop of 0.125% pilocarpine.

Due to supersensitivity of the nerve fibers associated with this condition, a tonic pupil would constrict with diluted pilocarpine; however, a normal pupil would not.[1,2]

It is important to note that in addition to the anisocoria, Virginia also had a supraduction deficit and mild ptosis of the right eye. Both of these can be features of either dorsal midbrain syndrome or aberrant regeneration of cranial nerve III. Dorsal midbrain syndrome is caused by damage to the dorsal aspect of the midbrain, most commonly by tumors of the midbrain or pineal gland, hydrocephalus, or stroke. It usually results in bilateral light–near dissociation because the tectum of the midbrain carries pupillary fibers that innervate both eyes. In addition to light–near dissociation, patients with dorsal midbrain syndrome commonly display a bilateral upgaze palsy, eyelid retraction (Collier sign), and convergence retraction nystagmus (on attempted upgaze the eyes converge and retract).[2,4] Virginia did not have a bilateral presentation or convergence retraction nystagmus, making dorsal midbrain syndrome unlikely.

Aberrant regeneration of cranial nerve III occurs due to miswiring of cranial nerve III fibers after damage to the nerve. There are multiple proposed mechanisms for how aberrant regeneration of cranial nerve III occurs. A commonly accepted theory is that both the nerve and the surrounding endoneurium (the connective tissue surrounding the myelin sheath) are disrupted. There is subsequent Wallerian degeneration distal to the injury site. Because the endoneurium is disrupted, as the nerve regenerates, it is no longer confined to its original structure and can create a new pathway. Aberrant regeneration of cranial nerve III is most commonly due to trauma or compression by a tumor, aneurysm, or hemorrhage.[5,6]

In addition to features of residual cranial nerve III palsy, aberrant regeneration of cranial nerve III has several pathognomonic features. The most common presenting sign is vertical motility restriction. This can be from residual deficits from a cranial nerve III palsy or it can be from co-contraction of the superior and inferior rectus muscles with or without globe retraction. To determine if it is due to co-contraction, intraocular pressure can be checked in primary gaze and upgaze. If there is an increase of intraocular pressure in upgaze in the affected eye, this would suggest co-contraction. A more recognizable feature of aberrant regeneration of cranial nerve III is eyelid retraction with ductions. This is due to synkinetic innervation of the levator palpebrae superioris muscle with the medial rectus, inferior rectus, inferior oblique, and/or superior rectus. Although the synkinesia with the eyelid can occur with any of the extraocular muscles controlled by cranial nerve III, it is easiest to see with adduction and infraduction. On infraduction, the eyelid elevation is called pseudo-Von Graefe sign as it can look similar to the eyelid elevation in thyroid eye disease. Finally, on attempted adduction, infraduction, or supraduction, there can be pupillary constriction due to a synkinesia with the extraocular muscles and postganglionic parasympathetic fibers to the pupillary sphincter. Because the pupil may have a poor reaction to light from the previous cranial nerve III palsy, the reaction to near may be greater due to the developed synkinesia on adduction (convergence) causing a light–near dissociation.[5,6]

Virginia had several features of aberrant regeneration of cranial nerve III, including a supraduction deficit, eyelid synkinesa on adduction and infraduction, light–near dissociation, and a cover test pattern consistent with a partial cranial nerve III palsy. Specifically, she had a reversing hyper deviation (left hyper on up gaze and right hyper on down gaze) and an increasing exodeviation away from the vertically limited eye (left gaze).[5]

Virginia had a significant event of head trauma, which is a frequent cause of aberrant regeneration as discussed earlier. Despite this, a magnetic resonance imaging (MRI) and magnetic resonance angiography (MRA) of the brain are still necessary to rule out an intracranial mass or aneurysm compressing the nerve and causing this presentation.[5,6] Virginia had an MRI and MRA of the brain, which only demonstrated a right zygomatic arch fracture (unrelated to her aberrant regeneration). Her MRA was unremarkable. In cases of significant head trauma, physical damage to cranial nerve III is not usually visible on MRI unless there is significant edema or mass effect.

It is important to note that aberrant regeneration can never be due to an ischemic cause, because there has to be a physical disruption of the nerve for aberrant regeneration to occur. In a vasculopathic cranial nerve III palsy, there is a reduction in the blood flow that is supplying the nerve. Despite the lack of blood flow, the continuity of the axon is maintained and the nerve can continue on its normal course to the eye once blood flow is returned. Therefore, if a patient is diagnosed with a vasculopathic cranial nerve III palsy and aberrant regeneration occurs a few months later, further workup must be immediately pursued to determine the etiology.[6]

From an ocular standpoint, Virginia's double vision can be treated with prism or occlusion if the patient is symptomatic. If it is an acute presentation, it would be better to treat with a Fresnel prism and/or a bangarter filter (for occlusion) to see how the misalignment may change over time. Prism can also be challenging as the ocular misalignment is frequently noncomitant, varying in direction in multiple positions of gaze. However, the goal is to provide clear, single, binocular vision in most positions of gaze. Botox injections and strabismus surgery are other treatment options; however, the results are usually unpredictable.[6]

CLINICAL PEARLS

- If the pupils do not react well to light, the clinician must check for a pupillary reaction to a near target.

- A diagnosis of light–near disassociation narrows the differential down to 1 of 5 conditions: a blind eye, Argyll Robertson pupil, tonic pupil, dorsal midbrain syndrome, or aberrant regeneration of cranial nerve III.

- Aberrant regeneration is not caused by ischemic vasculopathy.

REFERENCES

1. Gross JR, McClelland C, Lee MS. An approach to anisocoria. *Curr Opin Ophthalmol.* 2016;27(6): 497-492.
2. Kawasaki AK. Diagnostic approach to pupillary abnormalities. *Continuum.* 2014;20(4):1008-1022.
3. Thompson HS, Kardon RH. Argyll Robertson pupil. *J Neuro-Ophthalmol.* 2006;26:134-138.
4. Skarbez K, Danciullo L. Metastatic melanoma from unknown primary presenting as dorsal midbrain syndrome. *Optom Vis Sci.* 2012;89:e112-e117.
5. Sayed SA, Rabea M. Misdirection (aberrant regeneration) of the third cranial nerve. *J Egypt Ophthalmol Soc.* 2013;106:150-152.
6. Weber ED, Newman SA. Aberrant regeneration of the oculomotor nerve: implications for neurosurgeons. *Neurosurg Focus.* 2007;23(5):E14.

3.17 Optic Nerve Drusen

Ryan Bulson

Ali, a 26-year-old Caucasian female, presented due to bilateral visual field loss that had been incidentally discovered while sitting as a practice subject for her husband, a second year optometry student. She did not notice the visual field defects in everyday life and reported no other visual concerns. Ocular and systemic histories were unremarkable. Family ocular history was positive for a maternal aunt who had glaucoma.

Clinical Findings

Unaided distance VA	OD: 20/15; OS: 20/15
Color vision (Ishihara)	OD: 10/10 plates; OS: 10/10 plates
Pupil evaluation	PERRL; no RAPD
Extraocular motilities	Full and comitant OU
Refraction	OD: +1.00 sph; OS: +1.00 sph
Slit-lamp examination	Unremarkable OD and OS
Intraocular pressures (GAT)	OD: 24 mm Hg; OS: 24 mm Hg at 2:32 PM
Pachymetry	OD: 586 micrometer; OS: 581 micrometer
Fundus examination (Figure 3.17-1)	OD: 0.1/0.1 CD ratio; pallor of the neuroretinal rim tissue inferiorly with distinct disc margins; fovea flat and dry; trifurcation of retinal blood vessels; periphery flat and intact
	OS: 0.1/0.1 CD ratio; pallor of the neuroretinal rim tissue inferiorly with distinct disc margins; fovea flat and dry; trifurcation of retinal blood vessels; periphery flat and intact
Visual fields (Humphrey 30-2 SITA-standard, Figure 3.17-2)	OD: dense superior nasal arcuate defect respecting the horizontal midline with minimal crossing of the vertical meridian in both eyes
	OS: dense superior nasal arcuate defect respecting the horizontal midline with minimal crossing of the vertical meridian in both eyes
Autofluorescent imaging (Figure 3.17-3)	Hyperautofluorescence mainly localized to the inferior disc OD and OS
B-scan ultrasonography	Bilateral hyperreflectance on the optic nerve head on both high and low gain
Nerve fiber layer OCT (Figure 3.17-4)	Symmetric bilateral nerve fiber layer loss inferiorly

Abbreviations: CD, cup to disc; GAT, Goldmann applanation tonometry; OCT, optical coherence tomography; OD, right eye; OS, left eye; OU, both eyes; PERRL, pupils equal, round, reactive to light; RAPD, relative afferent pupillary defect; sph, sphere; VA, visual acuity.

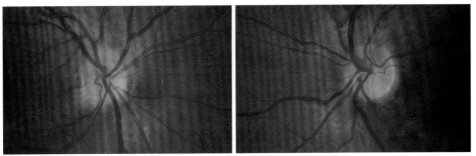

Figure 3.17-1 Fundus images showing inferior pallor or the right and left optic nerve.

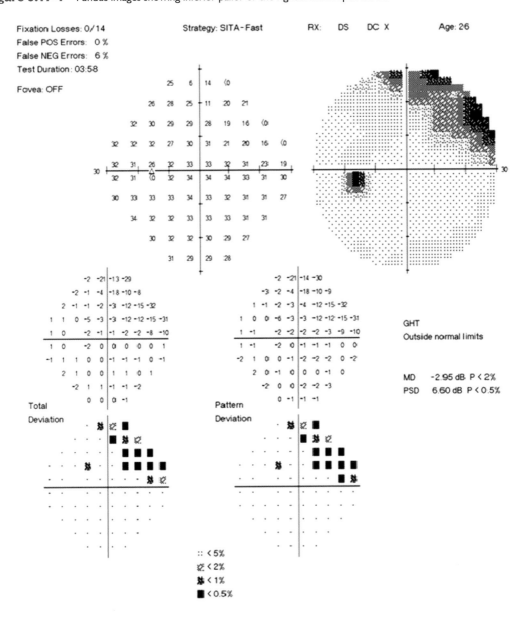

Figure 3.17-2 Visual field demonstrating bilateral superior nasal scotomas respecting the horizontal midline A, left eye; B, right eye.

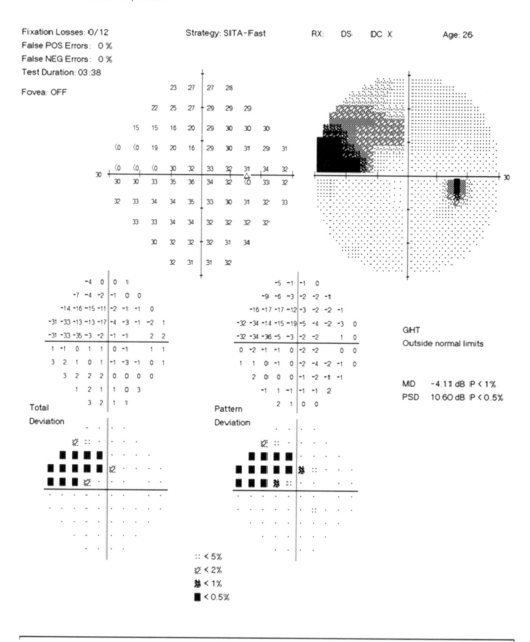

Fixation Losses: 0/12   Strategy: SITA-Fast   RX: DS·   DC X   Age: 26·

False POS Errors: 0 %

False NEG Errors: 0 %

Test Duration: 03:38

Fovea: OFF

GHT

Outside normal limits

MD   -4.11 dB   P < 1%

PSD   10.60 dB   P < 0.5%

Total Deviation

Pattern Deviation

:: < 5%

∷ < 2%

※ < 1%

■ < 0.5%

B

Figure 3.17-2   (Continued)

Discussion

Ali was diagnosed with buried optic nerve head drusen causing superior nasal visual field loss in both eyes. Visual field loss associated with optic nerve drusen typically causes slowly progressing arcuate defects, identical to that found with glaucoma. Patients are commonly asymptomatic and the differentiation between optic nerve drusen and glaucoma based on visual fields alone is difficult. With Ali, there was a suspicion of glaucoma due to the arcuate nature of the visual field defects, ocular hypertension, and family history of glaucoma. At subsequent visits, the intraocular pressures (IOPs) remained high, between 22 and 25 mm Hg, but they did not fluctuate diurnally. Pachymetry was thicker than average, and her

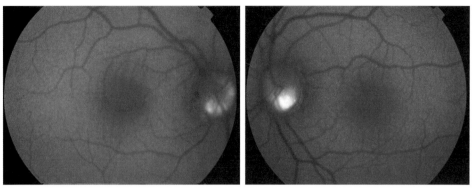

Figure 3.17-3   Autofluorescence imaging shows hyperautofluorescence involving the right and left optic nerve.

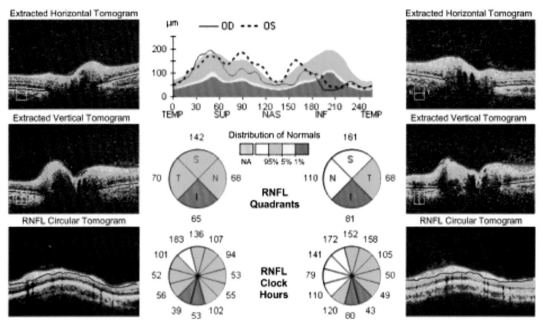

Figure 3.17-4   Nerve fiber layer optical coherence tomography showing significant thinning of the retinal nerve fiber layer inferiorly on both eyes (right eye data shown on the left and left eye data shown on the right).

cupping was minimal. She was educated on the possibility of initiating brimonidine tartrate 0.1% for both anti-ocular hypertensive and potential neuroprotective benefits. Ali declined initiating the medication but agreed to consider treatment if changes were observed in either the visual field or optical coherence tomography (OCT) nerve fiber layer analysis testing in the future. The visual field and OCT abnormalities remained stable over a period of nearly 3 years.

Optic nerve head drusen, or disc drusen, is often an incidental finding on routine ocular examination. Disc drusen are congenital,

acellular, calcific bodies commonly found bilaterally and associated with small, crowded optic nerves. Optic nerve drusen is associated with abnormal axonal metabolism, as well as axonal transport alterations. The prevalence in the general population has been estimated at approximately 0.4%; however, histological studies have reported prevalence as high as 2.4%.[1] The condition can occur sporadically or in an autosomal dominant fashion, and there is a strong predilection for Caucasians and females.[2]

In young patients, optic nerve drusen will present as an elevated optic disc with indistinct borders (buried drusen) due to the drusen being deeply embedded in the papilla. With age, the drusen become more evident ophthalmoscopically as yellow excrescences on the disc surface. They enlarge due to calcium apposition and move anteriorly within the nerve head. The disc is elevated, and optic nerve cupping is usually not present. Patients with disc drusen often have anomalous vascular patterns, including arterial or venous trifurcation (Figure 3.17-1). They may also have the appearance of an increased number of vessels on the disc, abnormal or premature branching, tortuosity, vascular loops, or cilioretinal vessels.

Visual field defects secondary to optic nerve drusen occur in 24% to 87% of adults.[1] This is likely due to impaired axonal transport leading to gradual nerve fiber layer loss, direct compression of prelaminar nerve fibers by drusen, or ischemia within the optic nerve head. While numerous types of visual field defects are associated with optic nerve drusen, arcuate defects are the most common.

B-scan ultrasonography continues to be the gold standard for detecting disc drusen. Here disc drusen are highly reflective on both high and low gain levels. Other noninvasive ocular imaging technology, such as fundus autofluorescence imaging and OCT, is becoming an increasingly important tool for diagnosing optic nerve drusen. With fundus autofluorescence, optic nerve drusen will appear as bright areas on the optic nerve. Enhanced depth OCT has the ability to detect the drusen themselves, allowing more ability to assess the structure and location. Optical coherence tomography is also useful in following the progression of retinal nerve fiber layer (RNFL) loss.

There are a number of conditions, including optic nerve drusen, that can be confused with papilledema because they look like bilateral swollen optic nerves (pseudopapilledema). Other conditions that can mimic papilledema include hypoplastic optic nerves, myelinated RNFL, high hyperopia, and vitreopapillary traction. Cases of pseudopapilledema must be differentiated from the more ominous diagnosis of papilledema because inappropriate referrals may result in timely and expensive neuroimaging studies that expose healthy patients to unnecessary radiation.

There are various methods for using OCT to differentiate optic nerve drusen from true optic nerve edema. Optic nerve drusen will present with a bumpy internal contour and an abrupt ending to the subretinal hyporeflective space around the nerve. In contrast, optic nerve edema will show a smooth internal contour with a tapering of the subretinal hyporeflective space that leads to a characteristic "lazy V" pattern. A number of studies have found that quantitative values may be better than subjective data in differentiating disc drusen from edema. Using a spectral domain OCT, Flores-Rodrguez[3] found that an average RNFL thickness cutoff of 116 micrometer gave a 91% sensitivity and 97% specificity in differentiating the 2 conditions. Anything thicker than 116 micrometer was likely to be papilledema. Anything thinner than 116 was more likely to be disc drusen. In a different study, Lee[4] found something similar, but he demonstrated that the nasal RNFL thickness measurement was most valuable in differentiating edema from pseudoedema. He found that a cut off of 78 micrometer in the nasal area provided 80% sensitivity and 89% specificity.

There is currently no universally accepted treatment for optic nerve drusen. It is reasonable to closely monitor the patient for changes in visual field, nerve fiber layer analysis, and clinical appearance of the optic nerve. While there has been speculation that the nerve fiber layer may be more susceptible to elevated or even normal intraocular pressure, it is not clear whether topical antihypertensive medications are indicated. These patients should be monitored closely with serial visual field testing, nerve fiber layer analysis, and optic nerve photos.

The topical alpha-2 adrenergic agonist brimonidine has demonstrated potential neuroprotective benefits in patients with ischemic optic neuropathies.[5] Although the exact mechanism of neuroprotection remains unclear, brimonidine has demonstrated 3 out of 4 criteria required to demonstrate neuroprotective effects: receptors on target tissue, adequate penetration to the retina, and induction of intracellular changes that enhance neuronal resistance to insult in animal studies. To date, brimonidine has yet to satisfy the fourth criterion, that is, demonstrated efficacy in human clinical trials.

Visual field loss associated with optic nerve drusen is typically slow. Lee and Zimmerman[6] found the average rate of visual field loss was 1.6% over 36 months. Visual field loss occurs at a significantly higher rate in ocular hypertensive eyes.[7] Despite visual field loss central visual acuity (VA) is generally spared, and the patient remains asymptomatic.

CLINICAL PEARLS

- Optic nerve head drusen is often discovered incidentally on clinical examination; since central visual acuity is generally spared, these patients are typically asymptomatic.

- Peripheral visual field defects are common with optic nerve head drusen, most often following a superior or inferior arcuate pattern that can mimic glaucoma.

- Although there is no universally accepted treatment for optic nerve head drusen, appropriate diagnosis and differentiation from true papilledema are critical.

REFERENCES

1. Morris RW, Ellerbrock JM, Hamp AM, Joy JT, Roels P, Davis CN. Advanced visual field loss secondary to optic nerve head drusen: case report and literature review. *Optometry.* 2009;80:83-100.
2. Mansour AM, Hamed LM. Racial variation of optic nerve diseases. *Neuroophthalmology.* 1991;11:319-323.
3. Flores-Rodriguez P, Gili P, Martin-Rios. Sensitivity and specificity of time-domain and spectral-domain optical coherence tomography in differentiating optic nerve head drusen and optic disc oedema. *Ophthalmic Physiol Opt.* 2012;32:213-221.
4. Lee KM, Woo SJ, Hwang JM. Differentiation of optic nerve head drusen and optic disc edema with spectral-domain optical coherence tomography. *Ophthalmology.* 2011;118:971-977.
5. Saylor M, McLoon LK, Harrison AR, Lee MS. Experimental and clinical evidence for brimonidine as an optic nerve and retinal neuroprotective agent: an evidence-based review. *Arch Ophthalmol.* 2009;127:402-406.
6. Lee AG, Zimmerman MB. The rate of visual field loss in optic nerve head drusen. *Am J Ophthalmol.* 2005;139:1062-1066.
7. Grippo TM, Shihadeh WA, Schargus M, et al. Optic nerve head drusen and visual field loss in normotensive and hypertensive eyes. *J Glaucoma.* 2008; 17:100-104.

3.18 Demyelinating Optic Neuritis

Erin M. Draper

Jack, a 33-year-old male, presented to the emergency clinic with concerns of blurry vision in his right eye for the past week. He reported that a little over a week ago he was hit in the right eye by his 3-year-old son's hand while playing, but the vision loss did not start until a few days later. He felt that his vision had become progressively worse over the past week, and he noticed pain when he moved his eyes. He denied the presence of flashes, floaters, diplopia, or light sensitivity. This was his first eye examination.

Medical history was remarkable for depression and bipolar disorder. He reported being stabbed in the back of the neck 1 year ago. He also reported a history of dizziness and vertigo over the past 7 months. Current medications included lithium, bupropion (Wellbutrin), and sertraline hydrochloride (Zoloft). He smoked cigarettes but denied any drug or alcohol abuse.

Clinical Findings

Unaided distance VA	OD: 20/50 (no improvement with pinhole); OS: 20/20
Confrontation visual fields	OD: central scotoma temporal to fixation OS: full to finger counting; no central scotoma
Pupil evaluation	PERRL; grade 2 right RAPD
Color testing (Ishihara)	OD: 11/14 plates; OS: 14/14 plates
Brightness sense	40% decreased sensation of brightness in the right eye compared to left eye
Ductions	OD: full and smooth with pain on adduction OS: full and smooth with no pain
Distance cover test	4Δ exophoria in primary gaze; comitant in all positions of gaze
Slit-lamp examination	OD: Grade 1 nasal conjunctival injection; otherwise unremarkable with no evidence of cells or flare in the anterior chamber OS: Grade 1 nasal conjunctival injection; otherwise unremarkable with no evidence of cells or flare in the anterior chamber
Intraocular pressure (GAT)	OD: 13 mm Hg; OS: 11 mm Hg at 3:44 PM
Fundus examination	OD 0.3/0.3 CD ratio; healthy rim tissue with distinct disc margins; fovea flat and dry; normal vasculature; no evidence of inflammation; periphery intact OS 0.35/0.35 CD ratio; healthy rim tissue with distinct disc margins; fovea flat and dry; normal vasculature; no evidence of inflammation; periphery intact
Visual field (24-2 SITA-standard, Figure 3.18-1)	OD: generalized reduction, with central depression, that does not respect the horizontal or vertical midlines OS: superior edge defects are likely an eyelid artifact

| Neuroimaging (Figures 3.18-2 and 3.18-3) | MRI of the brain with contrast demonstrated findings consistent with optic neuritis and demyelinating disease |

Abbreviations: CD, cup to disc; GAT, Goldmann applanation tonometry; MRI, magnetic resonance imaging; OD, right eye; OS, left eye; PERRL, pupils equal, round, reactive to light; RAPD, relative afferent pupillary defect; VA, visual acuity.

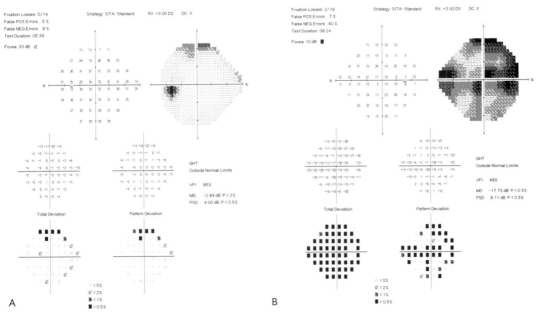

Figure 3.18-1   Visual field demonstrating mild superior visual field loss, likely from lid artifact, in the left eye (A) and overall depression with central scotoma in the right eye (B).

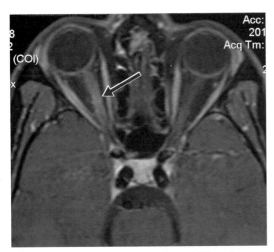

Figure 3.18-2   Gadolinium-enhanced T1 axial magnetic resonance imaging cut through the optic nerves. The right optic nerve (arrow) is hyperintense compared to the left optic nerve indicating enhancement following gadolinium administration.

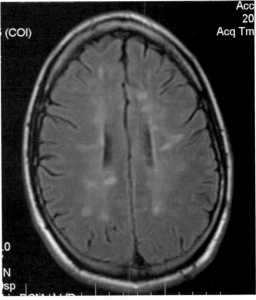

Figure 3.18-3   Axial fluid-attenuated inversion recovery magnetic resonance imaging with white matter lesions consistent with demyelinating disease.

Comments

Jack was diagnosed with retrobulbar optic neuritis and was treated with intravenous methylprednisolone for 5 days with an oral taper of prednisone. He was asked to return to the clinic in 1 month to assure resolution. In addition, he was referred to a neurologist, diagnosed with multiple sclerosis (MS), and started on the immunomodulator treatment glatiramer acetate (Copaxone).

Follow-up Visit (1 Month Following the Initial Examination)

Best-corrected distance VA	OD: 20/25+2; OS: 20/20
Confrontation visual fields	Full to finger counting; no central scotoma OD and OS
Pupil evaluation	PERRL; grade 1 right RAPD
Color testing (Ishihara)	OD: 10/14 plates; OS: 14/14 plates
Fundus examination	OD: 0.3/0.3 CD ratio with mild temporal pallor of neuro retinal rim; otherwise unremarkable OS: 0.35/0.35 CD ratio with intact and pink neuro retinal rim; otherwise unremarkable

Abbreviations: CD, cup to disc; OD, right eye; OS, left eye; PERRL, pupils equal, round, reactive to light; RAPD, relative afferent pupillary defect; VA, visual acuity.

Discussion

A clinician triaging a patient complaining of decreased vision after trauma is likely to have traumatic uveitis or retinal detachment as leading differential diagnoses. In Jack's case, as there were no clinical findings consistent with uveitis or retinal detachment, further analysis was necessary.

On examination, all measures of the afferent visual system of the right eye were found to be compromised. These included decreased visual acuity, decreased color vision, confrontation visual field defects, decreased sense of brightness, and, most importantly, the presence of a relative afferent pupillary defect (RAPD). The latter is the only objective measurement of the afferent visual system and therefore does not rely on input from the patient. The presence of an RAPD with a normal appearing retina should immediately alert the practitioner that the lesion is likely to involve the optic nerve or optic tract. In this case, optic neuropathy was the most likely diagnosis, but fundus examination showed the optic nerve head to have a completely normal appearance. One should not be fooled by this observation. Fundus examination only allows the detection of anterior optic neuritis or papillitis. The RAPD and other decreased measures of the afferent visual system, together with the normal fundus appearance, are indicative of retrobulbar optic neuritis. Additionally, Jack complained of pain on eye movements, which is a classic symptom of demyelinating optic neuritis. The pain occurs because the sheaths of the medial and superior rectus muscles are connected to the optic nerve sheath. With eye movement, the muscles pull on the inflamed nerve leading to pain.

Optic neuritis is an inflammation that can occur at any point on the optic nerve. The intraocular portion of the optic nerve, which is the portion that can be viewed during fundus examination, represents only 1 mm of the approximately 5 cm total length of the nerve. Therefore, it is not surprising that the majority (approximately two-thirds) of optic neuritis presentations are retrobulbar and therefore will not be detected during fundus examination. Only about one-third of cases present with papillitis. Even if disc edema is visible, peripapillary hemorrhages are rare in demyelinating optic neuritis. Therefore, the presence of hemorrhages can help differentiate between demyelinating optic neuritis and other causes of papillitis such as anterior ischemic optic neuropathy. Another distinguishing feature of demyelinating optic neuritis is timing. Patients typically notice a gradual decrease in vision over a few days to 2 weeks. These patients generally experience significant improvement in visual acuity within 2 to 3 weeks from the onset.[1]

Demyelinating optic neuritis most often occurs in patients 18 to 50 years of age and has a high association with MS. Diagnosis of optic neuritis can be made on clinical findings alone, but a gadolinium-enhanced magnetic resonance imaging (MRI) is often performed to confirm the diagnosis and aid in assessment of prognosis and treatment decisions. Fifteen-year follow-up data from the Optic Neuritis Treatment Trial (ONTT) found that 25% of patients who had no MRI abnormalities consistent with MS at the time of the episode of optic neuritis still went on to develop MS. In addition, 50% of patients with 1 or more MRI lesions but no other symptomology went on to develop MS in 5 years, and 72% of patients with 1 or more MRI lesions developed MS in 15 years.[2]

The severity of vision loss during an episode of optic neuritis varies from 20/20 to no light perception. Fortunately, the prognosis for visual acuity recovery is very good. The ONTT found that 5 years after an episode of acute optic neuritis, mean visual acuity was 20/25 or better in 87% of affected eyes and only 3% had acuity of 20/200 or worse.[3] Further, visual function, including visual acuity, contrast sensitivity, and visual field, was worse in patients diagnosed with MS compared to those not diagnosed with MS.

Based on the findings of the ONTT, if a patient's acuity is worse than 20/40 during the first 8 days after onset of visual symptoms, treatment with intravenous methylprednisolone followed by oral prednisone should be considered. Treatment was found to hasten visual recovery, although the final visual acuity was similar to that of untreated patients. In addition, patients with abnormal MRI findings who were treated with intravenous methylprednisolone had a 2-year protective benefit against developing MS.[4]

If a patient's characteristics are inconsistent with those typically found in optic neuritis, such as being outside the expected age range or having poor visual recovery, causes of atypical optic neuritis should be considered.[5] These include neuromyelitis optica, infectious optic neuropathy, inflammatory optic neuropathy, Leber hereditary optic neuropathy, and other autoimmune optic neuropathies.

The pathology of demyelinating optic neuritis is similar to that of acute MS plaques in the brain. Unlike other cranial nerves, which are covered by Schwann cells, the optic nerves are myelinated by oligodendrocytes, the same myelination found in the central nervous system. Therefore, oligodendrocytes of the optic nerve are susceptible to attacks of inflammation and demyelination resulting in optic neuritis and optic atrophy. Although the exact mechanism is not yet understood, there is believed to be a systemic T-cell activation that leads to the release of cytokines and other inflammatory agents. These agents attack the oligodendrocytes that create the myelin sheath around the axons of the central nervous system. The attacks lead to the demyelination of axons, which impair the ability of the nerve fiber to conduct impulses at expected frequencies. Additionally, these nerve fibers may have abnormal excitation. Due to these changes, patients with demyelination may experience focal or generalized paresthesias, sudden brief electric-like sensations radiating down the spine or extremities (Lhermitte's sign), facial myokymia, or photopsia induced by eye movement.[6] Demyelination also makes the nerves more susceptible to temperature changes. Therefore, when the body temperature rises after exercise or a warm shower, nerve fiber conduction is further impaired creating temporary production or exasperation of MS symptoms (Uhthoff's phenomenon).

CLINICAL PEARL

- The pupils do not lie. If the optic nerve head and retina appear healthy on clinical examination, but the patient has an afferent pupillary defect, you should be suspicious of a retrobulbar optic nerve disorder.

REFERENCES

1. Shams PN, Plant GT. Optic neuritis: a review. *Int MS J*. 2009;16:82-89.
2. Volpe NJ. The optic neuritis treatment trial: a definitive answer and profound impact with unexpected results. *Arch Ophthalmol*. 2008;126:996-999.

3. Optic Neuritis Study Group. Visual function five years after optic neuritis: experience of the Optic Neuritis Treatment Trial. *Arch Ophthalmol.* 1997;115: 1545-1552.

4. Beck RW, Cleary PA, Anderson MM, et al. A randomized, controlled trial of corticosteroids in the treatment of acute optic neuritis. The Optic Neuritis Study Group. *N Engl J Med.* 1992;326:581-588.

5. Malik A, Ahmed M, Golnik K. Treatment options for atypical optic neuritis. *Indian J Ophthalmol.* 2014;62:982-984.

6. Miller NR, Newman NJ, Biousse B, Kerrison JB, eds. *Walsh & Hoyt's Clinical Neuro-Ophthalmology.* 6th ed. Philadelphia, PA: Lippincott Williams & Wilkins; 2005.

3.19 Nonarteritic Anterior Ischemic Optic Neuropathy

Alana M. Santaro and Andrew J. Di Mattina

Howard, a 57-year-old white male, presented with sudden onset reduced vision in his left eye. The reduced vision had started approximately a week prior to presentation. He also reported a transient, dull ache in the left temporal area and around the left eye. He denied jaw claudication or scalp tenderness. There were no other associated symptoms.

Ocular history was significant for an elevated benign choroidal nevus of the right eye and refractive error previously correctable to 20/20 in each eye. Medical history was significant for hyperlipidemia and erectile dysfunction. He was controlling the hyperlipidemia with diet modification and was taking tadalafil (Cialis) for the past 10 months for erectile dysfunction.

Clinical Findings

Habitual distance VA	OD: 20/20; OS: 20/40 (no improvement with pinhole)
Extraocular motilities	Full, smooth, and accurate with no pain noted OD and OS
Pupil evaluation	PERRL; positive left RAPD
Color vision (Ishihara)	OD: 7/7 plates; OS: 3/7 plates
Slit-lamp examination	OD: trace nuclear sclerosis; otherwise unremarkable
	OS: trace nuclear sclerosis; otherwise unremarkable
Intraocular pressure (GAT)	OD: 20 mm Hg; OS: 20 mm Hg at 4:45 PM
Fundus examination (Figure 3.19-1)	OD: 0.10/0.10 CD ratio; healthy rim tissue with distinct disc margins; fovea flat and dry; normal vasculature; periphery intact
	OS: 0.10/0.10 CD ratio; edematous and hyperemic rim tissue greater temporally with indistinct disc margins; splinter hemorrhages surrounding disc superiorly and inferiorly; fovea flat and dry; periphery intact
Visual field (Humphrey 30-2 SITA-standard, Figure 3.19-2)	OD: good reliabilty; mild depression, greater inferiorly that respects the vertical midline
	OS: good reliabiilty; overall depression not respecting the horizontal or vertical midlines
Urgent laboratory testing	ESR, CRP, CBC with platelet count were within normal limits

427

| Additional laboratory testing | Fasting glucose and HbA1c were within normal limits; lipid panel showed normal triglyceride and high density lipoprotein cholesterol levels but high total cholesterol (237 mg/dL, normal 0-200 mg/dL) and low-density lipoprotein cholesterol (135 mg/dL, normal 0-129 mg/dL) |

Abbreviations: CBC, complete blood count; CD, cup to disc; CRP, C-reactive protein; ESR, erythrocyte sedimentation rate; GAT, Goldmann applanation tonometry; OD, right eye; OS, left eye; PERRL, pupils equal, round, reactive to light; RAPD, relative afferent pupillary defect; VA, visual acuity.

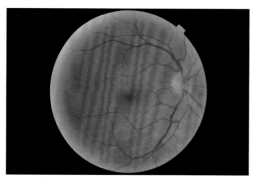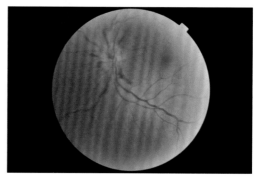

Figure 3.19-1 The right eye showed a small optic nerve with minimal cupping. Disc edema is evident in the left eye.

Discussion

Based on the presentation of sudden onset, painless decreased vision with an associated swollen optic nerve, reduced color vision, and relative afferent pupillary defect, our main differential diagnoses were nonarteritic anterior ischemic optic neuropathy (NAION) and arteritic anterior ischemic optic neuropathy (AAION). After receiving normal erythrocyte sedimentation rate (ESR) and C-reactive protein (CRP) results, Howard was diagnosed with an NAION. He was referred to his primary care physician where he was started on atorvastatin (Lipitor) 40 mg daily to better control his cholesterol levels. We also recommended that he discontinue Cialis.

At the 2-month follow-up visit, vision had recovered to 20/25 in the left eye, and his color vision was 7/7 plates in each eye. His nerve displayed diffuse pallor without edema.

Ischemic optic neuropathy is a potentially visually devastating disease that affects middle-aged to elderly patients. Loss of vision from the optic neuropathy can manifest as reduced visual field, loss of visual acuity (VA), or both. If disc edema is visible with ophthalmoscopy, it is considered anterior optic neuropathy, whereas posterior optic neuropathy affects the orbital, canalicular, or intracranial portions of the optic nerve. Nonarteritic anterior ischemic optic neuropathy is a noninflammatory hypoperfusion of the optic nerve. Ischemia associated with AAION is secondary to vasculitis, most commonly due to giant cell arteritis.[1]

Nonarteritic anterior ischemic optic neuropathy is the most common acute optic neuropathy in individuals older than 50 years and is more common in white individuals compared with African American or Hispanic populations. The etiology of NAION is presumed to be vascular insufficiency to the optic nerve, and it has been associated with hypertension, hyperlipidemia, diabetes, and smoking. It is unclear whether obstructive sleep apnea is causative or a coexisting condition in these patients. Phosphodiesterase inhibitors, such as sildenafil and tadalafil, used for the treatment of erectile dysfunction, have been implicated in the development of NAION. Likewise, amiodarone, used for arrhythmia treatment, is associated with bilateral NAION. However, it is unclear whether the optic neuropathy associated with

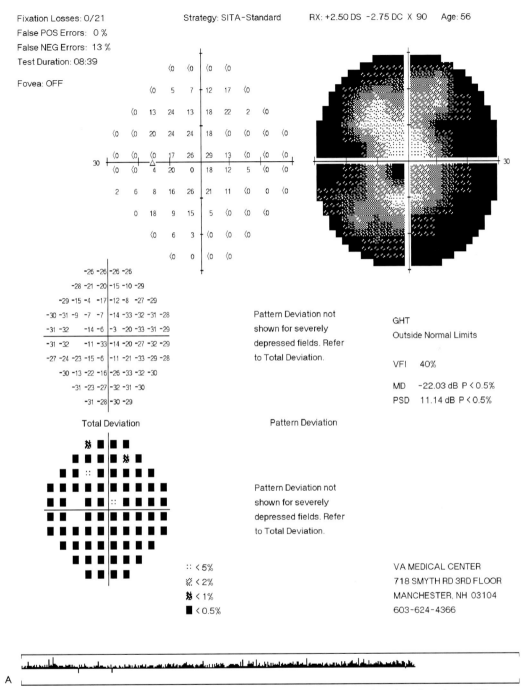

Figure 3.19-2 Visual field showing overall loss in the left eye (A) and mild loss inferiorly in the right eye (B).

these medications is coincidental in this at-risk age group. In patients younger than 50 years, consider hypercoagulable states as a possible etiology, as these conditions are associated with a significantly increased incidence of NAION.[2]

Patients with NAION generally present with painless, monocular vision loss. This is most commonly noted on awakening. Visual acuity can be variable, from 20/20 to no light perception, but two-thirds of patients retain

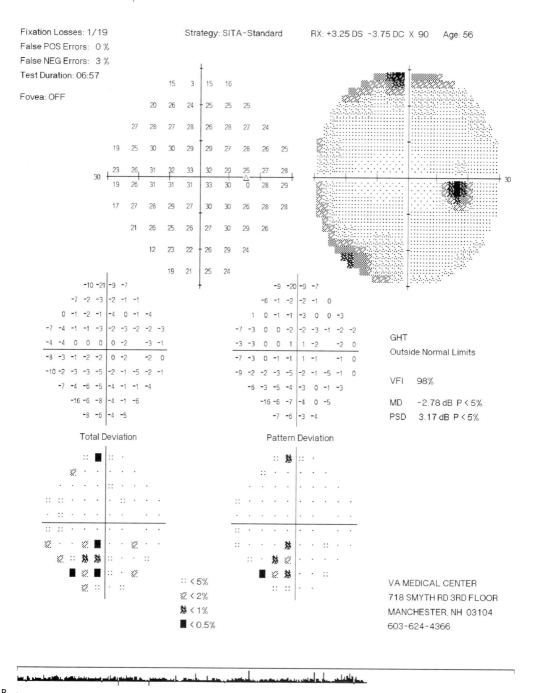

Fixation Losses: 1/19   Strategy: SITA-Standard   RX: +3.25 DS -3.75 DC X 90   Age: 56

False POS Errors: 0 %

False NEG Errors: 3 %

Test Duration: 06:57

Fovea: OFF

GHT
Outside Normal Limits

VFI   98%

MD   -2.78 dB P < 5%

PSD   3.17 dB P < 5%

Total Deviation

Pattern Deviation

:: < 5%

▨ < 2%

🐾 < 1%

■ < 0.5%

VA MEDICAL CENTER

718 SMYTH RD 3RD FLOOR

MANCHESTER, NH 03104

603-624-4366

B

Figure 3.19-2 (Continued)

vision better than 20/200.[3] On examination, the fellow eye may display a "disk at risk", defined as a small diameter, crowded optic disc with a small cup. Acutely, the optic nerve has optic disc edema and peripapillary flame–shaped hemorrhages. Altitudinal visual field loss is the most common pattern of visual field loss, but overall loss or an arcuate defect can occur. Color vision and visual field are lost after an episode of NAION and the nerve develops diffuse or segmental pallor 4 to 6 weeks after the event.[3]

Laboratory testing is not necessary to make the diagnosis of NAION, but an urgent complete blood count (CBC), ESR, and CRP should be ordered to rule out giant cell arteritis. Neuroimaging is not indicated unless the case demonstrates atypical findings, such as pain, lack of disc at risk in the contralateral eye, progressive vision loss after 1 to 2 weeks, or persistent optic nerve edema lasting more than 6 weeks.

There is currently no standard treatment regimen for an acute NAION. Disc edema resolves in 6 to 8 weeks without treatment. Visual acuity may improve within the first 6 months.[4] Medical and surgical options have been proposed and trialed with no clear benefit found. Surgical intervention in the form of optic nerve decompression has been attempted but was not beneficial in improving final acuity.[5] Hayreh found some effect on vision with 80 mg of prednisone within 2 weeks of an acute NAION. However, the results have not been uniformly accepted, and the potential benefits may be outweighed by the risk of steroid-induced complications in these patients with vasculopathy, including diabetes.[5,6]

Over 5 years, the risk of NAION in the contralateral eye is approximately 15%.[3] Therefore, it is important to treat vasculopathic risk factors and recommend avoidance of potential associated substances, such as erectile dysfunction drugs. To minimize nocturnal hypotension, blood pressure medication should not be taken before bed.

Giant cell arteritis is a vasculitis of medium and large vessels with an average age of onset of 70 years. This vasculitis results in AAION, which can cause rapidly progressive, bilateral blindness if left untreated in 15% to 20% of those affected. Patients may present with symptoms of headache, scalp tenderness, jaw claudication, malaise, anorexia, fever, and weight loss. However, 25% of patients with AAION due to giant cell arteritis have no systemic symptoms.[6] Transient vision loss or diplopia may precede permanent vision loss.

Vision loss is generally more severe in AAION compared to NAION, leaving more than half of patients unable to count fingers.[6]

The swollen disc is often pale, and a disc at risk is not necessarily present with AAION.

On suspicion of ischemic optic neuropathy, laboratory testing should be obtained immediately to help differentiate AAION from NAION. Specific laboratory testing should include a CBC, platelet count, ESR, and CRP. The combination of the ESR and CRP is 97% specific for giant cell arteritis when they are both elevated.[4] If the clinical suspicion for AAION is low and the laboratory testing is normal, no further workup is required. Howard had no systemic symptoms of giant cell arteritis, vision loss was not severe, and laboratory tests were normal. For these reasons, the diagnosis of giant cell arteritis was excluded.

If the ESR and CRP are elevated, a temporal artery biopsy should be performed to confirm the diagnosis of giant cell arteritis. On biopsy, inflammation in the vessel wall will confirm the diagnosis of giant cell arteritis. Two to 3 cm sections bilaterally should be studied as inflammation may be missed from discontinuous arterial involvement, known as skip lesions, resulting in a false negative result.

Treatment with high dose oral steroids should be initiated immediately on elevated ESR and CRP levels, as a biopsy may not be immediately available.[4] Systemic symptoms are very responsive to steroid treatment. Unfortunately, even with treatment, vision loss is usually profound and permanent. Without treatment, the contralateral eye becomes involved in more than half of cases, making AAION one of the true ophthalmic emergencies.[6]

CLINICAL PEARL

- All patients older than 55 years who present with transient vision loss, persistent vision loss, or diplopia should be sent for an urgent ESR and C-reactive protein testing to rule out giant cell arteritis.

REFERENCES

1. Hayreh S, Zimmerman MB. Nonarteritic anterior ischemic optic neuropathy. *Ophthalmology*. 2008;115:298-305.
2. Cestari D, Gaier E, Bouzika P, et al. Demographic, systemic, and ocular factors associated with

nonarteritic anterior ischemic optic neuropathy. *Ophthalmology*. 2016;123:2446-2455.

3. Atkins E, Bruce B, Newman N, Biousse V. Treatment of nonarteritic anterior ischemic optic neuropathy. *Surv Ophthalmol*. 2010;55:47-63.

4. Chacko JG, Chacko JA, Salter M. Review of giant cell arteritis. *Saudi J Ophthalmol*. 2015;29:48-52.

5. Ischemic Optic Neuropathy Decompression Trial Research Group. Optic nerve decompression surgery for nonarteritic anterior ischemic optic neuropathy (NAION) is not effective and may be harmful. *JAMA*. 1995;273:625-632.

6. Biousse V, Newman NJ. Ischemic optic neuropathies. *N Engl J Med*. 2015;372:2428-2436.

3.20 Idiopathic Intracranial Hypertension

Caroline M. Ooley

Sarah, a 30-year-old Caucasian female, presented with headaches and blurred vision in both eyes, which began 4 weeks ago. The headaches were located behind both eyes and became worse when reclining and getting out of bed in the morning. Sarah reported seeing triangular shapes in the temporal field of each eye, which caused words to disappear, and she described hearing a whooshing sound in both ears. Each of these symptoms began at the same time as the headaches.

Sarah was seen in our office 18 months ago. The examination was unremarkable other than asymptomatic lattice degeneration. She had no history of trauma or family history of eye disease. She had gained 15 pounds over the past 3 to 6 months. She denied any recent illness or travel and was not a current smoker.

Current medications included methylphenidate (Concerta) for attention deficit disorder, paroxetine (Paxil) for anxiety disorder, methocarbamol for pain and muscle relaxation, and hydrocodone 5 mg/acetaminophen 325 mg (Vicodin) for back pain following a recent car accident.

Clinical Findings

Habitual distance VA	OD: $20/20^{-1}$; OS: $20/20^{-1}$
Present Rx	OD: −2.75 −0.75 × 171 OS: −3.25 −0.75 × 175
Cover test	Orthophoria distance and near
Color vision (Ishihara)	OD and OS: 10/10 plates
Pupil evaluation	PERRL; no RAPD
Slit-lamp examination	OD: mild punctate epithelial erosions OS: unremarkable
Intraocular pressure (GAT)	OD: 13 mm Hg; OS: 15 mm Hg at 11:15 AM
Fundus examination (Figure 3.20-1)	OD: 0.1/0.1 CD ratio; elevated margins with scattered peripapillary hemorrhages; fovea flat and dry; slightly dilated veins; peripheral lattice degeneration OS: 0.1/0.1 CD ratio; elevated margins with scattered peripapillary hemorrhages; fovea flat and dry; slightly dilated veins; periphery intact
Nerve fiber layer OCT (Figure 3.20-2)	OD: significant optic disc swelling with elevated RNFL thickness (average thickness 391 μm); hyporeflective subretinal space present surrounding the optic disc OS: significant optic disc swelling with elevated RNFL thickness (average thickness 352 μm); hyporeflective subretinal space present surrounding the optic disc

Visual field (SITA-standard 24-2, Figure 3.20-3)	OD: good reliability; enlarged blind spot OS: good reliability; enlarged blind spot, mild inferior depression

Abbreviations: CD, cup to disc; GAT, Goldmann applanation tonometry; OCT, optical coherence tomography; OD, right eye; OS, left eye; PERRL, pupils equal, round, reactive to light; RAPD, relative afferent pupillary defect; RNFL, retinal nerve fiber layer; Rx, prescription; VA, visual acuity.

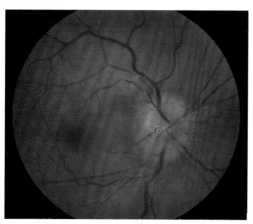 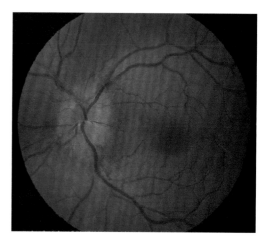

Figure 3.20-1   Optic nerve edema is evident in both eyes.

Comments

Sarah presented with recent onset headaches, temporal scotomas, and pulsatile tinnitus. This presentation, along with recent weight gain, bilateral disc edema, and bilateral enlarged blind spots, is suspicious for idiopathic intracranial hypertension, a subset of papilledema. The patient was sent to the emergency department for an urgent magnetic resonance imaging (MRI) of the brain with and without contrast, as well as a magnetic resonance venography (MRV). Both were unremarkable. A lumbar puncture was subsequently performed revealing an opening pressure of 370 mm H_2O with clear cerebral spinal fluid (CSF). She was prescribed acetazolamide (Diamox) 250 mg orally twice per day. She was discharged the same day with the advice to lose weight.

Sarah was followed every 2 to 3 months until her symptoms and optic disc appearance returned to normal. She struggled with losing weight and had a relapse of her symptoms requiring an increase in acetazolamide to 500 mg twice per day. Eventually, she was able to lose weight, return to an acetazolamide dosage of 250 mg twice per day, and ultimately discontinue the medication once all subjective and objective findings subsided. We continue to follow her every 6 months.

Discussion

The pia, arachnoid, and dura mater that make up the meninges in the brain also surround the intracranial and intraorbital optic nerve. Because the subarachnoid space surrounding the brain is continuous with the subarachnoid space surrounding the optic nerve, an increase in intracranial pressure will cause compression of the optic nerves, leading to impaired axoplasmic flow and papilledema.

Not all optic disc edema is papilledema. The term papilledema is reserved for conditions where the CSF pressure surrounding the brain and spinal column is increased. Papilledema that occurs despite normal CSF composition and without an anatomical reason for the increased intracranial pressure is termed primary pseudotumor cerebri or idiopathic intracranial hypertension. This typically occurs in young females of childbearing age who have an elevated body mass index or have recently

ONH and RNFL OU Analysis:Optic Disc Cube 200x200   OD ● | ● OS

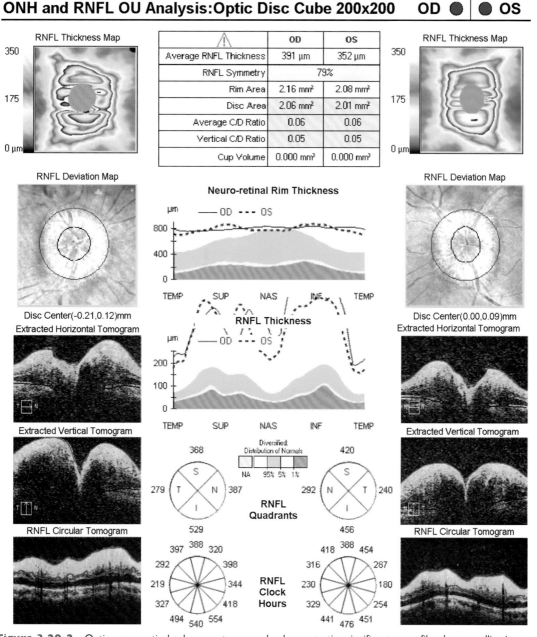

	OD	OS
Average RNFL Thickness	391 μm	352 μm
RNFL Symmetry	79%	
Rim Area	2.16 mm²	2.08 mm²
Disc Area	2.06 mm²	2.01 mm²
Average C/D Ratio	0.06	0.06
Vertical C/D Ratio	0.05	0.05
Cup Volume	0.000 mm³	0.000 mm³

Figure 3.20-2   Optic nerve optical coherence tomography demonstrating significant nerve fiber layer swelling in both eyes.

gained weight.[1] More than 90% are female, and more than 90% are overweight.[2]

The exact etiology of idiopathic intracranial hypertension is not well understood. Any process increasing CSF production by the choroid plexus within the ventricles, decreasing CSF absorption by the arachnoid villi, or inhibiting normal venous circulation can lead to an increase in intracranial pressure. Proposed mechanisms include abnormal vitamin A metabolism, endocrine factors, stenosis of the venous sinuses, and venous hypertension.

Headache is the most common symptom associated with papilledema, occurring in 84% of patients.[3] The headache is often pulsatile and not localized to a specific region. It worsens

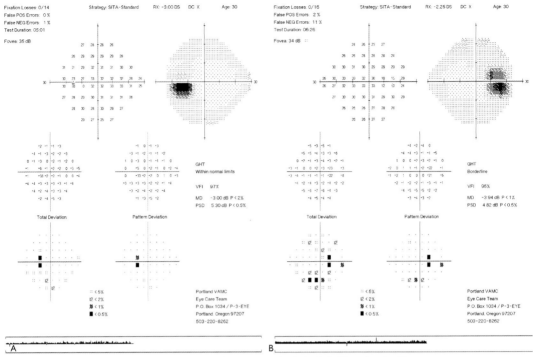

Figure 3.20-3 Visual fields show an enlarged blind spot in both the left (A) and right (B) eyes.

with changes in posture or other activities that increase cerebral venous pressure like Valsalva maneuver or coughing. Other symptoms include nausea and vomiting, pulsatile tinnitus, transient visual obscurations lasting seconds to minutes, photophobia, and horizontal diplopia secondary to a cranial nerve 6 palsy.

Most patients with papilledema present with normal visual acuity (VA). Only 10% to 25% of patients present with vision worse than 20/20.[3] Color vision is generally normal, and there is usually no relative afferent pupillary defect (RAPD) since the condition is bilateral. Visual field loss is typically seen before a decline in VA and will show an enlarged blind spot in 92% of patients.[1,4,5] Disc edema associated with papilledema is typically bilateral and symmetric. Spontaneous venous pulsation, seen as subtle narrowing and widening of retinal veins, is absent in cases of papilledema. It is thought that spontaneous venous pulsation is present only when the intracranial pressure is less than 200 mm H$_2$O. However, only 80% of normal patients exhibit spontaneous venous pulsation, so the absence of spontaneous venous pulsation does not indicate increased intracranial pressure.

Conditions, including optic disc drusen, hypoplastic optic nerves, myelinated nerve fiber layer, and vitreopapillary traction, can have a similar appearance to papilledema despite not being associated with true optic disc edema. These conditions are called pseudopapilledema. It is important to differentiate these conditions from true papilledema to save the patient costly medical testing. Optical coherence tomography (OCT) is valuable in differentiating true disc edema from pseudopapilledema (see Chapter 3.17). In addition, circumferential peripapillary retinal folds or a gray halo surrounding the disc are commonly seen with papilledema but not pseudopapilledema.

Urgent neuroimaging is necessary to rule out other more devastating causes of increased intracranial pressure, including an intracranial mass, cerebral venous sinus thrombosis, meningitis, or subarachnoid hemorrhage. An MRI of the brain with and without contrast is preferred, although a computed tomography (CT) scan can be performed if magnetic imaging is contraindicated. Magnetic resonance venography, looking for cerebral venous sinus thrombosis, should be performed on patients suspected of having idiopathic intracranial hypertension, especially patients who do not fit into typical categories for this condition, that is, males, children, and nonobese women. Patients with cerebral venous sinus thrombosis are at a much higher risk for stroke so it is important to diagnose this correctly. An MRV should also be considered for patients who are postpartum, taking oral contraceptives, or who have known coagulopathy.

Although neuroimaging in patients with idiopathic intracranial hypertension should not show a mass or meningeal enhancement, there are specific neuroimaging findings suggestive of idiopathic intracranial hypertension. For example, an empty sella may occur due to compression of the pituitary gland or enlargement of the sella turcica. Flattening of the posterior globe may be present due to mechanical forces on the globe that occur due to the increased CSF pressure surrounding the optic nerve. Increased CSF in the subarachnoid space around the optic nerve can also lead to distention of the optic nerve sheath. Stenosis of the cerebral venous sinuses is a common finding in idiopathic intracranial hypertension. It is unclear whether the venous stenosis is caused by the increased intracranial pressure or whether the stenosis causes the increased intracranial pressure.

If no cause of papilledema is found on neuroimaging, a lumbar puncture is necessary to make the diagnosis of idiopathic intracranial hypertension. The upper limit for opening pressure in adults is 200 mm H_2O. A normal value of 200 to 250 mm H_2O is considered borderline, and greater than 250 mm H_2O is considered abnormal. In addition to the opening pressure, the composition of the cerebrospinal fluid should be analyzed for protein level, cell count, and glucose level.[4,5]

The first line of treatment for idiopathic intracranial hypertension is acetazolamide, a carbonic anhydrase inhibitor, which reduces sodium ion transport across the choroid plexus, thereby reducing the production of cerebrospinal fluid. Acetazolamide is generally prescribed as 250 to 500 mg orally twice daily and increased gradually to a maximum of 2 to 4 g per day. Side effects include rash, paresthesia, metallic taste sensation, nausea, vomiting, and fatigue.

Weight loss is very important for these patients. Even a 6% reduction in body weight is effective at reducing intracranial pressure. The Idiopathic Intracranial Hypertension Treatment Trial (IIHTT) concluded that acetazolamide along with a low sodium, weight reduction diet was better than weight loss alone at improving visual field, reducing disc edema, decreasing intracranial pressure, and improving quality of life measures.[1,3]

Headaches should be comanaged with a neurologist. Topiramate is a popular choice for headache treatment and has the added benefit that it often produces weight loss. Nonsteroidal anti-inflammatory agents may also be helpful.

Referral for surgical treatment may be necessary if vision loss progresses despite medical treatment. Surgical options include optic nerve sheath fenestration, ventriculoperitoneal or lumboperitoneal shunt, and venous sinus stenting. Optic nerve sheath fenestration involves an incision into the meninges surrounding the optic nerve to relieve the cerebral spinal pressure. A ventriculoperitoneal shunt is a surgically inserted tube that drains excess CSF from the ventricles of the brain into the abdomen where the CSF can be reabsorbed. A lumboperitoneal shunt is similar, although it diverts CSF from the arachnoid space in the lumbar spine into the abdomen for reabsorption. These techniques aim to reduce the pressure of increased CSF on the optic nerve. Venous sinus stenting is reserved for cases of papilledema due to narrowing of the venous sinuses determined from an MRV. Here, a stent is placed into the narrowed venous area to decrease buildup of CSF in the brain and relieve pressure on the optic nerve.

With treatment, symptoms typically improve or stabilize in 6 to 12 months, but patients may not fully recover and permanent vision loss can occur.[1,3,4]

CLINICAL PEARLS

- The term papilledema can only be used if the optic disc edema is due to elevated CSF.

- Papilledema can be differentiated from other types of optic disc edema by its bilateral nature and the fact that in most cases there is only a minimal impact on VAs, visual fields, and color vision.

REFERENCES

1. Wall M, McDermott M, Kieburtz K, et al. The idiopathic intracranial hypertension treatment trial clinical profile at baseline. *JAMA Neurol.* 2014;71(6):693-701.

2. Chen J, Costello F, Kardon R. Sex disparities in neuro-ophthalmologic disorders. *Curr Eye Res.* 2015;40(2):247-265.

3. Wall M, McDermott M, Kieburtz K, et al. Effect of acetazolamide on visual function in patients with idiopathic intracranial hypertension and mild visual loss: the idiopathic intracranial hypertension treatment trial. *JAMA.* 2014;311:1641-1651.

4. Friedman D, Grant L, Digre K. Revised diagnostic criteria for the pseudotumor cerebri syndrome in adults and children. *Neurology.* 2013;81(13):1159-1165.

5. Friedman D, Jacobson D. Diagnostic criteria for idiopathic intracranial hypertension. *Neurology.* 2002;59(10):1492-1495.

3.21 Minocycline-Induced Pseudotumor Cerebri

Marcelline A. Ciuffreda and Kenneth J. Ciuffreda

Kelly, a 20-year-old Caucasian female, presented on a late Friday afternoon with a chief concern of blurry vision and diplopia. Approximately 2 weeks ago, she noticed that her vision would occasionally become blurred. One week ago, she started noticing intermittent, horizontal diplopia in the distance that resolved on closing either eye. The diplopia was worse when she looked to the left. Blinking eliminated the diplopia during the day, but at night or when fatigued, she was unable to control it. Kelly also reported having headaches 3 to 4 times per week over the past 2 weeks. She had no long-standing history of headaches, although there was a similar episode of headaches with nausea approximately 6 weeks ago that resolved without treatment. She denied any recent eye or head trauma prior to her symptoms.

Kelly was an out-of-state college student who had never worn glasses. Her last vision examination was 3 years ago in her hometown. Ocular history was unremarkable. Medical history was remarkable for having acne and being slightly overweight. Current medications included naproxen for headaches and spironolactone and minocycline, which she had been taking for acne for the past 2 months. Kelly had an allergy to sulfonamides.

Clinical Findings

Unaided distance VA	OD: 20/20; OS: 20/20
Autorefraction	OD: +0.25 sph; OS: +0.25 sph
Pupil evaluation	PERRL; no RAPD
Extraocular muscle motility	Full, extensive, smooth, and accurate OD; mild abduction deficit OS
Distance cover test	10Δ alternating, intermittent esotropia; the magnitude increased to 15Δ in left gaze and reduced to 6Δ in right gaze
Near cover test	4Δ esophoria
Confrontation visual fields	Full to finger counting OD and OS
Color vision (Ishihara)	14/14 plates OD and OS
Intraocular pressure (GAT)	OD: 20 mm Hg; OS: 20 mm Hg at 3:23 PM
Slit-lamp examination	OD: unremarkable
	OS: unremarkable
Fundus examination (Figure 3.21-1)	OD: 0.1/0.1 CD ratio; edematous optic nerve with indistinct disc margins; hemorrhages surrounding disc, greatest superiorly; fovea flat and dry; periphery unremarkable

Nerve fiber layer OCT (Figures 3.21-2 and 3.21-3)

OS: 0.1/0.1 CD ratio; edematous optic nerve with indistinct disc margins; small hemorrhages surrounding disc; fovea flat and dry; periphery unremarkable

OD: raised disc with surrounding nerve fiber layer thickening (average NFL thickness 196 μm); hyporeflective subretinal space visible at the disc margins

OS: raised disc with surrounding nerve fiber layer thickening (average NFL thickness 193 μm); hyporeflective subretinal space visible at the disc margins

Abbreviations: GAT, Goldmann applanation tonometry; NFL, nerve fiber layer; OCT, optical coherence tomography; OD, right eye; OS, left eye; PERRL, pupils equal, round, reactive to light; RAPD, relative afferent pupillary defect; VA, visual acuity.

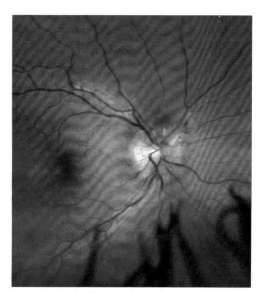
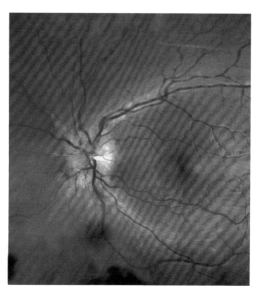

Figure 3.21-1   Fundus photos demonstrating optic disc edema in both eyes.

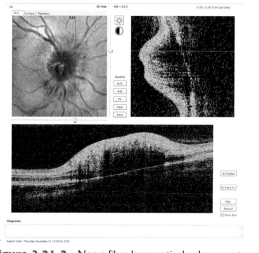
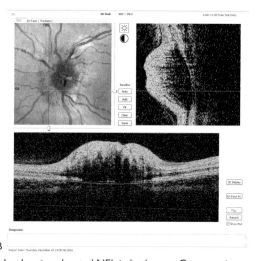

A   B

Figure 3.21-2   Nerve fiber layer optical coherence tomography showing elevated NFL in both eyes. Cross section of the right optic nerve (A) and left optic nerve (B).

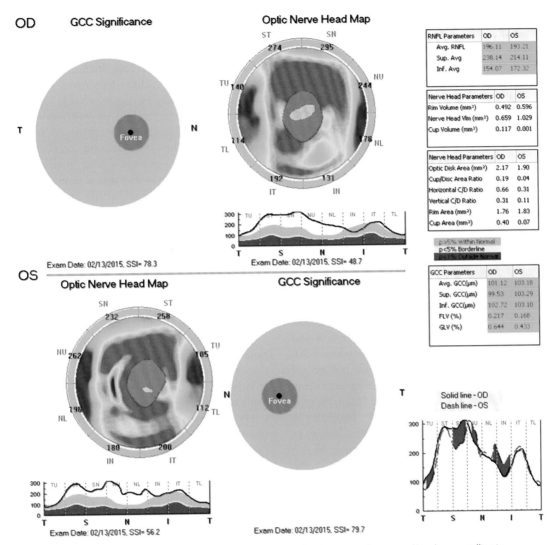

Figure 3.21-3 Nerve fiber layer optical coherence tomography demonstrating nerve fiber layer swelling in both eyes.

Discussion

Based on Kelly's signs and symptoms, she was diagnosed with bilateral optic nerve edema with associated left cranial nerve VI paresis. Because it was Friday evening, she was immediately referred to the local emergency department with explicit instructions to first perform a magnetic resonance imaging (MRI) of the brain with contrast, looking for any causes of papilledema. If the MRI results were normal, it was recommended that she then have a spinal tap with the opening pressure recorded, along with routine blood work. Neuroimaging was unremarkable, and on the lumbar puncture, her opening pressure was 280 mm H_2O with normal cerebral spinal fluid constituency.

These results, in combination with Kelly's history of taking minocycline, indicated a diagnosis of secondary pseudotumor cerebri. Her diplopia resolved immediately following the lumbar puncture, but her headache persisted. She was told to discontinue the minocycline and start oral acetazolamide (250 mg twice per day). It is important to note that the sulfa component in acetazolamide is different than that in sulfonamide antibiotics. Therefore, acetazolamide can be used in patients, such as Kelly, who have an allergy to sulfonamide antibiotics. At her 1-month follow-up, Kelly's headaches and visual symptoms had completely resolved. She discontinued the acetazolamide treatment, and it was recommended against restarting the minocycline.

As demonstrated in this case, the sixth nerve, or abducens nerve, can be affected by increased intracranial pressure (ICP). A cranial nerve VI palsy or paresis results in an eso deviation that is typically worse at distance and when gazing in the direction of the affected eye. In the present case, the cranial nerve VI paresis was attributed to the increased ICP due to the onset of diplopia coinciding with her other symptoms, as well as the diplopia resolving following the lumbar puncture. The sixth nerve is more vulnerable to damage with increased ICP than other ocular motor nerves due to its unique pathway from the brainstem to the eye. The nerve leaves the pontomedullary junction and travels up the clivus bone. It then takes a 90° turn at the ridge of the petrous portion of the temporal bone before traveling anteriorly toward the cavernous sinus. In addition, there is a point at the ridge where it passes beneath the petrosphenoidal ligament of Gruber. Changes in ICP can cause downward displacement of the brainstem, which can stretch the nerve at the pontomedullary junction or where it is anchored down at the ridge of the temporal bone.

Terminology for patients with papilledema is debated. Primary pseudotumor cerebri, which encompasses idiopathic intracranial hypertension, has no identifiable cause. Secondary pseudotumor has a known cause despite normal cerebral spinal fluid contents and a lack of anatomic cause for the papilledema on neuroimaging.

The diagnosis of pseudotumor cerebri is made based on several key findings: normal neurologic testing except for papilledema and possible cranial nerve VI palsy, elevated opening pressure on the lumbar puncture with normal cerebrospinal fluid constituency, and normal brain imaging.[1]

Possible causes of secondary pseudotumor cerebri include a variety of systemic conditions such as anemia, hypertension, pregnancy, Addison disease, chronic renal disease, sleep apnea, and thyroid disorders. Abnormalities of cerebral veins, such as cerebral venous sinus thrombosis or hypercoagulable state, can also result in secondary pseudotumor cerebri.[2]

Numerous medications are also associated with pseudotumor cerebri, including vitamin A analogues, tetracycline derivatives (tetracycline, minocycline, or doxycycline), lithium, growth hormones, use of or withdrawal of corticosteroids, and contraceptives.[3,4] In the present case, the pseudotumor cerebri was likely due to the patient's acne medication, minocycline, which is why it was promptly discontinued. The exact mechanism of how tetracycline derivatives cause an increase in ICP is unknown. A common hypothesis is that such medications impair the absorption of cerebrospinal fluid, possibly by affecting cyclic adenosine monophosphate at the level of the arachnoid granulations, which act as unidirectional valves to drain the cerebrospinal fluid from the subarachnoid space.[5]

One of the most important differential diagnoses, when papilledema is present, is an intracranial mass. Brain imaging must be performed to rule out a brain mass prior to performing the lumbar puncture. A lumbar puncture is relatively safe, but removal of cerebrospinal fluid from a patient with a tumor that is causing compression of intracranial structures can cause the brain to shift downward resulting in death. For this reason, neuroimaging should always be obtained before performing a lumbar puncture. Other emergent causes for papilledema that must be ruled out include cerebral venous sinus thrombosis, malignant hypertension, meningitis, and hydrocephalus.

The main goal of pseudotumor cerebri treatment is preventing permanent vision loss due to chronic papilledema. When secondary pseudotumor cerebri is suspected, it is critical to first find and treat the underlying cause. This includes discontinuing a medication or starting anticoagulant therapy. After the lumbar puncture, medication or other interventions are often still necessary to further decrease the ICP. Treatment options may include diuretic medications, such as carbonic anhydrase inhibitors, corticosteroids, weight management, and rarely, surgery. The most commonly used carbonic anhydrase inhibitor is oral acetazolamide, which acts to decrease cerebrospinal fluid production. Corticosteroids may be used only on an acute basis if there is progressive vision loss. If visual symptoms persist despite medical treatment, or if severe vision loss is present, surgical intervention may be warranted. Such surgeries include optic nerve sheath decompression, peritoneal shunting, and venous-sinus stenting.

In the aforementioned case, Kelly had a resolution of her symptoms with minimal treatment, which included acetazolamide and cessation of the implicated medication.

CLINICAL PEARLS

- Cranial nerve VI is the only ocular motor nerve affected by increased ICP from pseudotumor cerebri.

- When suspecting pseudotumor cerebri, it is crucial to obtain an MRI of the brain to rule out an intracranial mass before a spinal tap is performed.

- It is important to be aware of possible systemic medication effects on the visual system.

REFERENCES

1. Ehlers JP, Shah CP, eds. *The Wills Eye Manual*. 5th ed. Baltimore, MD: Lippincott Williams & Wilkins; 2008.
2. Ang ARG, Zimmerman JCC, Malkin E. Pseudotumor cerebri secondary to minocycline intake. *J Am Board Fam Med*. 2002;15(3):229-233.
3. Thon OR, Gittinger JW. Medication-related pseudotumor cerebri syndrome. *Seminars in Ophthalmology*. 2017;32(1):134-143.
4. Friedman DI. Medication-induced intracranial hypertension in dermatology. *Am J Clin Dermatol*. 2005; 6(1):29-37.
5. Chiu AM, Chuenkongkaew WL, Cornblath WT, et al. Minocycline treatment and pseudotumor cerebri syndrome. *Am J Ophthalmol*. 1998;126(1):116-121.

3.22 Pituitary Adenoma

Denise Goodwin

Jose is, a 46-year-old Hispanic male, presented for a brief office visit due to dry, irritated eyes throughout the day. This had been happening for years, but it had become significantly worse for a few weeks prior to the examination. He reported being diagnosed with a "carniosidad" (pterygium) several years ago. He had tried unknown eye drops, which gave him minimal relief from the irritation.

In addition to the dry, irritated eyes, Jose reported bilateral, frontal headaches. These had been occurring for years but had worsened over the past 2 to 3 weeks. The headaches were exacerbated by near work when he was not wearing his glasses. However, he stated that he rarely wore his glasses. Advil alleviated the headaches.

He had been seen in our clinic 4 years ago, but his last eye examination was 1 year ago at another facility. Other than the pterygium, his ocular history was unremarkable. He reported that he was in good health, and the only medication taken on a regular basis was Advil for headaches. Jose spoke minimal English, and an interpreter was not available.

Clinical Findings

Habitual distance VA	OD: 20/15; OS 20/30 (pinhole 20/30)
Present Rx	OD: +0.50 −1.75 × 170
	OS: +0.75 −1.00 × 125
	ADD: +1.00 OU (OD 20/20; OS 20/40)
Confrontation visual fields	Not performed at this brief office visit
Pupils	PERRL; no RAPD
Retinoscopy	OD: +1.00 −2.00 × 158
	OS: Pl −0.25 × 135
Subjective refraction	OD: +1.00 −2.25 × 145 (20/15)
	OS: +0.25 −1.00 × 125 (20/30)
Near ADD	+1.50 OU (20/20)
Slit-lamp examination	OD: pterygium nasally 1.5 mm onto cornea; otherwise unremarkable
	OS: pterygium nasally 1 mm onto cornea; otherwise unremarkable
Intraocular pressure (GAT)	OD: 14 mm Hg; OS: 15 mm Hg at 2:10 PM
Fundus examination	OD: 0.3/0.3 CD ratio; healthy rim tissue with distinct disc margins; fovea flat and dry; normal vasculature; periphery intact
	OS: 0.4/0.4 CD ratio; healthy rim tissue with distinct disc margins; fovea flat and dry; normal vasculature; periphery intact

Abbreviations: CD, cup to disc; GAT, Goldmann applanation tonometry; OD, right eye; OS, left eye; OU, both eyes; PERRL, pupils equal, round, reactive to light; Pl, plano; RAPD, relative afferent pupillary defect; Rx, prescription; VA, visual acuity.

Comments

Jose was diagnosed with pterygia in both eyes that were not within the pupil margin. He was educated regarding the importance of wearing sunglasses to protect from the wind and UV light. He was given a sample of rewetting drops to use 4 times daily. Although Jose would not normally have undergone a refraction during this brief office visit, there was concern about his headaches and decreased best-corrected acuity so a refraction was performed. This demonstrated minimal change in refraction, and the best-corrected visual acuity (VA) in the left eye remained at 20/30. Review of the records from 4 years earlier indicated that at that time, he was able to see 20/20 in that eye. Because the anterior and posterior segment examination did not provide any explanation for the decreased vision, dry eye or irregular astigmatism secondary to the pterygium was suspected as causing the decreased acuity. Jose was asked to return in 1 week for further testing, including corneal topography to rule out irregular astigmatism, optical coherence tomography of the macula to rule out occult maculopathy, and a visual field to rule out a neurologic lesion. In the meantime, the records from the examination 1 year earlier were obtained to determine the rate of VA change. In addition, he was asked to wear his glasses every day to see if the headaches improved.

Follow-up Visit (5 Weeks Following the Initial Examination)

Outside records were obtained indicating that 1 year prior Jose's visual acuities were 20/20 in each eye. Ocular health, pupils, and confrontation visual fields were reported to be within normal limits.

The patient did not show up for the scheduled 1-week appointment. He was contacted by phone, and he indicated that he could not afford to have further testing done. After agreeing to reduce the costs, he returned 5 weeks after the initial visit. At that time, Jose reported that the rewetting drops did help with the ocular irritation. Despite wearing the glasses regularly, he was still getting headaches.

In addition, he reported episodes of dizziness for which he had visited his primary care doctor 1 week prior after falling in the bathroom. He was given a medication for the dizziness, but he did not know the name.

Aided distance VA	OD: 20/15; OS: 20/40
Pupil evaluation	PERRL; no RAPD
Corneal topography (Figure 3.22-1)	OD: no irregular astigmatism or corneal abnormality present; 2.2 D of corneal astigmatism was found, consistent with the refractive astigmatism
	OS: no irregular astigmatism or corneal abnormality that would account for the decreased best-corrected acuity was present; 1.1 D of corneal astigmatism was found, consistent with the refractive astigmatism
Macular OCT (Figure 3.22-2)	OD: normal foveal architecture; no areas of abnormal thickness
	OS: normal foveal architecture; no areas of abnormal thickness
Visual field (30-2 SITA-standard, Figure 3.22-3)	OD: complete temporal visual field loss respecting the vertical midline
	OS: complete temporal visual field loss respecting the vertical midline

Abbreviations: D, diopters; OCT, optical coherence tomography; OD, right eye; OS, left eye; PERRL, pupils equal, round, reactive to light; RAPD, relative afferent pupillary defect; VA, visual acuity.

Discussion

Jose originally presented for an office visit due to dry eye. Decreased best corrected acuity prompted additional testing, which

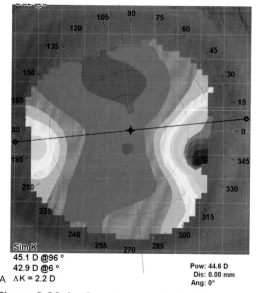
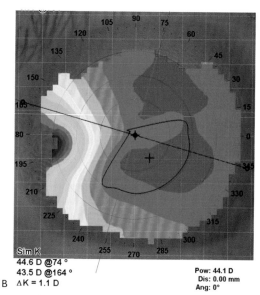

Sim K
45.1 D @96 °
42.9 D @6 °
A   ΔK = 2.2 D

Pow: 44.6 D
Dis: 0.00 mm
Ang: 0°

Sim K
44.6 D @74 °
43.5 D @164 °
B   ΔK = 1.1 D

Pow: 44.1 D
Dis: 0.00 mm
Ang: 0°

Figure 3.22-1   Corneal topography showing regular astigmatism in OD (A) and OS (B).

Abbreviations: OD, right eye; OS, left eye.

demonstrated a deep bitemporal hemianopia. After discussion with the patient's primary care provider (PCP), an urgent magnetic resonance imaging (MRI) with contrast was scheduled with emphasis on the chiasmal region. Neuroimaging demonstrated a large pituitary lesion pushing the chiasm upward (Figure 3.22-4A). The left optic nerve was being compressed by the lesion accounting for the poorer acuity in that eye (Figure 3.22-4B). Jose was sent to a local neurosurgery center and had surgery 1 week later. A biopsy at that time resulted in a diagnosis of a pituitary macroadenoma.

It would have been easy to assume the cause of Jose's decreased acuity was either dry eye or irregular astigmatism secondary to the pterygium. Decreased best-corrected acuity, regardless of the severity of loss, should never be ignored. Often, decreased best-corrected acuity is attributed to cataracts despite a lack of objective evidence. Before attributing the vision loss to any cause, assure that the findings are consistent with the observed level of acuity. Another common diagnosis used to account for decreased vision is amblyopia. To make such a diagnosis, there must be a reason that the visual system did not develop normally, such as uncorrected refractive error, anisometropia, or strabismus. Jose did have moderate astigmatism in both eyes; however, previous records confirmed

that he had normal acuity in that eye just 1 year earlier, thereby ruling out amblyopia. Rather, this was a relatively sudden change in vision. Visual fields can be critical in determining the cause of decreased best-corrected VA.

Pituitary adenomas are relatively common neoplasms, making up 10% to 15% of intracranial tumors.[1] They are generally benign, but up to half invade surrounding structures. Adenomas can be differentiated by size. Microadenomas are less than 10 mm while macroadenomas are larger than 10 mm. Many adenomas are asymptomatic, but some cause significant symptoms due to a mass effect on adjacent structures or secondary to changes in hormones released by the pituitary gland. Symptoms may include headache, visual field defects, galactorrhea, amenorrhea, decreased libido, and acromegaly. Rarely, an extraocular muscle palsy may occur if the tumor expands into the neighboring cavernous sinus.

Options for treatment include medical therapy, surgery, or radiation. Dopamine agonists, such as cabergoline or bromocriptine, or somatostatin analogues, such as octreotide, can aid in normalizing prolactin or growth hormone levels, respectively, and shrinking the tumor size.[1] With larger tumors that compress the chiasm, surgical treatment may be warranted. A transsphenoidal approach is considered safer

Macula Thickness : Macular Cube 512x128   OD ● | ○ OS

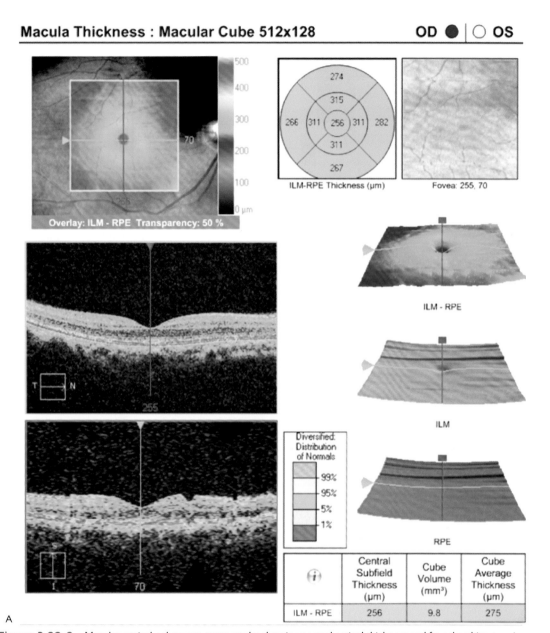

Figure 3.22-2 Macular optical coherence tomography showing normal retinal thickness and foveal architecture in both eyes.

Macula Thickness : Macular Cube 512x128   OD ○ | ● OS

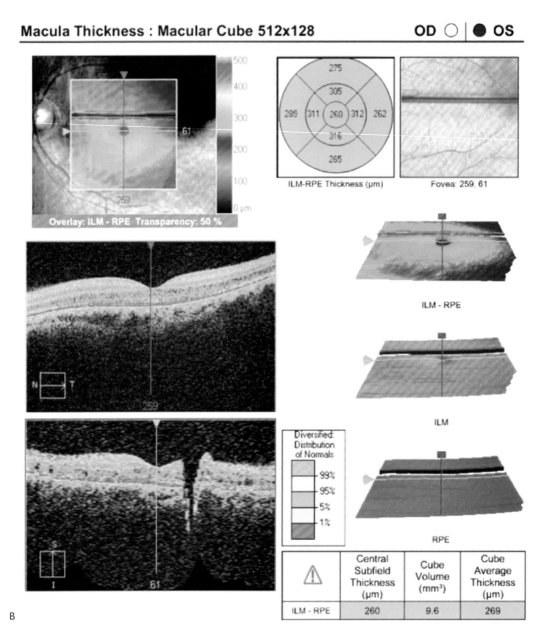

B

Figure 3.22-2   (Continued)

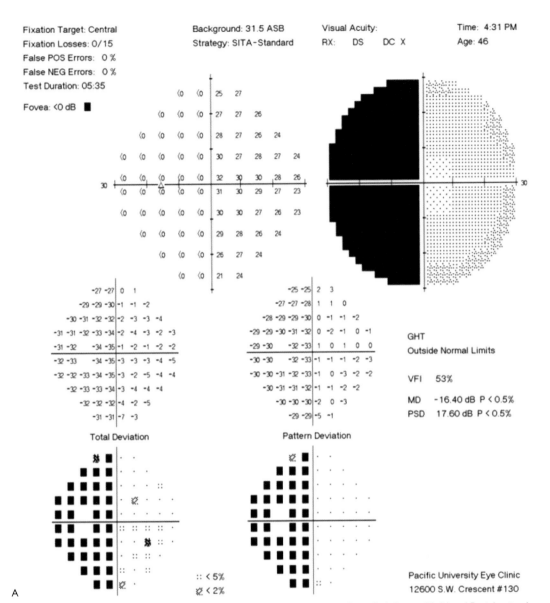

Fixation Target: Central
Fixation Losses: 0/15
False POS Errors: 0 %
False NEG Errors: 0 %
Test Duration: 05:35

Fovea: <0 dB ■

Background: 31.5 ASB
Strategy: SITA-Standard

Visual Acuity:
RX: DS   DC X

Time: 4:31 PM
Age: 46

Total Deviation

Pattern Deviation

GHT

Outside Normal Limits

VFI   53%

MD   -16.40 dB P < 0.5%
PSD   17.60 dB P < 0.5%

:: < 5%
⌀ < 2%

Pacific University Eye Clinic
12600 S.W. Crescent #130

A

Figure 3.22-3   Automated visual fields showing bitemporal visual field defects (A: left visual field and B: right visual field).

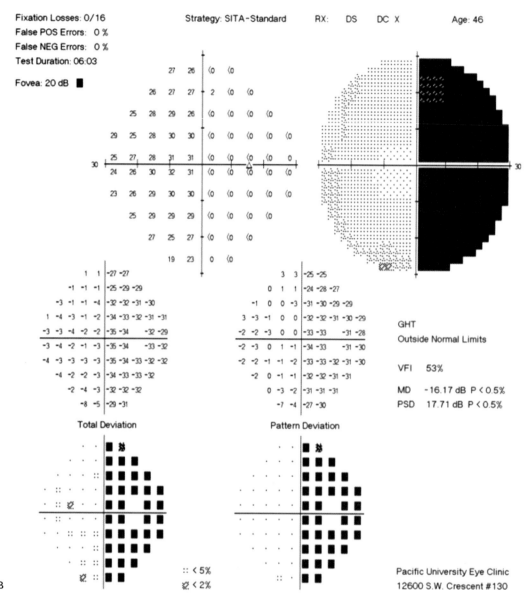

Fixation Losses: 0/16   Strategy: SITA-Standard   RX: DS   DC X   Age: 46
False POS Errors: 0 %
False NEG Errors: 0 %
Test Duration: 06:03

Fovea: 20 dB ■

Total Deviation

Pattern Deviation

GHT
Outside Normal Limits

VFI   53%

MD   -16.17 dB P < 0.5%
PSD   17.71 dB P < 0.5%

:: < 5%
⚅ < 2%

Pacific University Eye Clinic
12600 S.W. Crescent #130

B

Figure 3.22-3   (Continued)

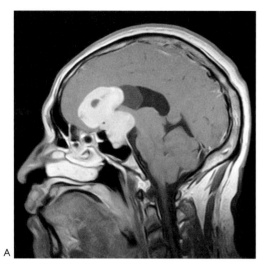
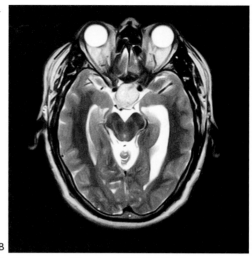

A   B

Figure 3.22-4   Sagittal T1 magnetic resonance imaging (MRI) with contrast (A) and axial T2 MRI (B) showing the pituitary macroadenoma.

than a transcranial approach, but if the tumor extends beyond the sellar region, craniotomy may be necessary.[2,3] Prompt treatment is critical if the pituitary lesion is affecting vision. A delay of more than a week after presentation can result in a poorer visual outcome.[2]

CLINICAL PEARL

- Never ignore unexplained, decreased best-corrected VAs.

REFERENCES

1. Di Ieva A, Rotondo F, Syro LV, Cusimano MD, Kovacs K. Aggressive pituitary adenomas—diagnosis and emerging treatments. *Nat Rev Endocrinol.* 2014;10(7):423-435.
2. Fraser CL, Biousse V, Newman NJ. Visual outcomes after treatment of pituitary adenomas. *Neurosurg Clin N Am.* 2012;23(4):607-619.
3. Kopczak A, Renner U, Karl Stalla G. Advances in understanding pituitary tumors. *F1000Prime Rep.* 2014;6:5.

3.23 Cranial Nerve III Palsy

Kirk L. Halvorson

Lincoln, a 63-year-old white male, presented with horizontal binocular diplopia that started 1 day earlier. He also complained of a diffuse headache on the right side that started about 2 weeks ago in which the pain was rated as 7 on a scale from 1 to 10. He experienced long-standing tinnitus but no other neurologic symptoms. Ocular history was unremarkable, but medical history was positive for type 2 diabetes (the patient was unsure of his blood glucose or HbA1c), esophageal reflux disease, and chronic back pain. He was taking glipizide, omeprazole, and ibuprofen.

Clinical Findings

Unaided distance VA	OD: 20/20^{-2}; OS: 20/20^{-2}
Pupil evaluation	PERRL; no RAPD
Confrontation visual fields	Full to finger counting OD and OS
Distance cover test (unaided)	Constant alternating 6Δ XT in primary gaze; 10Δ XT in left gaze; orthophoria in right gaze
Ocular motility	OD: 20% adduction deficit; all other gazes were full with no obvious vertical restriction OS: full and accurate
Upper eyelid margin to corneal reflex distance	OD: 3.0 mm; OS: 4.0 mm
Slit-lamp examination	OD: mild ptosis; otherwise unremarkable OS: unremarkable
Intraocular pressure (GAT)	OD: 15 mm Hg; OS: 15 mm Hg at 11:15 AM
Fundus examination	OD: 0.2/0.2 CD ratio; healthy rim tissue with distinct disc margins; fovea flat and dry with no clinically significant macular edema; normal vasculature with no intraretinal hemorrhage, exudates, or neovascularization; periphery intact OS: 0.2/0.2 CD ratio; healthy rim tissue with distinct disc margins; fovea flat and dry with no clinically significant macular edema; normal vasculature with no intraretinal hemorrhage, exudates, or neovascularization; periphery intact

Abbreviations: CD, cup to disc; GAT, Goldmann applanation tonometry; OD, right eye; OS, left eye; PERRL, pupils equal, round, reactive to light; RAPD, relative afferent pupillary defect; VA, visual acuity; XT, exotropia.

Comments

Lincoln had a noncomitant lateral deviation with only a mild adduction deficit and no vertical deviation. Although intranuclear ophthalmoplegia could not be completely ruled out, the patient did not exhibit nystagmus in the left eye on left gaze. However, a subtle ptosis was noted making a partial

452

cranial nerve III palsy a more likely diagnosis. Past laboratory work was reviewed immediately, which showed recent blood glucose values of 346, 289, and 311 mg/dL over the course of 6 months. All other laboratory results were unremarkable, including an erythrocyte sedimentation rate (ESR) performed 1 month ago. On further review of systems, the patient denied pain in the temporal region, jaw claudication, or fatigue. He did state that he had a cranial nerve III palsy on the left side a year ago which his previous provider said was due to uncontrolled diabetes. Neuroimaging was unremarkable at that time. We decided to retrieve previous neuroimaging results prior to ordering new neuroimaging. However, the patient returned to the clinic the next day saying the eyelid was now significantly droopy.

Follow-up Visit (1 Day Following the Initial Examination)

Unaided distance VA	OD: 20/20^{-2}; OS: 20/20^{-2}
Pupil evaluation	PERRL; no RAPD
Confrontation visual fields	Full to finger counting OD and OS
External examination (Figure 3.23-1)	Marked ptosis OD
Ocular motility (Figure 3.23-2)	OD: −4 adduction, −4 elevation, −3 depression, unrestricted abduction, normal intorsion with attempted depression OS: full and accurate

Abbreviations: OD, right eye; OS, left eye; PERRL, pupils equal, round, reactive to light; RAPD, relative afferent pupillary defect; VA, visual acuity.

Discussion

Lincoln originally presented with acute double vision. Initial findings were subtle, showing a noncomitant lateral deviation with a mild adduction deficit and subtle ptosis. Pupils were equal and responsive. Unfortunately, his condition deteriorated, and the next day he presented with a complete, pupil sparing

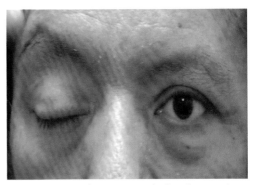

Figure 3.23-1   Severe ptosis displayed in complete right cranial nerve III palsy.

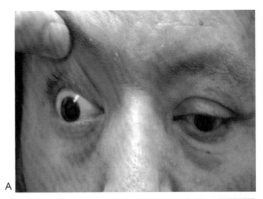

A

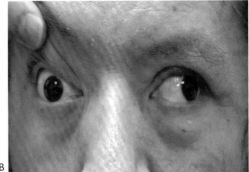

B

Figure 3.23-2   Limited downgaze (A) and adduction (B) of the right eye. The pupils are pharmacologically dilated.

cranial nerve III palsy exhibiting exotropia (XT) and hypotropia (down and out ocular posture), and advanced ptosis. Pupils were still responsive, and he showed no anisocoria. We obtained results from a magnetic resonance imaging (MRI) and magnetic resonance angiography (MRA) performed a year ago, which were unremarkable. Additional imaging was deferred at this point since the cause was most likely attributed to microvascular disease given his uncontrolled diabetes. Lincoln was told to monitor his pupils carefully to ensure they did not become involved. Over time, his signs and symptoms continued to improve until they resolved completely 2 months later.

Cranial nerve III, the oculomotor nerve, innervates several structures, including 4 extraocular muscles (superior rectus, inferior rectus, inferior oblique, and medial rectus) and the levator palpebrae superioris. It also carries parasympathetic fibers to the pupillary sphincter muscle and ciliary body.

A lesion involving the cranial nerve III nucleus within the midbrain nucleus will cause bilateral ptosis, contralateral superior rectus involvement, and ipsilateral involvement of other affected muscles. This unique presentation occurs due to the location of the cranial nerve III subnuclei. There is only 1 subnucleus that serves both levator muscles. Fibers from the superior rectus subnuclei cross to the contralateral side before traveling forward with the remaining fibers that originate from nuclei on the same side as the innervated eye.

Once the fibers leave the nucleus, a lesion will cause ipsilateral involvement of all involved ocular structures. From the nucleus, fibers travel anteriorly through the midbrain as the cranial nerve III fasciculus. Here, they travel near the superior cerebellar peduncle, red nucleus, and cerebral peduncles. A lesion in these areas will result in cerebellar ataxia, tremors, or hemiparesis, respectively. The nerve then exits the midbrain and travels anteriorly between the posterior cerebral and superior cerebellar arteries. It follows the posterior communicating artery briefly before reaching the cavernous sinus. Within the cavernous sinus, the nerve is in close proximity to the cranial nerves IV, the ophthalmic and maxillary branches of cranial nerve V, cranial nerve VI, and the sympathetic fibers traveling to the eye. From the cavernous sinus, the nerve enters the orbit. Lesions located in the orbit may cause other cranial nerve involvement including optic neuropathy.[1]

The majority of cranial nerve III palsies affect those older than 50 years. Approximately 35% are attributed to microvascular disease (eg, diabetes or hypertension) while only 16% are attributed to aneurysms.[2] Other causes of cranial nerve III palsies include trauma,

neoplasms/mass, inflammation, infection, and demyelination.[1,2,4]

Depending on the underlying cause and where the lesion is located, a cranial nerve III palsy may be isolated or associated with other neurologic symptoms. It may affect all (complete) or only a portion of the innervated muscles, and it may or may not involve the pupils.

Objectively, an isolated, complete cranial nerve III palsy presents with ptosis and a "down and out" eye posture. The patient will display reduced adduction, elevation, and depression on the affected side. Subjectively, the patient may complain of diplopia when the eyelid is not blocking vision.

For eye care providers, a cranial nerve III palsy that involves the pupil is one of the few true opthalmic emergencies, and an intracranial aneurysm must be ruled out immediately. Pupil involvement appears to be the most significant feature when clinically differentiating compressive (such as from an aneurysm or space-occupying lesion) from microvascular causes. As the nerve follows the posterior communicating artery, the parasympathetic pupillary fibers are situated along the outer area of the nerve. This arrangement causes the pupils to become involved first when there is compression of the nerve.

The pupils can have varying degrees of dysfunction, ranging from normal function (pupil sparing) to being fully dilated and non-reactive (pupillary involvement). Pupil abnormality does not always suggest a compressive lesion. Approximately 14% to 38% of microvascular cranial nerve III palsies affect the pupils, but anisocoria in these cases usually does not exceed more than 1 mm.[2-4] Conversely, some early aneurysms may not show pupillary involvement immediately. When anisocoria is present in aneurysm cases, it usually exceeds 2 mm.[2] It is important to monitor pupil sparing cranial nerve III palsies closely for the first week to ensure that they do not go on to exhibit anisocoria.

For most cases of complete cranial nerve III palsy with pupil sparing in patients older than 50 years, neuroimaging can be deferred since the majority have a microvascular etiology. Consultation with a primary care provider (PCP) and further evaluation of blood pressure along with blood work up (complete blood count [CBC] with differential, blood glucose, ESR, and C-reactive protein [CRP]) is recommended. Magnetic resonance angiography and MRI should be considered if there is no improvement in 6 to 8 weeks, the patient exhibits aberrant regeneration, or if the patient is younger than 50 years.[1] If the patient presents with an incomplete palsy, with or without pupil involvement, an MRI should be performed. An aneurysm needs to be ruled out with emergent MRA and MRI if there is a complete cranial nerve III palsy with pupil involvement, since there is a 50% chance of death if the aneurysm ruptures.[5] For patients diagnosed with an aneurysm, there should be an immediate referral to neurosurgery for possible clipping of the lesion or utilization of a coiling procedure to reduce blood circulation within the aneurysm.[1]

CLINICAL PEARLS

- A complete third nerve palsy that involves the pupil should be considered an aneurysm until proven otherwise and should be referred immediately for neuroimaging, including MR or CT angiography.

- A patient with an incomplete third nerve palsy, either sparing or involving the pupil, requires neuroimaging.

- A pupil sparing complete third nerve palsy should be followed closely to determine if the pupil becomes involved. Neuroimaging may be necessary to rule out nonischemic causes.

REFERENCES

1. Yanovitch T, Buckley E. Diagnosis and management of third nerve palsy. *Curr Opin Ophthalmol.* 2007;18(5):373-378.
2. Akagi T, Miyamoto K, Kashii S, et al. Cause and prognosis of neurologically isolated third, fourth, or sixth cranial nerve dysfunction in cases of oculomotor palsy. *Jpn J Ophthalmol.* January–February 2008;53(1):32-35.
3. Brazis PW. Isolated palsies of the cranial nerves III, IV, and VI. *Semin Neurol.* 2009;29(1):14-28.
4. Bruce BB, Biousse V, Newman NJ. Third nerve palsies. *Semin Neurol.* 2007;27(3):257-268.
5. Jacobson DM, Trobe JD. The emerging role of magnetic resonance angiography in the management of patients with third cranial nerve palsy. *Am J Ophthalmol.* 1999;128(1):94-96.

3.24 Cranial Nerve IV Palsy

Mark Rosenfield

Alan, a 52-year-old male, presented with difficulty when reading or working. He stated that these symptoms became significantly worse over the past 2 weeks, although work had been increasingly difficult over the past 3 to 4 months. Alan was a factory worker whose job required him to solder small electrical components onto circuit boards. This task was very demanding, as some of the components were less than 1 mm in size. The job was performed while seated at a bench, and a box of components was positioned down and to his right. At times, Alan had trouble identifying the correct elements. The typical viewing distance was approximately 35 cm. He wore 28 mm diameter, flat-top bifocal glasses full time (current prescription was 5 years old). The lenses were very scratched and the frame was in poor condition. Ocular history was unremarkable. Alan reported that he was in good health, and the only medication taken on a regular basis was olmesartan (Benicar) 20 mg once daily for hypertension.

Clinical Findings

Unaided distance VA	OD: 20/40; OS: 20/50
Present Rx	OD: +0.75 sph (20/20)
	OS: +1.25 sph (20/20)
	ADD: +1.75 OU (20/40)
Cover test (with current Rx)	1Δ EP, 3Δ left HP at distance
	4Δ XP, 3Δ left HP at near
Near point of convergence	11/14 cm; diplopia noted
Confrontation visual fields	Full to finger counting OD and OS
Pupil responses	PERRL; no RAPD
Retinoscopy	OD: +1.00 sph; OS: +1.25 sph
Subjective refraction	OD: +1.00 −0.25 × 90 (20/15⁻³); OS: +1.25 sph (20/20)
Distance oculomotor balance	1Δ eso, 3Δ left hyper
Near addition	+2.50 OU (near VA = 20/20)
NRA/PRA	+0.50/−0.50 relative to the near ADD
Near Maddox rod (primary gaze)	4Δ exo, 3Δ left hyper
Near Maddox rod (Figure 3.24-1)	2Δ exo, 5Δ left hyper in downward gaze
Intraocular pressure (GAT)	OD: 14 mm Hg; OS: 16 mm Hg at 3.30 PM
Slit-lamp examination	Unremarkable OD and OS
Fundus examination	Unremarkable OD and OS

Abbreviations: EP, esophoria; GAT, Goldmann applanation tonometry; HP, hyperphoria; NRA, negative relative accommodation; OD, right eye; OS, left eye; OU, both eyes; PERRL, pupils equal, round, reactive to light; PRA, positive relative accommodation; RAPD, relative afferent pupillary defect; Rx, prescription; sph, sphere; VA, visual acuity; XP, exophoria.

4Δ LH	3Δ LH	3Δ LH
5Δ LH	3Δ LH	4Δ LH
7Δ LH	5Δ LH	4Δ LH

Figure 3.24-1 Vertical oculomotor balance findings at near (40 cm), tested with a Maddox rod and trial frame in 9 cardinal gaze positions.

Discussion

A 52-year-old patient who presented with difficulties at near while wearing a 5-year-old prescription would initially lead one to assume that an increase in near addition is required. That was indeed the case here, but there were indications that other, more serious issues may have also been present. Although the patient was aware of the problem for some months, it had recently become significantly worse. While it is possible that the loss of range of clear vision had reached a critical point where the patient was no longer able to meet their visual requirements, a gradual loss of accommodative function is more typical. Furthermore, the patient reported difficulty seeing in a particular direction of gaze. This should raise the possibility of an incomitant deviation, and the practitioner should take care to assess the oculomotor function in this particular gaze position. It cannot be assumed that the measurements obtained in the primary position will represent the situation for all gaze angles. Testing for A- and V-patterns should be routine during customary motility testing.

Measurement of Alan's vertical deviation in the 9 cardinal gaze positions revealed a left hyper deviation that was largest when he looked down and right. This indicates an incomitant deviation where the diagnostic action field of the underacting muscle lies in the same direction as the maximum deviation (in this case down and right). Therefore, the primary affected muscle could either be the right inferior rectus or left superior oblique. Because a left hyper deviation is present, the affected muscle must either be a left depressor or right elevator. Accordingly, the primary affected muscle, in this case, must be the left superior oblique as this meets both criteria (ie, left depressor with diagnostic action field down and to the right).

Paresis of the superior oblique muscle is one of the most common isolated extraocular muscle palsies as cranial nerve IV is highly vulnerable to injury due to its long intracranial course.[1] A frequent cause of superior oblique paresis is closed head trauma, and a careful history must be completed to rule out this etiology.[2,3] It is critical that the practitioner determines whether this is a recent onset condition, which is an ocular emergency, or a long-standing condition, which can be dealt with over a longer time period.

Signs of a recent onset cranial nerve IV palsy include the presence of diplopia (often more exaggerated in 1 direction of gaze), a recently developed abnormal head posture, and the absence of amblyopia. Examination of old photographs can be a valuable way of determining whether a head tilt is long-standing or of recent origin.[2] Other possible signs of an acute cause (as opposed to decompensation of a long-standing deviation) may include symptoms from the underlying systemic condition or the presence of past-pointing. In the latter condition, a patient is asked to point his or her finger toward an object in the diagnostic action field of the paretic muscle while the unaffected eye is occluded. If past-pointing is present, the patient will point inaccurately, or "past" the object of regard, toward the diagnostic action field of the affected muscle. This inaccuracy is produced by excessive innervation to the paretic muscle interfering with egocentric localization (or false orientation).

Given that this patient presented with an incomitant deviation of apparently recent onset, referral for a neurologic assessment is warranted. Possible causes for the loss of cranial nerve IV function include trauma (this was not reported here, although patients should be questioned specifically about this), increased intracranial pressure, infection, demyelination, diabetic neuropathy, and pathology of the cavernous sinus. Although uncommon, pressure on the nerve from an aneurysm or tumor must also be ruled out. These are potentially life-threatening conditions, and further examination (including neuroimaging) should not be delayed.

Although the primary concern was ruling out any underlying systemic cause, Alan also had vertical diplopia, which was worse when looking down. Accordingly, he was provided with a pair of single-vision glasses to use for reading and near work (including his job) with the following prescription: OD +3.50 −0.25 × 90, 2.0Δ base-up; OS +3.75 sph, 2.0Δ base-down. This correction was demonstrated to the patient using a trial frame, and it was determined that he could maintain clear and single vision at near in downward gaze through this prescription.

CLINICAL PEARLS

- Assessment of the oculomotor status away from primary gaze is critical to test for the presence of an incomitant deviation.

- Any indication from the history or clinical assessment of an incomitant deviation must be accompanied by a comprehensive systemic evaluation to rule out a medical emergency.

REFERENCES

1. Latronico ME, Moramarco A, Russo L, Lasorella G. Superior oblique palsy: a review of 135 cases. *J Siena Acad Sci*. 2010;2:29-30.
2. Von Noorden GK. Superior oblique paralysis. *Aust J Ophthalmol*. 1979;7:45-48.
3. Helveston EM, Krach D, Plager DA, Ellis FD. A new classification of superior oblique palsy based on congenital variations in the tendon. *Ophthalmology*. 1992;99:1609-1615.

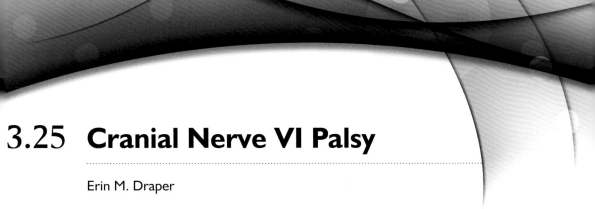

3.25 Cranial Nerve VI Palsy

Erin M. Draper

Montel, a 63-year-old male, presented with a chief concern of double vision and pain around his right eye. He reported that approximately 1 month ago he woke up and noticed diplopia. He described the diplopia as side-by-side, and it resolved if he closed 1 eye. He felt that the diplopia had been stable since onset. He found it very bothersome and as a result had stopped driving. Shortly after the double vision began, he started to experience pain around his right eye, which extended to his right ear. A large right head turn was noted on physical observation.

Montel's medical history was remarkable for hypertension and type 2 diabetes, which was diagnosed 18 years ago. At that time, he appeared to be having stroke symptoms and was rushed to the hospital. His blood glucose was measured at greater than 1000 mg/dL. He claimed that his blood glucose was now fairly well controlled with insulin. His most recent fasting blood glucose was 150 mg/dL, and he did not know his most recent HbA1c. His medications included atenolol, glimepiride, insulin, metformin, and ramipril.

Clinical Findings

Best-corrected distance VA	OD: 20/25^{+2}; OS: 20/25^{+2}
Pupil evaluation	PERRL; no RAPD
Color testing (Ishihara)	OD: 14/14; OS: 14/14
Confrontation visual fields	Full to finger counting OD and OS
Extraocular muscle motilities	Restricted abduction of the right eye at 50% of normal capacity (Figure 3.25-1); otherwise full and smooth movements with no pain OU
Distance cover test	Eso deviation which was greater on right gaze (Figure 3.25-2)
Forced duction test	Negative
Exophthalmometry	OD: 19 mm; OS: 19 mm with base of 98 mm
Slit-lamp examination	OD: clogged meibomian glands with punctate epithelial corneal defects; grade 1 nuclear sclerotic and cortical cataracts; otherwise unremarkable with no evidence of cells or flare in the anterior chamber
	OS: clogged meibomian glands with punctate epithelial corneal defects; grade 1 nuclear sclerotic and cortical cataracts; otherwise unremarkable with no evidence of cells or flare in the anterior chamber
Intraocular pressure (GAT)	OD: 18 mm Hg; OS: 17 mm Hg at 11:54 AM
Blood pressure	140/78 mm Hg RAS

Fundus examination	OD 0.4/0.4 CD ratio; healthy rim tissue with distinct disc margins; fovea flat and dry; large cotton wool spot and large retinal hemorrhage in posterior pole with a few other scattered dot hemorrhages; attenuated blood vessels; periphery intact
	OS 0.3/0.3 CD ratio; healthy rim tissue with distinct disc margins; few dot hemorrhages in macula and posterior pole but no macular edema present; attenuated blood vessels; periphery intact
Laboratory testing	Serum bloodwork included CBC with differential, serum glucose, HbA1c, lipid panel, ESR, CRP, Lyme titer, RPR, FTA-ABS, ACE, and ANA. Abnormal results included elevated serum glucose and HbA1c at 122 mg/dL and 8.7%, respectively.
MRI of brain and orbits	The MRI indicated small chronic bilateral cerebellar infarcts, chronic small vessel ischemia, and mild volume loss. No abnormalities were found along the pathway of cranial nerve VI.
Neurologic exam	Cranial nerves I to V and VII to XII intact bilaterally. Left cranial nerve VI intact. Motor, sensory, and coordination testing unremarkable.

Abbreviations: ACE, angiotensin converting enzyme; ANA, antinuclear antibody; CBC, complete blood count; CD, cup to disc; CRP, C-reactive protein; ESR, erythrocyte sedimentation rate; FTA-ABS, fluorescent treponemal antibody absorption; GAT, Goldmann applanation tonometry; MRI, magnetic resonance imaging; OD, right eye; OS, left eye; OU, both eyes; PERRL, pupils equal, round, reactive to light; RAPD, relative afferent pupillary defect; RAS, right arm sitting; RPR, rapid plasma reagin; Rx, prescription; sph, sphere; VA, visual acuity; XP, exophoria.

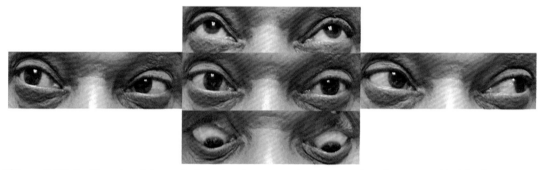

Figure 3.25-1 There is a slight eso deviation in primary gaze. In right gaze, the right eye is unable fully abduct.

	20 eso	
45 eso	30 eso	4 eso
	20 eso	

Figure 3.25-2 An incomitant eso deviation, worse in right gaze, was present.

Comments

After a thorough work up, Montel was diagnosed with an isolated right cranial nerve VI palsy. Due to the vasculopathic risk factor of poorly controlled type 2 diabetes, it was felt this was most likely of ischemic etiology. He was prescribed a 20 D base-out Fresnel prism over the right eye to alleviate symptoms of diplopia and referred to an endocrinologist for closer evaluation and control of his diabetes. A follow-up visit was scheduled 1 month after the initial examination.

Follow-up Visit (1 Month Following the Initial Examination)

Ductions	Greatly improved abduction ability estimated at 95% of normal abduction capacity
Cover test	Orthophoria in primary gaze with 3Δ esophoria in right gaze

Comments

Two months after the onset of diplopia, Montel had complete resolution of symptoms consistent with an isolated cranial VI palsy of vasculopathic etiology.

Discussion

A presentation of recent-onset diplopia can be intimidating to a clinician, but a stepwise clinical approach can help isolate the location of the lesion and determine the appropriate workup.[1] The first step is to assess ocular motility. Montel had esotropia in primary gaze, which worsened on right gaze, consistent with the large abduction deficit. He also exhibited a right head turn due to him trying to put his eyes in left gaze, the position with the least ocular misalignment. Not all deficits will be as obvious as Montel's, but performing a cover test in different positions of gaze and recognizing incomitant patterns of deviation will help to localize which cranial nerves are affected.

Having identified the affected nerve or muscle, the next step is to determine the specific location of the lesion. One must differentiate a restrictive process within the orbit from a lesion involving the nerve outside the orbit. Intraorbital lesions include a mass or enlargement of an extraocular muscle, which limits the ability of the eye to move in a particular direction of gaze. Exophthalmometry to test for proptosis is warranted. In addition, a forced duction test conducted in-office may help with the diagnosis. If the eye can be physically moved or pushed beyond the direction of the motility deficit, this is a negative forced duction test, which indicates the absence of a restrictive process.

Once a restrictive process is ruled out, an abnormality at the neuromuscular junction, such as myasthenia gravis should be considered. With such a condition, there may be variability in the amount and direction of ocular misalignment during the examination, as well as an associated ptosis.

If the lesion lies in or along cranial nerve VI, the entire nerve pathway from the pons to the lateral rectus must be evaluated. Brainstem lesions may affect other cranial nerves, which lie in close proximity, such as cranial nerves V, VII, and VIII. In addition, the patient may have contralateral paresis secondary to pyramidal tract involvement.[2] Lesions in the brainstem may be compressive, ischemic, or inflammatory. In a younger patient, demyelinating disease must be considered higher within the list of differential diagnoses.

After cranial nerve VI exits the brainstem, it follows a vertical course up the clivus within the subarachnoid space. Here it is susceptible to compression due to changes in intracranial pressure, infection (Lyme disease, syphilis), infiltration (sarcoidosis), or inflammation (lymphoma, carcinomas). Subsequently, it travels within Dorello canal where it can be injured by trauma or inflammation secondary to complicated otitis media.[2] It then enters the cavernous sinus and travels to the orbital apex. A wide variety of lesions may affect cranial nerve VI within these locations. However, lesions in these areas tend to involve multiple cranial nerves and may be accompanied by ipsilateral Horner syndrome or proptosis.

If there are no associated or localizing clinical signs or symptoms, the presentation may be considered an isolated cranial nerve VI palsy. In patients older than 50 years with risk factors such as hypertension, diabetes mellitus, or hypercholesterolemia, a microvascular ischemic etiology should be considered.[3] In these cases, the condition is typically self-limiting, and clinical improvement should be seen within 3 months of onset. The clinician should communicate with the primary care provider to further investigate and manage vasculopathic risk factors.

Recent studies recommend that even with cases of presumed microvascular etiology, additional testing should be considered.[4,5]

Early neuroimaging in the form of a magnetic resonance imaging (MRI) with contrast is recommended as a general guideline rather than waiting 2 to 3 months for spontaneous resolution to confirm the diagnosis of microvascular etiology. A high yield of other non-vasculopathic etiologies such as intracranial neoplasm, aneurysm, inflammation, infection, and brainstem infarctions have been reported, all of which benefit from an earlier diagnosis.[4,5]

Further evaluation with laboratory testing should be pursued in an older patient exhibiting symptoms that might suggest giant cell arteritis. Montel presented complaining of right temporal pain, which prompted laboratory testing, including complete blood count (CBC), erythrocyte sedimentation rate (ESR), and C-reactive protein (CRP). If one is highly suspicious of giant cell arteritis, a temporal artery biopsy is also warranted. In addition, in Montel's case, tests for Lyme disease, syphilis, sarcoidosis, and autoimmune conditions were also ordered.

CLINICAL PEARL

- When assessing cases of diplopia, use a stepwise approach to determine if one or more cranial nerves are involved. This will help localize the lesion and determine the etiology.

REFERENCES

1. Malloy KM, Draper EM, Maglione AK, Moody KL. A stepwise approach to evaluating diplopia and other ocular motility abnormalities. *Rev Optom.* 2016;153:94-102.
2. Azarmina M, Azarmina H. The six syndromes of the sixth cranial nerve. *J Ophthalmic Vis Res.* 2013; 8:160-171.
3. Kung NH, Van Stavern GP. Isolated ocular motor nerve palsies. *Semin Neurol.* 2015;35:539-548.
4. Tamhankar MA, Volpe NJ. Management of acute cranial nerve 3, 4, and 6 palsies: role of neuroimaging. *Curr Opin Ophthalmol.* 2015;26:464-468.
5. Tamhankar MA, Biousse V, Ying GS, et al. Isolated third, fourth, and sixth cranial nerve palsies from presumed microvascular versus other causes: a prospective study. *Ophthalmology.* 2013;120:2264-2269.

3.26 Internuclear Ophthalmoplegia

Ashley Kay Maglione

Kelly, a 69-year-old female, presented for further evaluation of a left nystagmoid movement on left gaze. Her history was difficult to obtain, and she would laugh uncontrollably at times. She complained of pain and pressure inside the right eye. She felt as though her right eye was being pushed outward and her eye would become "cockeyed" at times. The symptoms started approximately 1 month prior to her presentation.

Systemic history was significant for borderline diabetes controlled with diet, hypertension for 10 years, and osteoarthritis. Medications include losartan (Cozaar), nifedipine, alendronate sodium (Fosamax), vitamins A and E, calcium, magnesium, zinc, and potassium. Ocular history was remarkable for being a glaucoma suspect for approximately 18 years. Her social history was remarkable for smoking a maximum of 10 cigarettes per day since age 10 years, as well as occasional alcohol, and marijuana use.

Clinical Findings

Best-corrected VA	OD: 20/20; OS: 20/25^{+2}
Color vision	OD: 12/14 plates; OS: 14/14 plates
Pupil evaluation	PERRL; no RAPD
Confrontation visual fields	Full to finger counting with no red desaturation in any quadrant OU
Palpebral aperture	OD: 13 mm; OS: 13 mm
Exophthalmometry	OD: 22 mm; OS: 21 mm, base 100 mm
Ocular motilities (Figure 3.26-1)	50% normal adducting capacity OD with abducting nystagmus of the left eye on left gaze
Cover test at distance	Orthophoria in primary, up, and down gaze; 2Δ esophoria on right gaze; 20-25Δ exophoria on left gaze
Slit-lamp examination	OD: blepharitis and diffuse corneal punctate keratitis; otherwise unremarkable
	OS: blepharitis and diffuse corneal punctate keratitis; otherwise unremarkable
Intraocular pressure (GAT)	OD: 17 mm Hg; OS: 17 mm Hg at 11:34 AM
Fundus examination	OD: 0.8/0.85V CD ratio with thinning inferiorly; healthy rim tissue with no evidence of pallor and distinct disc margins; fovea flat and dry; normal vasculature; periphery intact
	OS: 0.85/0.90V CD ratio; healthy rim tissue with no evidence of pallor and distinct disc margins; fovea flat and dry; normal vasculature; periphery intact
Visual fields (Humphrey SITA-standard 24-2)	OD: superior nasal step OS: no defects

463

Neurologic examination	Cranial nerves V and VII through XII were intact; motor, sensory, and coordination testing were unremarkable
Laboratory testing	CBC with differential, platelet count, ESR (Westergren), CRP, serum folate, serum vitamin B12, Lyme titer, RPR, FTA-ABS, ACE, ANA (with reflex titer), methylmalonic acid, homocysteine, serum protein electrophoresis, and BUN/creatinine (in preparation for neuroimaging) were unremarkable
MRI of the brain and orbits with contrast	White matter signal changes involving the supratentorial white matter, pons, and left optic nerve

Abbreviations: ACE, angiotensin-converting enzyme; ANA, antinuclear antibody; BUN, blood urea nitrogen; CBC, complete blood count; CD, cup to disc; CRP, C-reactive protein; ESR, erythrocyte sedimentation rate; FTA-ABS, fluorescent treponemal antibody absorption; GAT, Goldmann applanation tonometry; MRI, magnetic resonance imaging; OD, right eye; OS, left eye; OU, both eyes; PERRL, pupils equal, round, reactive to light; RAPD, relative afferent pupillary defect; RPR, rapid plasma reagin; VA, visual acuity.

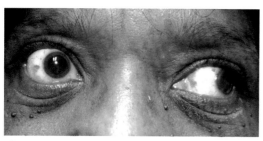

Figure 3.26-1 On attempted left gaze, the right eye is unable to fully adduct. The pupils are pharmacologically dilated.

Discussion

The most pertinent finding from Kelly's examination is her ocular misalignment, which demonstrated reduced adduction and an abducting nystagmus of the contralateral eye. This pattern is pathognomonic for an internuclear ophthalmoplegia (INO), a finding which warrants further workup into the underlying etiology.

To understand the pathology that gives rise to an INO, the anatomical pathway must be reviewed. The sixth nerve nucleus acts as the lateral gaze center. This nucleus controls movement of the ipsilateral lateral rectus and simultaneously facilitates contraction of the contralateral medial rectus as a yoked muscle. The medial longitudinal fasciculus (MLF) serves as the neuronal pathway for this process. The MLF exits the sixth nerve nucleus in the pons, immediately crosses the midline, and travels to the medial rectus subnucleus of the third nerve in the midbrain. Therefore, a lesion

of the MLF will result in an ipsilateral adduction deficit. The adduction deficit may range from a significant limitation to a subtle lag seen on saccades. If the lesion is at the level of the pons, as opposed to the midbrain, adduction may be preserved with convergence.[1]

Patients with an INO will exhibit a nystagmoid movement of the contralateral abducting eye. It is important to recognize that this is not a true nystagmus, as the involuntary, rapid movement is seen in only 1 eye. Nystagmoid movements with INO are thought to occur due to Hering's law of equal innervation. As increased signals are sent to compensate for the weak muscle, the fellow eye also receives increased innervation and consequently appears to have a nystagmoid movement.[2]

The INO is labeled based on the side with limited adduction. Therefore, Kelly exhibited a right INO due to a right adduction deficit and we would expect a lesion of the right MLF.

Patients who present with a unilateral INO are generally aligned in primary gaze. Therefore, most patients will not be symptomatic in primary gaze but will develop horizontal diplopia in lateral gaze. Kelly exemplified this with an orthophoric posture in primary gaze and only complained of becoming "cockeyed" on occasions.

Internuclear ophthalmoplegia may present bilaterally and be either symmetric or asymmetric. A subgroup of patients with bilateral adduction deficits exhibit exotropia in primary gaze. This syndrome, known as walleyed bilateral INO (WEBINO), often causes debilitating diplopia in primary gaze. Another variant of INO is one-and-a-half syndrome characterized by a gaze palsy (involving both eyes) in 1 direction (the one) and an adduction deficit in the other direction (the half). This is caused by a lesion involving both the abducens nucleus and the MLF. An INO may also be accompanied by a skew deviation and/or vertical gaze-evoked nystagmus.[1,3]

The most common causes of INO are multiple sclerosis or infarction depending on whether the patient is young or old, respectively. A bilateral INO is most commonly due to demyelination. Other causes of INO have been identified in just over one-quarter of patients and, therefore, should be considered.[4] These include trauma, infection, tumors, iatrogenic causes, drug overdose, inflammatory vasculitis, hydrocephalus, Arnold–Chiari malformation, neurodegenerative diseases, and hemorrhage.[1,4] In addition, clinicians must be cognizant of ocular myasthenia, which can mimic eye movement disorders of the central nervous system. In myasthenic patients, a "pseudo-INO" will be characterized by fatigability, which results in variation over time.[5]

Laboratory studies ruling out infectious and inflammatory etiologies are indicated along with neuroimaging, preferably magnetic resonance imaging (MRI), looking for intracranial lesions affecting the MLF in the pons or midbrain. It is of note that Kelly also exhibited an optic neuropathy, evidenced by loss of neuroretinal rim and a visual field defect in the right eye, in the setting of normal intraocular pressures. Therefore, her laboratory workup also included tests to rule out underlying non-glaucomatous etiologies of an optic neuropathy. Although it is possible that Kelly may have experienced an optic neuritis episode in the past, given the lack of optic nerve pallor, as well as the unremarkable laboratory tests, she was ultimately diagnosed with low-tension glaucoma and treatment with intraocular pressure lowering drops was initiated. The workup was remarkable for white matter changes on her MRI. Specifically, there were lesions within the pons,

which were the likely etiology of her INO. Kelly was subsequently evaluated by a neurologist and diagnosed with multiple sclerosis. Recall that Kelly had an inability to control her laughter during the case history. This is a neurologic sign known as pseudobulbar affect and was an indicator that her INO was likely associated with an underlying neurologic disorder, such as multiple sclerosis.

Treatment for an INO is often aimed at managing the underlying etiology. In Kelly's case, the treatment of choice would be aimed at controlling her multiple sclerosis. One study found that approximately half of patients with INO experience resolution within 12 months.[6] Fortunately, most patients with persistent INO are largely asymptomatic. In patients who are symptomatic from diplopia in primary gaze (such as those with WEBINO), prism, surgical, and Botox treatment can be considered.[3,7]

CLINICAL PEARL

- A lesion of the MLF will cause an ipsilateral adduction deficit with contralateral nystagmoid movements on abduction.

REFERENCES

1. Karatas M. Internuclear and supranuclear disorders of eye movements: clinical features and causes. *Eur J Neurol.* 2009;16(12):1265-1277.
2. Zee DS, Hain TC, Carl JR. Abduction nystagmus in internuclear ophthalmoplegia. *Ann Neurol.* 1987; 21(4):383-388.
3. Adams WE, Leavitt JA, Holmes JM. Strabismus surgery for internuclear ophthalmoplegia with exotropia in multiple sclerosis. *J Am Assoc Pediatr Ophthalmol Strabismus.* 2009;13(1):13-15.
4. Keane JR. Internuclear ophthalmoplegia. *Arch Neurol.* 2005;62(5):714.
5. Khanna S, Liao K, Kaminski HJ, Tomsak RL, Joshi A, Leigh RJ. Ocular myasthenia revisited: insights from pseudo-internuclear ophthalmoplegia. *J Neurol.* 2007;254(11):1569-1574.
6. Bolanos I, Lozano D, Cantu C. Internuclear ophthalmoplegia: causes and long-term follow-up in 65 patients. *Acta Neurol Scand.* 2004;110(3):161-165.
7. Murthy R, Dawson E, Khan S, Adams GG, Lee J. Botulinum toxin in the management of internuclear ophthalmoplegia. *J Am Assoc Pediatr Ophthalmol Strabismus.* 2007;11(5):456-459.

3.27 Intracranial Tumor

Kelsey L. Moody

Beverly, a 33-year-old African American woman, returned for an eye examination due to a tumor involving her right optic nerve. She was previously seen 2 years ago but then was lost to follow-up. Two years ago, she presented with progressive darkening of the vision in her right eye. At that time, her visual acuity was significantly reduced to 20/400 with dyschromatopsia, and she had a large central scotoma and a 1.8 log unit relative afferent pupillary defect (RAPD). Dilated fundus examination revealed mild diffuse pallor of the right optic nerve. A magnetic resonance imaging (MRI) performed at that time demonstrated a meningioma of the right sphenoid wing encasing the right optic nerve, chiasm, and cavernous and supraclinoid portions of the right internal carotid artery. She underwent a craniotomy and partial resection of the meningioma; however, residual tumor remained, encasing the internal carotid artery and adjacent cranial nerves. Due to the residual tumor, she was referred to radiation oncology but never proceeded with the treatment due to the risk of side effects. Following surgery, her visual acuity improved to 20/25 with normal color vision. Her RAPD decreased to 0.3 log units, and her visual field improved to a mild inferior temporal defect. The pallor of her right optic nerve remained.

Over the past 2 years, Beverly had not noticed any changes in her vision. She denied double vision, eye pain, or facial numbness. However, she had noted an increase in headaches over the past few months. The headaches were located on the right side of her head. She had attributed the headaches to working more and not eating well. She also had a seizure a few months ago and was put on anti-seizure medication. She had not followed up with neurosurgery for the past 2 years but had seen her primary care provider (PCP).

Beverly's general health was only remarkable for the history of the meningioma and recent seizure. Her medications included 2 seizure medications: levetiracetam and zonisamide. She did not smoke or use drugs or alcohol.

Clinical Findings

Aided distance VA	OD: 20/60 (pinhole 20/50); OS: 20/20
Cover test	Distance: 4Δ exophoria, which was comitant in up, down, right, and left gaze; near: 6Δ exophoria
Worth 4-dot	Fusion at distance and near
Confrontation visual fields	OD: central blur on facial description and peripheral temporal restriction with finger counting; red desaturation nasally
	OS: full to finger counting; red desaturation temporally
Pupil evaluation	PERRL; 1.2 log unit RAPD OD
Color vision (Ishihara)	OD: 10/14; OS: 14/14
Extraocular motilities	Full and smooth OD and OS
Intraocular pressure (GAT)	OD: 18 mm Hg; OS: 18 mm Hg at 2:13 PM

Slit-lamp examination	OD: unremarkable
	OS: unremarkable
Fundus examination (Figure 3.27-1)	OD: 0.3/0.3 CD ratio; 1 to 2+ diffuse and 2 to 3+ temporal pallor; distinct disc margins; fovea flat and dry; normal vasculature; periphery intact
	OS: 0.2/0.2 CD ratio; trace bow-tie pallor; distinct disc margins; fovea flat and dry; normal vasculature; periphery intact
Palpebral fissure width	OD: 10 mm; OS: 11 mm
Exophthalmometry	OD: 19 mm; OS: 19 mm (base: 95 mm)
Goldmann bowl perimetry (Figure 3.27-2)	OD: dense nasal loss with mild superior and inferior temporal constriction and a large central scotoma
	OS: superior temporal defect respecting the vertical meridian
Optic nerve OCT (Figure 3.27-3)	OD: small nerve with progressive superior, temporal and inferior RNFL thinning
	OS: small nerve with borderline temporal RNFL thinning at 3:00
Macular OCT (Figure 3.27-4)	OD: diffuse ganglion cell layer thinning
	OS: nasal ganglion cell layer thinning
MRI of the brain	Homogeneously enhancing lobulated extra-axial mass (5.2 × 5.5 × 4.1 cm) along the greater wing of the right sphenoid centered along the anterior clinoid, increased compared to previous study. A portion of the lesion extended into the sella. The mass extended along the right cavernous sinus but was not involving the actual cavernous sinus. There was mild regional mass effect on the right cerebral peduncle with mild left to right midline shift.

Abbreviations: CD, cup to disc; GAT, Goldmann applanation tonometry; MRI, magnetic resonance imaging; OCT, optical coherence tomography; OD, right eye; OS, left eye; PERRL, pupils equal, round, reactive to light; RAPD, relative afferent pupillary defect; RNFL, retinal nerve fiber layer; VA, visual acuity; XP, exophoria.

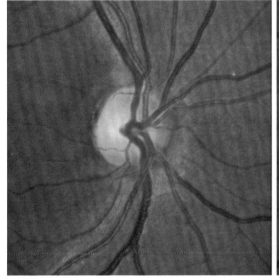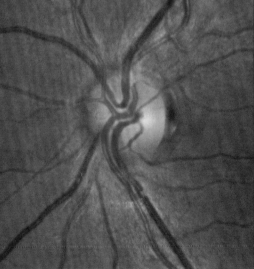

Figure 3.27-1   Fundus photos showing overall pallor of the right optic disc and bow-tie pallor of the left optic disc.

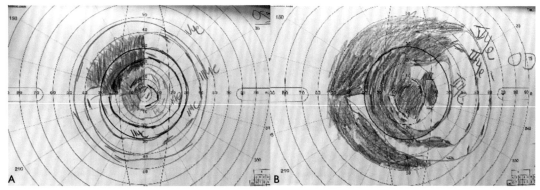

Figure 3.27-2 Goldmann visual fields demonstrating dense nasal loss with mild superior and inferior temporal constriction and a large central scotoma in the right eye (B) and superior temporal scotoma in the left eye (A).

Discussion

Beverly initially presented 2 years ago with reduced afferent function including reduced visual acuity, dyschromatopsia, visual field loss, and an afferent pupillary defect. A prompt workup revealed a meningioma of the anterior cranial base, specifically the sphenoid wing and anterior clinoid, which was compressing the right optic nerve. Although her optic nerve initially demonstrated optic nerve pallor, it was very mild. Due to this, she was able to significantly regain afferent function after surgery, emphasizing the importance of expedient intervention and treatment.

Meningiomas account for 20% to 30% of all intracranial tumors and 4% of intraorbital tumors.[1] The overall incidence rate is roughly 4.52 per 100 000, although this number may be higher as most meningiomas are found incidentally.[2] Meningiomas are more common in women than men (2:1) and their incidence increases with increasing age, peaking in the seventh and eighth decade of life. In addition to age, other risk factors include exposure to ionizing radiation and possibly other environmental, lifestyle, and genetic influences.[1,2]

Meningiomas arise from meningothelial cells of the arachnoid and are usually histologically benign (approximately 90%).[1] Meningiomas are graded according to the World Health Organization (WHO) classification system: benign tumors are grade I, atypical tumors are grade II, and anaplastic tumors are grade III.[1,3] Beverly's tumor was a WHO grade I meningioma. Although benign, meningiomas

can reoccur, particularly if the meningioma is only partially resected, like in our case, or if the tumor has high proliferative activity.[4] This risk can be decreased with adjunct radiotherapy.[1]

Meningiomas can compress ocular structures, including the optic nerve, visual pathway, and cranial nerves. Initially, only Beverly's right optic nerve was affected, but due to regrowth of the tumor both anteriorly and posteriorly, her optic chiasm and optic tract became affected as well. To better understand how this occurs, it is important to review the anterior visual pathway anatomy.

The visual pathway starts at the retina, where visual information travels to the optic nerve via the retinal nerve fiber layer (axons of the ganglion cells). The ganglion cell axons form the optic disc, leave the eye as the optic nerve, and travel to the optic chiasm. Here, nasal fibers, which represent the temporal visual field, from each eye cross to the opposite site. There are a few unique features of how the nasal fibers cross in the chiasm. Inferior nasal fibers cross more anteriorly and actually loop into the contralateral optic nerve, known anatomically as Wilbrand's knee, before traveling posteriorly. Nasal macular fibers are represented throughout the chiasm, but are most dense posteriorly.

The fibers leave the chiasm and form the optic tract. The optic tract traverses around the brainstem at the level of the midbrain until it reaches the lateral geniculate nucleus of the thalamus. Each optic tract contains temporal fibers from the ipsilateral eye and nasal fibers from the contralateral eye. This results in the

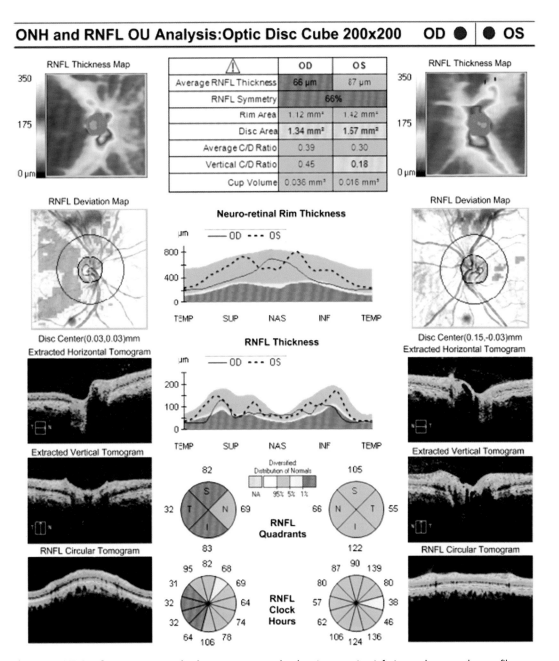

Figure 3.27-3 Optic nerve optical coherence tomography showing superior, inferior, and temporal nerve fiber layer loss of the right eye and borderline nerve fiber layer thinning at 3:00 in the left eye. Note that the neuroretinal rim thickness is normal indicating that the nerve fiber layer loss is due to optic atrophy rather than the optic disc cupping typically seen with glaucoma.

division of visual information for the right and left hemifield.[5]

If there is a lesion that damages the body of the chiasm, there will be a classic bitemporal defect that may be hemianopic or quandranopic. If there is a lesion at the anterior aspect of the chiasm, it can cause a central scotoma with overall field loss on the ipsilateral side and a superior temporal defect in the contralateral eye. This is called anterior chiasmal syndrome or junctional scotoma. There is often an RAPD on the ipsilateral side. A lesion

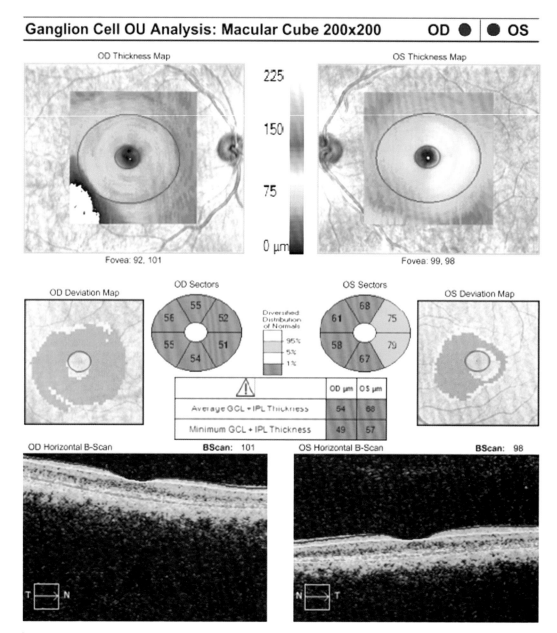

Figure 3.27-4 Ganglion cell analysis loss of the ganglion cells layer diffusely in the right eye but isolated to the nasal ganglion cells in the left eye.

affecting the posterior chiasm will have 1 of 3 visual field defects: a central bitemporal defect due to damage of the macular fibers, a classic bitemporal defect, or a non-congruous homonymous hemianopsia due to damage to the posterior optic chiasm and optic tract.[6]

An isolated complete optic tract lesion causes a characteristic clinical triad: a homonymous hemianopia, RAPD, and bow-tie

atrophy of the optic disc, all of which are contralateral to the damaged optic tract. The classic rule of congruity for homonymous hemianopic visual field defects states that the more posterior a lesion is in the visual pathway, the more congruous the visual field defect will be. However, this is only true for lesions of the optic radiations or occipital lobes. This rule is neither absolute, nor does it apply to optic tract lesions, of which 50% are congruous.[7]

The RAPD occurs in the eye contralateral to the optic tract lesion because more fibers cross at the chiasm than those that do not cross. This is due to the larger size of the temporal visual field compared to the nasal field.

The optic atrophy characteristic of an optic tract lesion is due to the organization of the retinal nerve fiber layer at the optic disc. Bow-tie atrophy involving the eye contralateral to the lesion occurs due to involvement of the fibers originating nasal to the disc and the nasal macular fibers located temporal to the disc, which cross in the chiasm. In the eye ipsilateral to the lesion, there will be diffuse pallor due to damage to the temporal fibers entering the superior and inferior disc.[6,7]

In addition to the pallor seen fundoscopically, retinal nerve fiber layer thinning can be seen on the optic nerve optical coherence tomography (OCT) or by evaluating the ganglion cell layer on a macular OCT. Specifically, there will be ganglion cell layer thinning that matches the distribution of the retinal nerve fiber layer thinning and optic disc pallor with the appearance of homonymous hemimacular thinning. On the eye contralateral to the optic tract lesion, there is temporal visual field loss that is mirrored by nasal ganglion cell layer thinning. On the eye ipsilateral to the optic tract lesion, there is nasal visual field loss that is mirrored by temporal ganglion cell layer thinning.[8]

Beverly's case was unique as her lesion grew both anteriorly and posteriorly, affecting her right optic nerve, optic chiasm, and optic tract. Initially, Beverly's right optic nerve was singularly affected despite its close proximity to other ocular structures. As the tumor regrew, it unfortunately affected the visual fibers of the contralateral eye causing a superior temporal field defect and optic disc pallor. The new visual field defect could be due to damage of either the anterior optic chiasm or the optic tract. The MRI report did note that the lesion was centered around the anterior clinoid. Additionally, she had central field loss in the ipsilateral eye and a superior temporal visual field defect in the contralateral eye, which could be consistent with a junctional scotoma. However, her visual field defect also represented a non-congruous homonymous hemianopsia and her MRI demonstrated mass effect on the cerebral peduncle, in the area of the optic tract. Although Beverly did not have contralateral upper or lower extremity weakness secondary to damage of the corticospinal tract, she did have a seizure episode. The optic tract is in close proximity to the temporal lobe, and lesions here could cause seizures or disturbances in memory.[7]

Likely both the optic chiasm and the optic tract were damaged in Beverly's case. Fortunately, after a second craniotomy and repeat resection, Beverly's visual acuity improved to 20/40, and her RAPD improved to 0.6 log units in the right eye. Her color vision and optic nerve pallor were unchanged. Although the incongruous homonymous hemianopsia remained, Beverly's visual field did improve as well. Although she initially declined radiation therapy, she is expected to undergo radiation treatment since the tumor did recur.

It is possible that Beverly would have maintained better visual function if she had returned for routine follow-up examinations. It is essential to routinely check both afferent and efferent function to assess for subtle changes suggesting tumor regrowth. Specifically, these patients require routine visual field testing, optic nerve and macular OCT, and dilated fundus examinations to check afferent function. Detailed sensorimotor examinations, including Worth 4-dot and cover test in multiple positions of gaze, are necessary to assess efferent function. Initially, patients should be seen every 3 to 4 months. If they remain stable, follow-up visits can occur every 6 to 12 months.

CLINICAL PEARL

- All patients with a history of a compressive mass along the visual pathway should be monitored closely for signs of tumor regrowth to prevent permanent damage to the afferent system.

REFERENCES

1. Malloy K, Chigbu DI. Anterior temporal choroid meningioma causing compressive optic neuropathy. *Optom Vis Sci.* 2011;88(5):645-651.
2. Barnholtz-Sloan JS, Kruchko C. Meningiomas: cases and risk factors. *Neurosurg Focus.* 2007;23(4):E2.
3. Backer-Grondahl T, Moen BJ, Torp SH. The histopathological spectrum of human meningiomas. *Int J Clin Exp Pathol.* 2012;5(3):231-242.
4. Abry E, Thomassen I, Salvesen OO, Torp SH. The significance of Ki-67/MIB-1 labeling index in human meningiomas: a literature study. *Pathol Res Pract.* 2010;206(12):810-815.
5. Rizzo, JF III. Embryology, anatomy, and physiology of the afferent visual pathway. In: Newman N. *Walsh & Hoyt's Clinical Neuro-Ophthalmology.* 6th ed. Vol 1. Philadelphia, PA: Lippincott Williams & Wilkins, 2005:22-42.
6. Levin, LA. Topical diagnosis of chiasmal and retrochiasmal disorders. In: Newman N. *Walsh & Hoyt's Clinical Neuro-Ophthalmology.* 6th ed. Vol 1. Philadelphia, PA: Lippincott Williams & Wilkins, 2005:503-509.
7. Fraser JA, Newman NJ, Biousse V. Disorders of the optic tract, radiation and occipital lobe. *Handb Clin Neurol.* 2011;102:205-221.
8. Romero RS, Gutierrez I, Wang E, Reder AT, Bhatti T, Bernard JT, Javed A. Homonymous hemimacular thinning: a unique presentation of optic tract injury in neuromyelitis optica. *J Neuroophthalmol.* 2012;32(2):150-153.

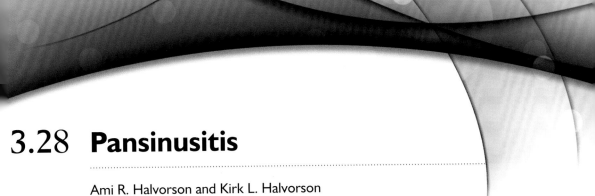

3.28 **Pansinusitis**

Ami R. Halvorson and Kirk L. Halvorson

Josh, a 38-year-old male, presented with intermittent diplopia that began approximately 1 month ago, although he stated that the symptoms had markedly worsened over the past week. The only additional symptom associated with the diplopia was periocular pain on the left side, which had started a few days ago. He denied headache, nausea, vomiting, dizziness, or fever, and he had no difficulties speaking or swallowing. He also denied any recent injury or trauma.

Medical history was positive for nonspecific back pain. He also reported a sinus and allergy history that first began 10 years ago, but he denied any current drainage. He was taking no medications. Allergies included dairy and wheat but no known drug allergies. Social history involved marijuana use twice per week.

Clinical Findings

Unaided distance VA	OD: 20/20; OS: 20/20
Present Rx	None
Cover test	5Δ left hypotropia and 10Δ left exotropia at distance; 7Δ left hypotropia and 12Δ left exotropia at near
Confrontation visual fields	Full to finger counting OD and OS
Pupil evaluation	PERRL; no RAPD
Extraocular muscles (Figure 3.28-1)	OD: full range of motion OS: marked restriction with adduction and elevation
Intraocular pressure (GAT)	OD: 14 mm Hg; OS: 12 mm Hg at 11:25 AM
Anterior segment examination	OD: 2 mm ptosis, no lagophthalmos; otherwise unremarkable OS: unremarkable
Fundus examination	OD: 0.25/0.25 CD ratio; healthy rim tissue with distinct disc margins; fovea flat and dry; normal vasculature; peripheral retina intact OS: 0.25/0.25 CD ratio; healthy rim tissue with distinct disc margins; fovea flat and dry; normal vasculature; peripheral retina intact
Blood pressure	127/82 mm Hg RAS
Additional cranial nerve testing	Normal sensation in all divisions bilaterally; normal orbicularis function bilaterally
Exophthalmometry	OD: 20 mm; OS 22 mm

| Forced ductions | Restricted movement of the right eye |
| Sinus palpitation | Tenderness over the frontal and maxillary sinuses on the left side |

Abbreviations: CD, cup to disc; GAT, Goldmann applanation tonometry; OD, right eye; OS, left eye; PERRL, pupils equal, round, reactive to light; RAPD, relative afferent pupillary defect; RAS, right arm sitting; Rx, prescription; VA, visual acuity; XT, exotropia.

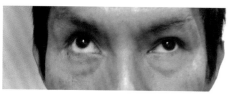

Figure 3.28-1 On upgaze, the patient demonstrated limited elevation left eye.

Discussion

Due to the forced duction testing and mild proptosis, Josh was felt to have a probable orbital lesion and was referred for a magnetic resonance imaging (MRI) of the orbits with contrast. The MRI revealed a large mucocele in the left frontal sinus that had eroded the frontal bone such that the mucocele was in contact with the orbital contents (Figure 3.28-2). He had evidence of chronic, bilateral frontal, maxillary, and ethmoid sinus disease, which were completely opacified on MRI. The patient was sent urgently to an ear, nose, and throat specialist for sinus evaluation. He was put on Augmentin, 875 mg bid, and prednisone, 40 mg for 7 days followed by 20 mg for 7 days. He was also scheduled

for sinus surgery. Three years later he had full range of motion in both eyes, and visual acuity remained 20/20 in each eye.

A sudden onset of diplopia in an otherwise healthy patient should raise a level of concern in a clinical setting. Paranasal sinuses surround the orbit on all but the lateral side. The frontal sinus is superior to the orbit, the maxillary sinus is inferior to the orbit, the ethmoid sinus is medial to the orbit, and the sphenoid sinus is posterior and medial to the orbit.

A mucocele is the most common sinus pathology affecting the orbit, followed by fibrous dysplasia, nasal polyp, neoplasm of the nasal cavity or paranasal sinus, and paranasal osteoma.[1] Mucoceles are mucus buildup in the paranasal sinuses that cause impaction and obstruction. A computed tomography (CT) scan can be a useful imaging technique to identify any changes to the boney structures surrounding the mucocele. The CT typically displays 3 characteristics: (a) homogeneous isodense mass, (b) clearly defined margins, and (c) patchy osteolysis around the mass.[3] Mucoceles can arise from several different etiologies, the most common being inflammation, allergies, trauma, fibrosis, previous lesion,

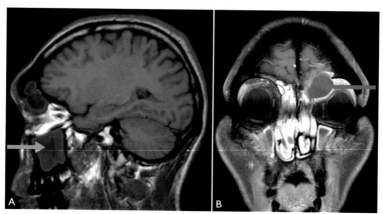

Figure 3.28-2 Sagittal (A) and coronal (B) magnetic resonance imaging with contrast shows impacted maxillary (blue arrow) and frontal (red arrow) sinuses. The frontal lesion has eroded the left orbital roof and is pushing on the globe.

or mass formation.[3] Mucoceles may erode the surrounding bone thereby extending into the orbit or intracranially.

Signs and symptoms may differ depending on the location of the mucocele. Proptosis, limited extraocular motility, swelling of the upper eyelid, and headaches are commonly found with frontal and anterior ethmoid sinus involvement.[2,3] Cranial nerve palsies or loss of vision from optic nerve compression may be seen in sphenoid or posterior ethmoid mucoceles.[2] Mucoceles are most frequently found in the fontal and ethmoid sinuses. Rarely, they can affect the sphenoid or maxillary sinuses.[2,3]

Treatment usually involves surgical removal of the mucocele, but the approach may differ depending on location and size of the lesion.[3] There is more urgency displayed if the optic nerve is compromised.

CLINICAL PEARL

- It is important to remember the anatomy of the paranasal sinuses to help identify the possible causes of extraocular muscle restriction with lid involvement.

REFERENCES

1. Samil KS, Yasar C, Ercan A, Hanifi B, Hilal K. Nasal cavity and paranasal sinus diseases affecting orbit. *J Craniofac Surg.* 2015;26(4):348.
2. Wang TJ, Liao SL, Jou JR, Lin LL. Clinical manifestations and management of orbital mucoceles: the role of ophthalmologists. *Jpn J Ophthalmol.* 2005;49(3):239-245.
3. Aggarwal SK, Bhavana K, Keshri A, Kumar R, Srivastava A. Frontal sinus mucocele with orbital complications: management by varied surgical approaches. *Asian J Neurosurg.* 2012;7(3):135-140.

3.29 Nonorganic Vision Loss

Kelly A. Malloy

Sarah, a 17-year-old girl and 12th grade student, had a 5-year history of keratoconus, for which she was wearing scleral contact lenses. These worked well for her for several years, historically helping her to achieve 20/30 vision in each eye. However, she noticed that her vision had been progressively worsening over the past 6 months. She also described some burning and stinging of her eyes. She tried lubricating drops, but they did not offer any relief. Sarah was in good health, with no known systemic health problems. She did not use any prescription medications.

Because of her blurry vision, Sarah initially returned for a contact lens evaluation. It was determined that her scleral lenses were still fitting well in each eye, and no improvement in vision could be obtained by making changes to the contact lenses. Therefore, she was referred for a neuro-ophthalmic evaluation. The results of that evaluation are as follows.

Sarah reported that she has been given accommodations at school because of her poor vision. Since she could no longer see the white board in class, she needed to use a personal computer. She was in a regular classroom with her peers, but rather than engage with her peers, she focused on her computer. She reported that this arrangement worked well for some time, but then she began having difficulty again. She had to keep increasing the magnification on the computer. Recently, she had increased the magnification to 500×. However, this too had been blurry for the last few weeks. She was currently using a magnification of 1350× and reported that she could barely see anything. In fact, she had not even gone to school for the last few days because of her poor vision.

A thorough history uncovered that Sarah felt isolated at school. She was teased when she was in 9th and 10th grade. She did not feel like she fit in so she did not talk to people. She reported that her counselor tried to get students to walk her to class as a sighted guide, but no one wanted to do it. She felt that she did not have many friends.

She hoped to attend community college after high school and then transfer to a 4-year college to pursue a career in forensic science. She was a bit concerned that her family may be moving to another state soon and that this may force her to change her plans. She did not want to move.

Clinical Findings

Entering distance VA (with habitual scleral contact lenses)	OD: hand motion; OS: hand motion
Color vision (Ishihara)	Unable to see any color plates with either eye
Confrontation visual fields	Hand motion in all quadrants OD and OS
Pupil evaluation	PERRL; no RAPD (pupils react briskly OU)
Ductions	Full in all positions of gaze OD and OS; no indication of nystagmus
Cover test	Unable to perform because patient could not see the target

Slit-lamp examination	OD: corneal stromal striae and mild pinpoint anterior stromal scarring, central corneal steepening/ectasia; scleral contact lenses well centered with adequate corneal clearance; otherwise unremarkable
	OS: corneal stromal striae and mild pinpoint anterior stromal scarring, central corneal steepening/ectasia; scleral contact lenses well centered with adequate corneal clearance; otherwise unremarkable
Fundus examination	OD: 0.6/0.6 CD ratio; healthy rim tissue with no evidence of edema or pallor; distinct disc margins; fovea flat and dry; normal vasculature; periphery intact
	OS: 0.55/0.55 CD ratio; healthy rim tissue with no evidence of edema or pallor; distinct disc margins; fovea flat and dry; normal vasculature; periphery intact
Macula OCT (Figure 3.29-1)	OD: no abnormalities; intact foveal contour
	OS: no abnormalities; intact foveal contour
Corneal topography	OD: stable keratoconus
	OS: stable keratoconus

Abbreviations: CD, cup to disc; GAT, Goldmann applanation tonometry; OCT, optical coherence tomography; OD, right eye; OS, left eye; PERRL, pupils equal, round, reactive to light; RAPD, relative afferent pupillary defect; VA, visual acuity.

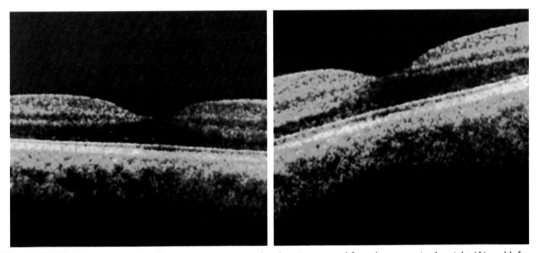

Figure 3.29-1   Macular optical coherence tomography showing normal foveal contour in the right (A) and left (B) eye.

Comments

Afferent visual function was retested with "special thick lenses" of a +20 and −20 D lens combination over her scleral contact lenses with the following results.

Visual acuity	OD: 20/40; OS: 20/40
Color vision (Ishihara)	OD: 14/14; OS: 14/14
Confrontation visual fields	Full to finger counting with no red desaturation OD and OS
Over-refraction (over habitual scleral contact lenses after discussing "special thick lenses")	OD: −0.50 −0.50 × 005 (20/40) OS: −0.25 −0.25 × 165 (20/40)

| ADD | +2.50 resulted in improved reading ability of 0.4/0.4 M (20/20) OU |

Abbreviations: OD, right eye; OS, left eye; OU, both eyes.

Comments

Sarah was prescribed her bifocals to be worn over her scleral lenses. She was told that the "special thick lenses" that helped her so much in-office could be ground to be much thinner so they would look like normal glasses. She did well with the glasses and returned to school without the need for everything to be magnified on her computer. She was again integrated with her peers.

Discussion

When Sarah presented with a complaint of progressively worsening vision in the setting of a history of keratoconus, there was an initial concern that there were corneal changes related to the keratoconus. However, when her corneal appearance and corneal topography were unchanged, and her scleral contact lenses still fit well, the focus shifted to alternate etiologies.

Because the vision loss was bilateral and severe, there was a concern for a neuro-ophthalmic disease process, or less likely a retinal/macular process. However, with briskly reactive pupils, a normal optic disc and macula appearance, and unremarkable macular optical coherence tomography (OCT), these etiologies were thought to be unlikely. It may be thought that even without optic disc edema or pallor, there could still be a retrobulbar process, such as retrobulbar optic neuritis. However, she reported that her vision had been progressively worsening for the past 6 months. If there was a retrobulbar process affecting her optic nerves for the past 6 months, with a resultant visual acuity (VA) of hand motion, neuroretinal rim pallor would be present. It typically takes approximately 1 month for neuroretinal rim pallor to develop after insult to the optic nerve.[1]

Because there was no evidence of a pathologic process, an alternate process needed to be considered. Since we saw no evidence of an organic process, we had to consider a nonorganic process. Nonorganic vision loss is known by other names, such as psychogenic vision loss or functional vision loss. It often manifests as a problem with afferent visual function in either 1 or both eyes. Although less likely, manifestations of efferent abnormalities are also possible. Not all presentations of nonorganic vision loss are the same. In fact, it has been proposed that there are 4 characteristics that can describe those who present with nonorganic vision loss. The "deliberate malingerer" knowingly fakes the vision problem for personal gain such as attention or a lawsuit. The "worrying imposter" is concerned that they have a serious problem; they knowingly exaggerate their symptoms so their problem will not be overlooked and they will not miss out on any potential future benefits. The "impressionable exaggerator" thinks there is something wrong with their eyes; they want to help their doctor and make their symptoms easy to recognize. The "suggestible innocent" has convinced themselves of a problem with their eyes; they are not very concerned about the problem itself but cannot function properly because of reduced visual function.[2]

People who present with nonorganic vision loss often have a coexisting psychological or psychiatric disorder, such as anxiety, depression, or panic attacks. They could be going through difficulty with family or finances or be a victim of abuse. Nonorganic vision loss can be a type of conversion disorder, where some type of psychological stress is manifesting as a physical problem.[2]

Nonorganic vision loss should be considered when the examination findings do not correlate with the ocular health assessment or when the patient seems to have better vision than expected based on formal testing. For example, watch the patient in the waiting room to see if their cell phone use correlates with examination results. Also, indirectly test vision in ways that the patient would not suspect as being part of a vision examination. It may be necessary to find out if there are any underlying stressors or problems in the patient's life. It is also important to find out if the patient has any pending lawsuits, disability applications, or other reasons to suspect malingering. This may need to be done outside of the confines of the standard eye examination or by someone else in the office, especially when dealing with a "deliberate malingerer" who may try to keep that information hidden.

The most important test in dealing with someone with nonorganic vision loss, especially when it is unilateral, is pupil testing. That is the only test of the afferent visual system, which is an objective assessment. The lack of a relative afferent pupillary defect can be a very important finding. Of course, this is less helpful in a bilateral presentation. But, as in the case presented here, the bilateral, briskly reactive pupils do not correlate with hand motion vision in each eye.

To diagnose nonorganic vision loss, the examiner needs to demonstrate that vision is actually normal or at the level expected based on the ocular health. This can be done with various techniques, such as using special thick placebo lenses with minimal power, as was done in this case, or using placebo eye drops or foaming eyelid cleaners. In unilateral cases, fogging the good eye in the phoropter while checking bilateral acuity can aid in the diagnosis. If the VA and visual fields cannot be proven to be normal, then other pathologic causes need to be further excluded with additional workup, which may include neuro-ophthalmology consultation or neuroimaging.

Avoid giving the patient the impression that you think there is nothing wrong with them. Assure them that although their symptoms are real, their eyes are healthy, the prognosis is good, and vision should improve. They may need a way out; therefore, it may help to prescribe eyeglasses that they think are the same prescription as the "special thick placebo lenses" that you showed them. Tell the patient that the lenses can be made to look much thinner for cosmetic reasons. That is what was done in this case. Sarah obtained eyeglasses with the over-refraction prescription to wear over her scleral contact lenses. She did well with the glasses, no longer needed the accommodations at school, and was able to rejoin her peers. In addition, psychologic/psychiatric evaluation was recommended to assess any underlying treatable issues that may have played a role in her nonorganic vision loss. It is important to realize that this is not a vision problem but a psychological issue. Although eye care providers can both prove that the vision is at an expected level and raise the suspicion of a conversion disorder, we must defer to psychology/psychiatry for definitive diagnosis and treatment of any underlying mental health issues.

CLINICAL PEARLS

- Psychological health can be as important as physical health.
- Nonorganic vision loss is a diagnosis of exclusion.

REFERENCES

1. Optic Neuritis Study Group. The clinical profile of optic neuritis: experience of the optic neuritis treatment trial. *Arch Ophthalmol*. December 1991;109(12):1673-1678.
2. Thompson HS. Functional visual loss. *Am J Ophthalmol*. 1985;100:209-213.

3.30 Primary Open Angle Glaucoma

Lorne Yudcovitch

Albert, a 60-year-old African American male, presented with a concern of constant bloodshot and irritated eyes over the past few months. He also reported having mildly watery eyes for the past year and difficulty with night vision. Ocular history included trichiasis with subsequent epilation of upper and lower lashes of both eyes. Review of past records indicated that there was a suspicion of glaucoma in both eyes due to borderline high intraocular pressures (IOPs; 22 mm Hg in each eye) and large optic nerve cupping in both eyes. When questioned, the patient stated that he had taken eye drops for glaucoma in the past but was later told that he did not have glaucoma, so he had been instructed to discontinue the medication.

Personal systemic history was positive for kidney transplantation and ongoing kidney dialysis. He also had hypertension. Medications included mycophenolate mofetil, prednisone, and cyclosporine to prevent organ rejection, valganciclovir to prevent viral infection, omeprazole for gastroesophageal reflux disease, and metoprolol, minoxidil, and clonidine for hypertension. The patient reported no medication allergies and was a current everyday alcohol drinker and smoker.

Clinical Findings

Habitual distance VA	OD: 20/30−; OS: 20/50−
Present Rx	OD: plano −1.25 × 170; OS: plano −1.25 × 015
	ADD: +2.50 OU
Extraocular motilities	Full, smooth, and equal in all fields of gaze OU
Confrontation visual fields	Full to finger counting OD and OS
Screening visual field (N-30-5 FDT, Figure 3.30-1)	OD: single, mild nasal defect above the horizontal midline OS: severe overall visual field constriction
Pupil evaluation	Round and reactive to light; left pupil 0.5 mm larger than right in bright and dim illumination; positive RAPD OS
Subjective refraction	OD: plano sph (20/20−); OS: +0.75 −1.00 × 015 (20/30−)
	ADD: +2.50 (20/25 OU at near)
Intraocular pressure (GAT)	OD: 20 mm Hg; OS: 28 mm Hg at 4:18 PM
Blood pressure	175/84 mm Hg RAS
Slit-lamp examination	OD: 1+ nuclear sclerotic cataracts; otherwise unremarkable
	OS: 1+ nuclear sclerotic cataracts; otherwise unremarkable
Fundus examination	OD: 0.65v/0.6h CD ratio; thin rim tissue superiorly with distinct disc margins; deeply excavated cup with lamina cribrosa and central retinal stalk exposure; no Drance hemorrhage or peripapillary atrophy; fovea flat and dry; normal vasculature; periphery intact

OS: 0.8v/0.85h CD ratio; thin rim tissue superiorly and inferiorly with distinct disc margins; deeply excavated cup with lamina cribrosa and central retinal stalk exposure; no Drance hemorrhage or peripapillary atrophy; fovea flat and dry; normal vasculature; periphery intact

Nerve fiber layer OCT (Figure 3.30-2)

OD: significant thinning of superior RNFL

OS: significant thinning of superior and inferior RNFL

Macular OCT (Figure 3.30-3)

OD: normal macula and foveal thickness and contour

OS: significant macular thinning and flattened contour

Visual field (30-2 SITA-standard, Figure 3.30-4)

OD: inferior arcuate scotoma with suggestion of inferior nasal step; glaucoma hemifield test outside normal limits

OS: overall depression except for central point; glaucoma hemifield test outside normal limits

Pachymetry

OD: 462 micrometer; OS: 481 micrometer

Gonioscopy

OD: open to ciliary body 360°; flat iris approach; no pigmentation of the trabecular meshwork; no angle recession

OS: open to ciliary body 360°; flat iris approach; no pigmentation of the trabecular meshwork; no angle recession

Abbreviations: CD, cup to disc; FDT, frequency doubling technology; GAT, Goldmann applanation tonometry; h, horizontal; OCT, optical coherence tomography; OD, right eye; OS, left eye; OU, both eyes; RAPD, relative afferent pupillary defect; RAS, right arm sitting; RNFL, retinal nerve fiber layer; Rx, prescription; sph, sphere; v, vertical; VA, visual acuity.

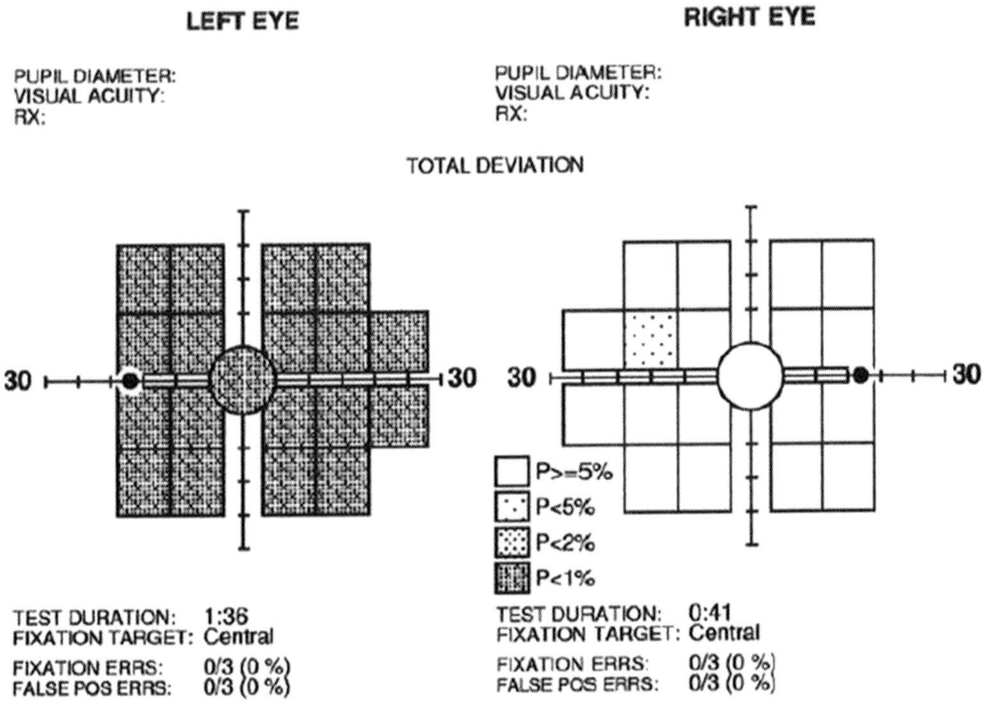

Figure 3.30-1 N-30-5 Frequency doubling technology screening visual fields showing overall constriction in the left eye and mild superior nasal defect in the right eye.

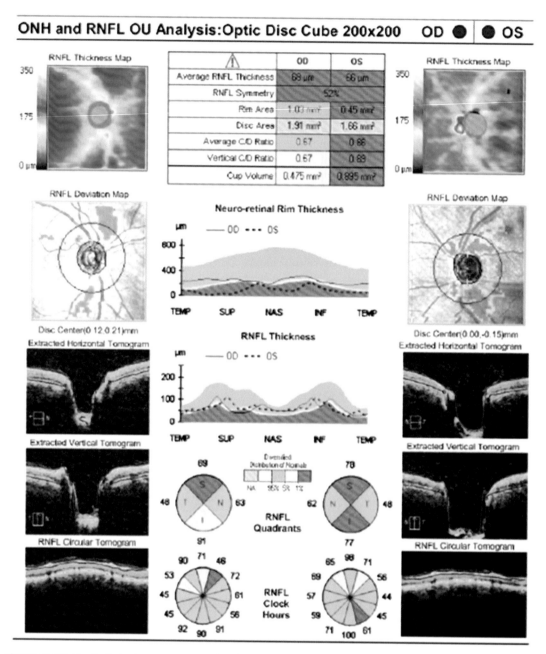

ONH and RNFL OU Analysis:Optic Disc Cube 200x200   OD ● | ● OS

⚠	OD	OS
Average RNFL Thickness	69 µm	66 µm
RNFL Symmetry	52%	
Rim Area	1.03 mm²	0.45 mm²
Disc Area	1.91 mm²	1.66 mm²
Average C/D Ratio	0.67	0.88
Vertical C/D Ratio	0.67	0.89
Cup Volume	0.475 mm²	0.895 mm²

RNFL Thickness Map

RNFL Deviation Map

Disc Center(0.12,0.21)mm
Extracted Horizontal Tomogram

Extracted Vertical Tomogram

RNFL Circular Tomogram

Neuro-retinal Rim Thickness
µm —— OD - - - OS

TEMP   SUP   NAS   INF   TEMP

RNFL Thickness
µm —— OD - - - OS

TEMP   SUP   NAS   INF   TEMP

Overmlied Distribution of Normals
NA   95% 5% 1%

RNFL Quadrants

RNFL Clock Hours

Disc Center(0.00,-0.15)mm
Extracted Horizontal Tomogram

Extracted Vertical Tomogram

RNFL Circular Tomogram

Figure 3.30-2 Optical coherence tomography of the nerve fiber layer showing significant retinal nerve fiber layer thinning in the superior and inferior quadrant of both eyes.

Discussion

Due to Albert's significant risk factors for glaucoma (African ethnicity, older age, increased IOPs, large cup to disc ratio with excavated cupping, thinned neuroretinal rim tissue, visual fields defects, and reduced corneal thickness), along with no secondary findings of pigment, neovascularization, pseudoexfoliation, or narrow anterior chamber angles, the diagnosis of primary open-angle glaucoma (POAG) was made. This diagnosis is complicated by the patient's systemic health conditions of hypertension and dialysis with kidney transplantation, for which he is taking oral prednisone to prevent organ rejection. Based on the patient's prior history

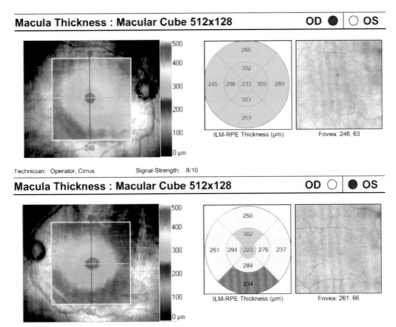

Figure 3.30-3   Macular optical coherence tomography of the right eye (top) and left eye (bottom) showing normal thickness of the right macula and moderate to severe thinning of the left macula.

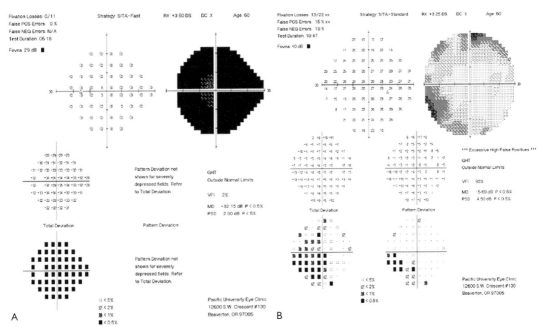

Figure 3.30-4   Threshold visual fields show overall constriction of the left eye (A) and an inferior arcuate scotoma with a nasal step in the right eye (B).

of boxing, the possibility of angle recession glaucoma in the left eye was also considered. Fortunately, no angle recession was present.

Due to the severity of Albert's vision loss, travoprost (Travatan Z) ophthalmic drops were

prescribed for both eyes, 1 drop at bedtime, as well as brinzolamide (Azopt) ophthalmic drops were prescribed for morning and late afternoon use, 1 drop both eyes. A beta-blocker (such as timolol) was avoided as the patient was already taking a systemic β-blocker (metoprolol) for his hypertension. Communication to the patient's primary care provider and nephrologist regarding the patient's blood pressure and prednisone use in light of his glaucoma was also made. The patient was promptly referred to a glaucoma surgeon for subsequent laser trabeculoplasty in the right eye and incisional trabeculectomy with filtration bleb in the left eye. Following the surgical procedures, he continues to take the prescribed glaucoma eye drops, with the addition of brimonidine (Alphagan) ophthalmic drops both eyes 1 drop twice daily.

Glaucoma is considered the leading cause of irreversible blindness in the world and the second leading cause of blindness worldwide next to cataracts.[1,2] Due to the often slow and painless damage to the retinal nerve fiber layer (RNFL), at least half of those with glaucoma are unaware that they have the condition. Some studies have shown no symptomatology or measured visual field loss despite half or more of the approximately 1.2 million retinal nerve fibers being lost.[3,4]

There are several types of glaucoma, divided broadly into primary (originating on its own) and secondary (originating from another pathologic source) forms, as well as open and closed angle forms. Here we concentrate on POAG, the most common form of glaucoma. Secondary and narrow angle forms of glaucoma will be covered in other areas of the book (Chapters 3.31 and 3.32).

There is still debate regarding the specific process by which POAG occurs. Three classic theories of why glaucoma occurs are (a) direct mechanical damage to the retinal nerve fibers, affecting internal organelles and axoplasmic flow, (b) ischemia of the optic nerve due to reduced blood flow to the optic nerve, and (c) apoptosis, or programmed cell death, which may have a genetic propensity.

Several risk factors for POAG have been identified. One key risk factor is the patient being of black race, as there is a much higher risk of development and progression of glaucoma. Patients elder than 40 years are at higher risk for POAG than younger patients. Although a family history of glaucoma is a variable in these patients, there is usually a greater risk

for developing POAG if a patient's sibling has been diagnosed with glaucoma. Vascular disease may also be a relative risk factor.[5] Patients with diabetes, hypertension, hyperlipidemia, Reynaud's syndrome, or other systemic vascular disease should be looked at more closely. Smoking and excess alcohol use may also be factors to consider.

Glaucoma was traditionally defined as a disease of elevated IOP, leading to specific optic nerve damage and visual field loss. Currently, eye pressure has been removed from the definition, as patients with normal untreated eye pressure (typically between 10 and 21 mm Hg) can have glaucoma. Although IOP is no longer considered part of the definition of glaucoma, the measurement of IOP remains the most direct way of determining if treatment is effective. The hope is that lowered IOP will help to reduce nerve fiber layer loss and subsequent visual field loss. As such, tonometry is critical at each visit.

Diurnal and nocturnal IOP variations may complicate IOP measurements. Intraocular pressure is usually higher in the early morning, lowering during the course of the day, and early evening until bedtime, where the IOP rises again during sleep. Patients with glaucoma tend to have greater diurnal fluctuation than patients without glaucoma, making IOP monitoring challenging.[6] Serial tonometry (taking multiple IOP measurements across an entire day or over several days) may be necessary to determine highest IOP readings. Follow-up visits may need to be scheduled at that peak baseline IOP time to determine treatment effectiveness.

Regardless of the type of glaucoma, the commonality is gradual RNFL loss and accompanying neuroretinal rim thinning of the optic nerve. This results in characteristic thinning of the optic disc rim tissue (typically starting inferiorly, then superiorly, temporally, and finally nasally) and exposure of the lamina cribrosa. Other signs may be present, such as notching of the neuroretinal rim tissue, bayoneting of retinal vessels over the neuroretinal rim, newly visible laminae striae, alpha and beta peripapillary atrophy, and (in the case of normotensive glaucoma) splinter or Drance hemorrhages near the optic disc. Pallor of the disc is very unusual in glaucoma and helps differentiate this from other neuropathies, such as chronic optic neuritis, toxic neuropathy, and ischemic neuropathies.

Glaucomatous visual field loss is characterized by early paracentral isolated defects between 10° and 20° from fixation. These defects eventually coalesce to form an arcuate scotoma that does not cross the nasal horizontal midline (nasal step). Eventually, the arcuate scotomas expand above and below the horizontal midline to create severe field constriction.

A glaucomatous OCT will show thinning of the superior and inferior peripapillary NFL. The temporal and nasal NFL will become involved in advanced stages. Ganglion cell analysis will show thinning within the macular region, associated with retinal nerve fiber death.

Normal central corneal thickness as measured with pachymetry is in the range of mid-500 micrometers. Thinner corneas (less than 530 micrometers, for example) may cause falsely low IOP readings, whereas thicker corneas (greater than 570 micrometers, for example) may cause falsely high IOP readings. Pachymetry readings should be considered 1 potential factor in the overall management of controlling IOP.

Indications to initiate treatment include any of the following:

- Established glaucoma
- Glaucoma in 1 eye and ocular hypertension in the other eye
- Rising IOP
- Risk factors and ocular hypertension
- IOP >21 mm Hg with a history of retinal vascular occlusion

Although future treatments such as neuroprotection, stem cell implantation, and gene therapy hold promise for novel ways to treat glaucoma, reduction of IOP remains the mainstay clinical treatment. This can be accomplished by a combination of medical and surgical treatment. Table 3.30-1 lists the main categories of pharmaceutical treatments.

Treatment is complicated by many factors, including drug cost, convenience of instillation, side effects, drug–drug interactions, and lifestyle changes. Several studies have shown that compliance with taking glaucoma drops reduces significantly with increased dosage or types of medication. The goal is to slow or halt progression of the disease over the course of a patient's lifetime with a minimum amount of treatment and the least side effects.

Based on a comprehensive history and testing, target pressures should be established. Ideally, this should be a range (eg, mid-teens) rather than a single number (eg, 17 mm Hg) because diurnal curves, treatment compliance, and other measurement elements usually factor into variations in IOP readings. Generally, the more severe the nerve damage or visual field loss, the lower the target pressure should be. A typical target pressure for early glaucoma may be a 20% reduction from baseline. A 30% reduction may be indicated if nerve damage or field loss is more severe. Target IOP may be raised or lowered at any time depending on examination findings.

Current accepted first-line medicinal treatment of glaucoma is prostaglandin analogues, usually instilled in the affected eye at bedtime. Should target IOP not be reached and/or structural damage or visual field loss is noted, a once daily β-blocker is added, usually in the morning. If target IOP is still not reached, the β-blocker dose may be increased to twice daily—morning and late afternoon. Evening β-blocker use is not recommended due to decreased effectivity in the evening, as well as the risk of hypotensive events and nocturnal breathing problems. Patients should have their blood pressure and pulse evaluated regularly when taking glaucoma medications—in particular, β-blockers. Patients who are taking β-blockers should also be questioned if they are experiencing any breathing problems, fatigue, depression, or other symptoms, and discontinuance should occur if there is a strong correlation of these symptoms with the timing of the medication.

If the patient does not sufficiently respond to the prescribed glaucoma drugs, or they have reactions/contraindications, carbonic anhydrase inhibitors or alpha-2 agonists can be used. These may be used in place of the β-blocker as adjunct treatment with the prostaglandin. Like the β-blocker, alpha-2 agonists should

Table 3.30-1 Main Categories and Examples of Pharmaceutic Treatments for Glaucoma, Including Typical Dosages and Potential Side Effects

Drug Category	Generic name Examples	Trade Name Examples	Dosage	Potential Side Effects
Alpha-adrenergic antagonist	Epinephrine Dipivefrin	Propine	Twice daily	Pupillary dilation Initial IOP increase Cystoid macular edema Tachycardia/arrhythmia Conjunctival deposits
Beta-blockers	Timolol Metipranolol Betaxtolol Levobunolol Carteolol	Timoptic Optipranolol Betoptic S Betagan Ocupress	Once daily or twice daily	Bradycardia Restricted breathing Dyslipidemia Sedation/lethargy Depression
Carbonic anhydrase inhibitors	Dorzolamide Brinzolamide	Trusopt Azopt	Twice daily or three times daily	Corneal endothelial toxicity Sulfa allergy
Alpha-2 agonist	Brimonidine Apraclonidine	Alphagan P Iopidine	Twice daily or three times daily	Ocular allergy Tachyphylaxis (apraclonidine) CNS depression (young patients)
Prostaglandin analogues	Latanoprost Bimatoprost Travaprost Tafluprost	Xalatan Lumigan Travatan Z Zioptan	Nightly	Lash lengthening/thickening Iris pigmentation (hazel eyes) Conjunctival injection Cystoid macular edema Uveitis Periorbitopathy
Docosanoid/ prostamide	Unoprostone	Rescula	Twice daily	Similar to prostaglandin analogues
Cholinergic agonist	Carbachol Pilocarpine	Isopto-Carb AK-Pilo	Three times daily- four times a day	Miosis/nyctalopia Headache/browache Pseudomyopia/difficult focusing Retinal tears (high myopes) Pupillary block
Combination medications	All except Simbrinza have timolol as 1 part	Cosopt Combigan Simbrinza Krytantek	Once daily- three times daily	Side effects based on individual drugs in the combination

Abbreviations: CNS, central nervous system; IOP: intraocular pressure.

be avoided in the evening. This is due more to effectiveness rather than safety reasons. Carbonic anhydrase inhibitors can be used in the evening if desired.

Should single-drug treatments not be achieving the target goals, combination glaucoma drops may be the next step. As dorzolamide hydrochloride/timolol maleate (Cosopt) is currently the only generically available form, this may be the most economical approach. Cosopt may be used once in the morning, in place of the single β-blocker. It can be increased to twice daily (again, avoiding evening use) if necessary. Combigan (if no β-blocker contraindication) or Simbrinza (if there is contraindication to beta-blocker) may be used similarly to Cosopt. Pilocarpine would be a much later choice as an additive drop if all other combinations fail. Dipivefrin (Propine) and unoprostone (Rescula) are far less prescribed compared to other glaucoma medications but may be used as alternative treatments once prior options have been explored.

Surgical treatment of glaucoma may be indicated if there is minimal IOP reduction, progression, or advanced glaucoma despite maximal pharmaceutical therapy, or if there is poor compliance with medicinal treatment. In general, the younger the patient with glaucoma, the more likely the need for surgical treatment to maintain vision throughout their life. Often, medicinal treatment continues after surgical treatment is performed. Although surgery can reduce IOP, the amount may not be significant enough to halt progression.

Surgical treatment options, including the following techniques, primarily serve to lower IOP by increasing aqueous outflow:

- Peripheral iridotomy/iridectomy (PI)
- Argon laser trabeculoplasty (ALT) or selective laser trabeculoplasty (SLT),
- Microinvasive glaucoma surgery (MIGS) involving microscopic trabecular stents
- Incisional trabeculoplasty with conjunctival filtration blebs/reservoir implants/tubes
- Cyclodestruction of the ciliary body through laser or cryotherapy
- Cataract extraction (to deepen the anterior chamber and widen the drainage angle)

Almost all of the major landmark glaucoma studies have shown that, even with treatment, glaucoma can still progress. Of those studies, currently only 1 (the Advanced Glaucoma Intervention Study) showed halting of visual field progression if IOP was kept under 18 mm Hg, with an average of 12 mm Hg.[7] Although this may be challenging, and particularly confounding in patients with normotensive glaucoma where the IOP is already low, other studies have shown that each millimeter lowering of IOP may slow the progression of glaucoma over 5 years by at least 10%.[8,9] This emphasizes the importance of continuing to lower eye pressure in glaucoma patients.

Once treatment has reduced IOP to at or below the target pressure, IOP checks are ideally done quarterly to determine stability. Evaluation of the optic nerves with stereoscopic biomicroscopy should also be performed at each visit. If Drance hemorrhages are noted, more aggressive treatment may be needed. Visual fields, if reliable and either clear of defects or showing only mild defects, should be monitored at least biannually. Retinal nerve fiber analysis should be performed annually. If any treatment modifications are made, the patient should be followed between 2 weeks to a month to ensure effectiveness.

CLINICAL PEARLS

- High IOP, thin corneas, age, black ethnicity, steroid use, sleep apnea, and systemic vascular disease have been linked as risk factors for POAG.

- The diagnosis of POAG is often confirmed through the combination of several tests (visual fields, stereoscopic optic nerve head evaluation, gonioscopy, IOP, pachymetry, RNFL, ganglion cell complex analysis) rather than 1 single test.

- Current POAG management involves using the most effective, convenient, and safe treatment to lower IOP to a target level that ideally achieves stability of visual function and ocular structure over time.

REFERENCES

1. Kingman S. In focus: glaucoma is second leading cause of blindness globally. *Bull World Health Organ.* November 2004;82(11):887-888.
2. Cook C, Foster P. Epidemiology of glaucoma: what's new? *Can J Ophthalmol.* June 2012;47(3):223-226. doi:10.1016/j.jcjo.2012.02.003.
3. Quigley HA, Addicks EM, Green WR. Optic nerve damage in human glaucoma. III. Quantitative correlation of nerve fiber loss and visual field defect in glaucoma, ischemic neuropathy, papilledema, and toxic neuropathy. *Arch Ophthalmol.* 1982;100:135-146.
4. Holmin C. Optic disc evaluation versus the visual field in chronic glaucoma. *Acta Ophthalmol.* 1982;60:275-283.

5. Fingeret M, Mancil GL, Bailey IL, et al. Optometric clinical practice guideline: care of the patient with open angle glaucoma. *Am Optom Assoc*. 2011: 1-161.

6. Liu JK, Zhang X, Kripke DF, Weinreb RN. Twenty-four-hour intraocular pressure pattern associated with early glaucomatous changes. *Invest Ophthalmol Vis Sci*. April 2003;44(4):1586-1590.

7. The AGIS Investigators: The Advanced Glaucoma Intervention Study (AGIS): 7. The relationship between control of intraocular pressure and visual field deterioration. *Am J Ophthalmol*. 2000;130:429-440.

8. Early Manifest Glaucoma Trial Group. Reduction of intraocular pressure and glaucoma progression: results from the Early Manifest Glaucoma Trial. *Arch Ophthalmol*. October 2002;120(10):1268-1279.

9. Canadian Glaucoma Study Group. Canadian Glaucoma Study: 3. Impact of risk factors and intraocular pressure reduction on the rates of visual field change. *Arch Ophthalmol*. October 2010;128(10):1249-1255.

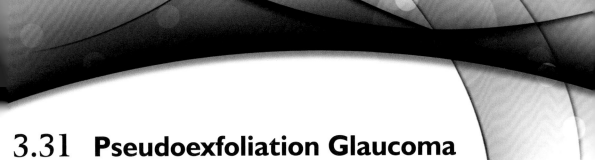

3.31 Pxeudoexfoliation Glaucoma

3.31 Pseudoexfoliation Glaucoma

Priscilla A. Lenihan and Kyla S. Duchin

Robert, a 68-year-old Caucasian male, presented for a diabetic eye examination. His only concern was fluctuating vision in both eyes since he was started on insulin 1 year ago. Robert's last eye examination was 6 years ago. He reported a history of amblyopia in the left eye and strabismus surgery at the age of 35 years. He had no known family history of ocular disease and denied a history of ocular trauma. Systemic conditions included type 2 diabetes (HbA1c tested one month ago was 8.3%), hypertension, and hyperlipidemia. He was taking insulin, metformin, losartan, amlodipine, atorvastatin, furosemide, vitamin D, and cyanocobalamin.

Clinical Findings

Habitual distance VA	OD: 20/20; OS: 20/30 (no improvement with pinhole)
Habitual Rx	OD: $-1.00 -1.00 \times 026$; OS: $-0.50 -1.00 \times 016$
	ADD: $+2.00$ (OD: 20/20^{-1}; OS: 20/30^{-2})
Pupil evaluation	PERRL; no RAPD
Confrontation fields	Full to finger counting OD and OS
Extraocular muscles	Smooth, accurate, full, and extensive OD and OS
Cover test with habitual Rx	10Δ intermittent, alternating exotropia at distance and near
Subjective refraction	OD: $-0.75 -1.00 \times 020$ (20/20); OS: $-0.25 -1.00 \times 005$ (20/25^{-2})
	ADD: $+2.25$
Intraocular pressure (GAT)	OD: 12 mm Hg; OS: 24 mm Hg OS at 10:44 AM
Central corneal thickness	OD: 490 μm; OS: 498 μm
Slit-lamp examination	OD: mild nuclear sclerotic cataracts; otherwise unremarkable
	OS: mild nuclear sclerotic cataracts; white, flaky material in a bull's eye pattern on the anterior surface of the lens (Figure 3.31-1); otherwise unremarkable
Fundus examination	OD: 0.4/0.4 CD ratio; healthy rim tissue with distinct margins; clear and flat fovea without clinically significant macular edema; few small scattered dot hemorrhages in all 4 quadrants; no holes, tears, or detachments
	OS: 0.6/0.6 CD ratio; thinned rim tissue superiorly and inferiorly with distinct disc margins; flat fovea with few fine hard drusen, no clinically significant macular edema; few scattered small dot hemorrhages in all 4 quadrants; no holes, tears, or detachments

| Nerve fiber layer OCT (Figure 3.31-2) | OD: borderline thinning of the superior and inferior RNFL |
| | OS: thinning of the superior and inferior RNFL with reduced average RNFL thickness |

Abbreviations: CD, cup to disc; GAT, Goldmann applanation tonometry; OCT, optical coherence tomography; OD, right eye; OS, left eye; RAPD, relative afferent pupillary defect; RNFL, retinal nerve fiber layer; Rx, prescription; VA, visual acuity.

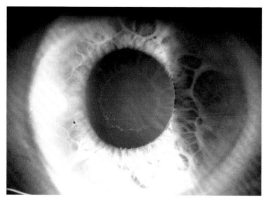

Figure 3.31-1   Pseudoexfoliation seen on the crystalline lens.

Comments

Robert was diagnosed as a glaucoma suspect due to the presence of pseudoexfoliation in the left eye, elevated and asymmetric intraocular pressure (IOP), thin central corneal thickness, asymmetric cup to disc (CD) ratio, and retinal nerve fiber layer (RNFL) thinning of the left eye with optical coherence tomography (OCT). In addition, he had mild non-proliferative diabetic retinopathy in both eyes. Although he did have mild nuclear sclerotic cataracts in both eyes, his history of amblyopia with strabismus surgery in the left eye led us to believe this was the cause of the decreased best-corrected visual acuity (VA). We asked him to return in 6 weeks for visual field, repeat IOP measurements, and gonioscopy.

Follow-up Visits and Supplemental Testing (6 Weeks Following the Initial Examination)

| Distance visual acuities | OD: 20/20; OS: 20/25⁻¹ |
| Intraocular pressure (GAT) | OD: 14 mm Hg; OS: 29 mm Hg at 11:15 AM |

Gonioscopy	OD: open to ciliary body 360° with mild pigment in the trabecular meshwork
	OS: open to ciliary body 360° with 2+ pigment in the trabecular meshwork
Visual fields (SITA-Fast 24-2; Figure 3.31-3)	OD: reliable; unremarkable
	OS: reliable; inferior arcuate scotoma and superior temporal defect extending from the blind spot

Abbreviations: GAT, Goldmann applanation tonometry; OD, right eye; OS, left eye.

Comments

Based on these findings, Robert was diagnosed with pseudoexfoliation glaucoma in the left eye. Although the glaucoma was currently manifesting in the left eye only, pseudoexfoliation typically becomes a bilateral disease. We discussed the benefits of monocular versus binocular therapy and decided to start binocular therapy. We initiated treatment with latanoprost ophthalmic solution 1 drop in both eyes at bedtime. We informed Robert of potential side effects of latanoprost and asked him to return in 6 weeks to check his IOP.

Robert returned 6 weeks later. His IOPs at that point were 11 mm Hg OD and 15 mm Hg OS with Goldmann applanation tonometry (GAT) at 8:30 AM. We instructed Robert to continue latanoprost in both eyes every night and return for a follow-up in 3 months.

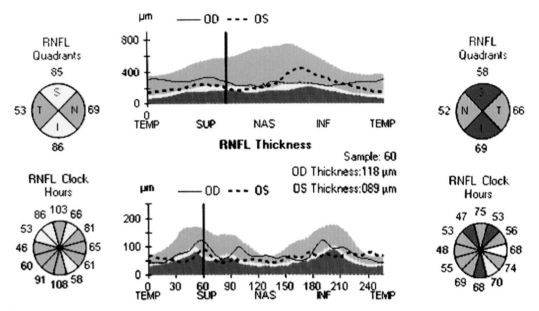

Figure 3.31-2   Nerve fiber layer optical coherence tomography demonstrating significant nerve fiber layer thinning superiorly and inferiorly in the left eye. The superior and inferior nerve fiber layer of the right eye has borderline thinning. Right eye findings is on the left and left eye findings are on the right.

Discussion

Pseudoexfoliation syndrome is a systemic condition characterized by the progressive deposition of extracellular fibrogranular material throughout the body. Pseudoexfoliative material accumulates over many tissues including the eyes, lungs, skin, liver, heart, kidney, and gallbladder; however, only in the eye is pseudoexfoliation known to have a direct effect on normal function. Some studies have shown a link between cardiovascular disease, cerebrovascular disease, aortic aneurysm, and dementia with pseudoexfoliation syndrome, but this association has not been supported in other population-based and case–control studies.[1] In the eye, pseudoexfoliative material is produced by various cell types in the anterior segment including the preequatorial lens epithelium, corneal endothelium, vascular endothelium, and iris.[2]

The reported prevalence of pseudoexfoliation syndrome ranges from 6% to approximately one-third of the population with the highest rate in Scandinavian countries and the Arizona Navajo population.[1,3,4] Pseudoexfoliation syndrome increases with age and is twice as common in women than men.[5]

Pseudoexfoliative glaucoma is the most common secondary glaucoma, and the presence of pseudoexfoliative material increases the risk of glaucoma development 2 to 3 times.[1] It is, therefore, important to closely evaluate and monitor for elevated pressures and glaucoma in these patients. Pseudoexfoliative material and iris pigment collects in the trabecular meshwork and impedes normal outflow of aqueous humor. This leads to secondary glaucoma in 2% to 15% of patients with pseudoexfoliation.[1]

A detailed ocular history, slit-lamp examination, and gonioscopy are essential in the clinical diagnosis of pseudoexfoliation. Pseudoexfoliative material is seen in the anterior segment of the eye as white flaky deposits along the pupillary border and anterior surface of the lens. Lens deposits typically collect in a bull's eye pattern with a clear intermediate zone due to rubbing of the iris on the lens. Dilation is necessary to view this pattern. Other signs include white flaky material on the corneal endothelium, as well as iris transillumination defects near the pupillary margin, and atrophy of the iris along the pupillary ruff, likely the cause of poor pupillary dilation seen

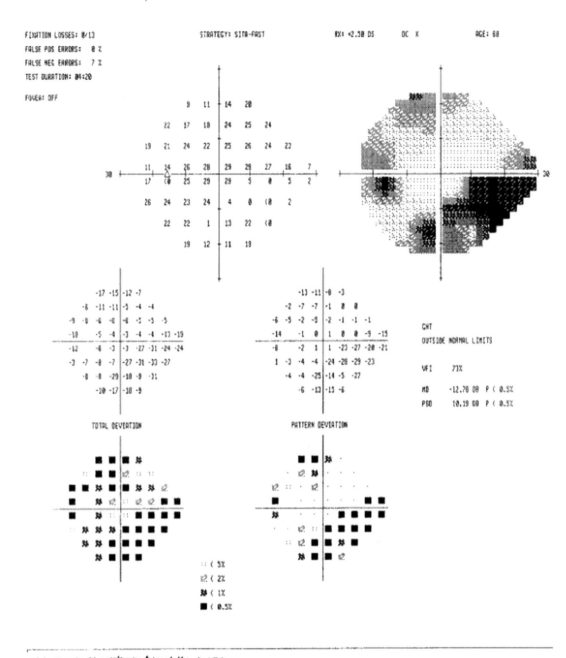

Figure 3.31-3   Visual field showing inferior arcuate defect in the left eye.

with pseudoexfoliation syndrome. Gonioscopy will reveal irregular dark pigment deposition in the trabecular meshwork, as well as pigment anterior to Schwalbe line (Sampaolesi line).[6] Findings are typically bilateral. Unilateral cases likely represent a subclinical asymmetric presentation as many patients over time develop pseudoexfoliation in the initially uninvolved eye.[7] Patients with pseudoexfoliation are likely to present with elevated IOP and often have greater fluctuations in IOP than those without pseudoexfoliation. High IOP and development of glaucoma are more dependent on the amount of pigment in the trabecular meshwork than the amount of pseudoexfoliative material in the angle.[1]

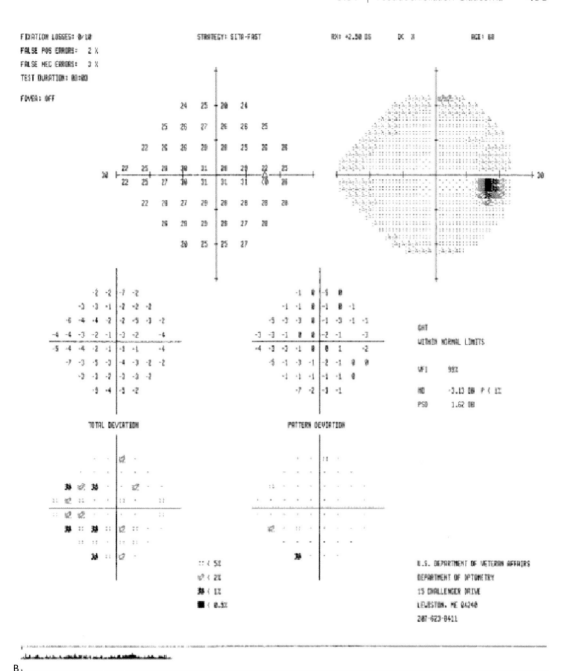

Figure 3.31-3 (Continued)

The differential diagnosis for pseudo-exfoliation is true exfoliation, which is the result of heat or infrared changes to the anterior lens capsule. Other differentials to consider are those that lead to asymmetric IOP as pseudoexfoliation glaucoma may present in 1 eye before the other. This includes angle recession, angle closure, neovascularization of the anterior chamber angle, uveitis, and ocular ischemic syndrome.

Pseudoexfoliative glaucoma can be a challenging disease to manage. Patients are more likely to present with higher IOP and more advanced visual field defects than patients with primary open-angle glaucoma.[3] Medical management with antiglaucoma drops may be enough to effectively control IOP; however, the ability of drops alone often becomes insufficient over time. A higher percentage of patients with pseudoexfoliative glaucoma fail with medical management compared to patients with primary open-angle glaucoma and therefore many patients with pseudoexfoliative glaucoma eventually require laser or surgical therapy.[8]

Another challenge in managing patients with pseudoexfoliation is cataracts. Although cataract surgery is considered safe, patients are more likely to experience complications than those without pseudoexfoliation. The pseudoexfoliative material that accumulates on the ciliary processes and zonules is thought to lead to zonular fragility and phacodonesis.[8] In patients with pseudoexfoliation, there is a higher incidence of capsular rupture, zonular dehiscence, and vitreous loss during cataract extraction.[3]

Thus far, Robert's glaucoma has been well controlled with latanoprost. We will continue to closely monitor his glaucoma with IOP measurements every 3 to 6 months and annual visual field testing and optic nerve evaluation.

CLINICAL PEARLS

- Patients with pseudoexfoliation syndrome need to be carefully followed looking for the development of ocular hypertension or glaucoma.

- A careful dilated slit-lamp examination is essential in finding the bull's eye pattern on the crystalline lens that is characteristic of pseudoexfoliation syndrome.

- Patients with pseudoexfoliative glaucoma are more likely to fail medical management compared to those with primary open-angle glaucoma.

REFERENCES

1. Anastasopoulos E, Founti P, Topouzis F. Update on pseudoexfoliation syndrome pathogenesis and associations with intraocular pressure, glaucoma and systemic diseases. *Curr Opin Ophthalmol.* 2015;26(2): 82-89.
2. Schlotzer-Schrehardt U, Naumann G. Ocular and systemic pseudoexfoliation syndrome. *Am J Ophthalmol.* 2006;141:921-937.
3. Ariga M, Nivean M, Utkarsha P. Pseudoexfoliation syndrome. *J Curr Glaucoma Pract.* 2013;7(3):118-120.
4. Desai MA, Lee RK. The medical and surgical management of pseudoexfoliation glaucoma. *Int Ophthalmol Clin.* 2008;48(4):95-113.
5. Arnarsson A, Damji KF, Sasaki H, Sverrisson T, Jonasson F. Pseudoexfoliation in the Reykjavik eye study: five-year incidence and changes in related ophthalmologic variables. *Am J Ophthalmol.* 2009; 148(2):291-297.
6. Ehlers JP, Shah CP. *The Wills Eye Manual.* 5th ed. Philadelphia, PA: Wolters Kluwer/Lippincott Williams & Wilkins; 2008:208-210.
7. Jeng SM, Karger RA, Hodge DO, Burke JP, Johnson DH, Good MS. The risk of glaucoma in pseudoexfoliation syndrome. *J Glaucoma.* 2007;16:117-121.
8. Plateroti P, Plateroti AM, Abdolrahimzadeh S, Scuderi G. Pseudoexfoliation syndrome and pseudoexfoliation glaucoma: a review of the literature with updates on surgical management. *J Ophthalmol.* 2015;2015:370371. doi:10.1155/2015/370371.

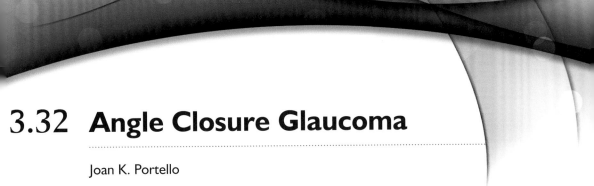

3.32 Angle Closure Glaucoma

Joan K. Portello

Suzette, a 52-year-old female, presented with concerns of blurry vision, especially in the left eye, at both distance and near and a headache over the left brow for the last week. She reported that the symptoms got worse at the end of the day. On the afternoon of the examination, the headache had progressively worsened to a 9 on a scale of 1 to 10 (10 being the worst). This prompted her to schedule the visit. She took 200 mg of ibuprofen (Advil), but this did not provide relief. In addition, Suzette reported that her eyes felt irritated and noticed redness and tearing, particularly in her left eye. Suzette's last eye examination was 1 year ago, and she reported that the ophthalmologist wanted to perform a procedure in his office, but she did not return. She could not remember the name of the procedure or why the doctor wanted to perform it. Suzette reported no medical conditions and was not taking any prescribed medications.

Clinical Findings

Habitual distance VA	OD: 20/20^{-2}; OS: 20/30 (no improvement with pinhole)
Present Rx	OD: +3.00 −0.50 × 165
	OS: +3.50 −0.50 × 150
	ADD: +2.00 OU (OD: 20/20^{-2}; OS: 20/30^{-2})
Ocular motility	Full and comitant OD and OS
Confrontation visual fields	Full to finger counting OD and OS
Pupil evaluation	OD: round and reactive to light
	OS: sluggish response to light
	No RAPD
Slit-lamp examination	OD: 1+ conjunctival injection; clear cornea; convex iris with grade 2 nasal and temporal Van Herick angle estimation; no anterior chamber cells or flare or posterior synechiae; trace nuclear sclerosis
	OS: 2+ conjunctival injection; microcystic corneal edema; convex iris with grade 1 nasal and temporal Van Herick angle estimation; no anterior chamber cells or flare or posterior synechiae; trace nuclear sclerosis
Intraocular pressure (GAT)	OD: 30 mm Hg; OS: 62 mm Hg at 11:00 AM
Undilated fundus examination	OD: 0.5/0.5 CD ratio; healthy rim tissue with distinct disc margins; fovea flat and dry; normal vasculature
	OS: 0.65/0.65 CD ratio; healthy rim tissue with distinct disc margins; fovea flat and dry; normal vasculature
Pachymetry	OD: 580 μm; OS: 583 μm

Gonioscopy	OD: Schwalbe line seen in the superior, nasal, and temporal quadrants; trabecular meshwork seen inferiorly; convex iris
	OS: no anterior chamber angle structures visible in any quadrant; convex iris
Anterior segment OCT (Figure 3.32-1)	OD: anatomically narrow angle; convex iris configuration confirmed
	OS: anatomically narrow angle; appositional angle closure noted; convex iris configuration confirmed

Abbreviations: CD, cup to disc; GAT, Goldmann applanation tonometry; OCT, optical coherence tomography; OD, right eye; OS, left eye; OU, both eyes; RAPD, relative afferent pupillary defect; Rx, prescription; VA, visual acuity.

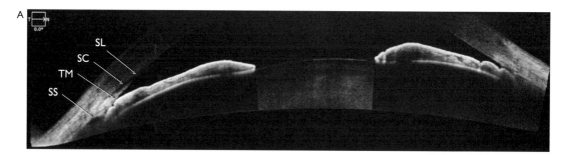

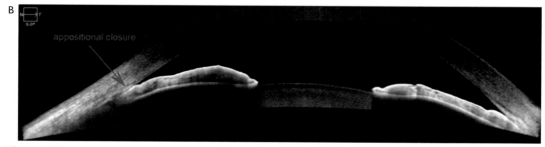

Figure 3.32-1   Anterior segment optical coherence tomography of the right (A) and left (B) eye showing significant iridocorneal touch in the left eye (red arrow). Scleral spur (SS) and Schwalbe line (SL) are shown posteriorly and anteriorly to the trabecular meshwork (TM), respectively. Schlemm canal (SC) is located outer to the TM.

Comments

Suzette was diagnosed with acute angle closure secondary to appositional closure and relative pupillary block due to the convex iris configuration in each eye. Antiglaucoma medications were administered immediately to lower the intraocular pressure (IOP) in each eye. She was given 2 tablets of 250 mg acetazolamide orally. Topical treatment included 1 drop brinzolamide 1%/brimonidine 0.2% suspension (Simbrinza) in each eye, 1 drop travoprost 0.004% solution (Travatan Z) in each eye, and 1 drop timolol 0.5% solution in each eye. After 30 minutes, an additional drop of all 3 medications was instilled into the left eye only. Intraocular pressure measurements 35 minutes after the first drop instillation were 18 mm Hg OD and 52 mm Hg OS. A second measurement of the left eye 60 minutes after the initial treatment yielded 42 mm Hg. One drop of pilocarpine 2% was then administered in the left eye. Intraocular pressure in the left eye approximately 90 minutes after the initiation of treatment was 34 mm Hg.

Suzette was given Simbrinza to be used twice daily in each eye and pilocarpine 2% to be used 4 times per day in the left eye only. She was advised to return to the clinic the next day to evaluate her IOP and was scheduled 3 days after the initial examination for a laser peripheral iridotomy (LPI) in each eye. Despite calls from the office, Suzette did not return for her 1-day follow-up.

Follow-up Visit (3 Days Following the Initial Examination)

History: Suzette presented for an LPI in both eyes due to the narrow-angle approach. She reported excellent compliance with both medications prescribed at the initial visit. She had a brow ache over the left eye since the instillation of pilocarpine, as well as blurry vision in the left eye and nausea.

Distance VA (with habitual Rx)	OD: 20/20; OS: 20/25
Pupil evaluation	OD: round and reactive to light
	OS: pharmacologically miotic pupil
	No RAPD on reverse swinging flashlight test
Intraocular pressure (GAT)	OD: 12 mm Hg; OS: 12 mm Hg at 9:00 AM

Abbreviations: GAT, Goldmann applanation tonometry; OD, right eye; OS, left eye; RAPD, relative afferent pupillary defect; Rx, prescription; VA, visual acuity.

Comments

The LPI procedure was performed in each eye by a staff ophthalmologist. Postoperative IOPs were 11 mm Hg OD and 11 mm Hg OS with GAT at 10:42 AM.

Follow-up Visit (2 Weeks Following the Initial Examination)

Intraocular pressure (GAT)	OD: 11 mm Hg; OS: 11 mm Hg at 11:00 AM
Visual field (24-2 threshold, Figure 3.32-2)	OD: unremarkable OS: nasal defect not respecting the horizontal midline
Optic nerve OCT (Figure 3.32-3)	OD: normal peripapillary RNFL thickness OS: superior, inferior, and temporal RNFL thinning

Ganglion cell complex OCT (Figure 3.32-4)	OD: no thinning of the ganglion cell layer OS: significant thinning of the ganglion cell layer

Abbreviations: GAT, Goldmann applanation tonometry; OCT, optical coherence tomography; OD, right eye; OS, left eye; RNFL, retinal nerve fiber layer.

Discussion

Angle closure has the potential to become visually devastating. Quigley et al[1] predicted that by 2020 the prevalence of primary open-angle glaucoma and angle closure glaucoma will be approximately 79.6 million people, with about 26% of these cases having angle closure glaucoma. In addition, approximately 3.9 million of the individuals with angle closure will have bilateral blindness.[1]

It is important to differentiate between angle closure and angle closure glaucoma. Angle closure occurs when there is contact between the iris and trabecular meshwork involving at least 180° of the anterior chamber angle. Apposition between the iris and trabecular meshwork impedes aqueous drainage causing increased IOP. Angle closure glaucoma is diagnosed when optic neuropathy is present. This involves loss of neuroretinal rim tissue, retinal nerve fiber layer, and visual field function. Hyperopia with short axial length, increased crystalline lens thickness, being older than 60 years, female gender, and East Asians or Inuit ethnicity are risk factors for angle closure due to decreased anterior chamber depth and volume. Suzette had 2 risk factors: being hyperopic and female.

The most common cause of angle closure is pupillary block, that is, contact between the anterior lens and posterior iris. When this occurs, aqueous is prohibited from moving from the nonpigmented ciliary epithelium, where it is produced, into the anterior chamber, where it exits the globe. When this occurs, a pressure difference is created between the anterior and posterior chambers causing the iris to bow forward bringing the peripheral iris into contact with the trabecular meshwork. Other causes

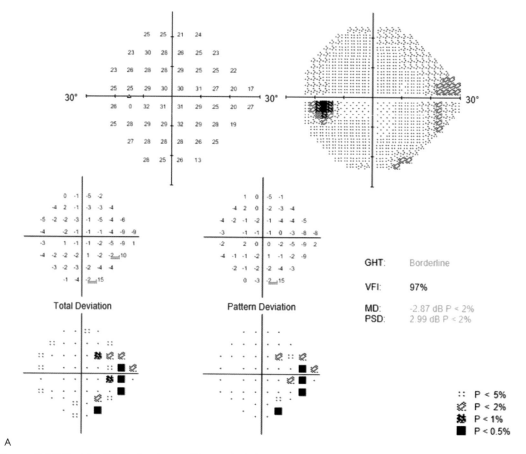

A

Figure 3.32-2   Visual fields showing nasal loss in the left eye (A). The right eye (B) is within normal limits.

of angle closure include a plateau iris configuration, increased lens thickness, and thickened peripheral iris stroma.

Angle closure may be acute, subacute, or chronic. The types can overlap and even occur in the same eye. Acute angle closure typically presents with blurry vision, halos around lights, unilateral headache, nausea, and vomiting. Subacute angle closure often has fewer symptoms compared with acute angle closure and may be asymptomatic. Subacute angle closure may be confused with migraine as it can present with unilateral headache, as well as nausea and visual symptoms similar to those of a migraine. Headaches associated with subacute angle closure generally last no more than 4 hours.[2] In chronic angle closure, the IOP gradually increases and symptoms are unusual until late in the process when vision is lost. For Suzette, the symptoms were not severe

enough to cause her to seek eye care sooner. In addition, she did not have the classical signs and symptoms despite experiencing an acute episode. This emphasizes the importance of listening to all of the patient's symptoms, and correlating these with examination findings, to complete the diagnosis.

Typical signs of acute angle closure include a shallow anterior chamber, conjunctival injection, corneal edema, a fixed mid-dilated pupil, and markedly elevated IOP. Glaukomflecken, focal infarcts of the crystalline lens epithelium characterized by small, gray-white, anterior opacities, may be present.[3] Suzette likely had intermittent angle closure for some time because her left eye exhibited the consequences of this with asymmetric optic nerve cupping, nerve fiber layer defects, and visual field loss.

Gonioscopy or anterior segment optical coherence tomography (OCT) is critical in the

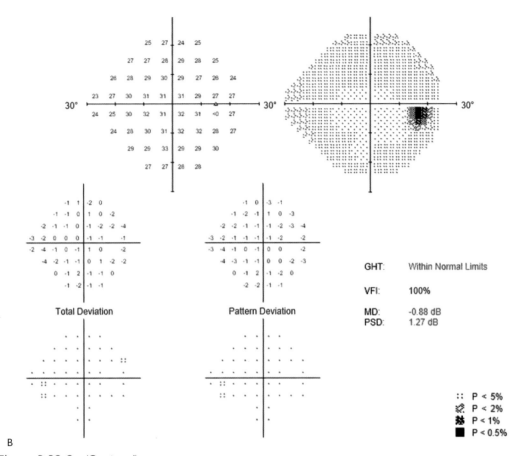

Total Deviation   Pattern Deviation

GHT: Within Normal Limits

VFI: 100%

MD: -0.88 dB
PSD: 1.27 dB

:: P < 5%
P < 2%
P < 1%
■ P < 0.5%

B

Figure 3.32-2   (Continued)

diagnosis of angle closure. Anterior synechiae are common sequela of angle closure. Synechiae can be differentiated from iridotrabecular contact by pressing on the central cornea with a gonioscopy lens that has a patient contact area smaller than the corneal diameter. This pushes aqueous into the peripheral angle. Doing this will open an appositionally closed angle; however, if synechiae are present, the iris and cornea will remain attached. The same technique can aid in lowering IOP following an angle closure event.

Anterior segment OCT provides a cross-sectional image of the anterior chamber angle (Figure 3.32-1A). The scleral spur lies at the junction between the higher reflective sclera and the lower reflective ciliary body. Schwalbe line is seen as a change of reflectivity at the termination of the corneal endothelium. The trabecular meshwork fills in the area between

the scleral spur and Schwalbe line, and Schlemm canal is an area of low reflectance outer to the trabecular meshwork.

The initial goal of treatment is to lower the IOP, generally using medications such as carbonic anhydrase inhibitors, β-blockers, alpha adrenergic agonists, prostaglandin analogs, and parasympathomimetics. It is then important to alleviate the cause of the angle closure by an LPI or cataract extraction. Carbonic anhydrase inhibitors and beta-adrenergic antagonists suppress aqueous humor production. Alpha-2 adrenergic agonists reduce aqueous humor formation and may also increase uveoscleral outflow. Prostaglandins, which increase uveoscleral outflow, take longer to lower IOP but have been shown to be useful in treating angle closure glaucoma.[4] When using oral acetazolamide, care should be taken to avoid the sustained release formulation because an

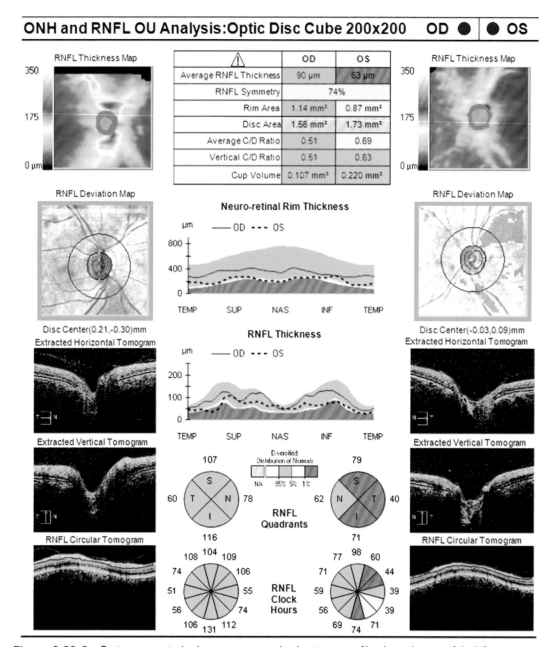

ONH and RNFL OU Analysis:Optic Disc Cube 200x200   OD ● | ● OS

⚠	OD	OS
Average RNFL Thickness	90 μm	63 μm
RNFL Symmetry	74%	
Rim Area	1.14 mm²	0.87 mm²
Disc Area	1.56 mm²	1.73 mm²
Average C/D Ratio	0.51	0.69
Vertical C/D Ratio	0.51	0.63
Cup Volume	0.107 mm³	0.220 mm³

Figure 3.32-3   Optic nerve optical coherence tomography showing nerve fiber layer thinning of the left eye.

immediate response is necessary. Pilocarpine causes contraction of the pupillary sphincter and ciliary body muscles, widening the angle. Pilocarpine should only be used when the IOP is below 40 mm Hg because at higher pressures the pupillary sphincter becomes ischemic and less responsive.

Laser peripheral iridotomy creates an opening in the iris, which decreases the pressure difference between the posterior and anterior iris. When this pressure difference is reduced, the iris flattens and the angle widens. Removal of the crystalline lens can also aid in widening the anterior chamber depth, opening the angle, and lowering the IOP. In fact, cataract extraction may be more efficacious and cost-effective than LPI.[5] Both eyes are often treated as many patients have bilateral disease.

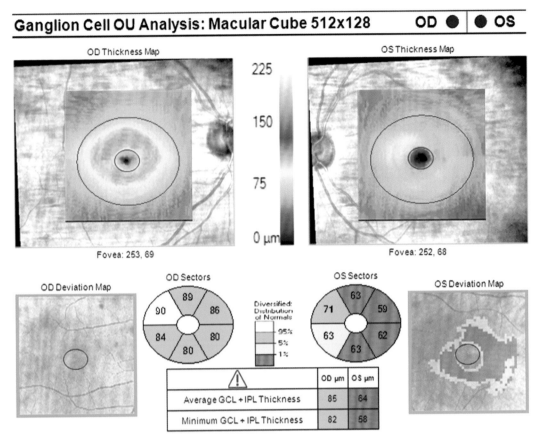

Figure 3.32-4   Ganglion cell analysis showing thinning of the ganglion cell complex of the left eye.

Because acute angle closure is more symptomatic and can lead to blindness, chronic or subacute angle closure can be more visually devastating because the lack of symptoms can delay the patient from presenting for diagnosis and treatment. Having a high suspicion for angle closure can prevent visual loss in these patients.

CLINICAL PEARL

- Surgical intervention of angle closure glaucoma changes the structure of the anterior angle, thereby lowering IOP and reducing the likelihood of structural damage to the optic nerve.

REFERENCES

1. Quigley HA, Broman AT. The number of people with glaucoma worldwide in 2010 and 2020. *Br J Ophthalmol*. March 2006;90(3):262-267.
2. Shindler KS, Sankar PS, Volpe NJ, Piltz-Seymour JR. Intermittent headaches as the presenting sign of subacute angle-closure glaucoma. *Neurology*. 2005;65:757-758.
3. See J, Aquino M, Chew P. Angle-closure glaucoma. In: Yanoff M, Duker JS, eds. *Ophthalmology*. 4th ed. Cambridge, MA: Elsevier Inc; 2014:1060-1069.
4. Sowka JW, Kabat AG. PGA ACG? Here's a look at prostaglandin analogs for the treatment of angle-closure glaucoma. *Rev Optom*. March 2011;15:139-140.
5. Azuara-Blanco A, Burr J, Ramsay C, et al. EAGLE study group. Effectiveness of early lens extraction for the treatment of primary angle-closure glaucoma (EAGLE): a randomized controlled trial. *Lancet*. 2016;388(10052):1389-1397.

3.33 Corneal Foreign Body

Lorne Yudcovitch

Jason, a 36-year-old Caucasian male, presented as a walk-in for evaluation of left eye irritation for the last 2 hours. He felt the irritation each time he blinked, and he had tearing and mild redness of the eye. Jason stated that the symptoms started while working on his car in the garage. Flushing with water under a sink tap at home did not relieve the irritation. He denied using any eye drops before or after the irritation. Systemic and ocular health were otherwise unremarkable, and he was taking no medications. He had no medication allergies. He smoked occasionally and drank alcohol socially.

Clinical Findings

Unaided distance VA	OD: 20/15; OS: 20/20^{-2}
Present Rx	None
Ocular motilities	Full, smooth, and equal in all fields of gaze OU; no diplopia was noted but irritation was noted in up and down gaze OS
Confrontation visual fields	Full to finger counting OD and OS
Pupil evaluation	PERRL; no RAPD
Intraocular pressure (noncontact tonometry)	OD: 17 mm Hg; OS: unable to test (patient squinting) at 11:15 AM
Slit-lamp examination (Figure 3.33-1)	OD: unremarkable OS: raised, mottled 1 mm × 1.2 mm metallic mass on the cornea at 1 o'clock within the pupil region, approximately 1 mm from the central pupil; the foreign body penetrated to the anterior corneal stroma; no signs of staining or pooling were noted with fluorescein; mild diffuse bulbar conjunctival injection noted around the limbus; no cells or flare
Fundus examination	OD: 0.2/0.2 CD ratio; healthy rim tissue with distinct disc margins; fovea flat and dry; normal vasculature; periphery intact; no intraocular foreign bodies noted
	OS: 0.2/0.2 CD ratio; healthy rim tissue with distinct disc margins; fovea flat and dry; normal vasculature; periphery intact; no intraocular foreign bodies noted

Abbreviations: CD, cup to disc; OD, right eye; OS, left eye; OU, both eyes; PERRL, pupils equal, round, reactive to light; RAPD, relative afferent pupillary defect; Rx, prescription; VA, visual acuity.

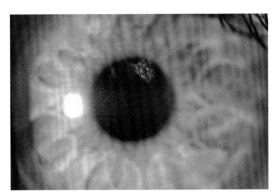

Figure 3.33-1   Metallic corneal foreign body on patient's left eye.

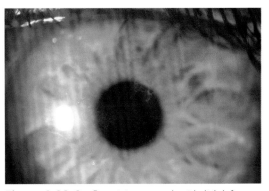

Figure 3.33-2   Remaining corneal epithelial defect (1 o'clock pupil edge) immediately post-foreign body removal. Trace fluorescein dye pooling is seen in the defect.

Discussion

Based on the clinical findings and patient symptoms, informed consent was obtained with recommendation for foreign body removal. Prognosis, alternatives (of treatment), risks, and questions (PARQs) were discussed, and Jason consented to in-office removal.

Initial in-office removal using sterile saline spray directed tangentially at the edge of the foreign body failed to lift it off the cornea. The decision was made to use a foreign body spud to remove the metal. The patient, doctor, and witness signed a completed informed consent form. One drop of fluorescein sodium/benoxinate (Fluress) was instilled in the left eye. This showed no other corneal epithelial defects and negative Seidel sign. A stainless steel surgical golf club spud was used to lift the foreign body off the cornea. After removal, Jason had a corneal epithelial defect of the same size and shape as the original foreign body (Figure 3.33-2). He showed negative Seidel sign and a deep anterior chamber. Noncontact tonometry of the left eye was 15 mm Hg at 11:39 AM. One drop moxifloxacin (Moxeza) was instilled, but Jason declined the use of a therapeutic bandage contact lens. He was discharged with instructions to use tobramycin/dexamethasone (Tobradex) 1 drop 4 times per day in the left eye and to return the next day for follow-up.

Jason returned the following day with resolved symptoms and a nearly fully healed corneal epithelium. Jason was instructed to continue the Tobradex drop regimen for 2 more days and encouraged to wear proper

eye protection when performing mechanical, garden, or other tasks that may result in eye injury.

Corneal foreign bodies are relatively common urgent visits in eye care practices and are commonly caused by high projectile particles (eg, dirt or dust from wind, grinding or drilling metal, sanding wood) or by rust, glass, or vegetative injury striking and embedding into the ocular tissue.

Symptoms of pain, redness, lacrimation, eyelid spasm, and sometimes blur, usually start immediately or very soon after the foreign body embeds in the cornea. On rare occasions, when the patient cannot open their eye, topical ophthalmic anesthetic may need to be instilled immediately to allow visual acuities (VAs) and proper evaluation of the eye.[1]

The foreign body often presents as an immovable object on the cornea. Objects that do not penetrate Bowman membrane are called superficial foreign bodies and can often be removed by irrigating tangentially on the edge of the object with ophthalmic saline to lift the object off. Objects that penetrate Bowman membrane are called embedded foreign bodies. These usually require a needle (usually 25 gauge, 5/8 in) or foreign body spud (smaller size is recommended) to physically lift the particle by its edge, off the cornea. Needles should be approached tangentially to the corneal surface, bevel side up. The Cockburn curve technique (bending the needle tip toward the bevel while inside its plastic jacket) may help reduce the risk of perforating the cornea while also

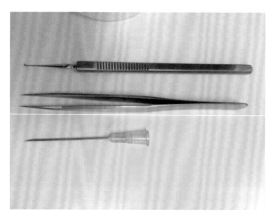

Figure 3.33-3 Examples of instruments used to remove corneal foreign bodies. Top to bottom: surgical "golf club" spud, precision jeweler forceps, 25-gauge needle.

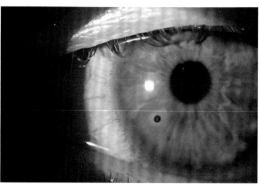

Figure 3.33-4 Rust ring (orange brown color) with surrounding Coat's ring (white) seen in another patient after metallic foreign body removal. The metallic foreign body was in the cornea for more than 48 hours.

providing more leverage to lift particles. Other instruments to remove foreign bodies include nylon (Bailey) loops, precision jeweler forceps (for larger foreign bodies), and saline moistened cotton-tipped applicators. Cotton-tipped applicators have more likelihood to abrade the corneal epithelium, as well as potentially embed the particle deeper into the cornea.[2] Instruments with strong magnets are also available for removing small superficial metallic foreign bodies.[3] Topical ophthalmic anesthetic should be used prior to utilizing the prescribed methods, although sterile saline spray may be used without anesthetic. Examples of instruments used in corneal foreign body removal are shown in Figure 3.33-3.

Infection is more likely with retention of foreign body material or the presence of a rust ring. Rust rings consist of oxidized ferrous material remaining in the cornea from a metallic foreign body (Figure 3.33-4). Usually, rust rings are orange-brown, follow the shape of the original metallic particle, and become more prominent if the particle exceeds 12 hours in the cornea. Any remaining foreign material or rust ring must be removed to ensure epithelial healing and reduce or prevent the chance of epithelial necrosis and infection. An algerbrush is often used to remove rust rings. The foreign body spud or sterile needle mentioned previously may also remove certain rust material.[4]

Ophthalmic antibiotic drops such as tobramycin, polymixin B/trimethoprim, or an ophthalmic fluoroquinolone (ie, moxifloxacin,

gatifloxacin, or besifloxacin) are usually prescribed several times per day for a few days after the injury to reduce bacterial infection risk. Suspicion of infection should be heightened if the eye continues to remain red and inflamed 3 days following the foreign body removal.

Vegetative injury is a concern due to greater risk of fungal infection. Often, fungal growth is insidious and slowly progressing. The infection may appear in a few days to more than a week after the initial injury. Follow-up on vegetative foreign bodies may necessitate an additional evaluation a week after removal of the particle, to ensure no mycosis is present.

On occasion, a white ring of corneal edema and infiltrative material surrounds the foreign body, called a Coats ring (Figure 3.33-4). This ring usually resolves within 2 weeks after the foreign body is removed. Rarely, the corneal endothelium may develop a ring immediately behind the foreign body, called annular keratopathy of Payreau. This finding may resolve after a few days.[5] Glass foreign bodies, due to their inert nature, generally do not produce a significant immune response.

Post-traumatic iritis, should it occur, usually happens within 24 to 72 hours after the foreign body injury. If the patient is light sensitive or cells or flare is seen in the anterior chamber, a cycloplegic eye drop is indicated for comfort and to reduce the inflammation. Topical ophthalmic steroid treatment several times daily is important to reduce the iritis, although steroids may be contraindicated if there is a vegetative injury and risk of fungal infection as this may potentiate the infection risk. Steroids may also be contraindicated if there is a large corneal epithelial defect, as steroids may reduce wound healing. Conversely, topical ophthalmic steroids may help lower the chance of corneal stromal scarring, as well as reduce ocular pain and redness. Combination of antibiotic–steroid drops may be useful in preventing bacterial infection while reducing inflammation.

Recurrent corneal erosions (RCEs) are a potential adverse effect from corneal foreign bodies. They occur more often from injuries that have larger (ie, greater than 1 mm diameter) epithelial defects. Bandage therapeutic contact lenses can be used over larger corneal epithelial defects after foreign body removal to reduce pain symptoms and allow corneal epithelial healing, reducing the chance of an RCE. The patient should be followed daily when a bandage contact lens is used to ensure no chance of infection and to determine when the lens should be removed or replaced. Bandage contact lenses should be used with caution and not used in cases of vegetative injury due to the potential risk of fungal growth. Despite complete wound healing, the patient should be informed that RCEs may occur days, weeks, months, or even years later, depending on the initial injury.

Depending on the location, depth, and extent of the foreign body, the patient should understand that permanent vision loss may occur despite treatment. Consideration of referral to a corneal specialist should be done if the foreign body:

1. is deeply penetrating or perforating the cornea;

2. is centrally located and significantly affecting vision;

3. may result in corneal scarring that is likely to reduce vision permanently;

4. leads to infectious keratitis not responsive to treatment; or

5. continues to cause symptoms long after removal.

Oral analgesics such as acetaminophen, ibuprofen, or naproxen are options to reduce initial pain. Opiate analgesics, such as hydrocodone or oxycodone, are rarely needed. In cases of extensive damage, protection of the affected eye with a fox shield and transfer to a corneal surgical center for potential keratoplasty may be necessary.

CLINICAL PEARLS

- Corneal foreign bodies can be effectively removed after close evaluation of the depth and extent of the foreign body is made.

- Proper management of a corneal foreign body includes removal using the least invasive method, judicious use of topical ophthalmic antibiotics and steroids, and occasionally a therapeutic bandage contact lens.

- Patients who present with a corneal foreign body should be informed of potential risk of infection, inflammation, scarring, iritis, RCEs, and permanent vision loss.

REFERENCES

1. Ehlers JP, Shah CP. Chapter 1: Differential diagnosis of ocular symptoms. In: *The Wills Eye Manual.* 5th ed. Philadelphia, PA: Lippincott Williams & Wilkins;2008:16-17.

2. Casser L, Fingeret M, Woodcombe HT. Chapter 44: Corneal foreign body removal. In: *Atlas of Primary Eyecare Procedures.* 2nd ed. Pennsylvania, PA: Mcgraw-Hill Medical;1997:164-169.

3. Kanski JJ. Chapter 23: Trauma. In: *Clinical Ophthalmology: A Systemic Approach.* 6th ed. New York, NY: Elsevier;2007:860-862.

4. Casser L, Fingeret M, Woodcombe HT. Chapter 45: Corneal rust ring removal. In: *Atlas of Primary Eyecare Procedures.* 2nd ed. Pennsylvania, PA: Mcgraw-Hill Medical;1997:170-175.

5. Catania LJ. Chapter 5: Diagnoses of the cornea. E. Foreign bodies. In: *Primary Care of the Anterior Segment.* 2nd ed. New York, NY: Appleton & Lange;1996:228-241.

3.34 Ocular Trauma

Navjit Kaur Sanghera

Michael, an 11-year-old African American male, presented with a chief concern of left eye blurriness, as well as a red, painful, tearing, and photophobic left eye. He reported trauma, which occurred 3 days ago while playing outdoors. He initially claimed his friend hit him in the eye with a pomegranate, but then he said the fruit was much smaller, possibly a crabapple. The pain was constant (9/10 at initial occurrence, now decreased to 5/10). He reported no self-treatment or alleviating factors. He reported liking to read, loving math, and having mostly A's and B's in school. His last eye examination was 2 years ago. He had glasses in the past, but they broke "a long time ago." His mother reported all developmental milestones and medical history to be normal. He was not taking any medications and had no allergies.

Clinical Findings

Unaided distance VA	OD: 20/200 (pinhole 20/30); OS: 20/400 (pinhole 20/30)
Unaided near VA	OD: 20/20; OS: 20/20
Pupil evaluation	OD: 4 mm in bright, 6 mm in dim; round, reactive to light
	OS: 6 mm in bright, 6.5 mm in dim; slow reaction to light
	No RAPD noted
Extraocular muscle evaluation	Full OU
Confrontation visual fields	Full to finger counting OD and OS
Intraocular pressure (GAT)	OD: 19 mm Hg; OS: 16 mm Hg at 10:00 AM
Slit-lamp examination	OD: unremarkable
	OS: no ecchymosis; diffuse 2+ conjunctival injection; corneal endothelial pigment dusting; 2+ cells and flare, with mild inferior hyphema; multiple tears in the area of the iris sphincter; no rosette cataract; no corneal staining or Seidel sign
Fundus examination	OD: unremarkable
	OS: no evidence of traumatic macular hole, Shaffer's sign, posterior vitreous detachment, or hemorrhage; periphery was flat and intact 360° with no retinal holes, retinal detachment or commotio retinae

Abbreviations: GAT, Goldmann applanation tonometry; OD, right eye; OS, left eye; OU, both eyes; RAPD, relative afferent pupillary defect; VA, visual acuity.

Comments

Michael was felt to have closed globe trauma secondary to a blunt object. There were no obvious lacerations or abrasions, and we carefully evaluated the vitreous and retina to rule out an intraocular foreign body. No relative afferent pupillary defect (RAPD) was present to indicate optic nerve involvement. There was no presence of ecchymosis or lid laceration, and extraocular motility movements were normal, which helped to rule out an orbital lesion. The cells and flare, as well as the pigment dusting on the corneal endothelium, hyphema, and lower intraocular pressure (IOP), were indicative of a traumatic iritis. Based on him seeing 20/20 at near in each eye, as well as having significantly improved acuity with pinhole, it was felt the visual acuity reduction was due to uncorrected refractive error rather than the injury itself.

Michael was prescribed a cycloplegic agent (atropine 1%, once daily OS) to help reduce pain and a steroid (prednisolone acetate 1%, 4 times per day OS) to reduce inflammation and improve comfort. He was also to use non-preservative artificial tears 6 times per day, at least 5 minutes after the other eye drops. The patient and his mother were educated that Michael was to sleep with the head elevated to help with blood settling. They were told to avoid aspirin or nonsteroidal anti-inflammatory drugs (NSAIDS) as these can increase the risk of a hyphema rebleed. He was asked to limit activity and take care to protect the injured eye with safety goggles. He was asked to return in 2 days to assess healing.

Follow-up Visits (2 Days, 1 Week, 2 Weeks, and 1 Month Following the Initial Examination)

Signs and symptoms steadily improved throughout this time. Michael was compliant with the atropine and prednisolone. He no longer experienced pain or photophobia. The conjunctival injection, hyphema, and anterior chamber inflammation had resolved by the 2-week follow-up; therefore, the patient was able to discontinue the atropine and taper the prednisolone (twice per day for 1 week, once per day for 1 week, then discontinue).

Intraocular pressure (at 2-week follow-up; GAT)	OD: 19 mm Hg; OS: 18 mm Hg at 10:00 AM
Refraction (at 2-week follow-up)	OD: −1.50 −0.25 × 097 (20/20)
	OS: −2.00 −0.50 × 104 (20/20)
Gonioscopy (at 1-month follow-up)	Angle recession greater than 270° (Figure 3.34-1) and a peripheral anterior synechiae (Figure 3.34-2)

Abbreviations: GAT: Goldmann applanation tonometry; OD, right eye; OS, left eye.

Discussion

The sudden nature of eye injury and the risk of potential sight loss can make eye trauma one of the most concerning clinical problems. Blunt ocular trauma is one of the most common and potentially vision-threatening ocular emergencies worldwide. It is the leading cause of

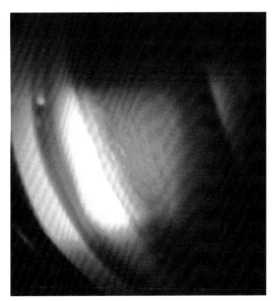

Figure 3.34-1 Angle recession following ocular trauma.

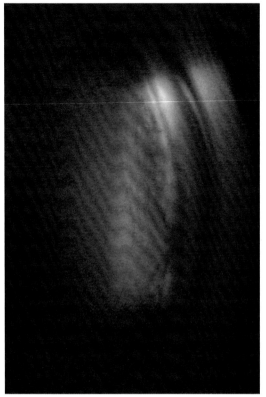

Figure 3.34-2   Anterior synechiae following blunt ocular trauma.

monocular visual disability and non-congenital unilateral blindness in children younger than 20 years.[1,2] In the pediatric population, eye trauma is the most common cause of mortality and morbidity. Injuries range from mild, non-sight threatening to extremely serious with potentially blinding consequences. It can occur in any setting including home, work, recreational, and motor vehicle accidents. The majority of ocular trauma cases are preventable with the simple use of eye protection.

Eye injury is the leading cause of monocular blindness in the United States today and is the most common reason for eye-related emergency department visits. In the United States, more than 2.5 million eye injuries occur annually. Worldwide, there are approximately 1.6 million people blind from eye injuries, 2.3 million with bilateral visual impairment, and 19 million with unilateral vision loss.[2] Although eye injury can affect anyone, young adults (52% of all trauma affects pediatric patients) and people older than 70 years are

at greatest risk. Males have a higher predilection until the age of 70 years, thereafter both sexes are at equal risk. Racial variations in rates of ocular injury have been observed but likely reflect variations in socioeconomic status and not race alone.

The etiology and setting of ocular injuries vary widely depending on the population under study (developed vs developing country), the source of data (eye trauma registry vs population-based survey), and the severity of the injury (penetrating injury vs all medically treated injuries).[3] There is no ideal classification of ocular trauma etiology. One classification is based on the source and nature of injury (eg, grinding, sharp instruments, falls, BB guns, or fireworks), while another classification is based on location and activity at the time of injury (eg, at work, in the home, during sports, or while commuting). In the adult population, work-related injuries are usually the most common cause of ocular trauma, followed by home-related injuries, and injuries from sports and recreation, assault, and travel. In the pediatric population, home is the leading site of trauma followed by injuries from sports and recreation.[3]

Due to the multi-structural effect of blunt trauma, a patient who presents in the acute phase should be evaluated systematically from anterior to posterior segment. In cases of acute trauma, the possibility of an open globe injury should always be ruled out first and foremost given its visually poor prognosis.

The assessment should aim to[3]:

- Understand the mechanism and nature of the injury.
- Identify associated injuries.
- Identify factors that could worsen outcome.
- Decide whether referral is necessary and, if so, the urgency of the referral.

Iris sphincter tears should be considered if pupil testing is unequal and the anisocoria is greater in light versus dim illumination, as in this patient.

During acute stages of trauma, IOP can remain normal, increase (intraocular hemorrhage, inflammation, lens subluxation in the anterior chamber, retinal detachment, or angle recession) or decrease (ruptured globe, retinal detachment, or iritis). The consequence of post-traumatic glaucoma should be considered with IOPs increasing immediately or months to years after trauma.

Gonioscopy should be performed on all patients who have sustained blunt ocular trauma to rule out an angle recession. Gonioscopy is contraindicated while a hyphema is present due to the increased risk of causing a rebleed. The presence of a peripheral anterior synechiae in this particular patient is due to inflammatory cells adhering the iris to the angle, which may reduce outflow of aqueous humor, and lead to increased IOP.

Michael had a grade 1 hyphema incorporating only the lower one-third of the cornea, which eliminated the need for surgical treatment. Hyphema is graded as follows: microhyphema (circulating red blood cells), grade 1 ($<\frac{1}{3}$ anterior chamber volume), grade 2 ($\frac{1}{3}$ to $\frac{1}{2}$ anterior chamber volume), grade 3 ($>\frac{1}{2}$ anterior chamber volume), and grade 4 (total anterior chamber volume or "eight ball").

Treatment of a hyphema is based on 3 factors: visual prognosis, risk of rebleed, and secondary hemorrhage. Stabilization of the eye to prevent a rebleed and facilitate resorption, normalization of the IOP, and reduction of associated inflammation all must be addressed. The use of cycloplegic agents and corticosteroids may be indicated. Cycloplegic agents can help immobilize the iris and ciliary body, which helps reduce further damage of blood vessels in the anterior chamber angle. Dilation can also reduce risk of pupillary block and synechiae. Corticosteroids address inflammation but also reduce the incidence of secondary hemorrhage by stabilizing the blood aqueous barrier. Surgical intervention is reserved for the most severe cases and, in general, is not advised for grade 1 or 2 hyphemas. All patients should be advised to avoid strenuous activity, rest with the head elevated, avoid NSAIDS and aspirin, and wear an eye shield.[4]

Child abuse should always be a consideration for children who present with blunt trauma. A detailed history that is consistent with the injury and repeatable is key. If child abuse is suspected, legally, it must be reported.

CLINICAL PEARLS

- Gonioscopy should be performed on all patients with a history of blunt ocular trauma but should be deferred in patients with an acute hyphema or open globe injury.

- The presence of a hyphema is concerning because it can lead to other complications, such as elevated IOP (due to blood cells and debris in trabecular meshwork [TM]), corneal blood staining (blood products being driven into the cornea), and rebleeding within 4 to 6 days post trauma.

- The consequence of post-traumatic glaucoma should be considered when IOP increases immediately or months to years after trauma.

- Angle recession is indicative of an increased risk of glaucoma. Continued follow-up care, at least yearly, is necessary.

REFERENCES

1. Tielsch JM, Parver L, Shankar B. Time trends in the incidence of hospitalized ocular trauma. *Arch Ophthalmol.* 1989;107:519.
2. Trauma. In: Kunimoto DY, Kanitkar KD, Makar MS, eds. *The Wills Eye Manual: Office and Emergency Room Diagnosis and Treatment of Eye Disease.* 4th ed. Philadelphia, PA: Lippincott Williams & Wilkins; 2004:14-39.
3. Ocular trauma. In: Heiberger MH, Madonna RJ, Nehmad L., eds. *Emergency Care in the Optometric Setting.* New York, NY: McGraw-Hill; 2004:81-116.
4. MacEwen CJ. Ocular injuries. *J R Coll Surg Edinb.* 1999;44:317-323.

3.35 Ocular Effects of Hypertension

Tamara Petrosyan

Don, a 49-year-old African American male, presented to the emergency clinic as a new patient with concerns of a red right eye. The redness was noted 2 hours prior to the visit when the patient looked in the mirror. The patient denied any associated pain, burning, itching, tearing, dryness, or change in vision. He had not exerted himself, was not constipated or coughing, and was taking no blood thinners, including aspirin, nonsteroidal anti-inflammatory drugs (NSAIDs), or nutraceuticals. He had not attempted any treatment and denied any recent trauma. He did note that he had a similar occurrence 2 years ago when he lifted something heavy. His last eye examination was 8 years ago, which he reported to be unremarkable. His last medical examination, including blood work, was 2 years ago at which time he was given a clean bill of health per the patient. Family history was unremarkable. He denied taking any prescription or over-the-counter medications.

Clinical Findings

Habitable distance VA	OD: 20/20; OS: 20/20
Habitual Rx	OD: −1.25 sph
	OS: −1.25 sph
Pupil evaluation	PERRL; no RAPD
Confrontation visual fields	Full to finger counting OD and OS
Extraocular muscle motility	Full and comitant OU
Blood pressure	183/85 mm Hg RAS
Slit-lamp examination (Figure 3.35-1)	OD: nasal subconjunctival hemorrhage with elevated, lobulated area in the center of the hemorrhage; otherwise unremarkable
	OS: Unremarkable
Intraocular pressure (GAT)	OD: 13 mm Hg; OS: 13 mm Hg at 6:04 PM
Fundus examination	OD: 0.4/0.4 CD ratio; healthy rim tissue with distinct disc margins; fovea flat and dry; normal vasculature with 2/3 artery to vein ratio; no holes or retinal detachment
	OS: 0.45/0.45 CD ratio; healthy rim tissue with distinct disc margins; fovea flat and dry; normal vasculature with 2/3 artery to vein ratio; no holes or retinal detachment

Abbreviations: CD, cup to disc; GAT, Goldmann applanation tonometry; OD, right eye; OS, left eye; OU, both eyes; PERRL, pupils equal, round, reactive to light; RAPD, relative afferent pupillary defect; RAS, right arm sitting; Rx, prescription; sph, sphere; VA, visual acuity.

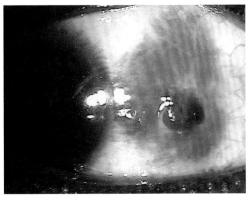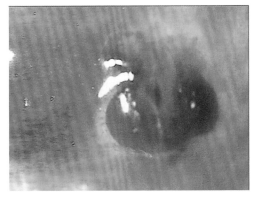

Figure 3.35-1   Anterior segment photograph of the subconjunctival hemorrhage in the right eye.

Comments

Don was diagnosed with a subconjunctival hemorrhage that was likely due to his high blood pressure. The patient was scheduled for an appointment the next day at the primary care provider's (PCP's) office for evaluation of the high blood pressure and a copy of the records was sent to the PCP's office. The patient was educated regarding the self-limiting nature of the condition but was told he could perform cold compresses to limit additional bleeding. He was asked to return to our clinic in 1 week to assure resolution of the subconjunctival hemorrhage.

Follow-up Visit (1 Week Following the Initial Examination)

The patient reported going to his PCP the day after his initial visit. He was diagnosed with hypertension and prescribed amlodipine to control his blood pressure. He reported that blood work showed an elevated HbA1c, and he was currently being evaluated for type 2 diabetes. Blood pressure was measured at 140/90 mm Hg at the follow-up visit, and the subconjunctival hemorrhage in the right eye was almost fully resolved. The blood-filled cyst in the center of the hemorrhage, caused by the elevated blood pressure, had resolved fully.

Discussion

A subconjunctival hemorrhage occurs when a capillary between the Tenon capsule and conjunctiva ruptures, appearing as a diffuse bright or dark red patch above the sclera.[1] There are usually no associated symptoms and the diagnosis is made based on clinical appearance and the absence of other findings. Despite its discernible appearance, subconjunctival hemorrhages are usually painless, spontaneous, benign, and self-resolving in 1 to 2 weeks as the blood is reabsorbed. Some patients report mild pressure around the eye or a sense of awareness of the eye.[1,2]

An isolated subconjunctival hemorrhage is often idiopathic or due to an elevation in venous pressure such as violent coughing or sneezing, straining, or vomiting.[3] It can be the result of an injury, including rough eye rubbing, contact lens wear, or ocular trauma, especially in younger patients. Subconjunctival hemorrhages may also occur in patients with advanced age due to changes in the structure of the aging blood vessels, increased microvascular dysfunction, and vascular hyperpermeability with age.[4]

Although a subconjunctival hemorrhage may be idiopathic, there are several systemic and medical causes that should be ruled out, especially in recurrent cases. Systemic vascular conditions, including diabetes, arteriosclerosis, and hypertension, increase the incidence of conjunctival vessel hemorrhaging due to damage and remodeling of the microvasculature.[3] Because patients with hypertension have microvascular changes caused by the disease itself, as well as concomitant aging changes, subconjunctival hemorrhage can result from uncontrolled hypertension but can also occur when the blood pressure is controlled.[5,6] Although there is no clear consensus regarding the workup for patients with an initial subconjunctival hemorrhage, there is general agreement that all patients with subconjunctival hemorrhage should be screened for hypertension.[1-3]

If a patient with hypertension presents with a subconjunctival hemorrhage, a fundus evaluation should be performed to rule out any posterior segment involvement. Ocular manifestations of hypertension include branch or central retinal artery or vein occlusion, anterior ischemic optic neuropathy, and hypertensive retinopathy.[6,7] Those with hypertensive retinopathy may experience symptoms (including blur, metamorphopsia, or visual field disturbances) depending on the severity and location of the retinopathy. Hypertensive retinopathy can be classified using the following Keith–Wagener–Barker Classification System[8]:

- Grade 1—mild retinal vascular changes and generalized arteriolar narrowing.

- Grade 2—more severe or tighter constrictions of the retinal arteries with arteriovenous crossing changes.

- Grade 3—signs of grade 2 plus retinal edema, microaneurysms, exudates, cotton-wool spots, or retinal hemorrhages.

- Grade 4—signs of grade 3 plus papilledema and macular edema with macular star formation.

Blood clotting disorders, as well as blood thinning medications (eg, warfarin and aspirin), increase the risk of subconjunctival hemorrhage due to poor blood clotting. Aside from prescription drugs, it is important to ask patients regarding the use of over-the-counter supplements, such as St. John's Wort, Ginkgo biloba, ginseng, vitamin E, coenzyme Q-10, and Omega-3 fatty acids, as they have blood thinning properties.[9,10]

Currently, there are no approved treatments to accelerate the resolution and absorption of subconjunctival hemorrhages. Because it is minimally symptomatic and self-resolving, treatment of subconjunctival hemorrhages is usually limited to lubrication (for comfort), cold compresses (for vasoconstriction and comfort), and time (for natural reabsorption). Over the 1- to 2-week reabsorption period, the hemorrhage will initially be red in appearance due to the iron-rich hemoglobin. As the hemoglobin breaks down and the blood is reabsorbed, the subconjunctival hemorrhage will become blue, green, orange, and finally yellow before fully resolving. The patient should be warned not to rub the eye, which can initiate a rebleed. Prescribed anticoagulation medications should not be stopped without first speaking with the prescribing physician.

Patients with a spontaneous, non-trauma-related subconjunctival hemorrhage, should be screened for hypertension as this is one of the more common causes for subconjunctival hemorrhage, especially in the elderly. If the patient is having recurrent subconjunctival hemorrhages without a known cause, he/she should be referred for laboratory work looking for a causative diagnosis. This may include a complete blood count (CBC) with differential, fasting blood glucose and HbA1c, and evaluation of clotting factors (prothrombin time, partial thromboplastin time, fibrinogen, and protein C and S).

A thorough systemic and medical history and clinical examination are required in patients with subconjunctival hemorrhage. Because subconjunctival hemorrhages can be idiopathic or related to trauma or contact lens wear, early diagnosis of systemic manifestations may lead to a more timely referral and appropriate management. By performing blood pressure evaluation on patients with subconjunctival hemorrhage and referring recurrent cases for proper comanagement, eye care providers play a critical role in the care of these patients.

CLINICAL PEARLS

- Eye care providers play a key role in a patient's overall health.

- A subconjunctival hemorrhage is not always a benign clinical finding but can be a sign of an underlying systemic condition, such as hypertension.

- It is critical that we know and understand potential visual and ocular side effects of systemic conditions and properly comanage patients with other health care providers.

REFERENCES

1. Sahinoglu-Keskek N, Cevher S, Ergin A. Analysis of subconjunctival hemorrhage. *Pak J Med Sci.* 2013;29(1):132-134.
2. Mimura T, Yamagami S, Usui T, et al. Location and extent of subconjunctival hemorrhage. *Ophthalmologica.* 2010; 224(2):90-95.
3. Tarlan B, Kiratli H. Subconjunctival hemorrhage: risk factors and potential indicators. *Clin Ophthalmol.* 2013;7:1163-1170.
4. Oakley R, Tharakan B. Vascular hyperpermeability and aging. *Aging Dis.* 2014;5(2):114-125.
5. Pitts JF, Jardine AG, Murray SB, Barker NH. Spontaneous subconjunctival haemorrhage – a sign of Hypertension? *Br J Ophthalmol.* 1992;76(5):297-299.
6. Tso MO, Jampol LM. Pathophysiology of hypertensive retinopathy. *Ophthalmology.* 1982;89(10): 1132-1145.
7. Klein R, Klein BE, Moss SE. The relation of systemic hypertension to changes in the retinal vasculature: the Beaver Dam Eye Study. *Trans Am Ophthalmol Soc.* 1997;95:329-350.
8. Heck AM, DeWitt BA, Lukes AL. Potential interactions between alternative therapies and warfarin. *Am J Health Syst Pharm.* 2000;57(13):1221-1227.
9. Norred CL, Brinker F. Potential coagulation effects of preoperative complementary and alternative medicines. *Altern Ther Health Med.* 2001;7(6):58-67.
10. Micieli JA, Easterbrook M. Eye and orbital injuries in sports. *Clin Sports Med.* 2017;36(2):299-314.

3.36 **Sarcoid Optic Neuropathy**

Ashley Kay Maglione

Michael, a 62-year-old African American male, was referred to our clinic for further evaluation of neuroretinal rim pallor of the right optic disc. He denied any specific ocular trauma but did box recreationally when he was younger. He denied any episodes of visual changes or loss, recently or even in the distant past.

Systemic history was remarkable for sarcoidosis, which was diagnosed 18 years ago. His initial symptom of the sarcoidosis was difficulty breathing, which led to the diagnosis after blood work and a lung scan. He had approximately 1 flare-up per year, been hospitalized multiple times, and was frequently treated with prednisone. He was also in remission from granulomatous mycosis fungoides, the most common form of cutaneous T-cell lymphoma, after treatment with 26 rounds of electron beam radiation.

Clinical Findings

Entering distance VA	OD: 20/20; OS: 20/20
Color vision (Ishihara)	OD: 13/14; OS: 13/14
Confrontation visual fields	Full to finger counting with no red desaturation OD and OS
Pupil evaluation	Equal and round, 2+ reaction to light OU; 0.3 log RAPD OD
Extraocular muscle motilities	Full in all positions of gaze OU
Cover test	2Δ XP at near, comitant in all positions of gaze
Intraocular pressure (GAT)	OD: 14 mm Hg; OS: 13 mm Hg at 10:46 AM
Slit-lamp examination	OD: upper and lower lid laxity; otherwise unremarkable
	OS: upper and lower lid laxity; otherwise unremarkable
Fundus examination (Figure 3.36-1)	OD: 0.65h/0.7v CD ratio; 1+ diffuse pallor and 2+ temporal pallor; distinct disc margins; fovea flat and dry; normal vasculature; periphery intact
	OS: 0.5h/0.6v CD ratio; healthy rim tissue with no pallor; distinct disc margins; fovea flat and dry; normal vasculature; periphery intact
Neurologic examination	Cranial nerves V and VII to XII intact
	Motor, sensory, and coordination testing unremarkable
External examination	Lesions on hands, arms, and neck reportedly similar in appearance to prior dermatologic lesions
Visual field (SITA-standard 24-2; Figure 3.36-2)	OD: inferior nasal step
	OS: no defects

Optic nerve OCT (Figure 3.36-3)   OD: superior and inferior RNFL thinning
OS: Borderline RNFL thinning inferiorly

Abbreviations: CD, cup to disc; GAT, Goldmann applanation tonometry; h, horizontal; OCT, optical coherence tomography; OD, right eye; OS, left eye; OU, both eyes; RAPD, relative afferent pupillary defect; RNFL, retinal nerve fiber layer; v, vertical; VA, visual acuity; XP, exophoria.

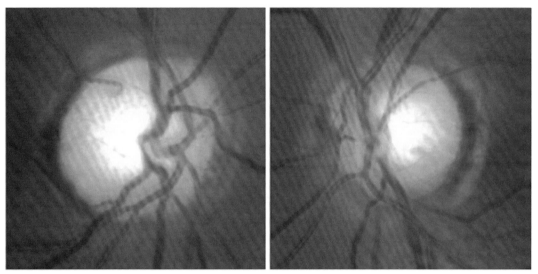

Figure 3.36-1   Diffuse pallor, greater temporally, of the right neuroretinal rim.

Comments

Michael had a right optic neuropathy evidenced by a relative afferent pupillary defect, optic disc pallor, and visual field defect. Because the cause of the optic neuropathy was unknown, laboratory testing and neuroimaging were obtained. Previous records were obtained, which indicated that the pallor was noted a year ago but not otherwise addressed.

Laboratory testing	Elevated hematocrit at 46.9% (normal 38.5-45.0%) and low mean corpuscular hemoglobin (MCHC) at 31.4 g/dL (normal 32.0-36.0 g/dL). CBC otherwise within normal limits.
	Platelet count, ESR, CRP, folate, vitamin B-12, Lyme titer, RPR, FTA-ABS, ACE, ANA, methylmalonic acid, homocysteine, serum protein electrophoresis, and BUN/creatinine (in preparation for neuroimaging) all within normal limits
MRI of the brain and orbits with and without contrast	No acute intracranial process, mild chronic small vessel ischemic changes, no intraorbital masses identified, no pathologic enhancement

Abbreviations: ACE, angiotensin converting enzyme; ANA, antinuclear antibody; BUN, blood urea nitrogen; CBC, complete blood count; CRP, C-reactive protein; ESR, erythrocyte sedimentation rate; FTA-ABS, fluorescent treponemal antibody absorption; RPR, rapid plasma reagin.

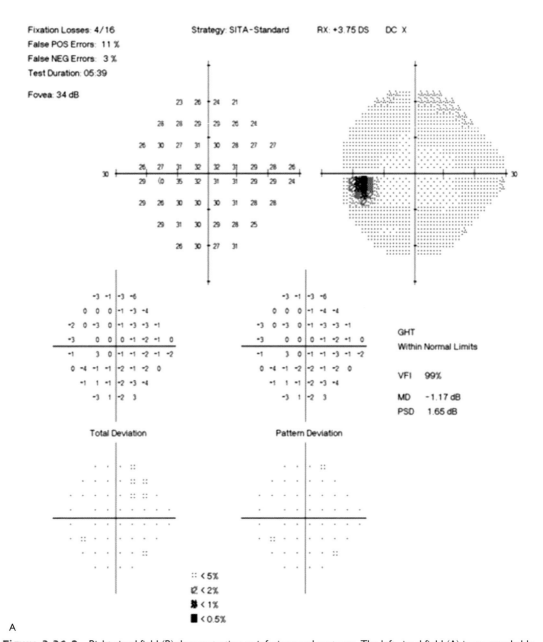

Fixation Losses: 4/16   Strategy: SITA-Standard   RX: +3.75 DS   DC X
False POS Errors: 11 %
False NEG Errors: 3 %
Test Duration: 05:39

Fovea: 34 dB

Total Deviation

Pattern Deviation

GHT
Within Normal Limits

VFI   99%

MD   -1.17 dB
PSD   1.65 dB

:: < 5%
∅ < 2%
⬚ < 1%
■ < 0.5%

A

Figure 3.36-2   Right visual field (B) demonstrating an inferior nasal scotoma. The left visual field (A) is unremarkable.

Discussion

Pallor of the optic nerve occurs when there is atrophy or death of the ganglion cell fibers anywhere along the pathway from the retina to the lateral geniculate nucleus. Generally, pallor indicates that the damage to the nerve has been present for more than 4 to 6 weeks. In addition, pallor of the optic nerve is atypical of glaucoma, the most common optic neuropathy. The presence of optic nerve pallor without a known cause necessitates further workup. Obtaining old records can be vital, but if these are not available or do not elucidate a cause, laboratory testing and/or neuroimaging may be necessary.

Although Michael's history of sarcoidosis and cutaneous T-cell lymphoma was a potential cause of the optic neuropathy, we could not

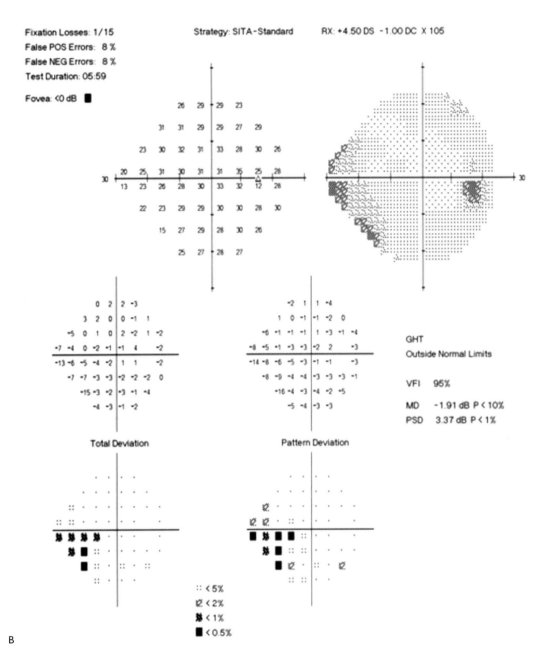

Fixation Losses: 1/15
False POS Errors: 8 %
False NEG Errors: 8 %
Test Duration: 05:59

Fovea: <0 dB ■

Strategy: SITA-Standard   RX: +4.50 DS -1.00 DC X 105

Total Deviation

Pattern Deviation

GHT
Outside Normal Limits

VFI   95%

MD   -1.91 dB P < 10%
PSD   3.37 dB P < 1%

:: < 5%
▨ < 2%
▩ < 1%
■ < 0.5%

B

Figure 3.36-2 (Continued)

conclude either was the definite etiology as he was asymptomatic and his presentation was long-standing. Therefore, further testing, including blood work and neuroimaging were indicated to rule out a treatable, non-glaucomatous etiology. Blood work did not reveal any underlying infectious, inflammatory, or nutritional process. Neuroimaging did not reveal any compressive lesion or structural abnormality related to either sarcoidosis or cutaneous T-cell lymphoma.

Ocular involvement from cutaneous T-cell lymphoma is uncommon. However, infiltrative optic neuropathies have been documented, and typically exhibit perineural enhancement of the optic nerve sheath on MRI.[1,2] The lack of abnormal enhancement on our patient's neuroimaging helped rule out cutaneous T-cell lymphoma as the cause of his optic neuropathy. In addition, the lack of optic nerve or leptomeningeal enhancement ruled out any

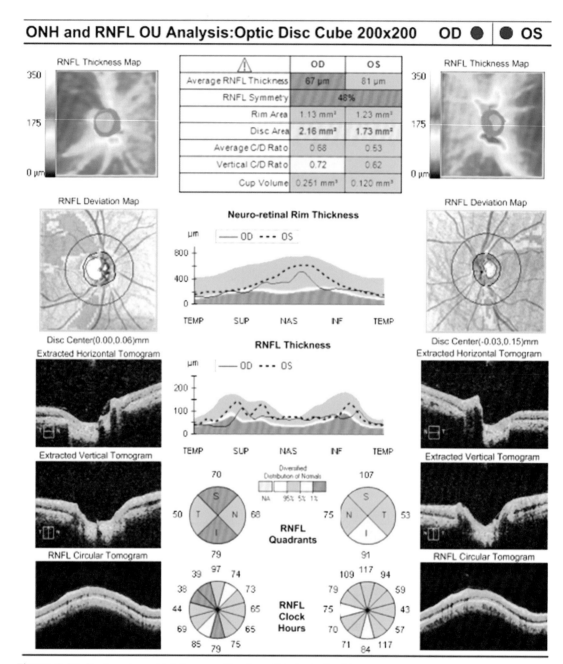

Figure 3.36-3 Superior and inferior nerve fiber layer thinning in the right eye.

active neurosarcoid involvement. Although there was no active optic nerve enhancement from sarcoidosis, this did not preclude a past episode of neurosarcoid, which was presumed to be the most likely etiology of the optic neuropathy.

Sarcoidosis is an autoimmune disorder that results in granuloma formation and fibrosis,

most commonly in the lungs, skin, lymph nodes, liver, and joints. The disease is more common in women than men, and there is a higher prevalence and more severe disease course in African Americans.[3] The age of onset varies but is most common in young adulthood.[3] The etiology of sarcoidosis is unknown. Possible environmental triggers, genetic factors, and infectious agents have been implicated, but no definite cause has been proven.[4]

Patients with sarcoidosis most commonly present with respiratory and constitutional symptoms, but they may be asymptomatic. Individuals may exhibit skin granulomas or lesions in the form of non-granulomatous red nodules in the lower extremities, known as erythema nodosum. Central nervous system involvement, including cranial nerve palsies (notably the facial nerve), encephalopathy, and optic nerve disease, occurs in 5% to 16% of patients and may be the initial manifestation.[5] Optic nerve involvement may follow 2 clinical courses: subacute optic disc swelling or progressive optic atrophy. There are multiple mechanisms of optic nerve disease in sarcoidosis including direct infiltration of the optic nerve, compression by an adjacent granulomatous mass, and meningeal inflammation, which leads to an optic perineuritis. Most commonly, the optic neuropathy is unilateral but may be bilateral (synchronous, sequential, or chiasmal in nature).

Recognizing that sarcoidosis may result in an optic neuropathy is vital as it may be the initial manifestation of an undiagnosed condition. In addition, optic nerve involvement is a sign of central nervous system involvement, which often requires aggressive and prompt treatment and a prolonged course of immunosuppressants.

Patients with sarcoidosis may have concurrent intraocular inflammation, most commonly an isolated uveitis. Classically, the anterior uveitis is characterized by mutton-fat keratic precipitates and Koeppe iris nodules. Intermediate uveitis with vitritis and snow banking may also occur. Periphlebitis seen as candle wax drippings and punched out choroidal lesions may also be seen funduscopically. Lacrimal gland and conjunctival granulomas are also a common finding in those with sarcoidosis.[5,6]

Diagnosis of ocular disease secondary to sarcoidosis is often a diagnosis of exclusion. As seen with Michael, other possible causes for optic neuropathy must be excluded. If a patient presents with intraocular inflammation, sarcoidosis but must be differentiated from other conditions that result in optic nerve inflammation, including multiple sclerosis, systemic lupus erythematosus, syphilis, tuberculosis, and toxoplasmosis. Furthermore, making the new diagnosis of sarcoidosis often requires multiple studies with correlation to clinical features. Serologic measurements of elevated angiotensin-converting enzyme (ACE) may be a sign of the disease; however, elevated ACE has been reported in other conditions including tuberculosis and diabetes mellitus. In addition, normal serum ACE levels, as was the case in our patient, do not exclude the diagnosis of sarcoidosis. Angiotensin-converting enzyme levels may vary with disease activity and may not be elevated, especially in patients with only ocular involvement or those on an ACE inhibitor. Radiographic studies, such as chest computed tomography (CT) or the less sensitive chest x-ray, are indicated to look for hilar adenopathy and interstitial lung disease. A gallium 67 scan, which utilizes a radioactive tracer that is preferentially taken up by inflamed tissues, may also be helpful. In patients with sarcoidosis, the sensitive but nonspecific "panda pattern" may be seen in which there is abnormal uptake of gallium in the salivary and lacrimal glands and the mediastinal and hilar lymph nodes. Finally, tissue biopsy, demonstrating noncaseating granulomas, from the lung or elsewhere is useful to differentiate sarcoidosis from infection and malignancy.

Treatment of sarcoidosis generally consists of a course of corticosteroids during exacerbations; however, additional immunosuppressant medications, such as methotrexate, may be indicated in steroid-resistant disease. Overall, sarcoidosis is a relatively benign disease with a good prognosis. However, patients may develop organ dysfunction. Contributing factors to a poorer prognosis include African American race, persistent disease, multiple organ involvement, and a childhood diagnosis. Ocular symptoms related to inflammation often resolve with proper treatment, but optic neuropathies, especially those with a progressive course, often respond less favorably.[3,6] Long-term follow-up is essential, and monitoring for exacerbations of sarcoidosis is warranted.

CLINICAL PEARL

- If pallor of the neuroretinal rim is present, consider a diagnosis other than glaucoma.

REFERENCES

1. Shunmugam M, Chan E, O'Brart D, Moonim MT, Stanford MR, Morley AM. Cutaneous γδ T-cell lymphoma with bilateral ocular and adnexal involvement. *Arch Ophthalmol*. 2011;129(10):1379-1381.
2. Levy Clarke GA, Greenman D, Sieving PC, et al. Ophthalmic manifestations, cytology, immunohistochemistry, and molecular analysis of intraocular metastatic T-cell lymphoma: report of a case and review of the literature. *Surv Ophthalmol*. 2008;53(3):285-295.
3. Rothova A. Ocular involvement in sarcoidosis. *Br J Ophthalmol*. 2000;84(1):110-116.
4. Semenzato G. ACCESS: a case control etiologic study of sarcoidosis. *Sarcoidosis Vasc Diffuse Lung Dis*. 2005;22(2):83-86.
5. Frohman LP, Grigorian R, Bielory L. Neuro-ophthalmic manifestations of sarcoidosis: clinical spectrum, evaluation, and management. *J Neuroophthalmol*. 2001;21(2):132-137.
6. Kidd DP, Burton BJ, Graham EM, Plant GT. Optic neuropathy associated with systemic sarcoidosis. *Neurol Neuroimmunol Neuroinflamm*. 2016;3(5):e270.

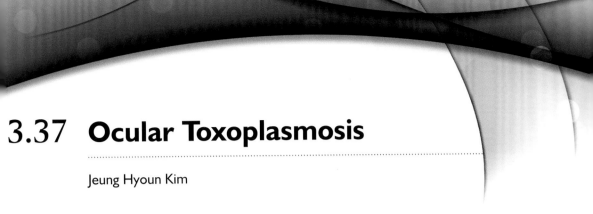

3.37 Ocular Toxoplasmosis

Jeung Hyoun Kim

Mario, a 9-year-old Hispanic male, presented for an annual comprehensive eye examination. He lost his glasses 3 months ago and complained of blurry vision, especially in his left eye. His last eye examination was 1 year ago. Ocular history was remarkable for ocular toxoplasmosis. His mother reported that he was otherwise in good health, and he was not allergic to any medications.

Clinical Findings

Unaided distance VA	OD: 20/200; OS: 20/400
Previous Rx	OD: −3.25 −0.75 × 180; OS: −3.50 −0.50 × 180
Pinhole distance VA	OD: 20/25; OS: 20/30
Cover test	Ortho at distance; 2 XP at near
Near point of convergence	To the nose
Confrontation visual fields	Full to finger count OD and OS
Pupil evaluation	PERRL; no RAPD
Subjective refraction	OD: −3.25 −1.00 × 180 (20/20); OS: −3.50 −1.00 × 180 (20/25)
Slit-lamp examination	OD: unremarkable
	OS: unremarkable
Intraocular pressure (GAT)	OD: 21 mm Hg; OS: 20 mm Hg at 9:30 AM
Fundus examination (Figure 3.37-1)	OD 0.25/0.25 CD ratio; healthy rim tissue with distinct disc margins; temporal peripapillary atrophy; Bergmeister papilla; fovea flat and dry; normal vasculature; 3 punched out chorioretinal scars along superior arcade about 1 DD from disc margin; 1 chorioretinal scar temporal to the macula outside of the arcade
	OS 0.3/0.3 CD ratio; healthy rim tissue with distinct disc margins; fovea flat and dry; normal vasculature; 2 punched out chorioretinal scars nasal to the optic disc associated with active inflammation; mild posterior vitreous cells

Abbreviations: CD, cup to disc; DD, disc diameter; GAT, Goldmann applanation tonometry; OD, right eye; OS, left eye; PERRL, pupils equal, round, reactive to light; RAPD, relative afferent pupillary defect; Rx, prescription; VA, visual acuity; XP, exophoria.

Comments

Mario was diagnosed with reactivated ocular toxoplasmosis in the left eye. He was comanaged with his pediatrician who prescribed trimethoprim 80 mg/sulfamethoxazole 400 mg (Bactrim)

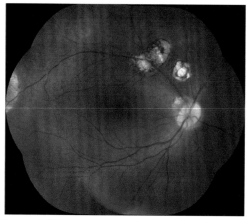
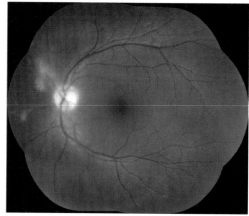

Figure 3.37-1 The right eye has multiple inactive chorioretinal scars. The left eye has an active toxoplasmosis lesion with overlying vitritis nasal to the disc.

1 tablet twice a day by mouth for 3 weeks. He was asked to return in 4 weeks.

Follow-up Visit (4 Weeks Following the Initial Examination)

Mario reported good compliance and tolerance with treatment. He also reported good vision through his new glasses that were prescribed at the previous visit.

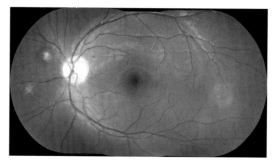

Figure 3.37-2 Following resolution of the active inflammation, multiple chorioretinal scars remain nasal to the disc.

Aided distance VA	OD: 20/20; OS: 20/20
Confrontation visual fields	Full to finger count OD and OS
Pupil evaluation	PERRL; no RAPD
Fundus examination (Figure 3.37-2)	OD: stable from previous visit OS: resolved posterior uveitis

Abbreviations: OD, right eye; OS, left eye; PERRL, pupils equal, round, reactive to light; RAPD, relative afferent pupillary defect; VA, visual acuity.

Discussion

Toxoplasmosis, which affects up to one-third of the world's population, is caused by the parasite *Toxoplasma gondii*. It is most commonly transmitted from contact with cats and exposure to their feces, ingestion of undercooked meat, or drinking contaminated water.

Congenital infections occur through the placental blood supply, but more commonly the parasite is transferred through the gastrointestinal tract resulting in acquired disease.[1] Based on the lack of macular scarring and absence of other associated findings, such as neurologic complications, the toxoplasmosis, in this case, was most likely acquired at an early age rather than being congenital.[2]

Ocular toxoplasmosis typically presents as necrotizing retinochoroiditis. During the dormant inactive stage, it remains as an atrophic chorioretinal scar. Once activated, focal fluffy white lesions will appear adjacent to a toxoplasmosis scar with overlying vitritis, which produces the classic "headlight in the fog" appearance. A granulomatous or nongranulomatous anterior uveitis, retinal vasculitis, or optic neuritis may also be present during the active stage. Cataract, epiretinal membrane, vitreous opacities, cystoid macular edema, retinal vascular occlusion, retinal detachment, secondary glaucoma, and subretinal neovascularization have also been reported as complications of ocular toxoplasmosis.[3]

Small lesions are often monitored without treatment. Significant posterior uveitis can be treated with oral or intravitreal corticosteroids in conjunction with anti-infective agents (generally pyrimethamine, sulfadiazine or azithromycin, and clindamycin).[4] In this case, the level of posterior involvement was minimal and was managed only by oral antibiotic treatment.

Retinal lesions recur in up to 79% of patients within 5 years despite treatment.[4] When a reactivated lesion is present one must consider the possibility that the patient is immunocompromised. This patient was closely monitored by his pediatrician who ordered a complete blood count to rule out immunodeficiency.[5]

CLINICAL PEARL

- Monitor patients with toxoplasmosis scarring for reactivated or vision-threatening lesions. When possible, the patient's general practitioner needs to comanage the systemic condition.

REFERENCES

1. Park Y, Nam H. Clinical features and treatment of ocular toxoplasmosis. *Korean J Parasitol.* 2013;51(4): 393-399.
2. Bowling B. *Kanski's Clinical Ophthalmology: A Systematic Approach.* 8th ed. Philadelphia, PA: Saunders; 2015.
3. Soheilian M, Sadoughi MM, Ghajarnia M, et al. Prospective randomized trial of trimethoprim/sulfamethoxazole versus pyrimethamine and sulfadiazine in the treatment of ocular toxoplasmosis. *Ophthalmology.* 2005;112(11):1882-1884.
4. Bosch-Driessen LEH, Berendschot TJM, Ongkosuwito JV, Rothova, A. Ocular toxoplasmosis. *Ophthalmology.* 2002;109(5):869-878.
5. Alexander LJ. *Primary Care of the Posterior Segment.* 3rd ed. New York, NY: McGraw Hill; 2002.

3.38 Thyroid Eye Disease

Len V. Koh and Tina Porzukowiak

Joe, a 66-year-old black male army veteran, presented for an ocular examination with concerns of binocular horizontal diplopia, as well as chronic blur, hyperemia, dryness, and photophobia in both eyes. Ocular history was remarkable for cataracts, dry eye syndrome, and presbyopia. He recently underwent bilateral orbital decompression. Medical history included degenerative intervertebral disc disease, hypertension, and secondary hypothyroidism following a radioactive iodine procedure. Current medications included lisinopril and levothyroxine. He had no known drug allergies. Family history was positive for cataracts. Joe was a former smoker, but he denied alcohol or illicit drug use.

Clinical Findings

Best-corrected VA	OD: 20/200⁻ (no improvement with pinhole); OS: 20/40⁻² (no improvement with pinhole)
Pupil evaluation	PERRL; 2+ right RAPD
Ocular motility	Restriction in all gazes with horizontal diplopia
Cover test	Distance: 5Δ right hypertropia and 8Δ left exotropia Near: 6Δ right hypertropia and 10Δ left exotropia
Color vision (Ishihara)	OD: 0/12 plates; OS: 9/12 plates
Exophthalmometry	OD: 25 mm; OS: 25 mm with 109 mm base
Anterior segment examination	OD: steatoblepharon of upper and lower eyelids; bulbar conjunctiva showed 1-2+ diffuse injection; cornea arcus; reduced tear breakup time; 2+ nuclear sclerosis; grade 2 Van Herick angles nasally and temporally OS: steatoblepharon of upper and lower eyelids; bulbar conjunctiva showed 1-2+ diffuse injection; cornea arcus; reduced tear breakup time; 1+ nuclear sclerosis; grade 2 Van Herick angles nasally and temporally
Gonioscopy	Ciliary body present 360° with slightly convex iris; trace pigmentation in the trabecular meshwork OD and OS
Intraocular pressure (GAT)	OD: 16 mm Hg; OS: 16 mm Hg at 9:15 AM
Fundus examination	OD: 0.5/0.5 CD ratio; significant temporal pallor of the rim tissue with distinct disc margins; fovea flat and dry; normal vasculature OS: 0.4/0.4 CD ratio; trace temporal pallor of the rim tissue with distinct disc margins; fovea flat and dry; normal vasculature
Visual fields (Figure 3.38-1)	OD: overall depression greater inferiorly OS: inferior temporal depression

Optic nerve OCT (Figure 3.38-2)	OD: temporal RNFL thinning OS: temporal RNFL thinning
MRI of the orbits (Figure 3.38-3)	Extremely enlarged extraocular muscle bellies with relative sparing of the tendons

Abbreviations: CD, cup to disc; GAT, Goldmann applanation tonometry; OCT, optical coherence tomography; OD, right eye; OS, left eye; PERRL, pupils equal, round, reactive to light; RAPD, relative afferent pupillary defect; RNFL, retinal nerve fiber layer; VA, visual acuity.

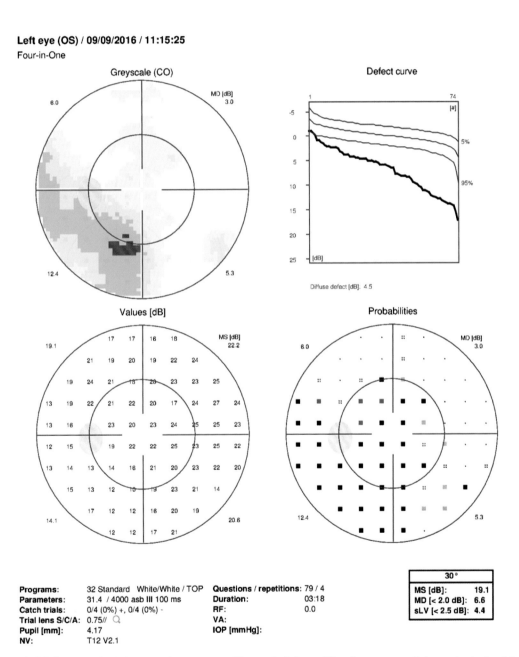

Figure 3.38-1 Visual field showing inferior temporal loss in the left eye (A) and severe overall depression in the right eye (B).

Right eye (OD) / 09/09/2016 / 11:10:06
Four-in-One

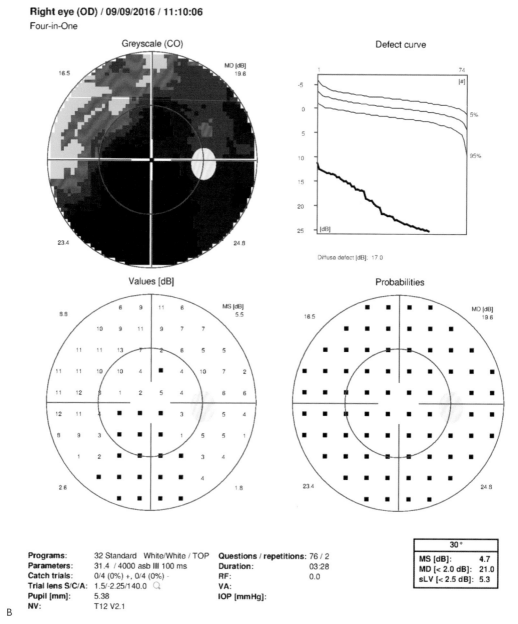

Programs:	32 Standard White/White / TOP	Questions / repetitions:	76 / 2
Parameters:	31.4 / 4000 asb III 100 ms	Duration:	03:28
Catch trials:	0/4 (0%) +, 0/4 (0%) -	RF:	0.0
Trial lens S/C/A:	1.5/-2.25/140.0	VA:	
Pupil [mm]:	5.38	IOP [mmHg]:	
NV:	T12 V2.1		

30°	
MS [dB]:	4.7
MD [< 2.0 dB]:	21.0
sLV [< 2.5 dB]:	5.3

B

Figure 3.38-1   (Continued)

Discussion

Joe had thyroid eye disease (TED). He had recently underwent bilateral orbital decompression because the extraocular muscles were compressing the optic nerve, but diplopia persisted following the surgery. He was prescribed 10Δ base-in Fresnel prism OS for distance and near over his current spectacle prescription. He was advised to use artificial tears every hour, as well as an ophthalmic lubricant ointment at night, in each eye. Joe was educated on the importance of avoiding tobacco use. He expressed understanding of the importance of regular eye examinations to monitor for TED that could pose a threat to his vision. Once the ocular inflammation had stabilized, Joe proceeded with new glasses that included

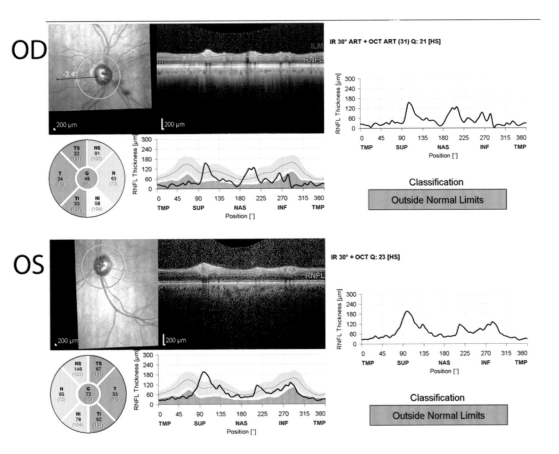

Figure 3.38-2 Thinning of the temporal retinal nerve fiber layer in both eyes.

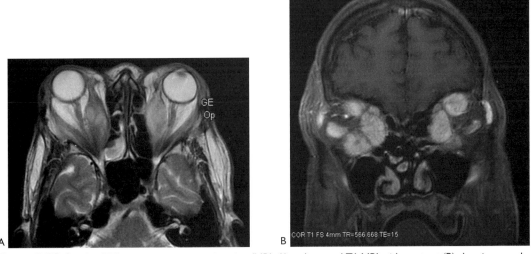

Figure 3.38-3 Axial T2 magnetic resonance imaging (MRI; A) and coronal T1 MRI with contrast (B) showing grossly enlarged extraocular muscles with sparing of the tendons in both the right and left orbit.

ground in prism. He was not interested in strabismus surgery at that time. The patient's primary care provider (PCP) and endocrinologist were informed of the ocular findings and advised to continue serologic monitoring.

Thyroid eye disease is the most common cause of orbital disease leading to unilateral and bilateral exophthalmos in North America. Although most TED cases are associated with hyperthyroidism (eg, Graves disease), 6% of those with TED have euthyroid, 3% have Hashimoto thyroiditis, and 1% have hypothyroid.[1] Furthermore, the latency of TED onset is variable with 20% of the cases being diagnosed simultaneously with thyroid dysfunction, while 60% of TED cases present within 1 year of the systemic diagnosis. In some cases, TED can show up years before or decades after the initial presentation of thyroid disease.[2]

Women are 4 times more likely to be affected by TED than men. A bimodal age of onset is observed in both genders, with the diagnosis in women most commonly occurring between 40 and 44 years and 60 to 64 years of age. In men, the diagnosis is most commonly made between 45 to 49 years and 65 to 69 years of age. The median age of diagnosis for all patients is 43 years, with a range from 8 to 88 years. In addition to age and gender as risk factors, a positive family history is found in 61% of TED patients.[2] Furthermore, cigarette smoking, low selenium levels, and stress are likely environmental risk factors for TED. Smoking is the worst culprit because it can accelerate the development and progression of TED and render treatment less effective. Smokers are twice as likely to develop Graves disease, and smokers with Graves disease are 7 times more likely to develop TED than nonsmoking Graves patients.[1]

The pathophysiology of TED has not been fully elucidated, but cumulative evidence supports the role of orbital fibroblasts as the primary cells responsible for orbital involvement. Orbital fibroblasts derive from neural crest cells that can differentiate into adipocytes and myofibroblasts, both of which are evident histologically in TED. Adipocyte differentiation and deposition commonly lead to compressive optic neuropathy, whereas myofibroblast differentiation enlarges the extraocular muscles resulting in restrictive myopathy. Furthermore, orbital fibroblasts are unique in being the only fibroblast in the body that carries CD40 receptors commonly found on B-cells. During inflammation, T-cells interact with CD40 receptors on orbital fibroblasts to produce pro-inflammatory cytokines that induce the synthesis of glycosaminoglycans (GAGs) and hyaluronic acid. Overproduction of these extracellular substances compound the congestion and edema of the orbital tissue.[3] In addition to the immunologic process mediated via CD40 receptors on orbital fibroblasts, autoantibodies against insulin-like growth factor 1 receptors and thyroid-stimulating hormone receptors also contribute to TED. Activation of these receptors generates cytokines and GAG deposition in orbital tissues.[4] Thyroid-stimulating immunoglobulin is the main thyroid-stimulating hormone receptor antibody that correlates directly with the activity and severity of TED.[5] Hence, thyroid-stimulating immunoglobulin could serve as a strong disease biomarker for many cases of TED.[6]

Clinical manifestations of TED consist of a variety of signs and symptoms depending on the severity of the condition (Table 3.38-1). Patients frequently present with dry eye.

Table 3.38-1   The Werner's NOSPECS Measures Clinical Severity Based on Clinical Manifestation of Thyroid Eye Disease[6]

Class 0	N	No signs or symptoms
Class 1	O	Only signs, no symptoms (upper eyelid retraction and stare, ±lid lag)
Class 2	S	Soft tissue involvement (edema of conjunctiva and eyelids, conjunctival injection)
Class 3	P	Proptosis
Class 4	E	Extraocular muscle involvement (usually with diplopia)
Class 5	C	Corneal involvement (primarily lagophthalmos)
Class 6	S	Sight loss (due to optic nerve involvement)

Other common concerns include photophobia, ocular discomfort, swelling of the eyelids, diplopia, and cosmetic concerns.

The most common early sign of TED is upper eyelid retraction, affecting up to 90% of patients. This occurs because of increased sympathetic stimulation of the Muller's muscle (thyroid hormone increases the responsiveness of cells to epinephrine and norepinephrine), contraction of the levator palpebrae superioris, and proptosis.[2] Dalrymple sign (widening of the palpebral fissure so that the inferior and superior sclera are exposed) and temporal flare (elevation of the temporal portion of the upper eyelid) may be seen. Exophthalmos is the second most common sign of TED. This is observed in 60% of patients and commonly results in punctate epithelial erosions.[7] Eyelid lag (elevation of the upper eyelid in downgaze) affects 50% of patients, and von Graefe sign (delayed descent of the upper eyelid during downgaze) may be present. Diplopia can arise secondary to restrictive extraocular myopathy in 40% of patients. The inferior and medial rectus muscles are most commonly affected, leading to hypotropia and esotropia, respectively.[8] Pain with eye movement manifests in 30% of patients. Compressive optic neuropathy, an ophthalmic emergency, can be found in 6% of patients. Joe presented with dyschromatopsia, visual field defects, and irreversible vision loss, consistent with compressive optic neuropathy. The optic nerve pallor indicates that this is long standing.

Two out of 3 clinical requirements, namely, laboratory testing, clinical signs, and radiographic evidence must be present for the diagnosis of TED. Laboratory evidence confirming Graves disease or Hashimoto thyroiditis includes thyroid-stimulating hormone, free T3 and free T4, thyroid-stimulating hormone receptor, thyroperoxidase, or thyroglobulin antibodies, or thyroid-stimulating immunoglobulin. Clinical signs include eyelid retraction, swelling of the eyelids that is worse in the morning, injection of the conjunctiva or caruncle, proptosis, restrictive strabismus, or compressive optic neuropathy. Radiographic evidence shows enlargement of the extraocular muscles with sparing of the tendons.[9]

Determination of the clinical activity score of TED is essential because the disease may be in an active or quiescent stage (Table 3.38-2). Visual acuity, color vision, exophthalmometry, orthoptic assessment, visual field testing, biomicroscopy, and fundus examination are helpful in evaluating TED. Active inflammation manifests as conjunctival injection and chemosis, swelling of orbital tissue and eyelids, or enlargement of extraocular muscles.

Conditions with similar presentations to TED include myasthenia gravis, orbital tumors, and carotid–cavernous fistula. Like TED, myasthenia gravis can present with diplopia, but it tends to be worse later in the day and better after rest. In contrast, the diplopia associated with TED is worse in the morning when fluid accumulates in the ocular tissue when the head is not raised. Ptosis is often associated with myasthenia gravis rather than the lid retraction observed in TED. Orbital tumors tend to be unilateral and rarely cause lid retraction or lid lag. A carotid–cavernous fistula may present with proptosis, pulsatile

---

Table 3.38-2 Clinical Manifestation of Thyroid Eye Disease Can Be Used to Find the Clinical Activity Score[9]

Initial Visit (1 Point Each)	Follow-up Visit (1 Point Each)
1. Spontaneous orbital pain in last 4 weeks 2. Gaze-evoked orbital pain in last 4 weeks 3. Eyelid swelling 4. Eyelid erythema 5. Conjunctival injection 6. Chemosis 7. Inflammation of caruncle or plica semilunaris	- Criteria 1-7 and 8. Increase in proptosis ≥ 2 mm 9. Decrease in uniocular motility in any 1 direction $\geq 8°$ 10. Decrease in visual acuity of 1 line on a Snellen chart
CAS $\geq 3 \rightarrow$ ACTIVE	CAS $\geq 4 \rightarrow$ ACTIVE

exophthalmos, dilated episcleral vessels, and elevated intraocular pressure (IOP), but does not cause eyelid retraction.

Management of TED requires a multidisciplinary approach. Because TED is an ocular manifestation of a systemic etiology, the first goal in management is smoking cessation and achieving a euthyroid state via comanagement with an internist or endocrinologist. Hyperthyroidism can be managed with systemic medications that block the production of thyroid hormones such as propylthiouracil and methimazole, or with radioactive iodine or thyroidectomy.[10]

The second goal in managing TED is to treat ocular symptoms and preserve vision. Corneal exposure secondary to eyelid retraction can be managed with ocular surface lubricants and topical medications such as ophthalmic cyclosporine 0.05% (Restasis), lifitegrast 5% (Xiidra), or loteprednol 0.5% (Lotemax). In severe cases, eyelid retraction can be managed with injection of hyaluronic acid gel fillers or botulinum toxin, or surgical implantation of an eyelid weight (ie, gold or titanium) into the upper lid. Diplopia in the active phase can be managed with Fresnel prism or monocular occlusion. Sleeping with the head elevated can decrease diplopia and as swelling of the eyelids. Strabismus surgery should be avoided in the active phase of the disease. Orbital decompression is needed for emergent cases of diplopia and compressive optic neuropathy, where irreversible vision loss is possible. In patients with diplopia, surgical decompression is followed by strabismus surgery, and cosmetic concerns should be addressed last.[11]

Systemic corticosteroids are necessary in the treatment of active TED because of the potent anti-inflammatory and immunosuppressive effects. High doses of oral prednisone (60-100 mg/d) or intravenous methylprednisolone infusions of 500 mg weekly for 6 weeks, followed by 250 mg weekly for a further 6 weeks) and then a slow taper is a typical dosage.[12]

Diagnosis of TED after the age of 50 years decreases the prognosis compared to those diagnosed at a younger age.[1] Early initiation of therapy is crucial in minimizing irreversible damage caused by TED.

CLINICAL PEARLS

- Smoking increases by 7 times the likelihood that patients will develop TED.

- Thyroid eye disease has the potential to cause vision loss due to exposure keratopathy or compressive optic neuropathy.

REFERENCES

1. Krassas GE, Wiersinga W. Smoking and autoimmune thyroid disease: the plot thickens. *Eur J Endocrinol.* 2006;154(6):777-780.
2. Bartley GB, Fatourechi V, Kadrmas EF, et al. Clinical features of Graves' ophthalmopathy in an incidence cohort. *Am J Ophthalmol.* 1996;121(3):284-290.
3. Kazim M, Goldberg RA, Smith TJ. Insights into the pathogenesis of thyroid-associated orbitopathy: evolving rationale for therapy. *Arch Ophthalmol.* 2002;120(3):380-386.
4. Tsui S, Naik V, Hoa N, et al. Evidence for an association between thyroid-stimulating hormone and insulin-like growth factor 1 receptors: a tale of two antigens implicated in Graves' disease. *J Immunol.* 2008;181(6):4397-4405.
5. Ponto KA, Zang S, Kahaly GJ. The tale of radioiodine and Graves' orbitopathy. *Thyroid.* 2010;20(7):785-793.
6. Douglas RS, Gupta S. The pathophysiology of thyroid eye disease: implications for immunotherapy. *Curr Opin Ophthalmol.* 2011;22(5):385-390.
7. Talke LM, Murchison AP. Globe subluxation: review and management. *Rev Ophthalmol.* 2007;14. https://www.reviewofophthalmology.com/article/globe-subluxationreview-and-management. Accessed April 6, 2018.
8. Dolman PJ, Cahill K, Czyz CN, et al. Reliability of estimating ductions in thyroid eye disease: an International Thyroid Eye Disease Society multicenter study. *Ophthalmology.* 2012;119(2):382-389.
9. Mourits MP, Prummel MF, Wiersinga WM, Koornneef L. Clinical activity score as a guide in the management of patients with Graves' ophthalmopathy. *Clin Endocrinol (Oxf).* 1997;47(1):9-14.
10. Bahn RS, Burch HB, Cooper DS, et al. Hyperthyroidism and other causes of thyrotoxicosis: management guidelines of the American Thyroid Association and American Association of Clinical Endocrinologists. *Thyroid.* 2011;21(6):593-646.
11. Jellema HM, Braaksma-Besselink Y, Limpens J, von Arx G, Wiersinga WM, Mourits MP. Proposal of success criteria for strabismus surgery in patients with Graves' orbitopathy based on a systematic literature review. *Acta Ophthalmol.* 2015;93:601-609.
12. Vannucchi G, Covelli D, Campi I, et al. The therapeutic outcome to intravenous steroid therapy for active Graves' orbitopathy is influenced by the time of response but not polymorphisms of the glucocorticoid receptor. *Eur J Endocrinol.* 2014;170(1):55-61.

3.39 Myasthenia Gravis

Doug Rett

Jerry, a 78-year-old white male, presented for his annual eye examination. He had been coming to the clinic for many years. At past eye examinations, he complained of fluctuating blurred vision when he moved his head, which was attributed to misalignment and maladaptation of his progressive addition lenses. However, he now stated that adjustment of the glasses did not help the problem. Also at the previous examination, he complained of horizontal binocular diplopia. Examination revealed a comitant, moderate angle exophoria that was intermittently breaking into a right exotropia. After ruling out giant cell arteritis as a causative factor with laboratory testing, he was diagnosed with a decompensated phoria and prescribed prism. At the current examination, Jerry presented wearing these glasses but stated that his diplopia had changed. He described the double vision as diagonal, binocular, intermittent, and worse after a long day at work. He was still working at an office job. He had been under a lot of stress recently, and the diplopia was certainly not helping.

Jerry had an ocular history of pseudophakia in the right eye (cataract surgery was performed 2 years ago). He had a visually significant cataract in his left eye. Medical history was significant for diabetes, hypertension, hyperlipidemia, and chronic obstructive pulmonary disease.

Clinical Findings

Habitual distance VA	OD: 20/15; OS: 20/30
Present Rx	OD: +0.50 −1.75 × 100; 2^Δ BI OS: +3.75 −1.50 × 100; 2^Δ BI ADD: +2.50 OU (OD: 20/20; OS: 20/25)
Cover test (with current Rx)	Distance: 4^Δ right exotropia and 3^Δ right hypertropia Near: 4^Δ right exotropia and 3^Δ right hypertropia Comitant in all gazes
Confrontation visual fields	Full to finger counting OD and OS
Ocular motility	Full and smooth OU
Pupil evaluation	PERRL; no RAPD
Retinoscopy	OD: +1.00 −2.00 × 095 OS: +3.50 −1.50 × 095
Subjective refraction	OD: +0.50 −1.75 × 100 (20/15) OS: +3.75 −1.50 × 100 (20/30)
Near ADD	+2.50 OU (OD: 20/20; OS: 20/25)
NRA/PRA (relative to the +2.50 ADD)	+0.50/−0.50
Intraocular pressure (GAT)	OD: 12 mm Hg; OS: 12 mm Hg at 10:00 AM

Slit-lamp examination	OD: mild ptosis present; clear, centered, and stable posterior chamber IOL; otherwise unremarkable
	OS: moderate ptosis present; 2+ nuclear sclerosis; otherwise unremarkable
Fundus examination	OD: 0.3/0.3 CD ratio; healthy rim tissue with distinct disc margins; fovea flat and dry; normal vasculature; periphery intact
	OS: 0.3/0.3 CD ratio; healthy rim tissue with distinct disc margins; fovea flat and dry; normal vasculature; periphery intact
Eyelid evaluation	Right upper eyelid: corneal reflex to lid margin distance 4 mm; positive Cogan lid twitch
	Left upper eyelid: corneal reflex to lid margin distance 2 mm; positive Cogan lid twitch; 3 mm worsening of ptosis following sustained upgaze for 60 s

Abbreviations: BI, base in; CD, cup to disc; GAT, Goldmann applanation tonometry; IOL, intraocular lens; NRA, negative relative accommodation; OD, right eye; OS, left eye; OU, both eyes; PERRL, pupils equal, round, reactive to light; PRA, positive relative accommodation; RAPD, relative afferent pupillary defect; Rx, prescription; VA, visual acuity.

Comments

Based on the new hypertropia and ptosis, as well as the presence of Cogan lid twitch and worsening of the ptosis with upgaze, myasthenia gravis (MG) was suspected, and Jerry was sent for laboratory testing. He was scheduled for a follow-up visit in 2 weeks to review the laboratory findings.

Follow-up Visit (2 Weeks Following the Initial Examination):

Jerry continued to have intermittent double vision, sometimes horizontal and sometimes diagonal. He reported that the diplopia was worse in the middle of the day and resolved in the afternoon and evening. This examination was performed at 3:00 PM.

Cover test (with current Rx)	Distance: 6$^\Delta$ right exotropia and 5$^\Delta$ right hypertropia
	Near: 8$^\Delta$ right exotropia and 5$^\Delta$ right hypertropia; Comitant in all gazes
Ocular motility	Full and smooth OU
Eyelid evaluation	Right upper lid: corneal reflex to lid margin distance 2 mm
	Left upper lid: corneal reflex to lid margin distance 0 (−2) mm

Laboratory testing	Anti-acetylcholine receptor (AChR) antibody test: 11 nmol/L (normal <0.30)

Abbreviations: OU, both eyes; Rx, prescription.

Discussion

In retrospect, Jerry's past concerns of fluctuating blurry vision and diplopia were likely not related to misalignment of the progressive addition lenses or a decompensating phoria but were more likely to be the first symptoms of extraocular muscle weakness from MG. Sometimes a patient with mild diplopia will notice ghosting of letters, where the images are split into 2 but overlap each other. Many patients will correctly identify this as double vision, but others will describe it as blur. This may have occurred in this case.

Myasthenia gravis is an autoimmune disorder that affects the number of available acetylcholine receptors on postsynaptic skeletal muscles.[1] In normal neuromuscular transmission, acetylcholine is stored in the presynaptic motor nerve terminus and released into the synaptic cleft when an action potential travels down the nerve. Acetylcholine then binds to nicotinic receptors on the postsynaptic muscle. This binding ultimately results in depolarization of the muscle and if the depolarization is large enough, muscle contraction. The process ends by acetylcholinesterase breaking down the acetylcholine so it can no longer bind to the muscle receptors.[2]

Patients with MG have antibodies that block or destroy acetylcholine receptors, making it much harder for a muscle to generate an action potential strong enough to cause muscle contraction. The hallmark features of MG are weakness and fatigability of the affected skeletal muscles. Muscles that are used often, such as the eyelid (both the levator and orbicularis), extraocular, facial, and proximal limb muscles, are generally affected early. Rarely, systemic symptoms progress to involvement of the thoracic diaphragm muscle, resulting in respiratory problems. Approximately 70% of cases involve the levator and extraocular muscles first, and these are eventually affected in 90% of MG cases.[3] Because the eyelids and extraocular muscles are commonly the first muscles affected, eye care practitioners will often be the first specialists to confront and diagnose the condition. Diagnosis of MG can be difficult because it can cause any pattern of extraocular muscle restriction. Pupil reflexes are spared because the iris sphincter and dilator muscles are composed of smooth, rather than skeletal, muscle.

Symptoms are usually better in the morning (or after a nap) and worse in the evening.[3] Interestingly, during the follow-up examination, Jerry stated that his double vision was better at night. This may seem counterintuitive for MG. However, note that while the diplopia worsened as the day progressed, the ptosis also worsened. At the 2-week follow-up examination (at 3:00 PM) the ptosis was covering his left pupil. This would have eliminated binocularity and thus the diplopia.

There are several in-office tests that aid in the diagnosis of MG. Cogan's lid twitch is a common phenomenon in MG. Here the patient looks down for 10 to 20 seconds, thereby relaxing the levator palpebrae superioris muscle and giving an opportunity for acetylcholine to build up in the synapse. Then, when the patient looks straight-ahead, the eyelid will overshoot the ptotic eyelid position before falling to the ptotic position.[4] Another important MG test is the extended upgaze test, which attempts to fatigue the levator muscle. A patient with MG will display a noticeable worsening of the ptosis following 60 to 120 seconds of continued upgaze. Other clinical tests include the rest test and the ice pack test. Both tests should show an improvement in ptosis after closing the eyes for 30 minutes or after 2 minutes of ice pack application to the closed eyelids, respectively.[5]

Diagnosis of MG is based on clinical history and examination findings but may be confirmed with laboratory, pharmacologic, or electrophysiologic tests. Laboratory testing looks for anti-acetylcholine receptor (AChR) antibodies, which are detectable in the serum of 85% of those with generalized MG but only 50% to 80% of those with isolated ocular MG.[6,7] The presence of these antibodies is essentially diagnostic for MG, but a negative test does not rule out the disease. Muscle-specific kinase (MuSK) and anti-low-density lipoprotein receptor-related protein 4 (LRP4) antibodies may also be found in patients with MG. Pharmacologic testing with intravenous edrophonium will cause a rapid reversal of muscle weakness by inhibiting acetylcholinesterase, which thereby increases the amount of acetylcholine at the synapse.[3] The effects typically last approximately 5 to 10 minutes. Finally, electromyography consists of repeatedly stimulating an affected nerve. The data can then be analyzed to determine if there is a reduced action potential amplitude over time.

In Jerry's case, the diagnosis of MG was suspected based on the clinical findings, and then confirmed by laboratory testing, which was positive for AChR antibodies. Jerry was referred to a neurologist who prescribed pyridostigmine (Mestinon), an oral anticholinesterase medication. A chest computed tomography (CT) was ordered to rule out a thymoma, which occurs in 10% of MG patients.[1] Over time, the symptoms worsened and the dose of Mestinon needed to be increased. Jerry underwent several rounds of intravenous immunoglobulin plasma exchange infusions, which lowers the function of AChR antibodies.[8] Symptoms stabilized sufficiently that a prescription for single-vision glasses with prism could be prescribed. Jerry had not manifested respiratory symptoms, which is critical given his preexisting chronic obstructive pulmonary disease. The relatively early diagnosis and treatment was brought about by clinical testing that eye care practitioners should be aware of and be quick to perform if MG is suspected.

CLINICAL PEARLS

- Do not ignore subtle symptoms.

- Symptoms of MG generally worsen as the day progress, but diplopia may be eliminated as the ptosis worsens and covers the pupil.

- Cogan lid twitch, worsening of ptosis with prolonged upgaze, and improved symptoms with rest or ice pack application over closed eyes are indicative of MG.

REFERENCES

1. Kasper DL, Braunwald E, Hauser S, et al. *Harrison's Principles of Internal Medicine*. 16th ed. New York, NY: McGraw-Hill; 2005:2518-2523.
2. Sieb JP. Myasthenia gravis: an update for the clinician. *Clin Exp Immunol*. 2014;175(3):408-418.
3. Newman NJ, Miller NR, Biousse V. *Walsh and Hoyt's Clinical Neuro-Ophthalmology: The Essentials*. 2nd ed. Philadelphia, PA: Lippincott Williams & Wilkins; 2008:407-417.
4. Singman EL, Matta NS, Silbert DI. Use of the Cogan lid twitch to identify myasthenia gravis. *J Neuroophthalmol*. September 2011; 31(3):239-240.
5. Meriggioli MN, Sanders DB. Autoimmune myasthenia gravis: emerging clinical and biological heterogeneity. *Lancet Neurol*. 2009;8(5):475-490.
6. Benatar M. *Neuromuscular Disease: Evidence and Analysis in Clinical Neurology*. New York, NY: Humana Press; 2006:311-336.
7. Vaphiades MS, Bhatti MT, Lesser RL. Ocular myasthenia gravis. *Curr Opin Ophthalmol*. 2012;23(6):537-542.
8. Gajdos P, Chevret S, Toyka K. Intravenous immunoglobulin for myasthenia gravis. *Cochrane Database Syst Rev*. January 23, 2008(1):CD002277.

3.40 Acute Leukemia With Roth Spots

Joanne Caruso

Jimmy, a 30-year-old white male, presented for an eye evaluation having noticed decreased central and wavy peripheral vision in the left eye for the past 2 days. He did report light sensitivity in both eyes for 2 days, but vision in the right eye was fine otherwise. He was a soft contact lens wearer and did not have usable glasses, as they were broken. Medical history was pertinent for frontal headaches over the past week, which he attributed to a persistent sinus infection. He was taking amoxicillin for the sinus infection and naproxen for headaches. He also had a history (2 years ago) of severe idiopathic alopecia.

Jimmy's last eye evaluation was 1.5 years ago. At that time, his vision was correctable to 20/20 in each eye, and ocular health was unremarkable.

Clinical Findings

Habitual distance VA (with contact lenses)	OD: 20/20; OS: 20/50 (pinhole 20/40⁻)
Habitual near VA (with contact lenses)	OD: 20/20; OS: 20/25
Habitual contact lens Rx	OD: −2.25 sph OS: −3.25 sph
Confrontation visual fields	Full to finger counting OD and OS
Pupil evaluation	PERRL; no RAPD
Amsler grid	OD: within normal limits OS: metamorphopsia centrally
Contact lens over refraction	OD: −0.25 sph (20/20) OS: +0.50 sph (20/40)
Subjective refraction	OD: −2.50 sph (20/20) OS: −3.50 sph (20/40)
Slit-lamp examination	OD: Unremarkable OS: Unremarkable
Contact lens evaluation	Stable, central fit with good movement OU
Intraocular pressure (GAT)	OD: 13 mm Hg; OS: 12 mm Hg at 10:10 AM
Fundus examination	OD: 0.2/0.2 CD ratio; healthy rim tissue with distinct disc margins; fovea flat and dry; multiple flame hemorrhages and Roth spots in posterior pole; periphery intact OS: 0.2/0.2 CD ratio; healthy rim tissue with distinct disc margins; subretinal fluid in macula; multiple flame hemorrhages and Roth spots in posterior pole; periphery intact

Abbreviations: CD, cup to disc; GAT, Goldmann applanation tonometry; OD, right eye; OS, left eye; OU, both eyes; PERRL, pupils equal, round, reactive to light; RAPD, relative afferent pupillary defect; Rx, prescription; sph, sphere; VA, visual acuity.

Comments

Jimmy was diagnosed with Roth spots and flame-shaped hemorrhages in both eyes, as well as macular edema in the left eye. He was scheduled with a retinal specialist the next day. He was told to follow-up with his primary care provider (PCP) as soon as possible, but he was in the process of switching doctors. He told us he would schedule an appointment as soon as possible with his new PCP.

Follow-up Visit With Retinal Specialist (1 Day Following the Initial Examination)

Habitual distance VA (with contact lenses)	OD: 20/20⁻¹; OS: 20/40⁺²
Macular OCT (Figure 3.40-1)	OD: trace subretinal macular edema OS: significant subretinal macular edema
Fundus examination	OD: 0.2/0.2 CD ratio; healthy rim tissue with distinct disc margins; fovea flat and dry; multiple flame hemorrhages and Roth spots in posterior pole; periphery intact OS: 0.2/0.2 CD ratio; healthy rim tissue with distinct disc margins; subretinal fluid in macula; multiple flame hemorrhages and Roth spots in posterior pole; periphery intact
Fluorescein angiography (Figure 3.40-2)	OD: blockage from Roth spots; pinpoint late leakage in the area of macular subretinal fluid OS: blockage from Roth spots; pinpoint late leakage in the area of macular subretinal fluid

Abbreviations: CD, cup to disc; OCT, optical coherence tomography; OD, right eye; OS, left eye; VA, visual acuity.

Comments

Jimmy was again instructed to see his PCP immediately to rule out an infectious or inflammatory cause for the Roth spots and flame-shaped retinal hemorrhages. He was asked to return to see the retinal specialist for follow-up in 1 week.

Follow-up Visit With Retinal Specialist (1 Week Following the Initial Examination)

Jimmy returned stating that his sinus infection had gotten worse. He went to see a doctor at a walk-in health care clinic who put him on a higher dosage of amoxicillin. He had not seen his new PCP or told the doctor at the walk-in clinic that he was having ocular issues that required further systemic evaluation. He felt that his vision had improved, and he was less sensitive to lights.

Habitual distance VA (with contact lenses)	OD: 20/50; OS: 20/30
Fundus examination (Figure 3.40-3)	OD: subretinal fluid in the macula; multiple flame shaped hemorrhages, Roth spots and cotton wool spots in the posterior pole OS: subretinal fluid in macula; multiple flame hemorrhages Roth spots and cotton wool spots in posterior pole
Macular OCT (Figure 3.40-4)	OD: subretinal macular edema OS: subretinal macular edema

Abbreviations: OCT, optical coherence tomography; OD, right eye; OS, left eye; VA, visual acuity.

Comments

Jimmy now had macular edema in the right eye as well. He was again urged to go immediately

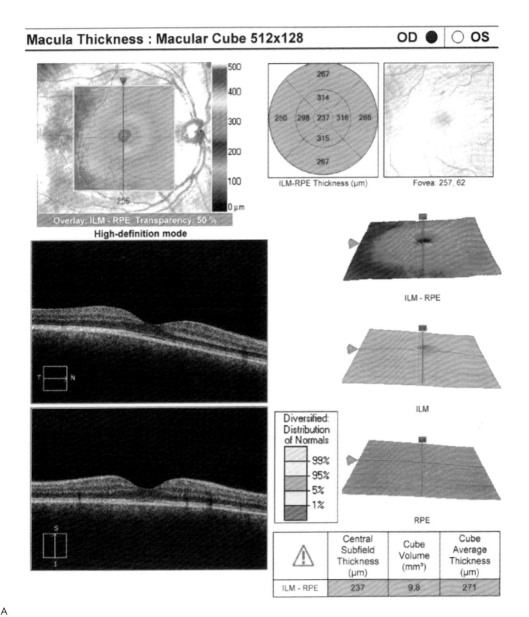

Macula Thickness : Macular Cube 512x128 OD ● ○ OS

High-definition mode

ILM-RPE Thickness (μm) Fovea: 257, 62

ILM - RPE

ILM

RPE

Diversified: Distribution of Normals
- 99%
- 95%
- 5%
- 1%

	Central Subfield Thickness (μm)	Cube Volume (mm³)	Cube Average Thickness (μm)
ILM - RPE	237	9.8	271

A

Figure 3.40-1 Macular optical coherence tomography at the 1 day follow-up examination showing subretinal fluid worse in the left eye (B) than the right eye (A).

to his PCP or the local emergency department. He finally went to his PCP 4 days later. Blood work was obtained, and he was diagnosed with acute myeloid leukemia. He was transferred to the hospital and treated with chemotherapy and a bone marrow transplant. Unfortunately, Jimmy passed away from complications of the acute myeloid leukemia less than 9 months after his initial eye evaluation.

Discussion

Jimmy presented for an eye evaluation because of decreased vision in his left eye. This was likely due to macular edema, but Roth spots were also detected in both eyes. A Roth spot is a retinal hemorrhage with a white spot in the middle. Named after Swiss Physician Dr. Moritz Roth, they were

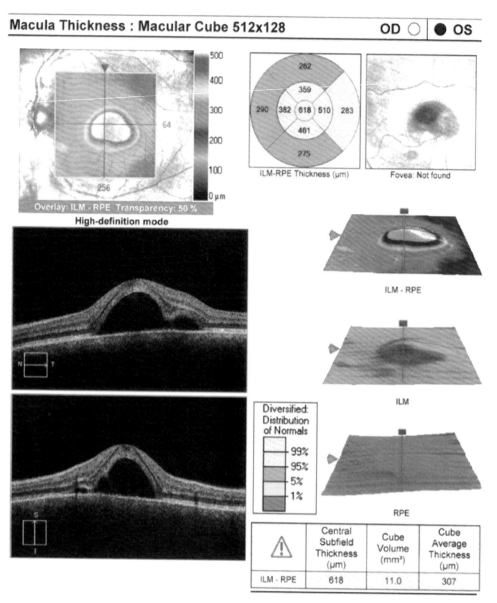

Macula Thickness : Macular Cube 512x128   OD ○ | ● OS

ILM-RPE Thickness (µm)   Fovea: Not found

Overlay: ILM - RPE Transparency: 50 %
High-definition mode

ILM - RPE

ILM

Diversified: Distribution of Normals
99%
95%
5%
1%

RPE

	Central Subfield Thickness (µm)	Cube Volume (mm³)	Cube Average Thickness (µm)
ILM - RPE	618	11.0	307

B

Figure 3.40-1   (Continued)

originally thought to be pathognomonic for subacute bacterial endocarditis. The white spot was thought to be an embolus from the bacterial abscess that lodged in the retina.[1,2] Roth spots are now thought to be a nonspecific sign caused by rupture of retinal capillaries, followed by aggregation of fibrin and platelets.[2,3] Roth spots are usually a sign of an infectious or inflammatory process. The white-centered hemorrhage can be due to focal accumulation of white blood cells in inflammatory vascular disease, cotton-wool spots surrounded by a hemorrhage, leukemic cell foci surrounded by a hemorrhage, or fibrin surrounded by a hemorrhage.[1] Diseases associated with Roth spots include subacute bacterial endocarditis, sepsis, toxoplasmosis, HIV, leukemia, diabetes, hypertension, vasculitis, severe anemia, rheumatologic disorders, and traumatic brain injuries in infants.[2-4] Roth

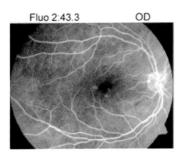 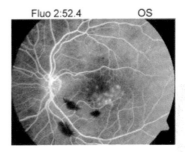

Figure 3.40-2 Late-stage fluorescein angiography demonstrating hypofluorescence in the areas of retinal hemorrhages. There is also pinpoint leakage in the macula of both eyes.

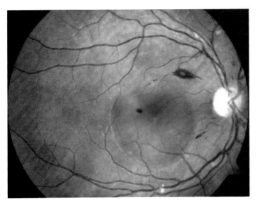 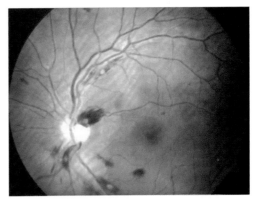

Figure 3.40-3 Subretinal macular fluid greater in the right eye, as well as scattered Roth spots and cotton-wool spots in the posterior pole of both eyes.

spots seen during an eye evaluation require the patient to be referred to their PCP for further medical testing as many of these conditions can be life threatening.

Leukemia is a neoplastic disorder involving the bone marrow and lymphatic system. There are several types of leukemia divided by their origin (myeloid or lymphoid) and the course of the disease (acute or chronic). The most common acute form of leukemia in adults is acute myeloid leukemia and the most common form in children is acute lymphoblastic leukemia.[5]

Normally blood stem cells are produced in the bone marrow. These stem cells will become either myeloid or lymphoid stem cells. A lymphoid stem cell will ultimately become a white blood cell, and a myeloid stem cell will become a red blood cell, white blood cell, or platelet. In acute leukemia (acute myeloid leukemia and acute lymphoblastic leukemia), abnormal

blast cells replace the normal bone marrow.[5] The abnormal cells move into the circulation to infiltrate other organs, including the eye. The acute disease process can progress quickly if not treated. Chronic leukemias (chronic myeloid leukemia and chronic lymphocytic leukemia) involve abnormal mature blood cells and are characterized by more indolent symptoms.[5]

Systemic symptoms of leukemia include fever, trouble breathing, easy bruising, fatigue, weight loss, and frequent infections. The symptoms are caused by infection, anemia, hemorrhage, or infiltration of organs. Ocular manifestations are seen in up to 90% of those with leukemia.[5] Studies have found a more aggressive disease and worse prognosis in those with retinal involvement.[5] Roth spots are evidence of direct infiltration of the leukemic cells. Other retinal signs include intraretinal hemorrhages, cotton-wool spots, vascular

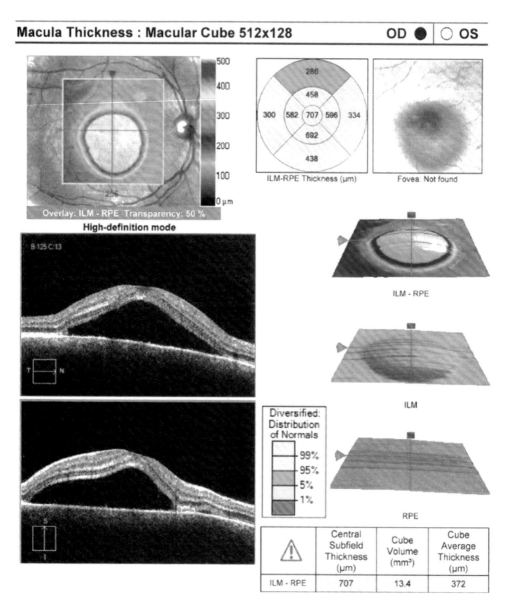

A

Figure 3.40-4 Macular optical coherence tomography showing subretinal macular edema in both eyes at the 1-week follow-up examination.

tortuosity, retinal vein occlusion, peripheral retinal microaneurysms, choroidal infiltration, retinal detachment, macular edema, and opportunistic infections. Nonretinal involvement may rarely be seen as conjunctival venous abnormalities, conjunctival tumors, iris infiltration, hypopyon, or hyphema.[5] In addition, leukemic cells may infiltrate the optic nerve or orbit.

Laboratory testing (including a complete blood count with platelets and differential), bone marrow biopsy, and genetic analysis will aid in diagnosis. If acute leukemia is suspected based on the laboratory testing, the patient should be referred immediately to the emergency department, hematologist, or oncologist. Those with chronic leukemia can be seen within 1 to 2 weeks. Jimmy

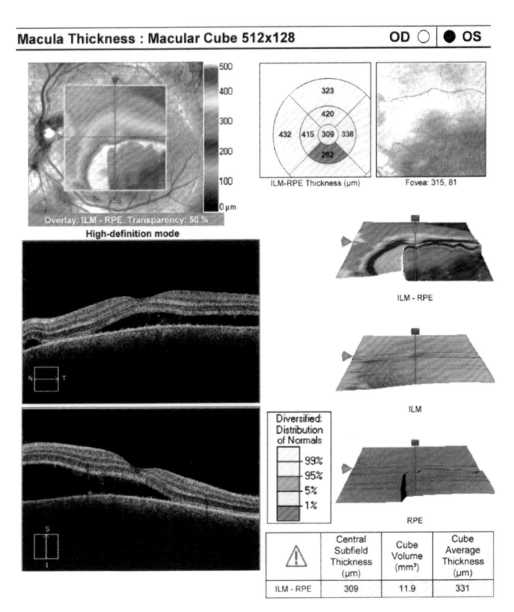

Macula Thickness : Macular Cube 512x128   OD ○ | ● OS

ILM-RPE Thickness (μm)   Fovea: 315, 81

High-definition mode

ILM - RPE

ILM

Diversified: Distribution of Normals

- 99%
- 95%
- 5%
- 1%

RPE

⚠	Central Subfield Thickness (μm)	Cube Volume (mm³)	Cube Average Thickness (μm)
ILM - RPE	309	11.9	331

B

Figure 3.40-4   (Continued)

needed to be seen immediately for laboratory testing but was not compliant with the instructions.

Treatment of leukemia involves chemotherapy and hematopoietic stem cell transplantation. With improved treatment regimens, acute myeloid leukemia can be cured in 35% to 40% of patients younger than 60 years.[6] Survival rates are lower in those older than 60 years.[6]

CLINICAL PEARLS

- Roth spots can be a presenting symptom of a serious medical condition. Eye care professionals play an important role in diagnosis and management of patients with life-threatening conditions.

- It is important to follow-up with patients and ensure that they follow through with your recommendations.

ACKNOWLEDGMENT

I would like to acknowledge the assistance of Torsten Wiegand, MD, Boston, Massachusetts with this case.

REFERENCES

1. Alexander L. *Primary Care of the Posterior Segment*. 3rd ed. New York, NY: McGraw Hill Medical; 2002:336-338.
2. Giovinazzo J, Mrejen S, Freund B. Spectral-domain optical coherence tomography of Roth spots. *Retin Cases Brief Rep*. 2013;7:232-235.
3. Kapadia RK, Steeves JH. Roth spots in chronic myelogenous leukemia. *Can Med Assoc J*. 2011;183(18): E1352.
4. Falcone PM, Larrison WI. Roth spots seen on ophthalmoscopy: diseases with which they may be associated. *Conn Med*. 1995;59:271-273.
5. Talcott KE, Garg RJ, Garg SJ. Ophthalmic manifestations of leukemia. *Curr Opin Ophthalmol*. 2016;27:545-551.
6. Medinger M, Lengerke C, Passweg J. Novel prognostic and therapeutic mutations in acute myeloid leukemia. *Cancer Genomics Proteomics*. 2016;13:317-330.

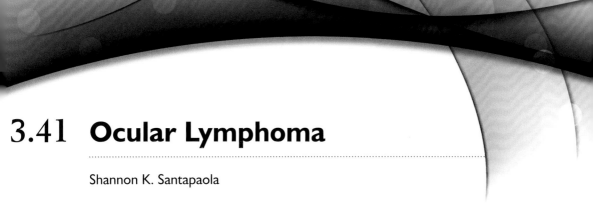

3.41 Ocular Lymphoma

Shannon K. Santapaola

Manuel, a 53-year-old black male, presented to the eye clinic for further evaluation of bilateral suspicious conjunctival lesions noted at an eye examination 6 months ago. The conjunctival lesions were detected during a routine vision examination, and at that time the patient was asymptomatic. Manuel was supposed to return for further evaluation after 1 month, but he was lost to follow-up. He did not report any changes in his vision and did not have any ocular complaints since his last eye examination, 6 months ago.

Ocular history was significant for normal tension glaucoma suspect and a peripheral atrophic retinal hole. Medical history was significant for type 2 diabetes, prostate cancer treated with radiation therapy, hepatitis C, nonfunctioning pituitary adenoma, hypertension, genital herpes, gout, heroin addiction, and tobacco use. The patient reported taking methadone for heroin addiction, metformin for diabetes, and an antihypertensive and gout medication for which he forgot the names.

Clinical Findings

Unaided distance VA	OD: 20/20; OS: 20/20
Present Rx	OD: Pl −1.00 × 080 (20/20); OS: −0.50 sph (20/20)
Pupil evaluation	Equal, round, and reactive to light with no relative afferent pupillary defect
Extraocular motilities	Full, smooth, and accurate OU
Slit-lamp examination (Figure 3.41-1)	OD: elevated, pink, fleshy lesion abutting the superior limbus and extending superiorly ~5-6 mm onto the bulbar conjunctiva; otherwise unremarkable
	OS: ~2 mm pink fleshy lesion with indiscriminate border on nasal bulbar conjunctiva extending from caruncle; otherwise unremarkable
Intraocular pressure (GAT)	OD: 12 mm Hg; OS: 12 mm Hg at 2:05 PM
Fundus examination	OD: 0.65v/0.6 CD ratio; healthy rim tissue with distinct disc margins; fovea flat and dry; normal vasculature; periphery intact
	OS: 0.7/0.7 CD ratio; healthy rim tissue with distinct disc margins; fovea flat and dry; normal vasculature; periphery intact
Visual fields (Humphrey SITA-standard 24-2)	OD: scattered defects not respecting the horizontal or vertical midlines
	OS: scattered defects not respecting the horizontal or vertical midlines

Abbreviations: CD, cup to disc; GAT, Goldmann applanation tonometry; OD, right eye; OS, left eye; OU, both eyes; Rx, prescription; sph, sphere; v, vertical; VA, visual acuity.

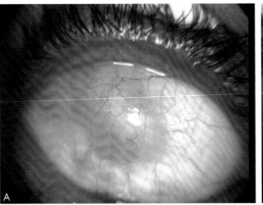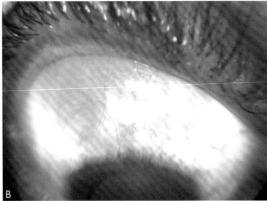

Figure 3.41-1 Conjunctival lesion at initial visit (A). Six months later the lesion had become diffusely enlarged and is now abutting the limbus (B).

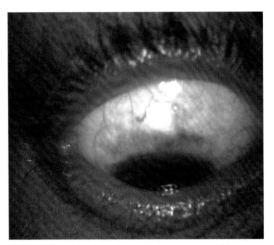

Figure 3.41-2 Resolution of the conjunctival lesion following treatment.

Comments

The patient's conjunctival, salmon-patch lesions were photodocumented 6 months ago (Figure 3.41-1A). On comparison, it was apparent that the conjunctival lesion in the right eye had progressed (Figure 3.41-1B). It was concerning that the lesion had grown in size and was now abutting the superior limbus. A corneal specialist was consulted and a biopsy was performed bilaterally.

Flow cytometry showed a clonal B cell population of the right conjunctival lesion. Immunostaining was positive for CD19 and CD20, negative for CD5, and negative for CD10. Unfortunately, the left eye specimen was crushed and unable to be analyzed. Based on these flow cytometry results, the patient was diagnosed with ocular adnexal lymphoma, specifically extranodal marginal zone lymphoma (EMZL) of the mucosa-associated lymphoid tissues. The patient was referred to the oncology service where laboratory testing was performed to rule out peripheral blood contamination.

Peripheral blood analysis	Serum protein electrophoresis, serum lactate dehydrogenase, peripheral flow cytometry, hepatitis B serology, coagulation testing, complete blood count, B2 microgluobulin, and a chemical profile were all within normal limits.
Positron emission tomography–computed tomography (PET-CT)	Increased fluorodeoxyglucose (FDG) uptake was present in the extraocular muscles, as well as adjacent to the inferior aspect of the right globe. It was felt that this may represent the patient's primary neoplasm. There was no evidence of FDG-avid disease in the chest, abdomen, or pelvis.
Chest x-ray	Unremarkable
Bone marrow biopsy	Patchy hypocellular erythroid predominant marrow. No morphologic evidence of involvement by a lymphoproliferative disorder.

Discussion

Manuel received bilateral orbital radiotherapy, a total of 16 fractions and 2400 cGy. He was followed regularly during and after radiation therapy. The lesions responded to treatment dramatically (Figure 3.41-2). Manuel complained of ocular surface dryness during radiation therapy. This was treated with artificial tears 4 times per day, which helped relieve symptoms. No recurrent lesions were seen 30 months post-radiation treatment.

Ocular adnexal lymphoma, a localized manifestation of systemic lymphoma, comprises approximately 2% of all non-Hodgkin's lymphomas.[1] Lymphoma is the most common orbital malignancy in older patients and represents 10% of orbital tumors.[2] Ocular adnexal lymphoma mostly occurs in the fifth to seventh decades of life.[4] It can be primary, where the lymphoma is isolated to the ocular tissue, or secondary, when the ocular manifestations have disseminated from systemic disease. The most common type of primary ocular adnexal lymphoma is EMZL, which includes mucosa-associated lymphatic tissue (MALT) lymphoma.[3]

The pathogenesis remains unknown; however, MALT lymphoma commonly arises in tissue that develops reactive lymphoid tissue secondary to chronic inflammation.[4] Those with autoimmune disorders or chronic inflammatory conditions are at an increased risk for EMZL. In addition, microbial pathogens such as *Helicobacter pylori* and *Chlamydia pneumoniae* have been associated with MALT lymphoma.[4]

The most common site of ocular lymphoma involvement is the orbit, followed by the conjunctiva, lacrimal gland, and eyelid.[4] Patients may be aware and symptomatic of a conjunctival lesion, complaining of swelling, irritation, proptosis, diplopia, or a visible mass. However, they may present completely asymptomatic, as in this case. A painless pink firm mass (salmon-pink patch) overlying the bulbar conjunctiva is the classical presentation of conjunctival lymphoma.[4] Clinical signs that may support lymphoma include invasion of surrounding tissue, ulceration, rapid growth, and presence of feeder vessels.[3]

Differential diagnoses include pterygium, nodular scleritis, and chronic conjunctivitis. A pterygium presents as a fibrovascular, triangular-shaped lesion involving the nasal or temporal aspect of the cornea. Usually, a pterygium is soft, flat, and bilateral, although it may be asymmetric. Unlike conjunctival lymphoma, which is painless, nodular scleritis will often present with an intensely painful eye that worsens with eye movement. Chronic conjunctivitis that is poorly responsive to traditional therapies warrants further evaluation and biopsy. Any pink fleshy conjunctival mass can be a differential for conjunctival lymphoma and biopsy is essential to determine malignancy.

Fortunately, ocular adnexal lymphoma is localized in 85% to 90% of patients.[4] However, further diagnostic testing is crucial for determining the stage of the condition, ruling out systemic disease, and determining therapy regimens. Patients are typically comanaged with an oncologist. Work up includes a physical examination, laboratory testing, chest x-ray, positron emission tomography–computed tomography (PET-CT), and bone marrow biopsy. Fluorodeoxyglucose is a radioactive dye that is administered intravenously prior to PET-CT imaging to assess for abnormal glucose metabolism in tissues. This is can be useful when diagnosing and managing a variety of cancers and lymphomas.

The treatment of choice for localized conjunctival EMZL is low-dose external beam radiotherapy.[5] This has shown high control rates of 85% to 100% for localized disease.[4] Possible ocular side effects of treatment include cataract, dry eye, and radiation retinopathy.[3-5] Other treatment options include surgical resection, chemotherapy, and immunotherapy (eg, rituximab).

Overall, conjunctival lymphoma has a good prognosis[3-5]; however, continued eye care is imperative because of the risk of recurrence and disseminated disease. Recurrence usually involves the contralateral eye.[3] Approximately 20% of those with conjunctival lymphoma develop systemic dissemination.[3,4]

CLINICAL PEARLS

- Do not forget to look under the eyelids.

- Photo documentation can be critical when determining progression of pathology.

REFERENCES

1. Freeman C, Berg JW, Cutler SJ. Occurrence and prognosis of extranodal lymphomas. *Cancer.* 1972;29:252-260.

2. Shields JA, Shields CL, Scartozzi R. Survey of 1264 patients with orbital tumors and simulating lesions: The 2002 Montgomery Lecture, part 1. *Ophthalmology.* 2004;111:997-1008.

3. Pallavi R, Popescu-Martinez A. More than meets the eye: the "pink salmon patch." *BMJ Case Rep.* Published online: January 10, 2016. doi:10.1136/bcr-2014-204357.

4. Stefanovic A, Lossos IS. Extranodal marginal zone lymphoma of the ocular adnexa. *Blood.* 2009;114:501-510.

5. Kirkegaard M, Coupland S, Prause J, Heegaard S. Malignant lymphoma of the conjunctiva. *Surv Ophthalmol.* 2015;60:444-458.

3.42 Human Immunodeficiency Virus Retinopathy

Alia N. Khalaf

Ed, a 22-year-old Hispanic male, presented for a comprehensive eye examination after moving to the country from Ecuador 3 months ago. He was referred by his primary care doctor because of a HIV diagnosis 4 months ago. When Ed had his initial visit with his primary care provider (PCP) at the Community Health Center, his laboratory testing revealed a CD4 count of 662 cells/mL (normal 500 to 1600 cells/mL) and his viral load was 110 186 copies/mL (normal is undetectable). He had started treatment with oral Genvoya (a combination drug of 150 mg of elvitegravir, 150 mg of cobicistat, 200 mg of emtricitabine, and 10 mg of tenofovir alafenamide) once per day, 1 month prior to his eye examination. His medical health otherwise was unremarkable.

Ed complained of blurry vision in both eyes at distance and near. His last eye examination was 6 months ago, but he reported that he did not see well with his most current glasses. He was interested in contact lenses. Ed did not speak English and was accompanied by a Spanish-speaking interpreter.

Clinical Findings

Habitual distance VA	OD: 20/40^{-2} (pinhole 20/30); OS: 20/20^{-2} (pinhole 20/20)
Habitual Rx	OD: −3.25 −6.00 × 180
	OS: −3.00 −6.00 × 169
Cover test	2$^\Delta$ XP at distance; 4$^\Delta$ XP at near
Confrontation visual fields	Full to finger counting OD and OS
Pupil evaluation	PERRL; no RAPD
Keratometry	OD: 43.00/49.13 @ 090
	OS: 43.00/48.00 @ 090
Retinoscopy	OD: −2.00 −5.50 × 180
	OS: −2.50 −5.00 × 180
Subjective refraction	OD: −3.25 −6.00 × 005 (20/30)
	OS: −3.00 −5.75 × 165 (20/20)
Slit-lamp examination	OD: unremarkable with no anterior chamber cells or flare
	OS: unremarkable with no anterior chamber cells or flare
Intraocular pressure (GAT)	OD: 11 mm Hg; OS: 11 mm Hg at 3:41 PM

Fundus examination (Figure 3.42-1A and B)	OD: 0.4/0.4 CD ratio; slight pallor inferiorly with distinct disc margins; a large cotton wool spot was present inferior temporal to the optic nerve head with underlying retinal fibrosis and traction; traction overlying the macula; periphery was intact
	OS: 0.5/0.5 CD ratio; healthy rim tissue with myelinated nerve fiber layer at the superior nasal disc margin; fovea was flat and dry; normal vasculature; posterior pole was unremarkable with no cotton wool spots or hemorrhages; periphery was intact
5-Line Raster OCT (Figure 3.42-2)	OD: intraretinal inflammation with overlying traction
	OS: thickened nerve fiber layer in the area of myelinated nerve fibers

Abbreviations: CD, cup to disc; GAT, Goldmann applanation tonometry; OCT, optical coherence tomography; OD, right eye; OS, left eye; PERRL, pupils equal, round, reactive to light; RAPD, relative afferent pupillary defect; Rx, prescription; VA, visual acuity; XP, exophoria.

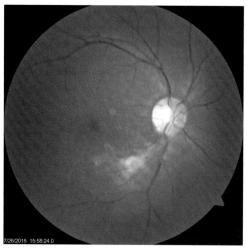 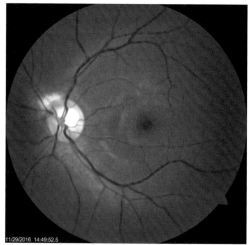

7/26/2016 15:58:24.0   11/29/2016 14:49:52.5

Figure 3.42-1 Fundus photos showing retinal infarction and traction in the right eye and a small area of myelinated nerve fiber layer superior to the optic disc in the left eye.

Comments

Ed was diagnosed with noninfectious microvasculopathy secondary to HIV in both eyes. The reduced visual acuity (VA) in the right eye was most likely due to macular traction. An extensive amount of time was spent educating Ed on the importance of adhering to his medication regimen and attending follow-up visits with his PCP. He was told his vision would likely improve as the CD4 levels normalized. A prescription for glasses was released, but due to the possibility that Ed's weakened immune system could put him at higher risk for opportunist infections with contact lens wear,[1] it was recommended he should wait for his CD4 count to improve before discussing the option of contact lenses.

After having all his questions answered, Ed seemed reassured as he left the office. A follow-up examination was scheduled in 8 weeks, and all findings were communicated to his primary care doctor.

Twenty minutes after Ed left the office a call was received from Ed's social worker within the building. She reported that Ed was in her office weeping because he believed he was going blind. Through the social worker, Ed was assured he would not go blind. With Ed's permission, all findings were explained to the

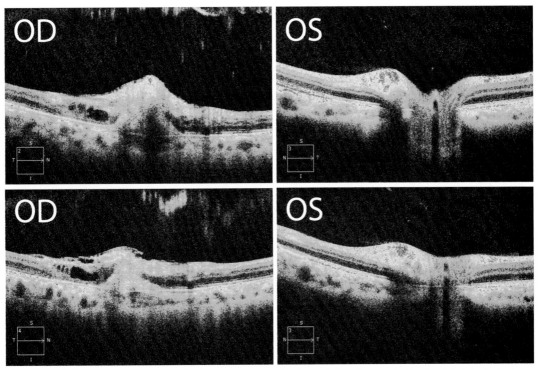

Figure 3.42-2 Five-line raster optical coherence tomography imaged directly over the focal point of the lesion in the right eye and the myelinated nerve fiber layer in the left eye at the initial visit (top) and at the 24-week follow-up examination (bottom).

social worker, and she was able to reassure him that everyone at the Community Health Center was doing their best to take care of him. The social worker later reported that Ed left in a much improved mood after he was able to let his emotions and worries out to her. Ed was overwhelmed being in a new country away from his friends and family, learning a new language, and dealing with the recent HIV diagnosis.

Follow-up Visits (at 8 and 16 Weeks Following the Initial Examination)

At his scheduled follow-up visits, Ed reported excellent adherence to his antiviral medication. He was in a great mood and happy to be there. At the 8-week visit, his CD4 count was up to 773 cells/mL and his viral load was down to 130 copies/mL. This continued to improve at the 16-week examination, where his CD4 count was 1154 cells/mL and his viral load was undetectable. Ed was praised and encouraged to continue his excellent adherence to the antiviral therapy.

Habitual visual acuities had improved to 20/25^{-2} OD with habitual glasses. The retinopathy improved on fundus examination and optical coherence tomography (OCT). Ed again asked about the possibility of being fit with contact lenses. Ed's PCP was consulted regarding his immune system status. She felt he was responding well to the antiviral therapy but agreed that waiting for a few months more before allowing Ed to try contact lenses would be prudent.

Follow-up Visit (24 Weeks Following the Initial Examination)

At the 24-week follow-up, Ed was hopeful that he would be approved to try contact lenses. The CD4 count was 1200 cells/mL, and his viral load remained undetectable. Vision had improved to 20/20^{-2} OD. The retinopathy was significantly improved on fundus examination and OCT (Figure 3.42-2). After discussion with the PCP, it was determined that Ed was ready to try contact lenses. He was fit with soft toric lenses, which eventually allowed VA of 20/25 OD and OS. Ed was very excited and hugged everyone on the way out.

Discussion

When the immune system is confronted with a virus, the body responds by activating specific processes of the immune system. A lymphocyte is a small white blood cell that plays a large role in defending the body against disease. There are 2 main types of lymphocytes: B-cells and T-cells. B-cells make antibodies that attack bacteria and toxins. T-cells help destroy infected cells but can attack the body's own cells when they have been taken over by a virus.[2]

When a virus is recognized in the body as foreign, it is delivered it to the lymph system, where it is ingested by a macrophage. The macrophage processes the virus and displays antigens for that particular virus on its own exterior. These antigens then signal helper T-cells. Helper T-cells read this signal and call for other parts of the immune system to respond. The B-cell responds to this call, reads the antigen from the surface of the macrophage, and then becomes activated, producing millions of antibodies that are specific to the antigen. These antibodies are released into the body to attach to the virus particles. The antibodies then send a signal to other macrophages and other immune cells to come, engulf, and destroy the virus. Once the number of virus particles has dropped significantly and the infection has resolved, the suppressor T-cell will signal the other cells of the immune system to rest.[3]

Human immunodeficiency virus infects 39.8 million people worldwide.[4] HIV is a retrovirus that disrupts the immune process by directly infecting helper T-cells. The body's initial immune response does get rid of a great deal of HIV, but some of the virus manages to survive and infect the helper T-cells. Once the infected helper T-cells are activated, they work to create new viruses. The virus elicits antibody formation yet these antibodies are not effective against preventing the spread of the disease. This infection results in cell-mediated immune suppression and susceptibility of life-threatening infections.[3]

Ocular manifestations are present in 50% to 75% of HIV-infected patients.[5] Noninfectious microvasculopathy of both the anterior and posterior segment of the eye is a consequence of HIV in patients with high viral loads. Cotton-wool spots and nerve fiber layer hemorrhages are seen in up to 70% of HIV-infected patients. With noninfectious HIV retinopathy, other retinal findings can include focal areas of non-perfusion, microaneurysms, telangiectatic vessels, and peripheral punctate hemorrhages. Human immunodeficiency virus retinopathy typically does not lead to permanent visual loss. There is no ocular treatment specific for the retinopathy but the retinopathy often improves with systemic antiviral therapy and increased CD4 counts.[6]

In patients who have CD4 counts that fall below 200 cells/mL, secondary opportunistic infections can arise because of the patient's weakened immune system. Cytomegalovirus retinitis is the most frequent opportunistic infection when the CD4 count falls below 50 cells/mL. Other secondary opportunistic infections include herpes simplex virus, herpes zoster, syphilis, candidiasis, cryptococcus, toxoplasmosis, and tuberculosis. These involve active infection and can manifest with symptoms of decreased vision and floaters secondary to an active inflammation of the vitreous. The retina will present with peripheral granular opacities, intraretinal hemorrhages, and possible retinal necrosis. These patients also have an increased risk of retinal detachments. Secondary opportunistic infections can lead to permanent visual loss. Treatment is specific for the type of infection present.[6]

Ed presented to the office believing that all he needed was a new pair of glasses to improve his blurry vision. Instead, Ed was informed that the HIV was affecting the back of his eye and was one of the reasons his vision was slightly decreased. It is overwhelming to hear that you are diagnosed with a chronic systemic disease such as HIV. Most patients at our Community Health Centers are immigrants from countries all over the world who do not share our language and have not had the means to obtain proper education or strong support systems. Caring for these patients and educating them on etiology, treatment, and management of a condition can be challenging.

Interprofessional collaboration is a way to approach this challenge. By working in partnership with the patient and health care professionals from different disciplines it can enhance the quality of care for patients with chronic conditions.[7] It was thought initially by the optometrist that Ed's visit was approached in an empathetic and educated manner. However, it was learned after the call from the social worker that with Ed's diagnosis, more resources were necessary. For patients with a chronic or complicated systemic diagnosis with ocular manifestations, the assistance of not only the PCP, but also the social work team should be involved. Working together enables heath care professionals to share their expertise and perspectives to benefit the patient's quality of life.[8]

CLINICAL PEARL

- Always approach a sensitive case with time and empathy. Involve the entire health care team to achieve an optimal quality of life for your patient.

REFERENCES

1. Chronister CL. Contact lens considerations for patients infected with HIV. *Optometry.* 2000;71(4):249-258.
2. Immune System 101. HIV.gov Web site. https://www.aids.gov/hiv-aids-basics/just-diagnosed-with-hiv-aids/hiv-in-your-body/immune-system-101/. n.d. Accessed April 14, 2017.
3. Manuselis G. Clinical virology. In: Mahon CR, Lehman DC, eds. *Diagnostic Microbiology.* 4th ed. Maryland Heights, MO: W.B. Saunders Company; 2011:729-730.
4. HIV Fact sheet. World Health Organization Web site. http://www.who.int/mediacentre/factsheets/fs360/en/. Updated November 2016. Accessed February 24, 2017.
5. Arévalo JF. Chapter 1: Retinal and choroidal manifestations of HIV/AIDS. In: *Retinal and Choroidal Manifestations of Selected Systemic Diseases.* New York: Springer Science + Business Media; 2013:1-21.
6. Ehlers JP, Shah CP. 12.10 Noninfectious retinal microvasculopathy/HIV retinopathy. In: *The Wills Eye Manual.* 5th ed. Baltimore, MD: Lippincott Williams & Wilkins; 2008:354.
7. Van Houdt S, De Lepeleire J, Driessche KV, Thijs G, Buntinx F. Multidisciplinary team meetings about a patient in primary care: an explorative study. *J Prim Care Community Health.* 2011;2:72-76.
8. Nisbet G, Dunn S, Lincoln M. Interprofessional team meetings: opportunities for informal interprofessional learning. *J Interprof Care.* 2015;29:426-432.

Index

Note: Page numbers followed by "*f*" and "*t*" refer to figures and tables, respectively.

A

AAION. *See* Arteritic anterior ischemic optic neuropathy (AAION)
Accommodative disorder/dysfunction, 75, 76, 107
  in children with Down syndrome, 159, 161
  vision techniques, 120*t*, 124*t*
Accommodative esotropia, 109
Accommodative excess, and pseudomyopia, 128
Accommodative infacility, 72*t*, 128
Accommodative insufficiency, 69–72, 72*t*
  and presbyopia, 9
Accommodative therapy, 80*t*
ACE. *See* Angiotensin-converting enzyme (ACE)
Acetaminophen, 227, 234, 505
Acetazolamide, 434, 437, 441–442, 496, 499
Acetylcholine, 532–533
AChR. *See* Anti-acetylcholine receptor (AChR)
Acne rosacea, 197
Acquired color vision deficiencies, 144–146, 145*f*
Acute angle closure, 496, 497, 499
Acute leukemia, 535–541, 537–538*f*, 540–541*f*
Acute lymphoblastic leukemia, 539
Acyclovir, 278, 280, 318
Adaptational issues, with progressive addition lenses, 33–35
Adenomas, 444–451, 446*f*, 447–451*f*
Adie tonic pupil, 410–411
Adrenocorticotropic hormone, 362
Adult inclusion conjunctivitis, 236–238
Aflibercept, 346, 353, 388
Age-Related Eye Disease Study 2 (AREDS 2) supplement, 340, 342, 346
Age-Related Eye Disease Study (AREDS) Research Group, 342
Age-related macular degeneration, 52–56
Aldara. *See* Imiquimod
Aleve. *See* Naproxen
Algerbrush, 504
Allergic conjunctivitis with eyelid involvement, 228
Allergic dermatitis, 228
Alpha-2 adrenergic agonists, 420, 485–486, 499
Alphagan. *See* Brimonidine
Alrex. *See* Loteprednol etabonate
Amblyopia, 5, 109–112, 148, 178, 446, 490
  and anisometropia, 12, 13

American National Standards Institute (ANSI)
  Z80.1 standards, 33
4-Aminoquinilone, 369
Amiodarone, 289–292, 428
  keratopathy, 290, 290*f*
  optic neuropathy, 292
Amniotic membranes, 246–247, 247*f*, 287
  graft, 224, 225, 277
Amoxicillin, 536
Amoxicillin-clavulanate, 214, 228, 229
Amsler grid, monitoring at home, 322, 340, 342, 345–346, 379
Analgesics, 17, 505. *See also specific analgesics*
Angioid streaks, 375–379, 376–377*f*
Angiotensin-converting enzyme (ACE), 519
Angle-closure glaucoma, 495–501, 496*f*, 498–499*f*, 500–501*f*
Angle recession, 269
Aniseikonia, 12, 117, 295
  and cataract surgery, 17
Anisocoria, 403*f*, 404, 411, 413, 454
Anisometropia, 11–13, 109, 295
  and amblyopia, 112
  and cataract surgery, 17
Annular keratopathy of Payreau, 504
Anomaloscope, 131, 134, 137, 138, 139, 142, 146
Anomalous trichromacy, 137
AN Series & EC Series Keystone Cards, 120*t*
ANSI. *See* American National Standards Institute (ANSI)
Anterior chiasmal syndrome, 469
Anterior herpetic uveitis, 319
Anterior uveitis, 318, 325, 327
Anti-acetylcholine receptor (AChR), 533
Antibiotics, 197–198, 260. *See also specific antibiotics*
Antibiotic-steroid drops, 281, 505
Anticoagulation, medications for, 512
Antihistamines, 246, 251. *See also specific antihistamines*
Anti-low-density lipoprotein receptor-related protein 4 (LRP4) antibodies, 533
Anti-suppression, vision techniques, 120*t*, 121, 124*t*
Anti-vascular endothelial growth factor (VEGF) agents, 349, 353, 378, 388
Aperture rule, 83*t*, 120*t*, 124*t*
Apraclonidine, 405
AREDS. *See* Age-Related Eye Disease Study (AREDS) Research Group

AREDS 2. *See* Age-Related Eye Disease Study 2 (AREDS 2) supplement
Argyll Robertson pupil, 410, 413
Arteritic anterior ischemic optic neuropathy (AAION), 428, 429
Artificial tears, 66, 197, 204, 205, 209, 224, 230, 234, 246, 251, 269, 272, 273, 290, 314
AS/NZS. *See* Australian/New Zealand (AS/NZS) eye protection standards
Aspheric soft multifocal contact lenses, 182
Aspirin, 507, 509, 512
Associated phoria, 91*f*, 92–93, 92*f*, 107, 108
Asthenopia, 108
Astigmatism, 3–6, 155, 181, 185, 200, 274, 275, 297, 298, 446
　against-the-rule, 4
Atkinson protocol, 154–155
Atopic keratoconjunctivitis, 314
Atorvastatin calcium, 428
Atrophic retinal holes, 396, 396*f*
Atropine, 19, 22, 112, 150, 507
Audiobooks, recommendation for, 55
Auditory-based feedback techniques, for congenital nystagmus, 99
Australian/New Zealand (AS/NZS) eye protection standards
　AS/NZS1336, 46, 47
　AS/NZS1337.6, 46
Autosomal dominant polycystic kidney disease, 405
Avastin. *See* Anti-vascular endothelial growth factor (VEGF) injection; Bevacizumab
AzaSite. *See* Azithromycin
Azelaic acid, 260
Azelastine, 278
Azithromycin, 237, 255, 259, 260, 523
　with pyrimethamine, 322
Azopt. *See* Brinzolamide

B
Bacitracin, 198
Bacterial conjunctivitis, 281
Bacterial infection, 504
Bactrim. *See* Trimethoprim-sulfamethoxazole
Bagolini striated lenses, 111
Bandage contact lenses, 287, 505
Bangarter filter, 415
Basal cell carcinoma, 201
Base-in (BI) prism correction, 102–104
B-cells, 550
B-dimension, 34, 35
Beading a string, 120*t*
BEB. *See* Benign essential blepharospasm (BEB)
Benign essential blepharospasm (BEB), 211
Benzoyl peroxide, 260
Besifloxacin, 504
Beta-adrenergic antagonists, 499
Beta-blockers, 291, 485
Betadine. *See* Povidone-iodine
Bevacizumab, 346, 353, 388
BI. *See* Base-in (BI) prism correction
Bifocal lenses, 38, 39, 128, 158*f*, 159, 161, 182
Bilateral, uncorrected astigmatism, 115

Bilateral exophthalmos, 528
Bilaterally nonreactive pupils, 408
Bilateral multifocal intraocular lenses, 305
Bilateral optic nerve edema, 441
Bilateral orbital decompression, 524
Bilateral posterior subcapsular cataracts, 303–305
Binocular accommodative facility, 80*t*
Binocular accommodative rock, 120*t*, 124*t*
Binocular cross-cylinder test, 8
Binocular Hart chart, 80*t*
Binocular horizontal diplopia, 524
Binocular sustained reading through plus lenses, 80*t*
Binocular therapy, 112, 490
　vision techniques, 120*t*
Binocular vision problems, 115–116, 117, 128
Binocular visual integration, 115–116
Bioptic driving, 63–64
Bioptic telescope for driving, 61–64
Bitemporal hemianopia, 446
Blepharitis, 197, 203–206, 255, 262, 279
Blepharospasm, 210–212
Blink analysis, 221
Blink exercises, 204, 206
Blood clotting disorders, 512
Blood-filled cyst, 511
Blood glucose, 352
Blood pressure, 511
Blood test, for subconjunctival hemorrhage, 270
Blood thinning medications, 512
Blue Mountains Eye Study, 304
Blunt ocular trauma, 507
　anterior synechiae following, 508*f*
Blur at near, 8, 71, 111, 181, 409
Botulinum toxin, 211–212, 530
Bowman membrane, 275, 503
Bow-tie atrophy of the optic disc, 470, 471
Brachytherapy, 330
Branch retinal artery occlusion (BRAO), 389–393, 390–391*f*
BRAO. *See* Branch retinal artery occlusion (BRAO)
Brimonidine, 420, 484
Brimonidine tartrate/timolol maleate, 486
Brinzolamide, 483
Brinzolamide/brimonidine, 486, 496
Brock string, 80*t*, 120*t*, 124*t*
Bromday. *See* Bromfenac
Bromfenac, 357
Bromocriptine, 446
Bruch membrane, 378, 379
Bull's eye pigment changes, 369

C
Cabergoline, 446
Cantharidin, 234
Capsular rupture, 358, 494
Carbonic anhydrase inhibitors, 442, 485–486, 499
Cardiff acuity cards (Good-Lite Co.), 149
Carotid artery dissection, 404–405
Carotid-cavernous fistula, 529–530
Carotid endarterectomy, 393
Cataracts, 16–17, 224, 294–296, 304, 494
　bilateral posterior subcapsular cataracts, 303–305

cortical cataracts, 295
  dense cataract, 334
  in geriatric patients, 66
  nuclear cataracts, 295
  posterior subcapsular cataracts, 295, 303–305
  traumatic cataract, 269
Cataract surgery, 16–17, 295, 399
  femtosecond laser-assisted, 16
  follow-up care after, 17
  refractive error, 17
CBC. *See* Complete blood count (CBC)
CCTV. *See* Onyx HD portable closed circuit
    television (CCTV)
CD4 counts, in human immunodeficiency virus (HIV)
    retinopathy, 550
CD4+ Th2 lymphocytes, and VKC, 245
CD40 receptors, 528
CDC. *See* US Centers for Disease Control and
    Prevention (CDC)
Central geographic atrophy, 342
Central nervous system, 519
Central retinal artery occlusion (CRAO), 392
Central retinal vein occlusion (CRVO), 386–388,
    386*f*, 387*f*
Central serous retinopathy, 361–364, 362*f*, 363*f*
Central ulcers, 282
Cephalexin, 199, 213, 214
Cephalosporins, 214, 229
Cerebral infarction, 405
Chalazia, 197, 198, 199–201, 255, 260
Cheiroscopic tracing, 120*t*, 124*t*
Childhood ocular rosacea, 257–261
Chlamydial conjunctivitis. *See* Adult inclusion
    conjunctivitis
Chlamydia pneumoniae, 545
Chlamydia trachomatis, 237
Chloroquine, 292, 369
Chlorpromazine, 292
Choroidal neovascularization, 342, 346, 378–379
Choroidal thickness, 364
Choroideremia, low vision management, 48–51
Chronic angle closure, 497
Chronic blur, 524
Chronic conjunctivitis, 545
Chronic leukemias, 539
Cicatricial ectropion, 208
Cidofovir, 234, 242
Ciliary body melanoma, 333–336, 335*f*
Ciprofloxacin, 278, 292
Circumscribed iris melanoma, 331
CISS. *See* Convergence Insufficiency Symptom
    Survey (CISS)
CITS. *See* Convergence Insufficiency Treatment
    Study (CITS)
CITT. *See* Convergence Insufficiency Treatment
    Trial (CITT)
Classic wet macular degeneration, 346
Clindamycin, 229, 260, 322, 523
  with dexamethasone, 322
Clinically significant macular edema (CSME), 352, 358
CLPU. *See* Contact lens peripheral ulcer (CLPU)
Coats disease, 165

Coats ring, 504
Cobblestone papillae, 244, 245*f*
Cocaine, 405
Cockburn curve technique, 503
Cogan's lid twitch, 533
Cold compresses, 234, 314
Collaborative Ocular Melanoma Study (COMS), 331
Colored filters, 134–135
Color vision deficiencies (CVDs), 132–140
  acquired, 144–146, 145*f*
  blue-yellow congenital deficiency, 137
  hereditary, 141–143
  red-green congenital deficiency, 137, 138, 140, 142
  testing. *See also* Color vision testing
Color vision occupational questions, 136
Color vision testing
  24 Plate Ishihara Test, 130, 132*t*, 133, 136, 137, 138*f*,
      139, 142
  anomaloscope, 131, 134, 137, 138, 139, 142, 146
  Anthony AI Test, 131
  book test, 133, 135
  cone contrast test, 141–143, 142*f*, 146
  desaturated D15 hue arrangement test, 146
  Fansworth D15 Test, 130–131, 133, 133*f*, 136, 137–
      138, 137*f*, 139
  Fansworth-Munsell 100 Hue Test, 132, 134,
      134*f*, 146
  Hardy Rand and Rittle Pseudoisochromatic Test, 130,
      131*f*, 133, 136, 137, 139, 146
  Lanthony D15 test, 133, 133*f*
  Oculus Heidelberger Multi-Color Anomaloscope, 141,
      143*f*, 146
Color visual-evoked potentials, 146
Combigan. *See* Brimonidine tartrate/timolol maleate
Complete blood count (CBC), 512
Complex task requirements, prescribing for, 36–39
Compressive optic neuropathy, 529
Computer Orthoptics vergence, 80*t*, 83*t*
Computer Orthoptics VTS3 & VTS4, 120*t*, 124*t*
Computer users, prescribing for, 40–42
COMS. *See* Collaborative Ocular Melanoma
    Study (COMS)
Cone contrast test, 141–143, 142*f*, 146
Cone dystrophy, 145, 145*f*, 342
Congenital aniridia syndrome, 311
Congenital ectropion, 208–209
Congenital Horner syndrome, 405
Congenital nystagmus, vision therapy for, 95–100
Conjunctival cysts, 265–266
Conjunctival granulomas, 519
Conjunctival laceration, 269
Conjunctival lesions, 272, 272*f*, 543, 544*f*
Conjunctival lymphoma, 545
Conjunctival nevus, 272
Conjunctival tarsal papillae, 194
Conjunctiva ruptures, 511
Conjunctivitis, 279
Conscious full blinks, 204, 206
Contact lenses, 111
  for anisometropia, 13
  aspheric soft multifocal contact lenses, 182
  for astigmatism, 4, 5

Contact lenses *(Cont.)*
  bandage contact lenses, 287, 505
  centration, 186
  for congenital nystagmus, 97
  hybrid multifocal contact lenses, 177
  -induced papillary conjunctivitis. *See* Giant papillary
    conjunctivitis (GPC)
  legislations regarding, 191, 192
  for myopia control, 19–22, 20*t*
  noncompliance, 190–195
  for presbyopia, 9
  -related ulcerations, 286
  soft contact lenses, 171–175
  soft multifocal contact lenses, 19, 20–21, 20*t*
Contact lens peripheral ulcer (CLPU), 283, 284
Contrast sensitivity, and sports vision, 25
Convergence excess, 74–76
Convergence insufficiency, 72*t*, 78–85, 107, 115
  management with prism, 101–104
  and presbyopia, 9
Convergence Insufficiency Symptom Survey (CISS), 81,
    102, 102*f*
Convergence Insufficiency Treatment Study
    (CITS), 85
Convergence Insufficiency Treatment Trial (CITT), 81
Convergence testing, 148, 149*f*
  in infants, 148
Cool compresses, 246, 269
Copaxone. *See* Glatiramer acetate
Copper, 342
Corneal astigmatism, 4
Corneal cross-linking, 187, 189
Corneal endothelium, 504
Corneal erosion, recurrent, 285–287, 286*f*
Corneal flattening, 191, 192
Corneal foreign body, 502, 503*f*
Corneal neovascularization, 245, 258*f*
Corneal sequela, 255
Corneal steepening, 185, 185*f*
Corneal topography, 5, 17
Corneal ulcer, 244
Cortical cataracts, 295
Corticosteroids, 225, 246, 313, 314, 322, 328, 358,
    442–443, 509. *See also specific corticosteroids*
Cosopt. *See* Dorzolamide hydrochloride/timolol maleate
Cotton-tipped applicator, 280
CPT perceptual speed, 124*t*
CPT visual search, 124*t*
Cranial nerve III, regeneration of, 414
Cranial nerve III palsy, 410, 452–455
Cranial nerve IV palsy, 456–458, 457*f*, 459–462, 460*f*
Cranial nerve VI palsy, 442
Cross-cylinder test, 75
CRVO. *See* Central retinal vein occlusion (CRVO)
Cryotherapy, 401
CSME. *See* Clinically significant macular edema (CSME)
Curettage, 231
CVDs. *See* Color vision deficiencies (CVDs)
Cyclopentolate, 149, 150, 246, 278, 321
Cycloplegia, 129, 283
Cycloplegic agents, 504, 509

Cycloplegic refraction, 11, 152, 154
Cycloplegic retinoscopy, 112
Cyclosporine, 206, 224, 225, 255, 328, 372
Cyclosporine A, 246
Cystoid macular edema, 355–359, 356–359*f*
Cytomegalovirus retinitis (CMV), 550

D
Dacryocystitis, 213–215, 214*f*
Dacryocystorhinostomy, 215
Daraprim. *See* Pyrimethamine
Decompensated exodeviation, 102
Decompensating phoria, 532
Demodex brevis, 255
Demodex folliculorum, 255
Demodex mite, 260
Demyelinating optic neuritis, 422–425, 423*f*
Dendrite of the corneal epithelium, 279, 279*f*
Dense cataract, 334
Desaturated D15 hue arrangement test, 146
Deuteranomalous color vision deficiency, 143
Deuteranomaly, 132–133
Deuteranopia, 137
DEWS (Dry Eye Workshop) I and II Reports, 218
Dexamethasone, 246, 262, 298, 322
Diabetes, 31
  classifications of, 350*t*
  diagnostic criteria, 351*t*
Diabetic macular edema (DME), 350
  management of, 353
Diabetic retinopathy, 290, 291*f*, 348–354, 349*f*,
    350*f*, 399
Diamox. *See* Acetazolamide
Dichromacy, 137
Diffractive multifocal intraocular lenses, 304
Diffuse iris melanoma, 331
Difluprednate, 325, 357, 358
Digital massage, 255
Dipivefrin, 487
Diplopia, 442, 454, 461, 464, 474, 529
Dipping, 62, 62*f*
Disc drusen, 419–420, 436
Disc edema, 428, 429, 435
Disorientation following prescription change, 30–32
Dispensing anomalies, 30–32
Dispensing issues with progressive addition
    lenses, 33–35
Disposable camera, 178
Disruption of corneal tissue, 269
Distance toric lenses, 177
Divergence excess, 87–89
  intermittent exotropia, 118–121
Divergence insufficiency, 75–76
DME. *See* Diabetic macular edema (DME)
Dome magnifiers, 58
Dorsal midbrain syndrome, 414
Dorzolamide hydrochloride/timolol maleate, 486
Dorzolamide-timolol, 316, 317, 318
Double vision, 8, 415, 453, 532
Down syndrome, 157–162
  and congenital ectropion, 209

Doxycycline, 198, 206, 237, 253, 255, 259, 260, 287
Doxycycline hyclate, 196–197
Drance hemorrhage, 484, 487
Driving
   bioptic telescope for, 61–64
   training with a certified driving rehabilitation
      specialist, 62–63
Drusen, 341
   optic disc drusen, 419–420, 436
   optic nerve drusen, 416–421, 417–418f, 419f
Dry age-related macular degeneration (ARMD), 339–
      342, 340f, 341f
Dry eye disease
   associated with secondary Sjögren syndrome,
      223–226
Dry eyes, 205, 230, 231
   and blepharospasm, 211
   and presbyopia, 9
Dry eye syndrome, 128, 290–291
Dry eye treatment, 216–221, 218f
   protocol, 220t
Dry mouth, 225
Dryness, 372, 524
Duane retraction syndrome, 122–125
   type I, 125t
   type II, 125t
Duloxetine, 227
Durezol. See Difluprednate
Dynamic retinoscopy, 158f

E
ECCE. See Extracapsular cataract extraction (ECCE)
Eccentric circles, 83t, 124t
Ectropion, 207–209, 208f, 208t
Ehlers-Danlos syndrome, 311, 378, 404
EKC. See Epidemic keratoconjunctivitis (EKC)
Electrocautery, 231
Embolism, 392
Emmetropization, of hyperopia, 153, 154, 155
EMZL. See Extranodal marginal zone lymphoma (EMZL)
Enbrel. See Etanercept
Enucleation, 165, 330
Epidemic keratoconjunctivitis (EKC), 239–243
   stages of keratitis in, 242t
Epiphora, 214, 215
Episcleritis, 313–315, 314f
Epithelial debridement with diamond burr polishing or
      phototherapeutic keratectomy, 287
Epithelial keratitis, 279
Equivalent viewing distance, 58
Erythema nodosum, 519
Erythematotelangiectatic rosacea, 259
Erythromycin, 198, 231, 236, 237, 260
4×13 Eschenbach Microlux monocular telescope, 58,
      58f, 59
Esophoria, 75, 76
Esotropia, 12, 112, 155
Etanercept, 368
ETDRS chart, 13
Exfoliation, 493
Exocin. See Ofloxacin

Exophoria, 8, 78, 92
Exotropia, 453
   intermittent exotropia, divergence excess type, 118–121
External hordeolum. See Hordeolum
Extracapsular cataract extraction (ECCE), 16–17
Extranodal marginal zone lymphoma (EMZL), 544, 545
Exudative retinal detachment, 400
Eye compresses. See Cool compresses; Warm compresses
Eye drop instillation, in elderly patients, 67
Eye injury, 508
Eyelid erythema, 255
Eyelid hygiene, 66, 197, 198, 204, 205, 206, 259,
      281, 313
Eyelid laxity, 208, 209, 283
Eyelid lesion, 230–231
Eyelid massage, 199, 205
Eyelid myectomy, 212
Eyelid papilloma, 230–232
Eyelid scrubs, 196, 197, 205, 255, 258, 259, 262, 313
Eyelid weight, surgical implantation of, 530
Eye masks, 205
Eye protection, 44–47, 379
   radial keratatomy, 190
Eye protectors, 44, 45f, 47f
Eyestrain, due to low vision, 51
Eylea. See Aflibercept

F
Fabry disease, 292
Face shields, 47
Face wrap, 32, 33
Falls, in elderly patients, 67
Fansworth D15 Test, 130–131, 133, 133f, 136, 137–138,
      137f, 139
Fansworth-Munsell 100 Hue Test, 132, 134, 134f, 146
FDA. See United States Food and Drug
      Administration (FDA)
Fibromuscular dysplasia, 405
Fibrovascular traction tissue, 349
Fitting height, 33
Fixation disparity, 90–93
Fixed-length corridor design, 34, 35
Flame-shaped hemorrhages, 536
Flap of torn retinal tissue, 395
Flat-top bifocals, 75
Flaxseed oil capsules, 204, 206
Flip-prism technique, 107–108
Floaters, 395, 400
Flomax-associated floppy iris syndrome, 358
Floppy eyelid syndrome, 283, 286
Flouromethalone, 206
Flow cytometry, 544
Fluctuating blurred vision, 531
Fluorescein evaluation, 191
Fluorescein sodium/benoxinate, 503
Fluorescein staining, 225
Fluorodeoxyglucose, 545
Fluoromethalone, 251
Fluoromethalone, 242, 246
Fluoroquinolones, 229, 283
Fluress. See Fluorescein sodium/benoxinate

FML Forte. *See* Fluorometholone
Focal laser, 353
Follicle stimulating hormone, 362–363
Foveal hypoplasia, 96f
Foveal reflex, loss of, 372
Free-form, optimized lenses, 31, 33
    progressive addition lenses, switching from conventional PALs to, 27–29
Fresnel prism, 104, 107, 415, 460, 526
Full-field flash ERG, 145
Fundus examination, 549
Fungal infection, 504
Furosemide, 291
Fusional instability, 115
Fusional vergence dysfunction, 72t

G
GAGs. *See* Glycosaminoglycans (GAGs)
Ganciclovir, 242, 280
Ganglion cell fibers, 516
Gardening tasks, eye protection during, 45–46, 46t
Gas-permeable (GP) contact lenses, 177
    alternating multi-focal lenses, 182
    aspheric front and back surface lenses, 182
    for astigmatism, 4, 5
    concentric multi-focal lenses, 182
    keratoconus management with, 184–189, 185f
    versus soft contact lenses, 171–175
GAT. *See* Goldmann applanation tonometry (GAT)
Gatifloxacin, 240, 504
Gaze viewing, 123, 125
Gene therapy, 384
Genetic testing of melanomas, 331–332
Gentamicin, 292
Geriatric patients, 65–67
Giant cell arteritis, 392, 393, 429
Giant papillae, 245–246
Giant papillary conjunctivitis, 194–195, 249–252, 251f
Glare-control issues, 50, 51
Glass foreign bodies, 504
Glatiramer acetate, 424
Glaucoma, 308, 319, 334, 418, 465
    angle-closure glaucoma, 495–501, 496f, 498–499f, 500–501f
    and diffuse iris melanoma, 331
    pharmaceutic treatments for, 486t
    primary open angle glaucoma, 480–487, 481–483f
    pseudoexfoliation glaucoma, 489–494, 490f, 491f, 492–493f
    uveitis glaucoma, 316
Glycosaminoglycans (GAGs), 528
Goldmann applanation tonometry (GAT), 507
Gonioscopy, 312, 509
GP. *See* Gas-permeable (GP) contact lenses
Gram-negative bacteria, 237
Gram-positive bacteria, 214
Granulomatous inflammation, 200
Granulomatous lesions, 327
Granulomatous uveitis, 318
Graves disease, 528, 529
Grid laser, 353

Ground prisms, 103
GTVT Chart & MFBF Perceptives, 120t, 124t

H
HAART. *See* Highly active antiretroviral therapy (HAART)
Halberg clips, 67, 103
Handedness, 178
Handheld (or pocket) magnifiers, 58
Hardy Rand and Rittle Pseudoisochromatic Test, 130, 131f, 133, 136, 137, 139, 146
Hashimoto thyroiditis, 529
HbA1c, 511
Head trauma, 414
Health Insurance Portability and Accountability Act (HIPAA), 66
Helicobacter pylori, 255, 545
Helper T-cells, 550
HEMA-based hydrogel contacts, 194
Hemispheric dome magnifiers, 58
Hemoglobin, 512
Hepatitis B, 314
Hereditary color vision deficiencies, 141–143
Herpes simplex, 314
Herpes simplex keratitis, 278–280
Herpes simplex virus, 279–280, 319
    HSV-1, 279
    HSV-2, 279
Herpes zoster, 314
Herpes zoster keratitis, 280
Herpes zoster virus, 280
Herpetic anterior uveitis, 316–319
Herpetic granulomatous anterior uveitis, 318
Herpetic infections, and trabeculitis, 319
Herpetic uveitis, 319
Heterophoria, 91–92
Highly active antiretroviral therapy (HAART), 234
High refraction, in infants, 152–155
HIPAA. *See* Health Insurance Portability and Accountability Act (HIPAA)
Hole in the hand/card test, 178
Homatropine, 282
Homocystinuria, 311
Homonymous hemianopia, 470–471
Hordeola, 255, 260
Hordeolum, 196–198, 200
Horizontal prism, 104
Horner syndrome, 402–405, 403f, 404f
Horner-Trantas dots, 245
Horseshoe tear, 394–395, 395f, 399f
Horticulture tasks, eye protection during, 45–46, 46t
Hot compresses, 204
HOTV symbols, 112
Hudson-Stahli line, 292
Human immunodeficiency virus (HIV) retinopathy, 547–551, 548f
Huygen-Fresnel principle, 304
Hyaluronic acid gel fillers, 530
Hybrid multifocal contact lenses, 177
Hydrocodone, 505
Hydroxyamphetamine, 405

Hydroxychloroquine, 292, 365–370, 366*f*, 367*f*, 368*f*
Hyperemia, 524
Hyperglycemia-induced retinopathy, pathways of, 351
Hyperopia, 109, 191
   emmetropization of, 153, 154, 155
   in infants, 147–150
Hypertension, ocular effects of, 510–512
Hypertensive retinopathy, 512
Hyperthyroidism, 528
Hypertonic ointments, 287
Hyphema, 269, 509
Hypotony, 400–401
Hypotropia, 453

I
Ibuprofen, 285, 505
Idiopathic intracranial hypertension, 433–437, 434*f*,
   435–436*f*
IEP. *See* Individualized Education Program (IEP)
Imaged-guided photocoagulation systems, 353
Imiquimod, 234
Incision and drainage surgery, for chalazia, 200–201
Individualized Education Program (IEP), 59
Indomethacin, 292
Infants
   high refraction in, 152–155
   hyperopia in, 147–150
   retinoblastoma in, 163–166
Infections
   bacterial infection, 504
   fungal infection, 504
   herpetic infections, 319
   preseptal cellulitis, 227–229
   pseudomonas infection, 283
Inferior palpebral conjunctiva, 263*f*
InflammaDry testing, 219*f*, 220*t*, 221
Inflammation
   blepharitis, 203–206
   chalazion. *See* Chalazia
   granulomatous inflammation, 200
   intraocular inflammation, 519
   lipogranulomatous inflammation, 200
Interferon Gamma Release Assays, 263, 264
Interleukin, 325
Interleukin-1a, 255
Intermediate age-related macular degeneration (ARMD),
   341–342
Intermittent exotropia, divergence excess type, 118–121
Intermittent Exotropia Control Scale, 120*t*
Internal hordeolum. *See* Hordeolum
Internal ocular examination, 153
Internuclear ophthalmoplegia, 463–465, 464*f*
Interpalpebral conjunctival hyperemia, 260
Intracranial tumor, 466–471, 467*f*, 468*f*, 469*f*, 470*f*
Intraocular inflammation, 519
Intraocular lenses (IOLs), 304, 312
   pseudophakia, 16, 17
Intraocular pressure (IOP), 308, 309–310, 507,
   508, 509
Intravitreal triamcinolone, 353
Involutional ectropion, 208
IOLs. *See* Intraocular lenses (IOLs)

IOP. *See* Intraocular pressure (IOP)
Iridotomy, 310
Iris cyst, 331
Iris melanoma, 329–332, 330*f*
Iris neovascularization, 334, 387–388
Iris nevus, 331, 332
Iris sphincter tears, 508
Iritis, 279
Irregular blood vessels growth, 346
Irvine-Gass syndrome, 358
Ischemia central retinal vein occlusion, 387
Ischemic optic neuropathy, 428
iTerminal 2 (Carl Zeiss Vision), 28

J
Jannelli clip, 67
Jetrea. *See* Ocriplasmin
JND. *See* Just noticeable difference (JND)
Jones Test 1, 214
Junctional scotoma, 469
Just noticeable difference (JND), 67

K
Keith-Wagener-Barker Classification System, 512
Keratitis, 208
Keratoconjunctivitis sicca, 314
Keratoconus, 478
   genetics, 187–188
   and interleukin-1, 187
   management with gas-permeable contact lenses,
      184–189, 185*f*
   topographical morphologies, 187
   with Vogt striae, 187, 187*f*
Keratoglobus, 187
Keratometry, 4, 5
Keratopathy
   annular keratopathy of Payreau, 504
   vortex keratopathy, 291–292
   whorl keratopathy, 290, 290*f*, 291, 292
Koeppe iris nodules, 519
Korb-Blackie lid seal test, 221
Korb Meibomian Gland Evaluator (MGE), 219–220

L
Lacrimal gland, 519
Lancing, 266
Lang I test, 148, 149*f*
Lang II test, 148
Lanthony D15 test, 131, 133, 133*f*
Laser ablation, 232
Laser peripheral iridotomy (LPI), 499
Laser photocoagulation, 401
LASIK, and blepharitis, 204, 205
Latanoprost, 494
Lattice, 399
   degeneration, 395, 395*f*
Lenses. *See also specific lenses*
   Bagolini striated lenses, 111
   bifocal lenses, 38, 39, 128, 158*f*, 159, 161, 182
   bilateral multifocal intraocular lenses, 305
   diffractive multifocal intraocular lenses, 304
   distance toric lenses, 177

Lenses. *(Cont.)*
  free-form, optimized lenses, 27–29, 31, 33
  intraocular lenses (IOLs), 16, 17, 304, 312
  minus addition lenses, for intermittent exotropia,
    119–120
  monocular lens sorting, 80*t*
  monocular loose lens rock, 80*t*
  monofocal intraocular lenses, 304
  monovision contact lenses, 176–178
  multifocal gas-permeable lenses, 180–182
  multifocal intraocular lenses, 303–305
  multifocal toric contact lenses, 177
  multifocal toric intraocular lens, 297–302, 299–302*f*
  opacified lenses, 295
  opacity, 297
  plano lenses, 51, 88
  plus lenses, binocular sustained reading through, 80*t*
  polycarbonate lenses, 67, 165, 190
  refractive intraocular lenses, 304
  scleral lenses, 173, 174*f*, 175, 177, 218
  single-vision lenses, 75
  subluxation of, 307–312, 308*f*, 309–310*f*, 311*f*
  tints, 23–25
  toric multifocal intraocular lens, 297–302, 299–302*f*
  Trivex lenses, 159
Lenticular astigmatism, 309
Leukemia, 539
Leukocoria, 166
Levothyroxine, 524
Lifesaver cards, 83*t*, 120*t*, 124*t*
Lifitegrast, 218, 221, 224, 530
Light-near dissociation, 411, 412–415, 413*f*
Lipid layer thickness, 220*t*, 221
LipiFlow vectored thermal pulse therapy, 218, 221
Lipitor. *See* Atorvastatin calcium
LipiView II, 218*f*
Lipogranulomatous inflammation, 200
Lisinopril, 291, 524
Lissamine green staining, 225
Logarithm of the minimum angle of resolution (LogMAR)
    size progression, 13
LogMAR. *See* Logarithm of the minimum angle of resolu-
    tion (LogMAR) size progression
Lotemax. *See* Loteprednol etabonate
Loteprednol, 246, 250, 251, 259, 530
Loteprednol etabonate, 242, 253, 259, 281, 313
Low-contrast sine wave grating, 98, 98*f*
Lower lid distraction test, 208
Low vision management, in patients with
    choroideremia, 48–51
  low vision device trials, 49–50
LPI. *See* Laser peripheral iridotomy (LPI)
LRP4. *See* Anti-low-density lipoprotein receptor-related
    protein 4 (LRP4) antibodies
Lubricators, 224, 251, 266, 282
Lucentis. *See* Ranibizumab
Lumboperitoneal shunt, 437
Lutein, 342
Lyme disease, 314
Lymphocytes, 325
Lymphoma, 545

M
Macrolides, 229, 260, 261
Macular degeneration
  age-related, 52–56
    dry age-related, 339–342, 340*f*, 341*f*
    wet age-related, 344–347, 345*f*
Macular disease, 369–370
Macular edema, 290, 291*f*, 352, 388
  cystoid macular edema, 355–359, 356–359*f*
Macular optical coherence tomography, 537–538*f*,
    540–541*f*
Maddox rod, 111
Magnification/magnifiers, 49–50, 51, 55–56, 58, 59*f*, 60,
    optelec dome magnifier
  handheld (or pocket) magnifiers, 58
  hemispheric dome magnifiers, 58
  Mattingly Advantage 4×12 D LED illuminated stand
    magnifier, 59
  video magnifier, 59
Mallett near vision unit, 91*f*, 92*f*, 93
MALT. *See* Mucosa-associated lymphatic tissue (MALT)
    lymphoma
Marfan syndrome, 311, 405
Marsden ball looping, 120*t*
Mast cell stabilizers, 246, 251
Matrix metalloproteinase-9 (MMP-9), 219*f*, 221,
    225, 255
Mattingly Advantage 4×12 D LED illuminated stand
    magnifier, 59
Maxidex. *See* Dexamethasone
Mechanical ectropion, 208
Medial longitudinal fasciculus (MLF), 464
Medrol. *See* Methylprednisolone
Meibography, 225
Meibomian gland dysfunction, 197, 198, 204, 205, 218,
    221, 225, 255, 259, 260, 372
Meibomian glands
  expression of, 225
  management of, 251
Meibomian glands yielding liquid secretion (MGLYS)
    score, 219, 220*t*, 221
Meige syndrome, 211
MEM. *See* Monocular estimation method (MEM)
Meningiomas, 468
Meridional amblyopia, bilateral, 4
Mestinon. *See* Pyridostigmine
Metamorphopsia, 347, 372, 378
Methadone, 543
Methicillin-resistant *Staphylococcus aureus* (MRSA),
    228, 229
Methotrexate, 519
Methylprednisolone, 317, 318, 424, 425, 530
Metronidazole, 260
MFBF. *See* Monocular fixation binocular field (MFBF)
mfERG. *See* Multifocal ERG (mfERG)
MG. *See* Myasthenia gravis (MG)
MGE. *See* Korb Meibomian Gland Evaluator (MGE)
MGLYS. *See* Meibomian glands yielding liquid secretion
    (MGLYS) score
Microbial keratitis, 283
  ulcers, 282

Microtropia, 112
Mild uveitic glaucoma, 318
Minocycline, 206, 260
  -induced pseudotumor cerebri, 439–443, 440f, 441f
Minus addition lenses, for intermittent exotropia, divergence excess type, 119–120
Mirror and correct-eye scope stereoscopes, 120t
Mixed vernal keratoconjunctivitis, 245
MLF. See Medial longitudinal fasciculus (MLF)
MMP-9. See Matrix metalloproteinase-9 (MMP-9)
Mohindra technique, 150, 153f
Molluscum contagiosum, 233–235, 234f
Monocular accommodative rock, 120t, 124t
Monocular diplopia, 309, 311
Monocular estimation method (MEM), 154, 161
Monocular fixation binocular field (MFBF), 120t, 124t
Monocular Hart chart, 80t
Monocular lens sorting, 80t
Monocular loose lens rock, 80t
Monofocal intraocular lenses, 304
Monovision contact lenses, 176–178
Monovision correction, 304
Moxeza. See Moxifloxacin
Moxifloxacin, 214, 246, 258, 265, 285, 503, 504
MRSA. See Methicillin-resistant Staphylococcus aureus (MRSA)
M&S Sports Performance software, 24
M&S system fixation disparity target, 108
Mucocele, 474–475
Mucosa-associated lymphatic tissue (MALT) lymphoma, 545
Muller's muscle, 529
Multifocal ERG (mfERG), 145
Multifocal gas-permeable contact lenses, 180–182
Multifocal intraocular lenses, 303–305
Multifocal toric contact lenses, 177
Multifocal toric intraocular lens, 297–302, 299–302f
Multiple sclerosis, 465
Munson's sign, 187
Muscle-specific kinase (MuSK), 533
Musicians, prescribing for, 36–39
MuSK. See Muscle-specific kinase (MuSK)
Mutton-fat keratic precipitates, 519
Myasthenia gravis (MG), 529, 531–532f, 531–534
Myopia, 128, 309, 399
Myopia control, 19–22
  factors determining desirable contact lens modality for, 20t

N
Naproxen, 505, 535
Near exophoria, 8, 102
Near/far Hart Chart, 124t
Near point blur, 70
Near tangent screen test, 53f
Negative relative accommodation (NRA), 8
Neovascularization, 349, 351, 353, 493
  choroidal neovascularization, 342, 346, 378–379
  corneal neovascularization, 245, 258f
  iris neovascularization, 334, 387–388
Nepafenac, 298

Neuro-optometric rehabilitation, of post-concussion patient, 114–117
Neuropathy, 514–519, sarcoid optic neuropathy
  arteritic anterior ischemic optic neuropathy (AAION), 428, 429
  compressive optic neuropathy, 529
  ischemic optic neuropathy, 428
  nonarteritic anterior ischemic optic neuropathy (NAION), 427–431, 428f, 429–430f
  optic neuropathy, 292, 428, 515, 519
Neurosensory retina, 399
Neurosyphilis, 413
Nevanac. See Nepafenac
Night blindness, 51
Nocturnal lagophthalmos, 286
Nodular scleritis, 545
No infrared (NoIR) fit-over sunglasses, 50, 51, 53f, 55
NoIR. See No infrared (NoIR) fit-over sunglasses
Nonarteritic anterior ischemic optic neuropathy (NAION), 427–431, 428f, 429–430f
Noncompliant patients, 190–195
Noncontact tonometry, 503
Non-cycloplegic retinoscopy, 154
Noninvasive tear breakup time, 219f, 220t, 221
Nonischemic central retinal vein occlusion, 387
Non-necrotizing nodular anterior scleritis, 325
Nonorganic vision loss, 476–479, 477f
Nonprescription eye protectors, 44
Non-proliferative diabetic retinopathy (NPDR), 351
Nonsteroidal anti-inflammatory drugs (NSAIDs), 314–315, 346, 358, 437, 507, 509
Non-variable tranaglyphs, 83t
Nott method, 161
NPDR. See Non-proliferative diabetic retinopathy (NPDR)
NRA. See Negative relative accommodation (NRA)
NSAIDs. See Nonsteroidal anti-inflammatory drugs (NSAIDs)
NSUCO test, 71
Nuclear cataracts, 295
Nystagmoid movements, 464

O
Occlusion test, prolonged, 89
Occult wet macular degeneration, 346
Occupational therapy, 62
Ocriplasmin, 374
OCT. See Optical coherence tomography (OCT)
Octeotide, 446
Ocular adnexal lymphoma, 544, 545
Ocular burning and irritation, 66
Ocular histoplasmosis syndrome, 320
Ocular hypertension, 316, 319
Ocular lymphoma, 543–545, 544f
Ocular prosthetics, 165–166
Ocular rosacea, 253–256, 254f, 314
  childhood, 257–261, 258f
Ocular surface squamous neoplasia (OSSN), 272, 275
Ocular toxoplasmosis, 521–523. See Toxoplasmosis
Ocular trauma, 399, 506–509, 507f
Oculocutaneous albinism, 57–60

Oculomotor
    balance at near, 123f
    dysfunction, 71, 72t
    vision techniques, 120t, 124t
Oculoplastic consultation, 209, 214, 230
Oculosympathoperesis. *See* Horner syndrome
Oculus Heidelberger Multi-Color Anomaloscope, 141,
        143f, 146
Ocutech 4X VES-K telescope, 61
Office-based vision therapy, 72, 78–79, 85, 88
Ofloxacin, 237, 298
Oligodendrocytes, 425
Olopatadine, 246, 247, 250
Olopatadine hydrochloride, 250
Omega-3 fatty acids, 204, 205–206, 224, 225, 255
Onyx HD portable closed circuit television (CCTV), 59
Opacified lenses, 295
Opera glasses, 52–53
Operculated retinal break, 396
Ophthalmic anesthetic, 504
Ophthalmic antibiotics, 504
Ophthalmic cyclosporine, 530
Ophthalmic fluoroquinolone, 504
Ophthalmic steroids, 504, 505
Ophthalmoscope, direct and indirect, 166
Ophthalmoscopy, direct and indirect, 150, 153
Opiate analgesics, 505
Optelec dome magnifier, 58, 59f
Optical coherence tomography (OCT), 111
Optic disc drusen, 419–420, 436
Optic disc edema, 434
Optic nerve, pallor of, 515, 516
Optic nerve drusen, 416–421, 417–418f, 419f
Optic nerve involvement, 519
Optic nerve sheath fenestration, 437
Optic neuritis, 424
Optic neuropathy, 292, 428, 515, 519
Optic tract lesion, 470
Optometric vision therapy, 123
Orbital cellulitis, 228
Orbital fibroblasts, 528
Orbital lesion, 474
Orbital tumors, 529
Orthokeratology, 19, 20t. *See also* Gas-permeable (GP)
        contact lens
OSSN. *See* Ocular surface squamous neoplasia (OSSN)
Osteogenesis imperfecta type 1, 405
Oxycodone, 505
Oxytetracycline, 206

P
Pachymetry, 418
Paget disease of bone, 378
Pallor of the disc, 484
Pallor of the optic nerve, 515, 516
Palpebral conjunctiva evaluation with eyelid eversion, 195
PALs. *See* Progressive addition lenses (PALs)
Pancoast syndrome, 404
Pan-retinal photocoagulation (PRP), 353
Panretinal photocoagulation (PRP) agents, 388
Pansinusitis, 473–475, 474f

Pantoscopic tilt, 32, 33
Papilledema, 420, 434–435, 437, 441, 442
Papilloma, 230–232, 233
Papillopustular rosacea, 259
Paralytic ectropion, 208
Parasympathetic system, and tonic pupil, 409
Paresis, 457
Pars plana vitrectomy, 349, 401
Pataday. *See* Olopatadine hydrochloride ophthalmic
        solution
Patanol. *See* Olopatadine
PDR. *See* Proliferative diabetic retinopathy (PDR)
Pediatric Eye Disease Investigator Group (PEDIG), 112
PEDIG. *See* Pediatric Eye Disease Investigator Group
        (PEDIG)
Pegboard rotator, 120t
Pelli-Robson contrast chart, 304
Pencil pushups, 80t
Pentacam corneal topography, 172f
"PEPSI," 378
Perceptual learning effect, and astigmatism, 4
Periocular erythema, 260
Peripheral corneal ulcer, 281–284, 282f
Peripheral retinal degenerations, 399
Peripheral retinal lesions, 394–396
Peripheral vision loss, 51
Periphlebitis, 519
Phacoemulsification, 16
Pharmacologic dilation, 410
Phenylephrine, 240, 315, 325, 405
Phlyctenular keratoconjunctivitis (PKC), 263–264
Phlyctenules, 262–264, 263, 263f, 264
Phoropter testing, prism bar ranges in, 119
Photophobia, 88, 111, 255, 524
    blepharospasm, 211
Photopsia, 400
Photosensitivity, 115
Phymatous rosacea, 259
Pigment mottling, 342
    within the macula, 341
Pilocarpine, 312, 410, 487, 499
Pinguecula, 271–273, 346
Pinhole test, 4
Pituitary adenoma, 444–451, 446f, 447–451f
Pituitary lesion, 446
PKC. *See* Phlyctenular keratoconjunctivitis (PKC)
Plano lenses, 51
    single-vision photochromic lenses, 88
Plastic frames, 67
Plateau iris configuration, and angle closure, 497
Pneumatic retinopexy, 398, 401
Pola mirror walkaways, 120t
Polycarbonate lenses, 67, 165, 190
Polymerase chain reaction testing, 322
Polymyxin B, 504
Polysporin, 196, 198, 234
Positive relative accommodation (PRA), 8, 70
Post-concussion patient, neuro-optometric rehabilitation
        of, 114–117
Posterior subcapsular cataracts, 295, 303–305
Posterior uveitis, 318

Posterior vitreous detachment (PVD), 395
Postganglionic Horner syndrome, 405
Post-laser refractive surgery dry eye, 204
Post-traumatic iritis, 504
Potassium hydroxide, 234
Povidone-iodine, 242
PPD. *See* Purified protein derivative (PPD) test
PRA. *See* Positive relative accommodation (PRA)
Pred Forte. *See* Prednisolone acetate
Prednisolone, 206, 246, 507
Prednisolone acetate, 268, 279, 280, 316, 317, 318
Prednisone, 321, 424, 431, 484, 530
Prentice's rule, 13
Presbyopia, 7–9, 42, 91, 102, 176, 178, 409
    laser vision correction, 178
Presbyopic convergence insufficiency patients, 103
Preseptal cellulitis, 227–229
Previous personal or family history of a retinal
    detachment, 399
Primary open angle glaucoma, 480–487, 481–483f
Prism controlled bifocals, 91
Prisms, 415
    base-in (BI) prism correction, 102–104
    convergence insufficiency management with, 101–104
    flip-prism technique, 107–108
    Fresnel prism, 104, 107, 415, 460, 526
    ground prisms, 103
    horizontal prism, 104
    sustained reading through, 80t, 83t
    for vertical heterophoria, 107–108
    vertical prism, 108
    yoked prisms, 97, 123
Prognosis, alternatives (of treatment), risks, and questions
    (PARQs), 503
Progressive addition lenses (PALs), 30–32, 33–34, 75, 91,
    103, 532
    adaptational issues with, 33–35
    dispensing issues with, 33–35
    free-form, switching from conventional to, 27–29
    general-purpose lenses, 37, 40, 41, 42
    variable-length corridor design, 34, 34f
Proliferative diabetic retinopathy (PDR), 350, 351–352,
    353–354
Proparacaine, 240
Prophylactic oral acyclovir, 279
Prophylaxis, 358
Propine. *See* Dipivefrin
Prostaglandins, 485, 499
Protanopia, 137
PRP. *See* Pan-retinal photocoagulation (PRP); Panretinal
    photocoagulation (PRP) agents
Pseudobulbar affect, 465
Pseudocyst, 374
Pseudoedema, 420
Pseudoexfoliation glaucoma, 489–494, 490f, 491f,
    492–493f
Pseudoexfoliation syndrome, 311, 491
Pseudogerontoxon lesions, 245
Pseudoisochromatic plate test, 138
Pseudomembranes, 240–241, 240f
Pseudomonas infection, 283

Pseudomyopia, 127–129
Pseudopapilledema, 420, 436
Pseudophakia, 15–17, 531
Pseudotumor cerebri, 442, 443
Pseudo-Von Graefe sign, 414
Pseudoxanthoma elasticum, 378, 379
Pterygium, 272, 274–277, 275f, 276f, 445, 545
Ptosis, 200, 414, 453, 529
Punctal occlusion, 255
Pupillary block, and angle closure, 497
Purified protein derivative (PPD) test, 264
PVD. *See* Posterior vitreous detachment (PVD)
Pyridostigmine, 533
Pyrimethamine, 321, 322, 523

R
Radial keratatomy, 190–191
Ranibizumab, 346, 353, 388
Ranitidine, 325
RAPD. *See* Relative afferent pupillary defect (RAPD)
RB1 gene, 166
RCEs. *See* Recurrent corneal erosions (RCEs)
Reading glasses, 49–50, 51
Recurrent corneal erosions (RCEs), 285–287, 286f, 505
Reepithelialization, 287
Refractive error, 9, 31, 111–112, 149, 153–155, 177
    and anisometropia, 12
    and cataract surgery, 17
Refractive intraocular lenses, 304
Relative afferent pupillary defect (RAPD), 387, 424, 435,
    470, 471, 507
Rescula. *See* unoprostone
Residual astigmatism, 298–299, 305
Restasis. *See* Cyclosporine
Retin-A. *See* Tretinoin
Retinal acuity meter, 16
Retinal artery occlusion, 389–393, 390–391f
Retinal detachment, 165, 318, 334, 392, 394–395
    rhegmatogenous, 398–401, 399f, 400f
Retinal ischemia, 387
Retinal lesions, 394–396
Retinal pigment epithelium (RPE), 341, 346, 369, 377,
    378, 381, 399–400
Retinal toxicity, 342, 369
Retinal tufts, 396, 396f
Retinal vein occlusion, 385–388, 386f, 387f
Retinitis, 279
Retinitis pigmentosa, 380–384, 381f, 382f, 383f
Retinoblastoma, in children, 163–166, 164f, 165f
Retinopathy, 550
    central serous retinopathy, 361–364, 362f, 363f
    diabetic retinopathy, 290, 291f, 348–354, 349f,
        350f, 399
    human immunodeficiency virus retinopathy,
        547–551, 548f
    hyperglycemia-induced retinopathy, pathways of, 351
    hypertensive retinopathy, 512
    non-proliferative diabetic retinopathy (NPDR), 351
    of prematurity, 399
    proliferative diabetic retinopathy (PDR), 350, 351–
        352, 353–354

Retrobulbar optic neuritis, 424, 478
Retroillumination, 308, 308f
Rhegmatogenous retinal detachment, 398–401,
    399f, 400f
Rheumatoid arthritis, 291
Right optic neuropathy, 515
Ring melanoma, 334
Rizutti's sign, 187
Rod photoreceptors, death of, 381
Rosacea, 253–256
ROSacea COnsensus (ROSCO) panel, 254
ROSCO. See ROSacea COnsensus (ROSCO) panel
Roth spots, 536, 537–539
RPE. See Retinal pigment epithelium (RPE)
Rust rings, 504, 504f

S
Saccadic dysfunction, 107
Salicylic acid, 234
Salmon-patch lesions, 544
Sarcoid optic neuropathy, 514–519
Sarcoidosis, 324–328, 326t, 327t, 518–519
Schirmer test, 225
Scleral buckle, 401
Scleral lenses, 173, 175, 218
    multifocal contact lenses, 177
    sodium fluorescein pattern of, 174f
Scleritis, 314, 315, 325
Sebaceous cell carcinoma, 201
Secondary glaucoma, 334
Secondary Sjögren syndrome, dry eye disease associated
        with, 223–226
Sectoral tissue excision, 330
Seidel sign, 503
Selenium, and thyroid eye disease, 528
Senaptec Sensory Performance software, 24
Serum angiotensin-converting enzyme, 327
Sheard's criterion, 8, 9, 104
Shield ulcer, 244, 245, 245f
Short-pulse lasers, 353
Short wavelength automated perimetry (SWAP), 146
Sickle cell disease, 378
SICS. See Small-incision cataract surgery (SICS)
Sildenafil, 428
Silver nitrate paste, 234
Simbrinza. See Brinzolamide/brimonidine
Single-surrounded Lea symbols, 112
Single-vision lenses, 75, 91
Singulair. See Sodium montelukast
Sinuses, 474
Sjögren syndrome, 224–226, 411
Slit-lamp biomicroscopy, 259
Small-incision cataract surgery (SICS), 17
Snap test, 208
Sodium chloride, 286
Sodium fluorescein, 221, 286
Sodium montelukast, 246
Sodium sulfacetamide, 260
Soft contact lenses
    versus gas-permeable lenses, 171–175
    multifocal lenses, 19, 20–21, 20t

Spectangle Pro/Optikam (HOYA Vision Care), 28
SPEED Questionnaire, 217f, 220f
Split quoit walkaways & alignment, 120t
Sports vision, 23–25
    M&S Sports Performance software test, 24
    Senaptec Sensory Performance software test, 24
Spotting, 62
Squamous papilloma, 230–232
Stainless steel surgical golf club spud, 503
Staphylococcal marginal keratitis, 258
Staphylococcus, 197–198, 263
Staphylococcus aureus, 228, 282
Staphylococcus epidermidis, 255
Stereoacuity, and amblyopia treatment, 112
Stereoacuity, and anisometropia, 12
Stereoscope cards, 120t
Sterile saline spray, 503
Steroids, 200, 201, 206, 280, 358, 505
Strabismus, and amblyopia, 111, 112
Stress, and thyroid eye disease, 528
Stromal keratitis, 279, 280
Stromal puncture, 287
Stye, 197
Subacute angle closure, 497
Subconjunctival hemorrhage, 268–270, 269f,
        511–512, 511f
Subjective refraction, 4
Subluxated lens, 307–312, 308f, 309–310f, 311f
Sulfadiazine, 322, 523
Sulfamethoxazole, 521
Sulfite oxidase deficiency, 311
Sulfonamide antibiotics, 441–442
Superficial foreign bodies, 503
Supraduction deficit, 414
Surgery
    for cataract. See Cararact surgery
    for chalazia, 200–201
    corneal, 191
    for glaucoma, 487
    for idiopathic intracranial hypertension, 437
    for intermittent exotropia, divergence excess type, 119
    for presbyopia, 9
    for pterygium, 275
Surgical "golf club" spud, 504f
Sustained reading through prism, 80t, 83t
SWAP. See Short wavelength automated perimetry (SWAP)
Synechiae, 498
Synkinesia, 414
Synoptophore testing, 111
Syphilis, 314, 405
Systemic corticosteroids, 530
Systemic vascular conditions, 511

T
Tacrolimus, 246, 251
Tadalafil, 428
Tamoxifen, 292
TB. See Tuberculosis (TB)
T-cell lymphoma, 517
Tear breakup time, 219f, 220t, 221
Tear film imaging, 225

Tear osmolarity, 225
Tear production testing, 225
TED. *See* Thyroid eye disease (TED)
Telangiectasia, 255, 260
Telescope, bioptic. *See* Bioptic telescope for driving
Tenon capsule, 511
Terrien marginal degeneration, 187
Tetracyclines, 206, 237, 255, 260, 261
Tetrahydrozoline hydrochloride, 285
Three dot (barrel) card, 80*t*
Thyroglobulin, 529
Thyroid, and episcleritis, 314
Thyroid eye disease (TED), 524
Thyroid-stimulating hormone, 363, 529
Thyroid-stimulating hormone receptor, 529
Thyroid-stimulating immunoglobulin, 528, 529
Thyroperoxidase, 529
Timolol, 308
TMP-SMX. *See* Trimethoprim-sulfamethoxazole (TMP-SMX)
TNF
    See Tumor necrosis factor (TNF), – alpha
Tobradex. *See* Tobramycin/dexamethasone
Tobramycin, 262, 281, 283, 292, 504
Tobramycin/dexamethasone, 240, 503
Tonic pupil, 407–411, 408*f*, 409*f*, 413–414
Topical cyclosporine, 221
Topiramate, 437
Toric multifocal intraocular lens, 297–302, 299–302*f*
Toxoplasma gondii, 522
Toxoplasmosis, 320–322, 321*f*. *See also* Ocular toxoplasmosis
Trabeculitis, and herpetic infections, 319
Tractional retinal detachment, 400
Transconjunctival approach, 200
Trauma
    and episcleritis, 314
    -induced pseudopterygium, 275
Traumatic brain injury, visual problems associated with, 107
Traumatic cataract, 269
Traumatic iridocyclitis, 268, 269
Traumatic lens subluxation, 307–312
Travatan Z. *See* Travoprost
Travoprost, 483, 496
Tretinoin, 234
Trial frame verification, 4, 5
Triamcinolone, 200, 349
Trichloroacetic acid, 234
Trifluridine, 242, 278, 279, 280
Trimethoprim, 504, 521
Trimethoprim-sulfamethoxazole (TMP-SMX), 229, 322
Trivex lenses, 159
Tuberculosis (TB), 262–264
Tumor necrosis, 334
Tumor necrosis factor (TNF)-alpha, 325
Tunnel vision effects, 181
24 Plate Ishihara Test, 130, 132*t*, 133, 136, 137, 138*f*, 139, 142
Tylenol. *See* Acetaminophen
Type 2 diabetes, 511

U
Ulster-Cardiff Accommodation Cube, 161
Ultraviolet A radiation, 187
Uncorrected astigmatism, 178
Uncorrected refractive error, 128
    and amblyopia, 111, 112
Unilateral exophthalmos, 528
Unilateral optic nerve hypoplasia, 112
United States Food and Drug Administration (FDA), 187
Unmedicated lubricant ointment, 204
Unoprostone, 487
US Centers for Disease Control and Prevention (CDC), 237
    recommendation for epidemic keratoconjunctivitis, 242
US Fairness to Contact Lens Consumers Act, 191, 192
U-shaped tear, 395
Usher's syndrome, 384
Uveal melanomas, 334
Uveitis, 268, 269, 280, 318, 399, 519
Uveitis glaucoma, 316
UV protection, 47

V
Variable-length corridor design, 34, 34*f*, 35
Variable tranaglyphs, 80*t*, 83*t*
Variable vectograms, 120*t*, 124*t*
Varicella zoster virus, 319
Vascular endothelial growth factor (VEGF), 346
Vectograms, 80*t*, 83*t*
VEGF. *See* Anti-vascular endothelial growth factor (VEGF) agents; Vascular endothelial growth factor (VEGF)
Venous sinus stenting, 437
Ventriculoperitoneal shunt, 437
Vergence, 107
    vision techniques, 124*t*
Vergence disorder, 75
Vergence therapy, 80–81*t*, 83*t*
Vernal keratoconjunctivitis (VKC), 244–247
    sequential treatment of, 246*t*
Vertex distance, 33
Vertical heterophoria, 106–108
Vertical motility restriction, 414
Vertical prism, 108
Vidarabine, 280
Video magnifier, 59
Vigamox. *See* Moxifloxacin
Viral conjunctivitis
    with eyelid involvement, 228
    with secondary eyelid swelling, 228
Viroptic. *See* Trifluridine
Visagraph nystagmus therapy, 98–99, 98*f*
Visine. *See* Tetrahydrozoline hydrochloride
VisiOffice 2 (Essilor), 28
Vision therapy, 76, 102, 104
    for congenital nystagmus, 95–100
    for intermittent exotropia, divergence excess type, 119–121
    for neuro-optometric rehabilitation, 115–116
    office-based, 72, 78–79, 85, 88
    optometric vision therapy, 123

Vision therapy *(Cont.)*
    phases, 115–116
    procedure, 80–81*t*, 83*t*
    for pseudomyopia, 128
Vistide. *See* Cidofovir cream
Visual automaticity, 116
Visual feedback techniques, for congenital
        nystagmus, 97–99
    low-contrast sine wave grating, 98, 98*f*
    Visagraph nystagmus therapy, 98–99, 98*f*
Visual stabilization, 115
Visual tracing, 124*t*
Visuoscopy, 111
Vitamins, 342
    vitamin A, 384
    vitamin B2 (riboflavin), 187
Vitrectomy, 353–354
Vitreomacular traction, 371–374, 372*f*, 373*f*
Vitreous detachment, 373
VKC. *See* Vernal keratoconjunctivitis (VKC)
Vortex keratopathy, 291–292

W
Walleyed bilateral internuclear ophthalmoplegia
        (WEBINO), 465
Warfarin, 512
Warm compresses, 66, 196, 197, 198, 199, 200, 205,
        213, 255, 258, 259, 262, 290
Wayne Saccadic Fixator, 124*t*
WEBINO. *See* Walleyed bilateral internuclear ophthalmo-
    plegia (WEBINO)

Wegener's granulomatous, 314
Weill-Marchesani syndrome, 311
Werner's NOSPECS measures clinical severity, 528*t*
Wet age-related macular degeneration (ARMD),
        344–347, 345*f*
Wheatstone double-mirror stereoscope, 83*t*
White-centered hemorrhage, 538
WHO. *See* World Health Organization (WHO)
Whorl keratopathy, 290, 290*f*, 291, 292
World Health Organization (WHO), 237
Wraparound fit-over shield, 61, 62*f*

X
Xerostomia, 225
Xiidra. *See* Lifitegrast
X-linked retinitis pigmentosa, 382

Y
Yoked prisms
    for congenital nystagmus, 97
    for duane retraction syndrome, 123

Z
Zantac. *See* Ranitidine
Zeaxanthin, 342
Zeiss ZCalc software, 298, 301*f*
Zinc, 342
Zonular dehiscence, 494
Zylet. *See* Tobramycin
Zymar. *See* Gatifloxacin